Handbook of Health Decision Science

Michael A. Diefenbach
Suzanne Miller-Halegoua
Deborah J. Bowen

Editors

Handbook of Health Decision Science

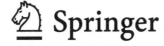 Springer

Editors
Michael A. Diefenbach
Behavioral Research, Department of
    Medicine and Urology
Northwell Health
Manhasset, NY
USA

Deborah J. Bowen
Department of Bioethics and Humanities
    Seattle
University of Washington
Seattle, WA
USA

Suzanne Miller-Halegoua
Fox Chase Cancer Center
Philadelphia, PA
USA

ISBN 978-1-4939-3484-3   ISBN 978-1-4939-3486-7   (eBook)
DOI 10.1007/978-1-4939-3486-7

Library of Congress Control Number: 2016942500

Printed on acid-free paper

This Springer imprint is published by Springer Nature
The registered company is Springer Science+Business Media LLC New York

Acknowledgments

M.A. Diefenbach thanks his wife Catherine for unwavering encouragement throughout the years, his children (Nicky, Franziska, Alexander) for making it all worthwhile, and his friends and colleagues, who challenge him in the pursuit of excellence.

S. Miller-Halegoua thanks her husband Isaak Halegoua, MD, for his professional insights and loving encouragement along with her children (Natasha and Nicolas Miller Benacerraf; Jason and Jamie Halegoua) for believing in this book and for showing her how decisions about health are not just personal but also interfamilial and intergenerational, and her colleagues for shining the light on the scientific and clinical roads to better medical choices. Dr. Miller also acknowledges her institutional grant NIH P30 CA06927.

D.J. Bowen would like to thank her partner and family for ongoing support and her colleagues for driving her to think harder.

We would also like to thank all of the patients, families, providers, and decision makers who have faced complex and important medical decisions and have provided us with data and insight about their processes. These insights are filtered through the volume.

Special thanks to Phapichaya Chaoprang Herrera, MS and John Scarpato, MS, and Sara Fleszar, MS for their organizational skills and calmness in a demanding situation. And finally, to Janice Stern from Springer for shepherding this complex endeavor from conception to publication.

Contents

Introduction

In this *Handbook of Health Decision Science*, we take an inclusive view of this area of scientific inquiry, based on our many discussions together of the state of the science in health decision-making. We were struck not only by the rapid growth of evidence-based theory and research, but also by its central position in the unprecedented and large-scale developments in healthcare practice and policy more broadly, both nationally and globally. At the same time, we realized that there was no unifying resource available that provided a systematic and comprehensive overview of the field.

This handbook was borne out of these discussions and was specifically conceived to respond to recent changes and challenges in healthcare law, ever expanding healthcare options, and the proliferation of preventive, diagnostic, treatment and medical management options. These developments have resulted in a dramatic shift in how healthcare decisions get made, with greater and greater responsibility falling on individual patients and families to chart and navigate their own course through often muddy medical waters in accordance with their own needs, goals, and values. Yet, many individuals, families, providers, and systems are still ill-equipped to take on this responsibility to produce outcomes that are satisfactory for everyone.

Research has convincingly demonstrated that most people, especially after a diagnosis of an unexpected life-threatening disease, show deficits in processing information, understanding their options, and reaching a quality decision. On the provider side, clinicians often do not have the time or training to follow recommended shared-decision protocols, despite their understanding of the importance of such approaches to care. Furthermore, systems for various policy or financial reasons do not always support the latest evidence-based measures, thus creating an environment that is not conducive to optimal decision-making and health outcomes.

Health decision-making pervades every aspect of life, yet individuals rarely notice the myriad decisions that they and those around them make throughout a given day, week, or year. With regard to their health, individuals often focus on the "big" and highly salient decisions that confront them, such as whether to have surgery or radiation treatment for prostate cancer or whether to forgo chemotherapy after breast cancer treatment. However, even seemingly small daily decisions, such as choosing food for breakfast in the morning or engaging in a routine exercise regimen, can have a long-term consequential impact on their health and well-being.

Since Tversky's and Kaheneman's (1974) seminal paper on decision biases, decision-making research has exploded rapidly in a number of non-medical, as well as medical, domains. Initial research efforts focused on the nature and determinants of choice behavior in the economic arena but quickly expanded to other decision areas, including health decision-making. Over time, the field has become increasingly clear that individuals and families in the medical context want to be involved in decision-making about their health. This has been especially true for preference-sensitive decisions, those decisions that entail in equivalent options for disease management from a medical standpoint but result in different consequences for patients at the personal level, such as the nature of their post-treatment symptoms and/or their quality-of-life and function. A prime example of a preference-sensitive decision is the choice between different prostate cancer treatments (surgery, radiation, active surveillance) with similar effects on recurrence and mortality but different effects on quality of life.

These decisional dilemmas have largely originated from basic science and clinical advances which have produced an increasing number of efficacious regimens across the spectrum of disease prevention, detection, and treatment. Combined with developments in computing capabilities and bioinformatics these advances have created an increasing number of complex choices for providers, patients, and family members. For example, a woman deciding on hormone replacement therapy following breast cancer treatment needs to consider not only the potential benefits in preventing a breast cancer recurrence but also weigh the potential side effects and the increased cardiovascular and ovarian cancer risk. In addition, she may consider the costs and benefits of not taking any action and compare the pros and cons of action versus inaction on the implications for her daily activities, quality of life, and quantity of life.

While being adequately informed about the pros and cons of different options is a key component of the decision-making process, the other and arguably more important component is how individuals process the information they receive. Specifically, decisions are largely determined by how individuals cognitively and affectively react to the information, how they connect the incoming data with prior experiences, and the social and cultural context in which they are embedded. Together these factors help to explain a number of seemingly "irrational" decisions, such as why individuals do not choose to uptake evidence-based cancer prevention and screening regimens, including quitting smoking or obtaining colonoscopy to detect colon cancer or the Papanicolaou (PAP) smear to detect cervical cancer. Clearly, health insurance status, access to care and lack of information have been shown to be negatively associated with screening uptake. However, emotional factors such as worry about "finding cancer," and cognitive factors such as inaccurate perceptions about the risk of disease or side effects of the procedure also significantly impact decisions about screening.

An additional challenge for individuals is that health decision-making usually occurs under conditions of uncertainty. Only rarely are all relevant data known and available. Consider the example of prostate cancer treatment decision-making. Patients diagnosed with prostate cancer not only have to cope with the emotional impact of a cancer diagnosis but also they have to deal with different treatment options with fairly equivalent outcomes, ranging from active surveillance, to different forms of radiation therapy, to different forms of surgical removal of the prostate. There is no clinical trial evidence base on which to draw to help guide choice of treatment; thus patients need to make treatment choices guided by estimations of future urinary and erectile functioning and their impact on quality of life. These estimates involve high levels of uncertainty but need to be factored into the decision-making process, which further compounds the anxiety-inducing nature of the process for many men.

It is now well-established that in cases of decision-making under uncertainty, most individuals resort to using heuristics or "cognitive shortcuts," that are activated, often automatically, to reduce the degree of decisional complexity. Understanding how heuristics and biases influence health decision-making and become incorporated into the cognitive-affective processing system is a key focus of inquiry for researchers. Elucidating this area of research is also relevant to the issue of why some individuals often fail to act in their own best interest by taking what seems to be logical and simple precautions to protect themselves. There are many examples of such behaviors in the literature, such as the patient who is urged to adopt a low-fat diet after heart surgery but decides not to do so, or the lung cancer patient who continues to smoke.

Other factors that influence decision-making directly or indirectly are literacy and health literacy factors. Health literacy goes beyond an individual's ability to read, write, or compute basic mathematical operations. Health literacy is commonly defined as the "degree to which individuals have the capacity to obtain, process and understand basic health information and services needed to make appropriate health decisions." Low health literacy affects all aspects of health-related functioning and has clear implications for decision-making, ranging from difficulties adopting healthcare recommendations, medication intake instructions, and understanding public health warning messages. Improving communication methods to assess and address health literacy demands is an ongoing field of research and of utmost relevance for the decision-making literature.

The aim of the current volume is to provide the state-of-the-science information geared towards the researcher, clinician, policy maker, and student of the decision-making field. The handbook is divided into sections corresponding to key areas of inquiry. We start out with "Basics First" with chapters that are designed to provide a solid foundation on the building blocks of the decision literature, such as the Pieterse and Stiggelbout chapter on values, utilities, and preferences and the chapter on research methods by Kiviniemi and Ellis. The chapter by Beck discusses the literature on modeling medical decisions and that by Hesse introduces concepts of decision architecture. Finally, the last chapter in this section, by Hsu and Chiong, presents a needed overview of decision dysfunction focusing on a translational approach that combines basic studies with applied outcomes.

The introductory section of the handbook is followed by the section that examines decision-making at the individual level. The majority of research has focused on individual decision-making and various theoretical approaches to decision-making are represented here (see Brust-Renck et al., Leventhal et al., Peters et al., and Rothman et al.). The chapter by

Han and colleagues discusses the concepts of uncertainty and ambiguity, factors that have the capacity to influence decision-making at all levels. The last two chapters in this section discuss decision-making across the life span. Halpern Felsher and colleagues focus on adolescents and young adults, whereas Dr. Lockenhoff reviews the literature on age-related differences in decision-making.

This part of the handbook is followed by sections Decision-Making on the Interpersonal Level and Applied Decision-Making. At the interpersonal level, we examine decision-making in the family (Siminoff and Thompson) and shared decision-making between patient and providers (Rowland and Politi). This section concludes with a primer on the legal aspects of decision-making in a changed healthcare environment. Chapters 17–21 describe various aspects of applied decision-making. Ramachandran and colleagues discuss specific requirements for decision tools for healthcare professionals and Knight reviews how the Veteran's Affairs system has incorporated such tools into their web-based patient portal to improve patient and physician communication. Noar and colleagues synthesize the large field of tailored communications and Waters and colleagues provide a hands-on approach to communicating risk effectively. The chapter by Col and Springmann addresses the question about the effectiveness of decision aids.

The penultimate section deals with decision-making at organizational, state, and national levels. Greenup and Peppercorn provide a critical review of the shared decision-making approach in the clinical practice. This leads to a discussion of how the transformation of the healthcare system has led to an emphasis on evidence-based medicine and its influence on healthcare policy (Cheely and Zaas). This section closes with a concise description of how the healthcare delivery system has been transformed in recent years (Weiner).

The Handbook closes with two chapters that speculate on the future of decision-making that is already upon us. Graham and colleagues describe the transformation that social media has brought to health decision-making with its ubiquitous availability of information. Sanderson and Schadt discuss the promises and potential consequences of whole genome sequencing on individual decision-making.

This Handbook highlights progress in the discovery of how we make medical and health decisions in an ever more complex world. We believe that the chapters in this Handbook lay the groundwork for future research and the development of supportive decisional interventions. We hope that through this volume we have assembled a case for the field of decision-making that will resonate long after you have finished reading.

Reference

Tversky, A. & Kahneman, D. (1974). Judgment under uncertainty: Heuristics and biases. *Science, 185*(4157), 1124–1131.

Part I
Basics First

What Are Values, Utilities, and Preferences? A Clarification in the Context of Decision Making in Health Care, and an Exploration of Measurement Issues

Arwen H. Pieterse and Anne M. Stiggelbout

Introduction

Values are omnipresent in health-related decision-making—be it values of patients, professionals, policy-makers, or the general public. The term value is generally loosely described as something to strive for, something desirable or important, but in that respect may be just as meaningless as the term quality, another contemporaneous buzz word. Value is sometimes used in a quite specific sense, when meaning valuation, and thereby resembling the term *utility*, which is a synonym for a very specific form of value. Value is sometimes also used interchangeably with *preference*, causing further confusion. In this chapter, we will distinguish the various conceptions and misconceptions of these terms and illustrate the contexts in which the terms are, or should be used. We will further explain what the role values, utilities, and preferences play at different levels of decision-making in health care and describe the ways they can be assessed. We will conclude with key areas for future research.

A.H. Pieterse (✉) · A.M. Stiggelbout
Medical Decision Making, Leiden Quality of Care Institute, Leiden University Medical Center, PO Box 9600, 2300 RC Leiden, The Netherlands
e-mail: a.h.pieterse@lumc.nl

A.M. Stiggelbout
e-mail: a.m.stiggelbout@lumc.nl

Conceptualizing Values, Utilities and Preferences

Values

From a psychological perspective, various theoretical definitions of the concept of values exist. Schwartz and Bilsky (1987) identified five features common to many definitions. Values are (a) concepts or beliefs, (b) about desirable end states (i.e., terminal goals) or behaviors (i.e., instrumental goals), (c) that transcend specific situations, (d) guide the selection or evaluation of behaviors or events, and (e) are ordered by relative importance. Schwartz and Bilsky theorized that values stem from universal human requirements reflected in biologically based needs of the organism, social motives relating to social interactions, and social institutional demands for group welfare and survival. They further proposed that it is through cognitive development that individuals become able to represent these requirements consciously as goals or values. In other words, the value system is a meaning-producing super-ordinate cognitive structure, and this cognitive structure is affectively charged (Rohan 2000). An important empirical finding is that the *structure* of the human value system is universal and there are a finite number of universally important value *types* (e.g., power, hedonism, benevolence, and security). People differ rather in terms of their value *priorities* (Schwartz 1994).

© Springer Science+Business Media New York 2016
M.A. Diefenbach et al. (eds.), *Handbook of Health Decision Science*,
DOI 10.1007/978-1-4939-3486-7_1

In health-related decision-making and the evaluation of health care delivery in particular, more specific definitions of values are usually considered, which generally depend on the levels of decision-making. Three levels are generally distinguished (Sutherland and Till 1993). The first is the health care or macro-level, where in the case of limited resources budget allocation choices have to be made among programs. The second, or meso-level, pertains to policy making at the patient group or hospital level, at which decisions have to be made for defined groups of patients with the same symptoms or disease, and for which evidence-based guidelines or protocols are to be developed. The third is the micro-level and applies to decision-making for an individual patient. The term value refers to different entities in these contexts, resulting in different elicitation processes. For each of these levels, we prefer to reserve the term "values" for abstract, trans-situational judgments.

Utilities

Utility is a summary measure of the extent to which each outcome of each choice option achieves each of our ultimate goals (Baron 2008, p. 233). Health state utilities play an important role in health care decision-making and health economics. The most important applications of utilities are in expected utility decision analysis, in which the expected utility for each possible strategy is calculated by combining the utilities for all possible resulting health states (outcomes) with the probabilities of these states occurring. The utility of a health state is a cardinal measure of the strength of an individual's preference for particular outcomes when faced with uncertainty (Torrance and Feeny 1989). This concept of utilities dates back to the 1940s when a normative model for decision-making under uncertainty, expected utility theory, was developed (Von Neumann and Morgenstern 1944). In most decisions in health care, outcomes may occur with a certain probability, and the decision problem is thus a problem of choice under

uncertainty and expected utility theory applies. An important application of utilities is the QALY, or quality adjusted life year, in which each year spent in a health state is multiplied by its utility, and the thus adjusted life years are summed. QALYs are mostly used in cost-effectiveness ratios, based on expected utility decision analyses in which the numerator is expressed in costs (Dollars or Euros) and the denominator (effectiveness) in QALYs.

Preferences

There is no consistent definition of preferences in health care, but there is convergence in the notion that health care preferences can be defined as "statements made by individuals regarding the relative desirability of a range of health experiences, treatment options or health states" (Brennan and Strombom 1998, p. 259). Individual preferences exist as the relatively enduring consequences of values (Brennan and Strombom 1998). Differently from values, preferences are object-focused and relate to specific options, or attributes of options, in a specific decision context.

Health-related preferences have been described in relation to a variety of domains. In recent studies, the term has been used to describe, for example, choice among a set of treatment options (Alolabi et al. 2011), treatment aspects (Pfützner et al. 2012), or health professionals (Bishop et al. 2013); the desirability of procedural aspects of screening (Blom et al. 2012) or treatment (Vela et al. 2012); the desirability of sources (Gaglio et al. 2012), amount (Ter Hoeven et al. 2011), or kind of information (Ormond et al. 2009); and the desirability of participating in health-related decision-making (Davison and Breckon 2012). Patient preferences—and this is true for health care provider or significant others' preferences too—vary further widely with respect to stability and clarity (Street et al. 2012). Individual preferences can be quite steady but need not. Preferences can vary as a function of disease severity, can evolve as individuals learn new information or gain new experiences, or have had more opportunity to explore thoughts, feelings, and values relevant to the clinical situation. For example, Feldman-Stewart et al. (2004) found that 82 % of early stage prostate cancer patients who had already discussed their condition with their oncologist and who were thinking through their treatment options, changed which attributes affected their decision, and 72 % changed how much they valued the treatment options as a whole, as they were going through a patient decision aid (see section "Values Clarification Methods" on decision aids).

From Basic Values to Articulated Utilities and Preferences: A Constructive Process

Conceptualizations of values differ in the extent to which they are articulated (Fischhoff 1991). On the one end of the continuum, people are seen to hold *articulated* or well-differentiated, "complete" values that can be elicited if one asks the right question (Gregory et al. 1993). On the other end, people are seen to hold only *basic* values, that is, lack well-differentiated values for all but the most familiar issues, and that preferences need to be constructed (constructive preferences) from basic values at the time of decision-making (Payne et al. 1999). In this partial perspective, people could respond with values that are not at stake if they miss nuances of the question asked. Articulated values most often exist when decisions are personally familiar; with few consequences; implying no conflicting roles; and formulated in a familiar fashion (Fischhoff 1991, Table 3). Complex decisions in health care—such as allocation of resources or choice of treatment, often are new to decision makers; have more than a few consequences; and many of these consequences are not commensurable, such as trading treatment convenience (e.g., pills versus injections) for treatment effectiveness. Further, values may be conflicting because options on offer cannot achieve both the goals of, for example, lengthening life and improving quality

of life (Epstein and Peters 2009). For health care decision-making, the basic values paradigm thus seems most appropriate. Utilities and preferences are usually being constructed as a function of the specific decision options and the context in which the utility or preference is being elicited (Payne et al. 1992).

Measurement of Utilities at the Macro- and Meso-Level

Utilities are mostly used at the macro- and meso-levels of health care decision-making, and the level determines whether they should be assessed from the general public or from patients. In cost-utility analyses from a societal perspective, i.e., for macro-level decision-making, Gold et al. (1996) have recommended the use of society's preferences, that is, from a representative sample of fully informed members of the general public. In guideline development, the meso-level, the use of utilities obtained from actual patients is preferred. Members of the public who are asked to imagine experiencing health states assign lower utilities to those states than the patients who are actually experiencing these states (Stiggelbout and De Vogel-Voogt 2008), which resonate with the disability paradox; many people with serious disabilities report that they experience a good or excellent quality of life (Albrecht and Devlieger 1999). At the micro-level, with an individual patient, utility assessment is seldom used and if used, it is done in a constructive way and meant to serve as values clarification (e.g., Unic et al. 1998, and section "Values Clarification Methods").

Approaches to Utility Measurement

We can distinguish two different approaches to measuring utilities. The **holistic** approach requires the participant to assign values to each possible health state, where a state represents a combination of many attributes. The **decomposed** approach enables the investigator to obtain values for all health states without requiring the judge to assign values to each one. It expresses the overall value as a decomposed function of the attributes. This approach can also be used specifically to obtain the utilities of the attributes per se, in health services research.

Holistic Approaches to Utility Measurement

Holistic valuations of health states encompass valuations of the quality of life of those states, and the valuations are therefore sometimes called *preference-based* measures of quality of life, as distinct from *descriptive* measures of quality of life, using questionnaires such as the SF-36. The methods can be used either to have participants value hypothetical health states, or to have patients rate their own health. In the former case, the health states are described in a scenario, generally framed in terms of physical, emotional, and social functioning. Several methods exist to assess utilities for health states holistically (Stiggelbout and De Haes 2001). The **Standard Gamble (SG)** has long been seen as the gold standard, since it adheres to the axioms of expected utility theory. It is based on the principle that a person will be willing to accept a risk in order to obtain good health, if he or she feels that the health state under evaluation is undesirable. The participant is offered the hypothetical choice between the sure outcome (the health state to be valued, for one's remaining life expectancy) and a gamble, with probability p of obtaining the best possible outcome, set at 1 (generally optimal health, for one's remaining life expectancy) and a probability $(1 - p)$ of the worst possible outcome, set at 0 (usually immediate death). By varying p, the value is obtained at which the participant feels the sure outcome and the gamble to be equivalent. The utility for the sure outcome, the health state to be valued, is equal to the value of p at this point of indifference $(U = p \times 1 + (1 - p) \times 0 = p)$. Thus, for example, a woman is asked to rate the state "rheumatoid arthritis". If she is indifferent to the

choice between her remaining life in that state and a gamble with a probability of 0.90 that her remaining life will be in optimal health and a probability of 0.10 of immediate death, her utility for that health state is 0.90. The utility measured with a SG reflects not only the participants' preference for life in the health state, but also their attitude toward risk. The use of probabilities has proven to be a major drawback of the method, since participants have difficulties relating to probabilities. Moreover, they have been shown to transform probabilities; they tend to overweight small probabilities and underweight large probabilities (Tversky and Kahneman 1992). In most examples in health, small probabilities of bad outcomes (such as death) occur, which thus tend to be overweighted, leading to extremely risk averse answers, and too high utilities for the states under evaluation. Ceiling effects subsequently limit the ability of the SG to discriminate between health states. This has led researchers to use an alternative method, the time tradeoff method (**TTO**) (Wakker and Stiggelbout 1995).

In the **TTO,** a participant is asked to choose between her remaining life expectancy in the health state to be valued and a shorter life span in optimal health. In other words, she is asked whether she would be willing to trade years of her remaining life expectancy for an improved health. As an example, let us say a 65-year-old woman has a remaining life expectancy (according to national life tables) of 15 years. She is asked what length of time (X) in optimal health would be equivalent to 15 years in her state of rheumatoid arthritis, assuming that in each case death would follow immediately. The simplest and most common way to transform this optimal-health equivalent X into a utility (ranging from 0 to 1) is to divide X by 15. Thus, if she is willing to trade 3 years to obtain optimal health, her utility is 0.80 (12/15).

Both for the SG and TTO, elicitation becomes more complex when temporary states are to be valued (see, e.g., Jansen et al. 1998 for the details on the procedure).

In the TTO no uncertainty is involved, and it therefore does not adhere to expected utility theory, but in practice TTO-scores are generally considered utilities, since they are preference-based. This is in contrast with scores of the next method, the visual analogue scale.

A **Visual analogue scale (VAS)** is a rating scale, which can be self-administered, and therefore is often used to obtain valuations of health states in surveys. Participants are asked to rate the state by placing a mark on a 100-mm horizontal or vertical line, anchored by death (usually on the left or bottom) and optimal health (on the right or top). The preference is the number of millimeters from the "death" anchor to the mark, divided by 100. The VAS does not reflect any tradeoff that a participant is willing to make in order to obtain better health, neither in terms of risk nor in years of life. It can therefore not be considered a preference-based, or utility, method (Torrance et al. 2001). Transformations of VAS scores have been proposed to approximate true SG- or TTO utilities (Torrance 1976; Torrance et al. 1996).

To obtain utilities for policy making, the researcher needs to choose from SG, TTO, and VAS. The SG used to be considered as the gold standard, but due to biases in the method, especially probability transformation, the TTO is most frequently used nowadays. Further, patients generally find it an easier and more acceptable method. Little is known about the biases that may operate in the TTO (see Bleichrodt 2002, for a clear explanation of the possible biases operating in the SG and TTO). As described above, a VAS score is not a utility, but nevertheless the VAS is frequently used to assess utilities, due to its ease of administration. SG and TTO are preferably administered in an interview, to minimize inconsistent and incoherent responses, whereas a VAS can be administered in a questionnaire. The VAS is potentially influenced by basic psychological phenomena (Torrance et al. 2001), and its scores have been argued to be too low, since no tradeoff is involved. Therefore, transformations as described above are generally performed, although Abdellaoui et al. (2007) made a convincing case for an untransformed use of the VAS.

Decomposed Approaches to Utility Measurement

The decomposed methods to value treatments express the overall value as a decomposed function of the health state or treatment attributes. The best-known application of a decomposed method is that based on Multi-Attribute Utility theory (MAUT). Each attribute of a health state (or intervention) is given an importance weight. Next, participants score how well each health state (or treatment) does on each attribute. These scores are weighted by the importance of the attributes and then summed over the attributes to give an overall multiattribute score for each state (or treatment). For this summation, the theory specifies utility functions and the independence conditions under which they would be appropriate. For example, Chapman et al. (1999) provided a MAUT-model for metastatic prostate cancer. They predefined the five attributes such as pain, mood, sexual function, bladder and bowel function, and fatigue and energy to explain the state. Patients were asked to rate the relative importance of these attributes by dividing 100 points among them. Next, patients categorized their current level of health for each attribute. MAU-scores were computed by multiplying, for each attribute, the level by the attribute importance weight, and summing across the attributes.

Most decomposed methods assess valuations for health states or treatments and use regression models to infer the parameters of the attributes, assuming an additive linear process. In subsequent applications, the model thus estimated can be used to infer health state preferences from attributes. This approach has become widespread in the health state classification systems, which are used in cost-effectiveness analyses from a societal perspective, such as the EQ-5D (Dolan 1997) or the Health Utilities Index (Feeny et al. 1995), to generate utilities from the general public. Health state classification systems or health indexes are customarily composed of two components: a descriptive system and a formula for assigning a utility to the health states described by this system. The descriptive system consists of a set of attributes, and a health state is described by indicating the appropriate level of functioning on each attribute. For instance, in the EQ-5D the attributes are mobility, self-care, usual activities, pain/discomfort, and anxiety/depression. Each attribute is divided into three levels of severity (no problem, some problems, and extreme problems). By combining one level from each of the five attributes, a total of 3^5, that is, 243 EQ-5D health states are defined. The formula for assigning utilities to these states is based on utilities that have been obtained in a sample from the general public, in part from direct measurement and in part from application of MAUT (as in the Health Utilities Index) or statistical inference (as in the EQ-5D), to fill in values not measured directly. Based on this formula (for the EQ-5D, e.g., see Dolan 1997), premeasured utilities from the general public are thus available for these systems (Russell et al. 1996). In a cost-effectiveness study it suffices to map the treatment outcomes (the health states) onto the descriptive system—using a patient questionnaire based on the descriptive system—and to use the scoring formula to obtain utilities from the general public for the health states indicated by the patients. In this way, standardization over studies is obtained. All researchers use the same utility set, and cost-effectiveness ratios are comparable.

Whereas the aim of these decomposed techniques is mostly to assess holistic valuations of health states or treatments via decomposition, other techniques, such as conjoint analysis and discrete choice experiments, aim to measure how treatment or health state attributes are valued per se.

Conjoint Analysis, developed to examine consumer preferences in marketing is increasingly used in health to assess attribute preferences. Similar to the decomposition techniques described above, participants judge hypothetical cases (health states or treatments) that are described in terms of combinations of attributes at particular levels. Statistical analysis reveals the attribute level utilities (Ryan and Farrar 2000).

Most commonly, two cases or options (treatments or health states) are seen at a time (hence the name conjoint analysis) and a choice is made between them. *Adaptive* conjoint analysis cases are paired according to a set of stated attribute weights and responses to previous options—using special software (Pieterse et al. 2010). Analysis of the data is based on random utility theory. These methods have predominantly been used in health services research to assess correlates of preferences, such as sociodemographic characteristics of (potential) service users and to influence policy decision-making. The adaptive methods are finding their way in micro-level decision-making, to support values clarification, as described in the next section.

Measurement of Preferences at the Micro Level

Assessments of preference for specific options, rather than outcome states, are tailored to the clinical problem at hand and will reflect the real-life situation more than does the utility assessment. In health services research, at the meso-level, assessment of treatment preferences informs cut-offs in guidelines above or below which treatment is indicated. For example, patient preferences were incorporated in the decision to recommend chemotherapy at a benefit in overall 10-year survival of 5 % in the Dutch breast cancer treatment guidelines (Bontenbal et al. 2000). Alternatively, preferences can be assessed to define profiles of patients for whom a particular option is more germane than for others. At the micro or individual patient level, decisions about treatment and health care management ought to reflect individual patients' preferences (Kassirer 1994).

Treatment Tradeoff Method

The treatment or probability tradeoff method was developed to assess participants' strength of preference for one health management option relative to another, usually treatments. In this method, preferences for combined process-and-outcome paths are elicited in the following way. The patient is usually presented with two clinical options, for example, treatments A (e.g., no adjuvant treatment) and B (e.g., adjuvant chemotherapy), which are described with respect to (probabilities of) benefits (e.g., additional probability of 5-year survival) and side-effects (e.g., nausea, hair loss, and fatigue), and is asked to state a preference for an option. If treatment A is preferred, the interviewer systematically either increases the probability of benefit from treatment B, or reduces the probability of benefit from treatment A (and vice versa if treatment B is preferred at the outset). Which treatment aspects are altered and in which direction, is decided upon beforehand, according to the relevant clinical characteristics and the research question (Llewellyn-Thomas et al. 1996). The patient's willingness to accept side-effects of one treatment or forego benefits of the alternative treatment determines the patient's relative strength of preference. This general approach has been adapted to a variety of treatment decisions, including adjuvant chemotherapy in breast cancer (Levine et al. 1992), treatment of Lupus Nephritis (Fraenkel et al. 2002), and radiotherapy for rectal cancer (Pieterse et al. 2007). In all cases, preference strength is idiosyncratic to the original decision problem, that is, relative to the specific alternatives that were presented. The method can be used to support individual treatment decision-making and has been applied "at the bedside" using decision boards as visual aids (Levine et al. 1992).

Values Clarification Methods

At the micro-level, so-called patient decision aids have been developed to help individuals facing challenging health decisions make specific and deliberative choices (Stacey et al. 2011). As a part of these interventions, components referred to as "values clarification methods" (VCM) can be included to help elucidate individuals' health management preferences. The name is confusing as these interventions really are aimed at eliciting and clarifying *preferences*. VCM include any methods "that are intended to help patients evaluate the desirability of options or attributes of options within a specific decision context, in order to identify which option he/she prefers" (Fagerlin et al. 2013). These VCM can also be used to measure individual preferences (Fraenkel et al. 2006).

Many and very different types of VCM exist. In treatment-related decision-making, interventions described as VCM include balance scales (O'Connor et al. 1998); rating (Feldman-Stewart et al. 2006) or ranking (Sheridan et al. 2010) the importance of risks or benefits of options; indicating whether each piece of information pushes one toward or away from a given choice (Smith et al. 2010); or listing reasons (Abhyankar et al. 2011). They can also consist of having an open discussion about attributes of interest (Matheis-Kraft and Roberto 1997). Evidence on the effects of using VCM in the context of patient decision aids is still limited, but there are indications that it improves decision processes (Fagerlin et al. 2013).

There is a little evidence suggesting how patients actually clarify the personal importance they associate with different health management options, such as how they weigh pros and cons within a decision, and thus how best to support the process. Further, since preferences in health are deemed constructive, there is no way to measure "true" preferences since they are formed in the process of elicitation. From a cognitive psychological perspective, VCM should aim to facilitate one or more of the following processes: help optimize individuals' mental representations of the decision and the options; encourage individuals to consider all potentially appropriate options; delay the selection of an initially favored option; facilitate the retrieval of relevant values from memory; facilitate the comparison of options and their attributes; and offer time to decide (Pieterse et al. 2013). These recommendations were formulated based on commonalities between the four process theories of decision-making (differentiation and consolidation theory, image theory, parallel constraint satisfaction theory, fuzzy-trace theory), for which evidence has been gathered though mostly outside of the health care context.

Key Directions for Future Research

At the macro-level, most of the researches that are currently performed in utility assessment relate to the classification systems, such as the EQ-5D. This is likely because these have the most direct practical application in cost-utility analyses, which in turn are mandatory for reimbursement decisions in many health care systems around the world. The assessment of holistic utilities, for example using the TTO, is typically seen in purely scientific work, without direct practical application. The challenges for the EQ-5D mostly lie in improving the descriptive systems, for example, by adding levels to the attributes. A recurring issue is the actual content of the classification systems, and whether the traditional dimensions, generally based on the WHO definition of health and incorporating physical, psychological, and social functioning, should not be replaced by a capability approach or by dimensions of subjective well-being (Coast et al. 2008).

The elicitation of utilities is quite an abstract task, with which participants have been found to have difficulties (Edelaar-Peeters et al. 2014). Interviewer help is therefore generally needed, even though web-based administration would highly reduce costs. Future research should find ways to mimic the help that interviewers give as part of web-based administration.

Moreover, conventional approaches to the TTO are problematic when evaluating health states that are perceived to be worse than death. The TTO requires fundamentally different tradeoffs tasks for the valuation of states better and worse than death (Tilling et al. 2010). An alternative elicitation method, "lead time TTO" is currently under study as a way to possibly overcome the problem (Augustovski et al. 2013).

At the micro-level, research revolves around the evaluation of how effective the VCM are at clarifying preferences. A challenge at the micro-level for future research lies, therefore, in designing theory-based VCM and outcome measures—where the theory chosen should help in selecting outcome measures that the intervention is expected to affect (Pieterse et al. 2013).

Conclusion

Preferences refer to very different entities at the macro-, meso-, and micro-levels of health-related decision-making. At each of these levels, we recommend to save the term *value* for abstract, trans-situational judgments. The most adequate process of preference elicitation is a function of the goal of assessing individuals' health-related priorities and depends on the level of health care decision-making. Particularly at the level of the individual patient, more research is needed on the clarification of patient preferences.

> **Box 1. Definition of values, utilities and preferences in a health care decision context**
>
> **Values**
>
> Abstract, trans-situational judgments about intermediate or terminal goals that guide the evaluation of states or selection of behaviors and are ordered by relative importance
>
> **Utilities**
>
> Summary measures of how health states realize our ultimate values or goals; should be measured in specific ways resulting in a number between 0 and 1 and are most often applied in expected utility decision analyses and in cost-utility analyses at the macro and meso-decision-making level

> **Preferences**
> Relative desirability of a range of specific health experiences, health management options, attributes of options, or health states, in a specific decision situation; the assessment of preferences can inform decision-making at the meso- and micro-level of decision-making

References

Abdellaoui, M., Barrios, C., & Wakker, P. P. (2007). Reconciling introspective utility with revealed preference: Experimental arguments based on prospect theory. *Journal of Econometrics, 138*, 356–378.

Abhyankar, P., Bekker, H. L., Summers, B. A., & Velikova, G. (2011). Why values elicitation techniques enable people to make informed decisions about cancer trial participation. *Health Expectations, 14*(Suppl 1), 20–32.

Albrecht, G. L., & Devlieger, P. J. (1999). The disability paradox: High quality of life against all odds. *Social Science and Medicine, 48*, 977–988.

Alolabi, N., Alolabi, B., Mundi, R., Karanicolas, P. J., Adachi, J. D., & Bhandari, M. (2011). Surgical preferences of patients at risk of hip fractures: Hemiarthroplasty versus total hip arthroplasty. *BMC Musculoskeletal Disorders, 12*, 289–298.

Augustovski, F., Rey-Ares, L., Irazola, V., Oppe, M., & Devlin N. J. (2013). Lead versus lag-time trade-off variants: Does it make any difference? *European Journal of Health Economics, 14*(Suppl 1), S25–31.

Baron, J. (2008). *Thinking and deciding*. New York: Cambridge University Press.

Bishop, F. L., Smith, R., & Lewith, G. T. (2013). Patient preferences for technical skills versus interpersonal skills in chiropractors and physiotherapists treating low back pain. *Family Practice, 30*, 197–203.

Bleichrodt, H. (2002). A new explanation for the difference between time trade-off utilities and standard gamble utilities. *Health Economics, 11*, 447–456.

Blom, R. L., Nieuwkerk, P. T., Van Heijl, M., Bindels, P., Klinkenbijl, J. H., Sprangers, M. A., et al. (2012). Patient preferences in screening for recurrent disease after potentially curative esophagectomy. *Digestive Surgery, 29*, 206–212.

Bontenbal, M., Nortier, J. W., Beex, L. V., Bakker, P., Hupperets, P. S., Nooij, M. A., et al. (2000). Adjuvant systemic therapy for patients with resectable breast cancer: Guideline from the Dutch National Breast Cancer Platform and the Dutch Society for Medical Oncology. *Nederlands Tijdschrift voor de Geneeskunde, 144*, 984–989.

Brennan, P. F., & Strombom, I. (1998). Improving health care by understanding patient preferences: The role of computer technology. *Journal of the American Medical Informatics Association, 5*, 257–262.

Chapman, G. B., Elstein, A., Kuzel, T. M., Nadler, R. B., Sharifi, R., & Bennett, C. L. (1999). A multiattribute model of prostate cancer patients' preferences for health states. *Quality of Life Research, 8*, 171–180.

Coast, J., Smith, R. D., & Lorgelly, P. (2008). Welfarism, extra-welfarism and capability: The spread of ideas in health economics. *Social Science and Medicine, 67*, 1190–1198.

Davison, B. J., & Breckon, E. N. (2012). Impact of health information-seeking behavior and personal factors on preferred role in treatment decision making in men with newly diagnosed prostate cancer. *Cancer Nursing, 35*, 411–418.

Dolan, P. (1997). Modeling valuations for EuroQol health states. *Medical Care, 35*, 1095–1108.

Edelaar-Peeters, Y., Stiggelbout, A. M., & Van den Hout, W. B. (2014). Qualitative and quantitative analysis of interviewer help answering the time tradeoff. *Medical Decision Making, 34*, 655–665 (provisionally accepted).

Epstein, R. M., & Peters, E. (2009). Beyond information: Exploring patients' preferences. *JAMA, 302*, 195–197.

Fagerlin, A., Pignone, M., Abhyankar, P., Col, N., Feldman-Stewart, D., Gavaruzzi, T., et al. (2013). Clarifying values: An updated review. *BMC Medical Informatics and Decision Making, 13*, S8.

Feeny, D., Furlong, W., Boyle, M., & Torrance, G. (1995). Multi-attribute health status classification systems. Health utilities index. *Pharmacoeconomics, 7*, 490–502.

Feldman-Stewart, D., Brennenstuhl, S., Brundage, M. D., & Roques, T. (2006). An explicit values clarification task: Developmental and validation. *Patient Education and Counseling, 63*, 350–356.

Feldman-Stewart, D., Brundage, M. D., Van Manen, L., & Svenson, O. (2004). Patient-focussed decision-making in early-stage prostate cancer: Insights from a cognitively based decision aid. *Health Expectations, 7*, 126–141.

Fischhoff, B. (1991). Value elicitation: Is there anything in there? *American Psychologist, 46*, 835–847.

Fraenkel, L., Bogardus, S., & Concato, J. (2002). Patient preferences for treatment of lupus nephritis. *Arthritis and Rheumatism, 47*, 421–428.

Fraenkel, L., Gulanski, B., & Wittink, D. R. (2006). Preference for hip protectors among older adults at high risk for osteoporotic fractures. *Journal of Rheumatology, 33*, 2064–2068.

Gaglio, B., Glasgow, R. E., & Bull, S. S. (2012). Do patient preferences for health information vary by health literacy or numeracy? A qualitative assessment. *Journal of Health Communication, 17* (Suppl 3), 109–121.

Gold, M. R., Siegel, J. E., Russell, L. B., & Weinstein, M. C. (1996). *Cost-effectiveness in health and medicine*. New York: Oxford University Press.

Gregory, R., Lichtenstein, S., & Slovic, P. (1993). Valuing environmental resources—A constructive approach. *Journal of Risk and Uncertainty, 7*, 177–197.

Jansen, S. J., Stiggelbout, A. M., Wakker, P. P., Vliet Vlieland, T. P., Leer, J. W., Nooy, M. A., et al. (1998). Patients' utilities for cancer treatments: A study of the chained procedure for the standard gamble and time tradeoff. *Medical Decision Making, 18*, 391–399.

Kassirer, J. P. (1994). Incorporating patients' preferences into medical decisions. *New England Journal of Medicine, 330*, 1895–1896.

Levine, M. N., Gafni, A., Markham, B., & MacFarlane, D. (1992). A bedside decision instrument to elicit a patient's preference concerning adjuvant chemotherapy for breast cancer. *Annals of Internal Medicine, 117*, 53–58.

Llewellyn-Thomas, H. A., Williams, J. I., Levy, L., & Naylor, C. D. (1996). Using a trade-off technique to assess patients' treatment preferences for benign prostatic hyperplasia. *Medical Decision Making, 16*, 262–282.

Matheis-Kraft, C., & Roberto, K. A. (1997). Influence of a values discussion on congruence between elderly women and their families on critical health care decisions. *Journal of Women & Aging, 9*, 5–22.

O'Connor, A. M., Tugwell, P., Wells, G. A., Elmslie, T., Jolly, E., Hollingworth, G., et al. (1998). A decision aid for women considering hormone therapy after menopause: Decision support framework and evaluation. *Patient Education and Counseling, 33*, 267–279.

Ormond, K. E., Banuvar, S., Daly, A., Iris, M., Minogue, J., & Elias, S. (2009). Information preferences of high literacy pregnant women regarding informed consent models for genetic carrier screening. *Patient Education and Counseling, 75*, 244–250.

Payne, J. W., Bettman, J. R., & Johnson, E. J. (1992). Behavioral decision research: A constructive processing perspective. *Annual Review of Psychology, 43*, 87–131.

Payne, J. W., Bettman, J. R., & Schkade, D. (1999). Measuring constructed preferences: Towards a building code. *Journal of Risk and Uncertainty, 19*, 243–270.

Pfützner, A., Schipper, C., Niemeyer, M., Qvist, M., Löffler, A., Forst, T., et al. (2012). Comparison of patient preference for two insulin injection pen devices in relation to patient dexterity skills. *Journal of Diabetes Science and Technology, 6*, 910–916.

Pieterse, A. H., De Vries, M., Kunneman, M., Stiggelbout, A. M., & Feldman-Stewart, D. (2013). Theory-informed design of values clarification methods: A cognitive psychological perspective on patient health-related decision making. *Social Science and Medicine, 77*, 156–163.

Pieterse, A. H., Stiggelbout, A. M., Baas-Thijssen, M. C., Van de Velde, C. J., & Marijnen, C. A. (2007). Benefit from preoperative radiotherapy in rectal cancer treatment: Disease-free patients' and oncologists' preferences. *British Journal of Cancer, 97*, 717–724.

Pieterse, A. H., Stiggelbout, A. M., & Marijnen, C. A. (2010). Methodologic evaluation of adaptive conjoint analysis to assess patient preferences: An application in oncology. *Health Expectations, 13*, 392–405.

Rohan, M. J. (2000). A rose by any name? The values construct. *Personality and Social Psychology Review, 4*, 255–277.

Russell, L. B., Gold, M. R., Siegel, J. E., Daniels, N., & Weinstein, M. C. (1996). The role of cost-effectiveness analysis in health and medicine. *JAMA, 276*, 1172–1177.

Ryan, M., & Farrar, S. (2000). Using conjoint analysis to elicit preferences for health care. *BMJ, 320*, 1530–1533.

Schwartz, S. H. (1994). Are there universal aspects in the structure and contents of human values. *Journal of Social Issues, 50*, 19–45.

Schwartz, S. H., & Bilsky, W. (1987). Toward a universal psychological structure of human-values. *Journal of Personality and Social Psychology, 53*, 550–562.

Sheridan, S. L., Griffith, J. M., Behrend, L., Gizlice, Z., Jianwen, C., & Pignone, M. P. (2010). Effect of adding a values clarification exercise to a decision aid on heart disease prevention: A randomized trial. *Medical Decision Making, 30*, E28–E39.

Smith, S. K., Trevena, L., Simpson, J. M., Barratt, A., Nutbeam, D., & McCaffery, K. J. (2010). A decision aid to support informed choices about bowel cancer screening among adults with low education: Randomised controlled trial. *BMJ, 341*, c5370.

Stacey, D., Bennett, C. L., Barry, M. J., Col, N. F., Eden, K. B., Holmes-Rovner, M., et al. (2011). Decision aids for people facing health treatment or screening decisions. *Cochrane Database of Systematic Reviews, 10*, CD001431.

Stiggelbout, A. M., & De Haes, J. C. J. M. (2001). Patient preference for cancer therapy: An overview of measurement approaches. *Journal of Clinical Oncology, 19*, 220–230.

Stiggelbout, A. M., & De Vogel-Voogt, E. (2008). Health-state utilities: A framework for studying the gap between the imagined and the real. *Value in Health, 11*, 76–87.

Street, R. L, Jr., Elwyn, G., & Epstein, R. M. (2012). Patient preferences and healthcare outcomes: An ecological perspective. *Expert Reviews in PharmacoEconomics and Outcomes Research, 12*, 167–180.

Sutherland, H. J., & Till, J. E. (1993). Quality of life assessments and levels of decision making: Differentiating objectives. *Quality of Life Research, 2*, 297–303.

Ter Hoeven, C. L., Zandbelt, L. C., Fransen, S., De Haes, H., Oort, F., Geijsen, D., et al. (2011). Measuring cancer patients' reasons for their information preference: Construction of the Considerations Concerning Cancer Information (CCCI) questionnaire. *Psycho-Oncology, 20*, 1228–1235.

Tilling, C., Devlin, N., Tsuchiya, A., & Buckingham, K. (2010). Protocols for time tradeoff valuations of health states worse than dead: A literature review. *Medical Decision Making, 30*, 610–619.

Torrance, G. W. (1976). Preferences for health states: An empirical evaluation of three measurement techniques. *Socio-Economic Planning Sciences, 10*, 129–136.

Torrance, G. W., & Feeny, D. (1989). Utilities and quality-adjusted life years. *Journal of Technological Assessment in Health Care, 5*, 559–575.

Torrance, G. W., Feeny, D., & Furlong, W. (2001). Visual analog scales: Do they have a role in the measurement of preferences for health states? *Medical Decision Making, 21*, 329–334.

Torrance, G. W., Feeny, D. H., Furlong, W. J., Barr, R. D., Zhang, Y., & Wang, Q. (1996). Multiattribute utility function for a comprehensive health status classification system: Health utilities index mark 2. *Medical Care, 34*, 702–722.

Tversky, A., & Kahneman, D. (1992). Advances in prospect-theory—Cumulative representation of uncertainty. *Journal of Risk and Uncertainty, 5*, 297–323.

Unic, I., Stalmeier, P. F., Verhoef, L. C., & Van Daal, W. A. (1998). Assessment of the time-tradeoff values for prophylactic mastectomy of women with a suspected genetic predisposition to breast cancer. *Medical Decision Making, 18*, 268–277.

Vela, K. C., Walton, R. E., Trope, M., Windschitl, P., & Caplan, D. J. (2012). Patient preferences regarding 1-visit versus 2-visit root canal therapy. *Journal of Endodontics, 38*, 1322–1325.

Von Neumann, J., & Morgenstern, O. (1944). *Theory of games and economic behavior*. Princeton: Princeton University Press.

Wakker, P., & Stiggelbout, A. (1995). Explaining distortions in utility elicitation through the rank-dependent model for risky choices. *Medical Decision Making, 15*, 180–186.

Decision Architectures

Bradford W. Hesse

Introduction

At the core of many of the quality improvement initiatives spearheaded by the U.S. Institute of Medicine (IOM) was an assumption that medical communication and decision-making must be improved in order to achieve truc population benefits from evidence-based medicine. Medicine is an information-intensive enterprise, argued the authors of the IOM report *"Crossing the Quality Chasm: A New Health System for the 21st Century"* (Institute of Medicine 2001). The only sustainable way to improve patient outcomes is to reengineer the *systemic architectures of medicine* to ensure that the right information is delivered to the right people in the right way to improve the quality of care (Reid et al. 2005; Hesse and Shneiderman 2007). This was the rationale underlying passage of the Health Information Technology for Economic and Clinical Health (HITECH) Act of 2009, which sought to improve patient care by delivering better cognitive and decision support to health care providers, patients, and family caregivers. It was also the rationale underlying many of the provisions of the Affordable Care Act of 2010, which sought to reengineer incentives within

health care to emphasize prevention, patient engagement, continuity of care, and cost effectiveness (Hesse 2010; Stead and Lin 2009). The U.S. House Appropriations Committee added further reinforcement when it highlighted "health decision-making" as an important focus for ongoing research and development within the priorities of the National Institutes of Health (NIH) in 2011 (The Cancer Letter 2011; President's Council of Advisors on Science and Technology 2010).

Strains Within the System

The need for continued work in the area of supported decision-making sounds well and good, but what does it really mean to say that health systems researchers need to reengineer the systemic architectures of medicine? Isn't this what eight (+) years of advanced medical education in the classroom and residency programs, plus a plethora of up-to-date science articles in advanced medical journals, are supposed to accomplish? Aren't physicians and patients used to making effective decisions unassisted by decision aids or information technologies?

To be sure, training is an important and necessary part of medical judgment; but unaided decision-making is rapidly becoming insufficient in a world of information-intensive medicine. As hard as it may be to believe, the first Randomized Controlled Trial (RCT) in medicine was only

B.W. Hesse (✉)
Health Communication and Informatics Research, National Cancer Institute, Bethesda, MD 20892, USA
e-mail: hesseb@mail.nih.gov

© Springer Science+Business Media New York 2016
M.A. Diefenbach et al. (eds.), *Handbook of Health Decision Science*,
DOI 10.1007/978-1-4939 3486-7_2

published in 1952 (Daniels and Hill 1952). Staying abreast of the medical literature in 1952 when scientific publications from randomized controlled trials were few and far between may have been a reasonable task. By 2003, though, the U.S. National Library of Medicine estimated that it had been adding almost 10,000 new articles per week within its own online archives—a number that represented only about 40 % of all medical articles published worldwide in biomedical and clinical journals. To stay abreast of the exploding research base just within one specialty would require practitioners to read upwards of 20 articles per day, 365 days a year (Shaneyfelt 2001). That is an impossible task.

To complicate matters further, medical decision-making is by its nature becoming much more data intensive (Topol 2012). By one account, the average number of facts a physician would need to bear in mind when making a decision about a patient's treatment in 1990 was around five (Smith et al. 2012). These were decisions based on an evaluation of the clinical phenotype only; that is, decisions in which the medical practitioner's task would primarily be to evaluate the signs and symptoms accompanying a chief complaint and then to apply a type of one-size-fits-all formulary to match the hypothesized diagnosis with a population-based guess on treatment. Medicine is becoming much more predictive and personalized than that today (Culliton 2006; Collins 2010). Genomic indicators, functional expressions of DNA transcriptions, and molecularly precise assessments of treatment efficacy will create a reality in which the treating physician must take into account 1000 or more facts over the course of a patient's treatment. Cognitive research suggests that the number of facts a human information processor can manage at any given time hovers at around 7 ($\pm$2) (Miller 1956). Under the projections of precision medicine, it is difficult to consider a future that does not explicitly include the design of efficient decision architectures to improve the

ways in which clinical teams and their patients make ongoing judgments related to care (Institute of Medicine and McClellan 2008).

Failing to Support Patient Engagement in Decision-Making

Not only have strains in the system made it difficult to support physicians' decision needs, but it may also be failing to support patients' informed participation in their own care. In other sectors of the economy, consumers have been learning to interact with complex information systems in ways that are responsive, user-centered, and empowering. Whether relying on a seamless network of Automated Teller Machines and online bill paying to access their own money in any currency around the world, benefiting from the unparalleled safety records of an integrated air traffic control system, or simply reaching their own personal destinations with the help of a user-friendly Global Positioning System (i.e., GPS), consumers have come to depend on state-of-the-art information architectures to navigate the choices of their daily lives (Obama 2012). This has not necessarily been the case in health care.

Consider an all too familiar scenario. A patient waits until a medical problem has progressed to the point of extreme discomfort or reduced functioning before visiting a physician. If this is the patient's first visit to a physician's office, the receptionist may ask her to fill out a form listing all of the medications she may be currently taking; all of the medications she had previously taken; any remembered side effects or deleterious interactions from previous treatments; any persistent complaints or recollections of diagnosed conditions; blood type or other relevant biologic assessments; and a cursory explanation for the purpose of her visit. More often than not, these patients *will not* have brought their own records with them, and they will likely find it impossible to remember the technical names of pharmaceuticals they might have taken previous to the visit. They may even find it difficult to remember the names and prescribed dosages of medications they are taking currently.

After completing the intake forms, the patient is then escorted to an examination area where a few cursory measures of weight, height, blood pressure, and temperature are added to the patient's newly initiated file. The results are recorded, and the patient is instructed to disrobe and wait until the doctor is ready. After a few seemingly interminable moments the physician comes into the room, quickly peruses the chart and briefly asks a few clarifying questions, performs a focused physical examination, and then writes a prescription. To the patient, the prescription appears to be written in code, with abbreviated Latin terms for mode and frequency of administration (e.g., "p.o." for per os, or by mouth; "q 3 h" for quaque 3 hora, or "every three hours"). If there is accompanying literature, the formatted small print and technical jargon will look more like a legal disclaimer than a set of coherent, easy-to-follow instructions (McClellan 2008).

In the event the physician is not able to reach a firm diagnosis within the 15 min customarily allotted for a clinical encounter, the patient may be given instructions for visiting a laboratory or specialist. Responsibility for the handoff is frequently put on the shoulders of the patient with instructions to make the follow-up appointment, to request that the appropriate records be transferred, and to ensure that insurance will cover the extra expense. The patient will then proceed from one appointment to the next, repeating the chief complaint and brief history along the way. Office staff will take new notes and record them into an expanding chart, though the patient may not have any idea what information or how much information has been transferred between offices. The patient's files grow—with more insurance forms and more technically framed descriptions of

services—while at the same time the patient's sense of decisional control grows more tenuous (Taplin and Rodgers 2010).

The Consequences

The consequences of these systemic strains on the decision systems in medicine and health have become severe, especially when considered at the population level. Up until 1999, hospital staff intuitively knew that avoidable errors were occurring with some regularity within their system. In 1999, the Institute of Medicine put a population level count on the consequences of those errors by estimating that some 48,000–98,000 deaths occurred annually due to some type of avoidable medical error (Kohn et al. 2000). That figure exceeded the number of individuals dying from AIDS, breast cancer, or automobile accidents at the time it was reported. Actuarial data from 2008 suggested that the annual cost of measurable medical errors resulting in direct harm to patients as assessed through medical claims was $17.1 billion (Van Den Bos et al. 2011). The practice of medicine used to be "simple, largely ineffective, and relatively safe," argued Sir Cyril Chantler in an oft-quoted Lancet article. With advances in modern medical technology, medicine is rapidly becoming much more effective, but it is also becoming much more complex and extraordinarily dangerous (Chantler 1999).

Contrast these numbers with the number of avoidable deaths from an equally technology-dependent, complex system: aviation. On April 27, 2012, the U.S. National Transportation Safety Board (NTSB) reported that there were *zero fatalities* involving U.S. air carriers or commuter operations in 2011. According to the press release, 2011 was the second straight year in which no fatalities were observed from air travel among U.S. carriers (National Transportation Safety Board 2012).

This remarkable statistic was reported in spite of the fact that there was a small increase in the number of observed accidents or near misses in the industry overall in 2011. Even when factoring in deaths from previous years, the number of fatalities is astonishingly low in the airline industry. The NSTB had reported that the overall number of fatalities over the previous decade was about three deaths per 10 billion passenger miles traveled per year (Insurance Information Institute 2012). That makes a stark contrast to the 48,000–98,000 deaths from medical error estimated to occur annually during the same period (Kohn et al. 2000).

Why is there such a contrast between these two sectors of the economy? This is the question posed by Donald Berwick, Director of the Centers of Medicare and Medicaid from 2009 to 2011. He has concluded that there are significant differences in the contextual fabrics of medicine and aviation that account for these vast differences. In medicine, he observed, a perverse system of "fee-for-service" incentives has created a decentralized medical environment in which adherence to evidence-based approaches for treatment is spotty; the use of risky, and often unnecessary, treatments is prevalent; and an assessment of end-to-end quality control is infeasible (Berwick 2002; Berwick et al. 2008). National health care reform efforts are working to change those incentives while establishing the data infrastructure needed to track patients across health systems (President's Council of Advisors on Science and Technology 2010).

Another reason why the aviation system may be superior in its control of error is the investment it has made in understanding the psychology of human technology interaction, a field known historically as "human factors" research. There have been two antiquated cultures in modern times, reasoned human factors scientist Kim Vincente: one based on a mechanistic, engineering view of the world and one based on a very humanistic, social view of the world. The first view assumes that most problems can be solved through new and better technology—that the answer to bad technology is more technology; while the second assumes that the locus of all problems lies within people—that the way to fix problems is through more education, more rewards, or a culture of "blame and shame." Neither of these worldviews is sufficient on its own to guarantee safety and efficiency in a technology-dependent industry such as aviation or health care. Separated, they are leading to a hidden epidemic of error and chaos (Vicente 2003).

What human factors researchers discovered when performing root-cause analyses of accidents and near misses in aviation (i.e., using specialized analytic techniques to identify the originating cause, rather than symptom, of a critical error) was that the technological and human subsystems are *inextricably linked* and must be studied *together* to improve performance within systems. This combined, or transdisciplinary (Stokols et al. 2008), view is based on the observations: (a) that technical systems have social consequences; (b) that social systems have technical consequences; (c) that systems engineers do not create technologies, they create sociotechnical systems; and (d) that progress within these systems must be gained by understanding how people and technologies interact. In medicine this view is referred to as a sociotechnical perspective on health system redesign (Coiera 2004). Within the National Academy of Sciences, this focus has been referred to as *"Human System Integration"* (Committee on Human-System Design, N.R.C. 2007).

Nudging Best Practice: A Behavioral Economics Approach

Behavioral economists Thaler and Sunstein popularized the notion of improving the systemic architectures upon which individuals make day-to-day decisions in their book *"Nudge: Improving Decisions about Wealth, Health, and Happiness."* What these two authors were able to do was bring together decades of research in human factors, cognitive psychology, and social psychology to dispel the Cartesian notion popular in classical economics that human judgment

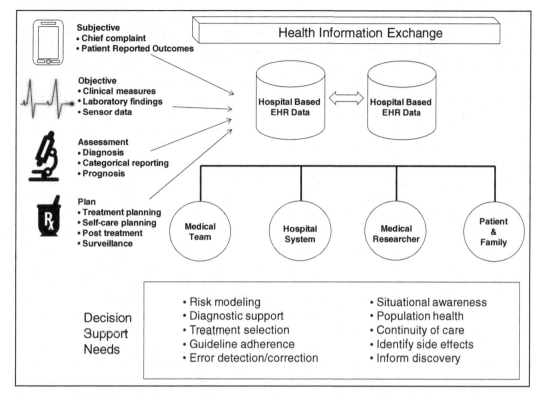

Fig. 2.1 Decision support within a fully connected, data-driven environment of care

is universally rational, logical, and deliberative; while at the same time suggesting how new supports could be constructed within systems to overcome those limitations and improve overall decision-making (Thaler and Sunstein 2009). Hesse et al. 2011 extended the architectural theme into the realm of contemporary health care by examining how a movement toward interconnected data systems could be marshaled to create a robust foundation for evidence-based practice.

Figure 2.1 offers an overview of what an interconnected data system in health care might offer decision makers. Once just a theoretical vision, these types of systems are becoming a reality in many health care systems around the world. In the United States, data from the Centers for Disease Control and Prevention show that adoption of Electronic Health Record (EHR) systems has risen above the 50 % penetration mark among all physicians. Penetration within Health Maintenance Organizations has

reached 100 % (Jamoom et al. 2012). At the left of Fig. 2.1 is a depiction of the various types of data signals that are available for compilation within an EHR system. The inputs are organized following the traditional SOAP notes format utilized in paper-based-charts; that is, with *subjective* and qualitative descriptions of the chief complaint included in the record along with *objective* measures from medical tests and laboratory findings, diagnostic conclusions and other professional *assessments*, and ongoing *plan* for treatment and in some cases long-term care or vigilance.

As these data are brought together, they can be made available—separately or jointly—to each of the stakeholders in an expanded view of the care team. According to a literature review sponsored by the Agency for Health care Research and Quality (AHRQ), data at the practice level can be harnessed for clinical decision support to: "(1) remind clinicians of things they need to do, (2) provide information when clinicians are unsure of what to do, (3) correct errors that clinicians have made, and (4) recommend that clinicians change their plans" as warranted by evidence (Berner 2009). Data at the hospital level can be harnessed by decision makers to: (1) guide quality improvement activities, (2) identify underserved patient populations for specialized outreach, (3) constrain costs, and (4) optimize workflow (Karsh 2009). Medical researchers can use the data to: (1) monitor for post-market side effects, (2) generate hypotheses, (3) update calculations for disease prevalence, and (4) improve the precision of care (McGinnis 2010). Although underappreciated currently, patients should benefit from clinical support around these same data to: (1) participate more directly in shared decision-making processes, (2) formulate more accurate mental models of their disease or condition, (3) improve their self-management skills with accurate feedback on physiological responsiveness, and (4) adhere more rigorously to recommended screening schedules and care plans (Goetz 2010).

Within the Thaler and Sunstein framework, there are six overarching dimensions to consider when constructing improved environments for decision-making. Each will be discussed in the context of a data-enabled, decision architecture as the foundation for evidence-based medicine.

Incentives

Incentives are a core aspect to consider in any view informed by behavioral economics. Understanding what motivates people in their day-to-day decision-making can go a long way in explaining some of the unanticipated consequences of policies or market forces within an economic sector. Berwick's observation that the traditional fee-for-service model may have led to a fragmented and error-prone system of care plaguing the U.S. medical system fits well in this regard. Many health economists have observed that if the current incentive structure is left unaltered it will continue to do even greater harm to patients while bankrupting social safety nets

(Cutler 2009). One of the express goals of the Accountable Care Act of 2010, then, was to use the purchasing power of the U.S. Medicare and Medicaid system—one of the largest consumers of medical services—to reassert influence back on the incentive structures in play within the medical marketplace.

Preparatory to passage of the Affordable Care Act, health care economists also noted that the incentives were not in place for medical decision makers to take full advantage of the electronic structures needed to improve care and capitalize on efficiencies (Cutler 2007). Speculations were that in a fee-for-service environment the participating entities who were digitizing records upstream were not necessarily the same parties who would gain maximum return on those investments downstream (Blumenthal 2009). To address this misalignment of incentives, Congress moved in 2009 to pass the Health Information Technology for Economic and Clinical Health (HITECH) Act (Title XIII of the American Recovery and Reinvestment Act). The HITECH Act offered monetary compensation for those who could demonstrate "meaningful use" of health information technologies to improve patient care initially, followed by penalties for failing to use these systems in meaningful ways subsequently in the program. *Meaningful use* was further defined as using Health I.T. to (a) improve the safety and efficiency of health care, (b) to promote patient engagement, (c) to encourage continuity of care, (d) to facilitate population health, and (e) to protect patients' privacy and confidentiality (Blumenthal and Tavenner 2010).

The "patient engagement" component of the meaningful use program resonated with existing research on the importance of patient activation as the first line of defense against chronic and acute conditions (Wagner 2004). University of Wisconsin researchers hypothesized that the health care system could be reengineered explicitly to do a better job at supporting patients' own internal incentives for becoming optimally involved in their own care. What these researchers found was that by adhering to psychological principles of intrinsic motivation (i.e., motivations that are internal rather than external to individuals), they were able to engineer decisional architectures to be more naturally empowering to patients. Specifically, the researchers were able to demonstrate greater patient activation by: (a) protecting a patient's sense of decisional autonomy or personal control, (b) offering resources to support mastery of new health behavior skills, and (c) providing a sense of reliable connection to supportive others (Hawkins et al. 2010).

Mental Models

Human information processing succeeds in guiding behavior because it is based on an intricate set of internal knowledge structures, developed both through formal education and through years of experience in complex social environments. These knowledge structures, or schema, serve to organize incoming information, establish parameters for rapid fire decision-making, and set the course for personal action (Morgan 2002). Human factors researchers have noted that many of the decision support structures developed throughout history have been created with the express objective of complementing these internal structures. Whether it was the evolution of human language (which elevated cognition through a system of symbolic abstractions) or the invention of writing, movable type, and now computers the purpose has been the same: to complement "knowledge in the head" with "knowledge in the world" to inform planning, decision-making, and action (Norman 2002; Hesse 2008).

In modern medicine, there are two types of knowledge structures that must converge to influence health outcomes. One is the general knowledge base that the biomedical community brings to the encounter as encapsulated through years of professional training, practice-based experience, and ongoing scientific discovery. The other is an ecologically valid model of the patient's current health condition as informed by the patient's previous health history, self-reports of functioning or chief complaint, physical measurement, and a cumulative set of professional assessments. Medical practitioners come to the clinical encounter imbued with their own, richly articulated mental models for diagnosing problems, for determining courses of treatment, for interacting within the patient-provider relationship, and for following up on care after treatment has been completed (Montgomery 2006). Patients and their families come into the medical encounter with their own "common sense models" of disease organized around understanding what a particular ailment might be, what its cause might have been, what its course (timeline) and consequences might be, and whether there is anything that can be done to control the ailment's outcomes (Cameron and Leventhal 2003). Both practitioners and patients will also bring a rich set of personal values to the encounter, which must also come into play when making decisions (O'Connor et al. 2009).

Much of the design work in decision support has focused on packaging information into a format that is interpretable from the perspective of an intended user's current mental model. Thus, risk communication brochures can be designed to be easily readable by patients with less than a college education and can be written to emphasize the specific links between a risk condition and the actions needed to reduce that risk (Morgan 2002). Information systems perform better when they conform to users' mental models (Shneiderman and Plaisant 2004). Group performance, a criterion of recent attention surrounding the importance of coordinated care teams, improves when the information provided to teams is transmitted in a way that conforms to shared mental models (Salas and Fiore 2004). The idea of using decision support technologies to build a sense of "situational awareness" among team members is relevant here. The goal of enhancing situational awareness is to improve the shared understanding of stakeholders in a patient's care by representing an ecologically valid model of the patient's history, status, and goals to the full team (Karsh 2009).

Defaults

Most decision architectures carry with them a default course of action, making it easier for users to interact with the system in a timely and cost-efficient way. Employees will either opt-in or opt-out of certain benefit programs at work, depending on the policies set by their organizations. Software users are accustomed to accepting default values when installing their systems or managing upgrades. When set appropriately, defaults can save decision makers a considerable amount of time while providing a course for action that has been calculated to benefit broader societal objectives. Something as simple as building green spaces into the architectural requirements of a new urban landscape can go a long way in making it easy for residents to stay active through walking.

Decision structures in medicine are no different, with default, easy-to-follow paths leading to more implicit endorsement than more effortful options. The difference between default and non-default paths became surprisingly clear to policy makers seeking to improve the rate at which their citizens volunteered to donate organs after death. Some countries have explicit "opt-in" policies for consent to organ donation. In those countries, citizens must go out of their way to indicate their willingness on a consent form to allow their organs to be harvested in the event of a fatal accident. In other countries, the default is different. Citizens are expected to offer their organs for the benefit of others in the event of a fatal accident, and must go out of their way to "opt out" if they are disinclined. Differences in donation rates based on the ways in which these two options are presented are dramatic. In countries with opt-out policies, donation rates usually exceeded 90 % of the population. In countries with opt-in policies, donation rates lingered below 15 % (Davidai et al. 2012).

The problem in modern health care has often been that an inattention to defaults has led to unanticipated negative consequences over time. A default policy suggesting that no one should be offered access to dependency services unless explicitly requested can easily push many would-be quitters away from trying to seek help. The end result is that more costs may be embedded in the system as unattended smoking addictions lead to serious chronic disease for patients in the long haul (Cancer Center Directors Working Group 2006). Similarly, a default hospital culture that makes it difficult for nursing staff to confront physicians about a missing laparotomy sponge upon closing an incision in surgery will increase the likelihood and frequency of medical errors. The consequences can then be terribly expensive, either in financial terms after fighting avoidable litigation or more lamentably in human terms through ruined lives and shattered careers (Berwick 2002). Needless to say, the opportunities for decision scientists to set new, healthier defaults within medical environments are abundant.

Feedback

The idea of integrating feedback into clinical care has been an important part of medicine for decades. It would be hard to imagine a contemporary operating theater that did not provide real time surveillance of blood pressure, O_2 content, heart rate, or operative progress through bioimaging. Ergonomics engineers have worked on these systems to ensure that they optimize team performance by offering continual surveillance of key physiological systems in the background, but then alerting the operating team when values go out of range. Outside of the operating room, precision measurements on physiological status will continue to provide feedback to the care team during post-operative recovery and long term healing. The use of a medical chart to record these measurements over the course of recovery makes it possible for all members of the care team to monitor feedback across situations and over time.

As the medical profession moves towards a model of engaged patient participation, new research will be needed to design the channels and presentations of feedback that can be motivating to patients and their proxies. The "know your number" campaign supported by the National Heart Lung and Blood Institute is a good example of a program designed to help patients keep track of their own cholesterol levels as feedback on their ongoing progress to keep hyperlipidemia in check. Building a record of laboratory tests into a patient's personal health record makes this type of biometric feedback accessible directly to patients as they adjust their diets and behaviors on a day-to-day basis (Krist and Woolf 2011). Psychological evidence suggests that this type of ongoing, biofeedback can be very to motivating to patients as they seek to regulate their own behaviors (Cameron and Leventhal 2003). Evidence from research on successful weight loss programs, for example, suggests that one of the most reliable predictors of dietary success is simply "weighing in" on a routine basis (Goetz 2010).

As the health system begins to record data from a burgeoning set of input channels—from mobile monitoring of input from personal sensors to the systemic integration of electronic health records over a life span—urgent work will be needed to create tools that are empowering and not overwhelming (Hesse and Shneiderman 2007). Hugo Campos, a presenter at a Ted[X] Cambridge conference and himself a heart patient, illustrated this need in a compelling way. At risk for myocardial infarction, Hugo had received a surgical implantation of a cardiac defibrillator. His specific model, Hugo knew, was sending wireless feedback to his care team. These signals were being interpreted by his care team through a set of well-designed, ergonomically supported decision interfaces. The problem was, (from Hugo's perspective) that everyone seemed to have access to these data except him: the one person who could make a difference in life-and-death decisions about personal activity. After fainting on a train platform, he petitioned to have access to the data, but was initially refused. When he finally did receive the information after much legal wrangling, what was delivered to him was a completely uninterpretable and unusable stack of raw data forms (TedX Cambridge 2012).

With stories such as these, the DHHS Office of the National Coordinator for Health Information Technology has made the transfer of data directly to patients a crucial part of the meaningful use requirements for financial remuneration under the HITECH Act of 2009. Moreover, giving data back to patients for their own consumption is not just a good idea, but according to the DHHS Office for Civil Rights it is an explicit obligation under the Health Insurance Portability and Accountability Act (HIPAA) of 1996. Those will only be useful, however, if they are presented in ways that are comprehensible and actionable for self-management.

Human Error

One of the most fundamental ways in which system designers can use a knowledge of human decision processes to improve the quality of health care is to begin with a scientific understanding of how error occurs, and then create robust architectures to compensate for the potential mistakes people may commit. The "undo" command on most word processing programs is a well-designed example of how software engineers were able to anticipate the situations in which users' writing decisions might lead them down unproductive paths. Other examples include the spelling and grammar checking routines that can help writers avoid common writing mistakes during the composition process along with the dialog boxes requiring users to confirm that an intention to delete or overwrite a file is fully intentional and not the result of a misplaced keystroke (Shneiderman and Plaisant 2004).

When considering ways of preventing errors through decision infrastructures in medicine it is useful to delineate the types of error that are likely to occur. Leap and colleagues aggregated common types of medical errors into four overarching categories: diagnostic errors, treatment errors, prevention errors, and other systemic errors (Kohn et al. 2000). Diagnostic errors, according to their typology, include errors or delays in diagnosis, failures to employ indicated tests, use of outmoded (and ineffective) tests or therapies, and failures to act on the results of monitoring or testing. Treatment errors include mistakes in the performance of an operation or procedure, errors in treatment administration, errors in administering the dose or method of using a drug, avoidable delays in treatment, or an inappropriate (not indicated or contraindicated) method of care. Preventive failures include a failure to provide prophylactic treatments or an inadequate monitoring or follow-up to treatment. Some of the failures they include in their broad "other" category include failures of communication, equipment failures, or other failures of a systemic nature. When Mazor and colleagues conducted critical incidence interviews with patients, she found that communication errors were especially prevalent sources of complaint from the patient's perspective (Mazor et al. 2012).

Efforts to prevent these errors through a redesign of decision contexts are beginning to show promise. In 2008, the World Health Organization endorsed checklists in set of pilot studies to improve surgical outcomes across cultures. "The magnitude of improvement demonstrated by the WHO pilot studies," according to one author, "was surprising." When implemented correctly, the checklists produced marked improvements in perioperative outcomes and have made significant contributions to patient safety worldwide (Walker et al. 2012). Other innovations that have shown promise in reducing error include the use of physician reminders triggered either by fully functional EHR systems or through paper-based administration records; computerized provider order entry systems (CPOEs), which will reduce variance between providers by offering standardization through pick-lists and by limiting choices to options already justified by evidence; electronic prescribing (eR$_X$), which can reduce writing/transcription errors while offering a hedge against dangerous drug by drug interactions or side effects; and bar-coded medication administrations (BCMA), which can prevent administration errors at point-of-care while keeping track of usage records across contexts (Institute of Medicine 2011).

Structured Decision-Making

Health-related decision-making is a process. Those involved in the decision process must acquire and interpret inputs, weigh alternatives against probabilities of success, consider course of action in light of personal values, and they must plan, execute, evaluate, and adjust a selected course of action. Patients who experience acute distress must identify symptoms as being out-of-the-ordinary, seek verification of the problem's cause and effect, decide on a course of action, adhere to that course of action until the symptoms and cause are ameliorated, and then take preventive measures to avoid experiencing similar problems in the future. Patients with chronic conditions must extend those processes over longer periods of time, and will need to engage in a protracted period of treatment and self-management. These patients will most likely want to gain an intricate knowledge of their disease so that they can figure out ways of living with it through multiple facets of their lives. They must make daily decisions over what to eat, over how to perform simple activities of daily living, how to work and how to play. They will also need to monitor their own conditions and know when to seek professional help.

Because decision-making is a process, it is useful to consider the ways in which choice architectures can be structured to support better outcomes from that process. Returning to the checklist example, inserting a procedure to evaluate actions against a pre-determined standard of care was an effective way of overcoming error by reorienting the team's attention to a predefined set of steps for effective surgical care. Many of the single-event decision aids for patients documented by the Cochrane Collaboration showed similar efficacy because they shaped a more effective decision process for considering personal values in conjunction with an understandable presentation of alternatives (O'Connor et al. 2009). On the flipside, decision aids that were not effective often failed to sequence the most important aspects of a decision in a way that was helpful or else created its own demands for structure (e.g., excessive data entry) that was not palatable to users or sustainable to systems (Stead and Lin 2009).

This latter point was reinforced in a review commissioned by the Agency for Health care Research and Quality (AHRQ). In that review, authors concluded that the incorporation of clinical decision supports into processes of care would frequently have a significant influence on overall workflow. In negative cases, the influence on workflow might create a backlog of appointments downstream or may inadvertently draw attention away from important decisional features. In the positive cases, the newly introduced decision architecture could improve workflow. Giving a patient material to read ahead of an appointment, and then reviewing the patients' understanding of crucial points for self-treatment, can work synergistically to promote adherence while making the best use of office time. More importantly, by thinking of shared decision-making as a process that occurs across multiple actors and across multiple settings over time, it is possible to construct new architectures that can improve the overall system of care across multiple interfaces (Karsh 2009).

Conclusion

As demands for precision medicine increase, so too will the needs for new ways of combining personal data with evidence-based recommendations to improve the quality of systemic care. For example, continuous, life sensitive EHRs will be needed to combine personally predictive health information with evolving epidemiologic models of risk to focus preemptive action on targets for primary and secondary prevention. Recorded histories of previous and current treatments can be used to improve pharmacovigilance and to collect valuable post-market data on treatment effectiveness and side effects. Ongoing data aggregation through health information exchanges can be used to improve situational awareness, and improve support for a coordinated mental model of the patient's condition as it evolves over different settings of practice.

A focus on decision architectures in this chapter should serve as a reminder that in the evolving ecology of health care there will be many opportunities for embedding a state-of-the science understanding of decision processes into the environment in which decisions will occur. The perspectives of behavioral economics, which are themselves a compilation of observations from the fields of human factors and social cognition, remind us that it is possible to overcome irrational tendencies and misperceptions by attending to user incentives, mental models, defaults, feedback, human error, and structured decision processes.

Decision Architectures: Implications for Application

Focusing attention on decision architectures changes the administrative vantage point for systems change. Rather than focusing on technologies or policies alone on one hand, or on people and training alone on the other, it recognizes that behavior and context are inseparably linked. Several programs have been retooled with this understanding in mind and present opportunities for action. Two concrete examples are listed below:

- Public Health. The Director of the CDC published a framework for health impact with a goal to "change the context to encourage healthy decisions" listed as a foundational activity in public health. Public health successes in this regard include: healthy defaults for clean air, water, and food; reduction in cardiovascular risk factors by changing from saturated to unsaturated cooking oils; offering healthy choices in school cafterias over high calorie choices; and promoting smoke-free public place policies.

• Clinical Practice. The decisional architecture approach is beginning to take
  hold in modern clinical care as practices
  and hospitals seek remuneration from
  the Center for Medicare and Medicaid
  Services for the "meaningful use" of
  health information technologies. As
  proposed by advisory councils to the
  Department of Health and Human Services, the criteria espouse many principles of behavioral economics: that is,
  they focus on (a) creating a safer environment in which decision-making
  must occur, (b) promoting patient
  engagement and system usability,
  (c) ensuring continuity of care across
  different actors, (d) managing outcomes
  at the population level, and (e) building
  safeguards for privacy and
  confidentiality.

References

Berner, E. S. (2009). *Clinical decision support systems: State of the Art*. Rockville, MD: Agency for Health-care Research and Quality.

Berwick, D. M. (2002). A user's manual for the IOM's 'Quality Chasm' report. *Health Affairs (Millwood), 21* (3), 80–90.

Berwick, D. M., Nolan, T. W., & Whittington, J. (2008). The triple aim: Care, health, and cost. *Health Affairs (Millwood), 27*(3), 759–769.

Blumenthal, D. (2009). Stimulating the adoption of health information technology. *New England Journal of Medicine, 360*(15), 1477–1479.

Blumenthal, D., & Tavenner, M. (2010). The "meaningful use" regulation for electronic health records. *New England Journal of Medicine, 363*(6), 501–504.

Cameron, L. D., and Leventhal, H. (2003). *The self-regulation of health and illness behaviour* (xii, 337 p.). London: Routledge.

Cancer Center Directors Working Group. (2006). *Accelerating successes against cancer*. Washington, DC: U. S. Department of Health and Human Services.

Chantler, C. (1999). The role and education of doctors in the delivery of health care. *Lancet, 353*(9159), 1178–1181.

Coiera, E. (2004). Four rules for the reinvention of health care. *BMJ, 328*(7449), 1197–1199.

Collins, F. S. (2010). *Transforming discovery into health*. In *NIH medline plus: The Magazine* (pp. 2–3). Bethesda, MD: National Institutes of Health and the Friends of the Naational Library of Medicine.

Committee on Human-System Design, N.R.C. (2007). *Human-system integration in the system development process: A new look*. R. W. Pew & A. S. Mavor (Eds.). The National Academies Press.

Culliton, B. J. (2006). *Extracting knowledge from science: A conversation with Elias Zerhouni*. Health Affairs (Millwood).

Cutler, D. M. (2007). The lifetime costs and benefits of medical technology. *Journal of Health Economics, 26* (6), 1081–1100.

Cutler, D. M. (2009). Will the cost curve bend, even without reform? *New England Journal of Medicine, 361*(15), 1424–1425.

Daniels, M., & Hill, A. B. (1952). Chemotherapy of pulmonary tuberculosis in young adults; an analysis of the combined results of three Medical Research Council trials. *British Medical Journal, 1*(4769), 1162–1168.

Davidai, S., Gilovich, T., & Ross, L. D. (2012). The meaning of default options for potential organ donors. *Proceedings of the National Academy of Sciences of the United States of America, 109*(38), 15201–15205.

Goetz, T. (2010). *The decision tree: Taking control of your health in the new era of personalized medicine* (xxiv, 294 p.). New York, NY: Rodale, Distributed to the trade by Macmillan.

Hawkins, R. P., et al. (2010). Mediating processes of two communication interventions for breast cancer patients. *Patient Education and Counseling, 81* (Suppl), S48–S53.

Hesse, B. W. (2008). Of mice and mentors: Developing cyberinfrastructure to support transdisciplinary scientific collaboration. *American Journal of Preventive Medicine, 35*(2S), S235–S239.

Hesse, B. W. (2010). Time to reboot: Resetting health care to support tobacco dependency treatment services. *American Journal of Preventive Medicine, 39*(6 Suppl 1), S85–S87.

Hesse, B. W., Ahern, D. K., & Woods, S. S. (2011). Nudging best practice: The HITECH act and behavioral medicine. *Translational Behavioral Medicine, 1* (1), 175–181.

Hesse, B. W., & Shneiderman, B. (2007). eHealth research from the user's perspective. *American Journal of Preventive Medicine, 32*(5 Suppl), S97–S103.

Institute of Medicine. (2001). *Crossing the quality chasm: A new health system for the 21st century* (xx, 337 p.). Washington, DC: National Academy Press.

Institute of Medicine. (2011). *Health IT and patient safety: Building safer systems for better care*. Washington, DC: Institute of Medicine.

Institute of Medicine (U.S.). Meeting (37th: 2007: Washington D.C.), & McClellan, M. B. (2008). *Evidence-based medicine and the changing nature of health care: 2007 IOM annual meeting summary* (xii,

190 p.). The learning healthcare system series. Washington, DC: The National Academies Press.

Insurance Information Institute. (2012). *Aviation.* [December 12, 2012]; Available from: http://www.iii.org/facts_statistics/aviation.html

Jamoom, E., Beatty, P., Bercovitz, A., Woodwell, D., Palso, K., & Rechtsteiner, E. (2012). Physician adoption of electronic health record systems: United States, 2011. *NCHS data brief, 98.*

Karsh, B. -T. (2009). *Clinical practice improvement and redesign: How change in workflow can be supported by clinical decision support.* Rockville, MD: Agency for Healthcare Research and Quality.

Kohn, L. T., Corrigan, J., & Donaldson, M. S. (2000). *To err is human: Building a safer health system* (xxi, 287 p.). Washington, DC: National Academy Press.

Krist, A. H., & Woolf, S. H. (2011). A vision for patient-centered health information systems. *JAMA, 305*(3), 300–301.

Mazor, K. M., et al. (2012). Toward patient-centered cancer care: Patient perceptions of problematic events, impact, and response. *Journal of Clinical Oncology, 30*(15), 1784–1790.

McClellan, M. B. (2008). *Evidence-based medicine and the changing nature of health care: 2007 IOM annual meeting summary* (xii, 190 p.). The learning healthcare system series. Washington, DC: The National Academies Press.

McGinnis, J. M. (2010). Evidence-based medicine— Engineering the learning healthcare system. *Studies in Health Technology and Informatics, 153*, 145–157.

Miller, G. A. (1956). The magical number seven, plus or minus two: Some limits on our capacity for processing information. *Psychological Review, 63*(2), 81–97.

Montgomery, K. (2006). *How doctors think: Clinical judgment and the practice of medicine* (viii, 246 p.). Oxford: Oxford University Press.

Morgan, M. G. (2002). *Risk communication: A mental models approach* (xi, 351 p.). Cambridge: Cambridge University Press.

National Transportation Safety Board. (2012). *Annual aviation statistics for 2011 released: No fatalities On U.S. airlines or commuters, general aviation accidents increased.* April 27, 2012 [cited 2012 December 11, 2012; Press Release]. Available from: http://www.ntsb.gov/news/2012/120427.html

Norman, D. A. (2002). *The design of everyday things* (1st Basic paperback. ed., xxi, 257 p.). New York: Basic Books.

Obama, B. (2012). *Building a 21st century Digital Government.* T. W. House (Ed.). Office of the Press Secretary.

O'Connor, A., et al. (2009). *Decision aids for people facing health treatment or screening decisions (review)*, ed. T.C. Collaboration. New York, NY: Wiley.

President's Council of Advisors on Science and Technology. (2010). *Realizing the full potential of health information technology to improve healthcare for Americans: The path forward.* Washington, DC: The White House.

Reid, P. P., et al. (2005). *Building a better delivery system: A new engineering/health care partnership* (xiv, 262 p.). Washington, DC: National Academies Press.

Salas, E., & Fiore, S. M. (2004). *Team cognition: Understanding the factors that drive process and performance* (1st ed., xi, 268 p.). Washington, DC: American Psychological Association.

Shaneyfelt, T. M. (2001). Building bridges to quality. *JAMA, 286*(20), 2600–2601.

Shneiderman, B., & Plaisant, C. (2004). *Designing the user interface: Strategies for effective human-computer interaction* (4th ed., xviii, 652 p.). Boston: Pearson/Addison Wesley.

Smith, M., et al. (2012). *Best care at lower cost: The path to continuously learning health care in America.* The National Academies Press.

Stead, W. W., & Lin, H. S. (Eds.). (2009). *Computational technology for effective health care: Immediate steps and strategic directions.* Washington, DC: National Academies Press.

Stokols, D., et al. (2008). The ecology of team science: Understanding contextual influences on transdisciplinary collaboration. *American Journal of Preventive Medicine, 35*(2 Suppl), S96–S115.

Taplin, S. H., & Rodgers, A. B. (2010). Toward improving the quality of cancer care: Addressing the interfaces of primary and oncology-related subspecialty care. *Journal of the National Cancer Institute Monographs, 2010*(40), 3–10.

TedX Cambridge. (2012). *Hugo Campos: Heart Patient.*

Thaler, R. H., & Sunstein, C. R. (2009). *Nudge: Improving decisions about health, wealth, and happiness* (Rev. and expanded ed., viii, 312 p.). New York: Penguin Books.

The Cancer Letter. (2011). *House appropriations boosts NIH by $1 billion in draft budget that cuts other HHS programs.* In *The Cancer Letter* (p. 1). Washington, DC: The Cancer Letter.

Topol, E. J. (2012). *The creative destruction of medicine: How the digital revolution will create better health care.* New York: Basic Books.

Van Den Bos, J., et al. (2011). The $17.1 billion problem: The annual cost of measurable medical errors. *Health Affairs (Millwood), 30*(4), 596–603.

Vicente, K. J. (2003). *The human factor: Revolutionizing the way people live with technology* (1st ed.). New York: Taylor and Francis Books.

Wagner, E. H. (2004). Chronic disease care. *BMJ, 328* (7433), 177–178.

Walker, I. A., Reshamwalla, S., & Wilson, I. H. (2012). Surgical safety checklists: Do they improve outcomes? *British Journal of Anaesthesia, 109*(1), 47–54.

Modeling Medical Decisions

J. Robert Beck

- In 2000, the International Society for Pharmacoeconomics and Outcomes Research (ISPOR) Task Force on Good Research Practices in Modeling Studies was formed. Continued methodological development led to a joint task force from ISPOR and the Society for Medical Decision-Making (SMDM) founded in 2010.
- A medical decision model is simply a representation of health care decision process with observable outcomes enabling health care decision makers to choose among competing courses of action.
- A best practice from the ISPOR-SMDM Task Force report highlights the need to develop a clear statement of the problem, objectives of the model, and scope.
- The credibility and value of a decision model depends largely on three components: the plausibility of the structure as measured against the problem concept, the quality of the data that feed the model parameters, and the validity of the outcome structure.
- Health decision models in use today include, decision trees, state-transition models (STM), and dynamic transmission models (DTM).
- Formal medical decision models are now almost exclusively represented as STMs which assume that an individual is always in one of a finite number of conditions (States) and events of interest to the problem are characterized as movements from one state to another (transition).
- Two common STMs are the Markov cohort, where a simulated group of patients begins in a particular health state and transitions within each time unit which are accomplished according to probabilities and the microsimulation, where a cohort of patients moves from state to state one at a time, using a random number based on probabilities to effect the state transitions.
- Adherence to best practices in model development, parameter estimation and analysis will enhance the validity as well as the transparency of STMs, and thus contribute to their value in health science decision-making.

The paper was supported by Award Number P30CA006927 from the National Cancer Institute. The content is solely the responsibility of the author and does not necessarily represent the official views of the National Cancer Institute or the National Institutes of Health.

J.R. Beck (✉)
Fox Chase Cancer Center, Philadelphia, PA, USA
e-mail: robert.beck@fccc.edu

© Springer Science+Business Media New York 2016
M.A. Diefenbach et al. (eds.), *Handbook of Health Decision Science*,
DOI 10.1007/978-1-4939-3486-7_3

The medical decision-making community has been built on a foundation of modeling. The rendering of complex human decisions in forms amenable to analysis dates to the middle of the 20th Century, with landmark work by Von Neumann and Morgenstern (1947) establishing the concept of outcome valuation ("utility") and a seminal *Science* article by Ledley and Lusted (1959) introducing formal approaches to uncertainty in medicine. Professors Howard Raiffa (1968) and Howard and Matheson (1983) developed decision analysis as a formal approach to modeling decisions under uncertainty in the 1960s; health sciences students taking their courses moved their techniques into medicine in the following decades. A special issue of the *New England Journal of Medicine* in 1975 summarized the field to that time, containing articles on decision modeling, cost-effectiveness analysis, and utility (Ingelfinger 1975). Journal articles employing techniques of decision modeling now number in the tens of thousands.

From the beginnings of the field, practitioners and critics have worried about the quality and fidelity of medical decision models. Polemics and philosophical arguments have forced decision scientists to study all aspects of the analytic process. In the past 20 years a number of efforts have been made to create tutorials and to establish guidelines and standards for health decision modeling. In 2000, the International Society for Pharmacoeconomics and Outcomes Research (ISPOR) Task Force on Good Research Practices in Modeling Studies was formed; it reported out in 2003 (Weinstein et al. 2003). Continued methodological development led to a joint task force from ISPOR and the Society for Medical Decision-Making (SMDM) founded in 2010. Their work on Modeling Good Research Practices was reported in a special issue of *Medical Decision-Making* in 2012 (Caro et al. 2012). This article draws heavily from the two task force reports, as well as from standard references and prior work of the author and colleagues. Its structure draws from the 2012 task force report.

Conceptualizing a Medical Decision Model

A model is simply a representation of a reality. It may be simple or complex; theoretical or data-driven. For the sake of this chapter a model is *normative*, that is, it is designed to prescribe an optimal course of action. Therefore the reality being modeled should constitute a health care decision process with observable outcomes. A useful or helpful model should enable health care decision makers to choose among competing courses of action. As several modeling techniques have been developed over the past few decades, a first step in the analytic process is to conceptualize the problem; this should lead to selection and conceptualization of the model.

Conceptualizing the problem. The first step in making a process tractable is to clarify the problem. Early decision models looked at clinical decision-making—either for a single patient or for a diagnostic or therapeutic dilemma. Over time such problems have faded in importance, to be replaced by clinical practice guideline development, reimbursement or funding decisions, or public health assessments. These are all characterized by the need to specify the population of interest, as well as the medical problems or choices faced by decision makers. Consultation with experts representing different aspects of the problem will be required to gain sufficient perspective to choose among competing models.

A best practice from the ISPOR-SMDM Task Force report highlights the need to develop a clear statement of the problem, objectives of the model, and scope (Roberts et al. 2012). The problem statement should constrain the clinical domain to a manageable subset (e.g., "early stage prostate cancer," not all prostate cancer, for a therapeutic decision model). The analytic perspective (clinical, patient, societal, payor, etc.), possible alternatives, and a full suite of outcomes of interest should also be part of the problem statement. In this chapter we will reanalyze a published hypothetical decision analysis of the cost-effectiveness of proton beam therapy in early stage prostate cancer (Konski et al. 2007). Following is a comprehensive problem statement for this analysis:

> The decision problem under study is the best course of initial treatment for men with intermediate risk adenocarcinoma of the prostate. The perspective is that of a payor for clinical services. Clinical interventions considered include intensity-modulated radiation therapy (IMRT) and proton beam therapy (PBT). Outcomes shall include freedom from biochemical failure (FFBF), life expectancy, and costs based on Ambulatory Payment Classification (APC) payment rates and resource-based relative value units. The two time horizons are FFBF period and patient lifetime.

The credibility and value of a decision model depends largely on three components: the plausibility of the structure as measured against the problem concept, the quality of the data that feed the model parameters, and the validity of the outcome structure. Notwithstanding the importance of data and outcomes, the model should be constructed primarily based on characteristics of the decision problem. The model must incorporate all of the key drivers of the decision, and omit no areas of controversy. On the other hand, there is no need to be completely comprehensive, if the decision problem is to evaluate a new approach against a current standard. That is the case in the chapter example: the issue at hand is to evaluate the costs and improvements expected with proton beam therapy to the current standard radiation treatment of IMRT. There is thus no need to model watchful waiting or surgery in this example, as would be the case if the problem under consideration were to select among all options for intermediate risk prostate cancer.

The time horizon of the decision model should be chosen to reflect both the available data and the relevant differences in outcomes among the strategies considered. Practically, however, it is difficult to find an endpoint that reflects all relevant outcomes. Thus most published decision models use patient lifetime as a convenient horizon. Note however that summarizing the remainder of a patient cohort's lifetime involves extrapolating outcomes, often beyond those reported from any study. Life expectancy models also ignore the prospect of qualitative advances in therapy, and thus may misestimate the benefit of one model approach.

The problem formulation must also consider the key variables in the decision, and take into account the feasibility of sensitivity analysis. Sensitivity analysis may involve model structure as well as all parameters; some problem formulations will require structural analysis and thus markedly increase the complexity of the decision problem.

Conceptualizing the model. Selecting the right mathematical and computational approach is based on the problem conceptualization (Roberts et al. 2012). Complex projects often bring together experts in modeling, the clinical domain, and policy analysis. A valuable first step with a mixed group is conducting a formal process of model design. This may involve tools not used in the analysis itself: concept maps (Ruiz-Primo and Shavelson 1996) and influence diagrams (Owens et al. 1997). These tools from behavioral decision-making are particularly valuable when an existing model is being adapted to new data or approaches. Going back to the problem formulation with a concept map may expose structural flaws in the existing model that appear when the new elements are introduced.

The choice of decision model is influenced by modeler preference as well as by the characteristics of the problem formulation (Roberts et al. 2012). Categories include individual and cohort models, and they may be deterministic or (usually) stochastic. The model types in use today include:

Decision trees: best used today for short time horizon problems with relatively complete characterization of the parameters and outcomes;

State-transition models (STMs): useful in long-term or lifetime horizon problems involving cohorts, with parameters that vary over time;

Discrete event simulation (DES): best applied to problems wherein individual variation drives the model and cohort simulation is infeasible;

Dynamic transmission models: the most complex formulations, wherein interactions between individuals and groups have impact on the model outcomes.

For the example in this chapter a state-transition model is most appropriate. One goal of the analysis is explicability, and trees and state models are easier to represent than the more complex DES and dynamic models. The desire to report life expectancy argues against a simple decision tree formalism.

Constructing a State-Transition Model

An STM provides a convenient way of modeling prognosis for clinical problems subject to ongoing risk (Sonnenberg and Beck 1993; Siebert et al. 2012). This model assumes that an individual is always in one of a finite number of conditions, in modeling language "states." Events of interest to the problem are characterized as movements from one state to another: "transitions." Under this broad scope there is room for substantial variation in STMs. Some admit interactions among groups, and others are entirely self-contained. Most clinical STMs incorporate the notion of time directly, although this is not a requirement. STMs can simulate a closed cohort of patients, or a dynamically changing population.

For this example we will construct two common STMs: a Markov cohort, and a microsimulation. These frameworks model a specific patient group, do not permit interactions between individuals, and have a discrete time interval. Transitions can vary. In a Markov cohort, a simulated group of patients begins in a particular health state and transitions within each time unit (or "cycle") are accomplished according to probabilities. In a microsimulation, a cohort of patients moves from state to state one at a time, using a random number (the Monte Carlo method) based on probabilities to effect the state transitions (Siebert et al. 2012). The principal tradeoff between the two formulations is the need for intermediate states in a Markov cohort to deal with nuances in the natural history, versus computational intensity in a microsimulation repeated many thousands of times.

For both the cohort and simulation model of our example we can use a single formulation. Figure 1.1 shows a simplified state-transition diagram for the decision to treat intermediate risk prostate cancer with IMRT or proton therapy. The blue circles on the left side of the figure reflect the choice in the problem: to use IMRT or PBT as initial treatment. In this model we assume the treatment has been completed as per plan; thus the labels "Post-IMRT" and "Post-PBT." Green arrows point to a light blue circle: "Biochemical

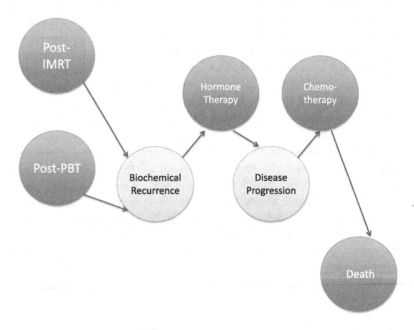

Fig. 1.1 Decision to treat intermediate risk prostate cancer with IMRT or proton beam therapy (PBT) (color figure online)

Fig. 1.2 State Transition Model with all possible transitions (color figure online)

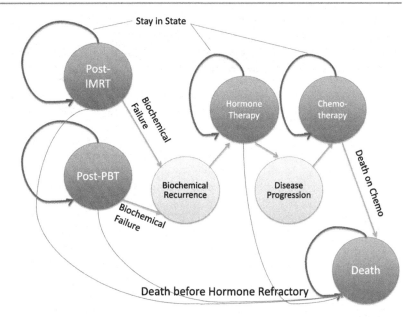

Recurrence." Other than staying in the Post-treatment state, the principal event is biochemical failure, which leads to androgen deprivation therapy (the blue circle "Hormone Therapy" in Fig. 1.1). Another green arrow points to "Disease Progression," which leads to the blue circle "Chemotherapy." Finally, there is a state entitled "Death," which represents mortality either from prostate cancer or other causes. In total there are five major states in the model represented by the darker blue circles, and two temporary states that lead immediately to specific downstream states, shown as lighter blue circles.

Figure 1.2 depicts the model with all possible transitions. The heavy blue arcs signify that for a cycle length of one month (chosen for the model to approximate clinical management), the most likely thing to happen to a patient is that he will stay in his current state of health. The green arcs shown in both Figs. 1.1 and 1.2 illustrate the state transitions due to biochemical failure, disease progression or death from disease while on chemotherapy. The light blue arcs show death while at an earlier stage of disease, either from a treatment complication or other causes. They are drawn lightly to signify that they are less likely transitions than the other possibilities.

Figure 1.3 illustrates the prostate STM as a Markov Cycle Tree, a formulation convenient for computer analysis (Sonnenberg and Beck 1993). The transitions are shown as branches on the tree, and the pathways terminate in a label that "sends" the model back to the beginning of the tree. As an example, the blue rectangular outlines illustrate a transition. Under the IMRT branch, at a given time the STM would be in the "Hormone Therapy" state branch. ("1" in Fig. 1.3). Assuming the patient doesn't die in that cycle ("2"), he experiences a hormonal treatment failure ("3"), leading to the "Chemotherapy" outcome ("4"), which would move the process to the "Chemotherapy" state branch (red outline, "5"). This wordy explanation illustrates why the Markov Cycle Tree formulation is conceptually less attractive than the state diagram, although it is easier to display model details within it.

Parameter Estimation and Valuation

All decision models have parameters that must be estimated. As the principles of evidence-based medicine have evolved over the past several decades, so have decision models matured in their approach to uncertainty. Formal methods of evidence synthesis should be used, including meta-analysis where possible, to populate an STM (Miller and Homan 1994; Owens et al.

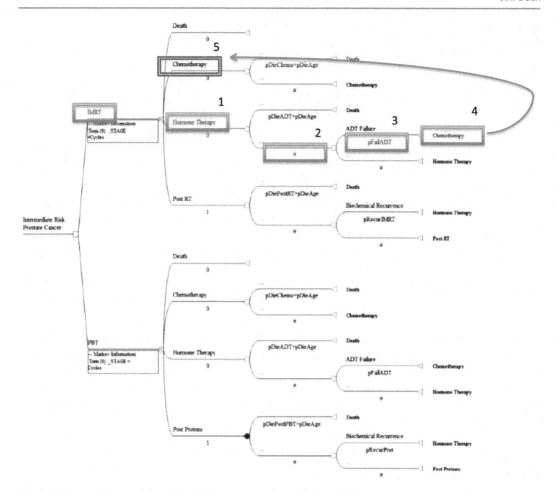

Fig. 1.3 Prostate State Transition Model as a Markov cycle tree (color figure online)

2010). Multiple sources must be considered, rather than basing an analysis on a single report. Where feasible, we can use the statistical distribution on which a probability value is based for uncertainty (sensitivity) analyses—see below.

In the example analysis used in this chapter, we have taken parameter estimates from the original paper (Konski et al. 2007) and updated as newer

data have become available. As this study was conducted to estimate theoretical cost-effectiveness, most of the parameters in the IMRT and PBT STMs are the same. The principal value that differs is the efficacy of treatment: what is the probability of remaining FFBF? Selected parameters, with their values and ranges used in the analysis, are presented in Table 1.

Table 1.1 Selected probabilities and costs used in the analysis

Name	Type	Baseline value	Range
FFBF, IMRT	5-yr probability	0.83	0.80–0.90
FFBF, PBT	5-yr probability	0.93	0.82–0.95
Failure, hormone therapy	Monthly probability	0.0335	0.02–0.05
Death on chemotherapy	Monthly probability	0.023	0.01–0.04
Cost, IMRT	Ambulatory payment	$33,700	
Cost, PBT	Ambulatory payment	$76,500	$50,000–80,000

Table 1.2 Initial cohort membership, IMRT STM

Stage	Post RT	Hormone	Chemo
1	0.99131	0.00309	0.00000
2	0.98270	0.00603	0.00010
3	0.00882	0.00882	0.00030
4	0.96570	0.01148	0.00059
5	0.95731	0.01401	0.00095
6	0.94899	0.01642	0.00139
7	0.94075	0.01870	0.00190
8	0.93526	0.02087	0.00247
9	0.92447	0.02293	0.00309
10	0.91644	0.02488	0.00377

One of the useful attributes of decision models is that the investigator can explore extreme ranges of variables to determine the behavior of the system at boundary conditions. For cost-effectiveness models the fact that parameters are varying in the numerator and the denominator can cause the systems to blow up and give ridiculous results. One therefore must be judicious in the development of sensitivity analyses.

Markov cohort analyses. Solving a Markov cohort analysis involves running a hypothetical cohort of subjects through the STM, and determining the expected values of cost and outcome (Sonnenberg and Beck 1993). Table 2 shows the first several iterations of the analysis for the post-IMRT arm in our sample problem. The entire cohort begins post-IMRT. After one Markov cycle (one month), 99.1 % are still in the post-IMRT state. However, 0.00309 (309 out of 100,000) have transitioned to hormone therapy.[1] After another cycle 0.6 % of the cohort is in hormone therapy, and now 0.01 % in chemotherapy. Note also that the sum of the cohort fraction is (0.9827 + 0.0060 + 0.0001), or 0.9888. Thus 1.12 % of the cohort has died in the first two cycles, due either to disease or other causes (much the more likely at the outset of the model). Running the model to completion

Table 1.3 Baseline Markov cohort model results

Strategy	Time FFBF (months)	Life expectancy (months)	Expected cost ($)
IMRT	102	134	44,260
PBT	109	148	83,700

generates the results shown in Table 3. PBT, on average, would yield seven more months FFBF, and 14 months of life expectancy, at a cost of $39,440. In terms of cost-effectiveness, PBT in this baseline analysis costs $5634 per additional month FFBF, and $33,800 per life-year gained.

To interpret a Markov cost-effectiveness analysis requires establishing norms, such as willingness to pay thresholds and cost-effectiveness acceptability curves for evaluating results (Briggs et al. 2012). This simplified analysis did not include discounting costs or life-years, include the cost and consequences of complications, and did not adjust the health states for quality of life—topics beyond the scope of this article, but covered in review articles and standard texts. However, the baseline analysis suggests that PBT might be an acceptable strategy, assuming the efficacy values are correct.

Microsimulation. Simulations can be of several types. In the simplest formulation, a patient moves through the Markov states, transitioning each cycle according to the model probabilities. This leads to a graph such as Fig. 1.4, where the costs and monthly survivals for 1000 patients are plotted, in blue for IMRT and in red for PBT. Note that many subjects generate no further costs

---

[1]This shows one of the challenges in model building—a simplified Markov model has transitions occurring with the first cycle. We could build a DES that delays this transition for a specified period of time, or we could make a more complex Markov model.

Fig. 1.4 The costs and monthly survivals for 1000 patients (color figure online)

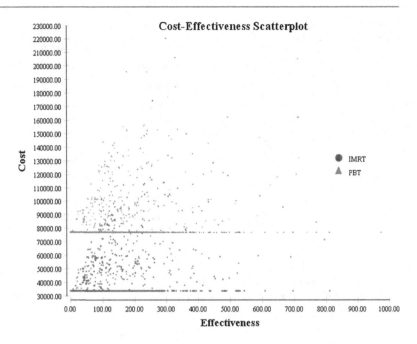

in this simplified model beyond the cost of their initial radiation therapy. This is shown as broken colored lines at the cost levels of IMRT and PBT. On the other hand, some post-IMRT patients run up a large additional expense as their disease progresses, as do some post-PBT subjects.

Sensitivity analysis. One of the most valuable aspects of formal medical decision modeling is that ability to vary parameters to gain insights (Briggs et al. 2012). This sensitivity analysis has two principal aspects. Real issues in the problem under consideration should motivate the clinical use of parameter variation. However, consistency checks of the model can be conducted by pushing variables to their extremes. We will illustrate these characteristics by an example.

Recent reports from several centers suggest that the differential efficacy between PBT and IMRT may not be as great as initially proposed eight years ago (Parthan et al. 2012; Mendenhall et al. 2014). We can explore this efficacy question by varying the parameter from 10 to 50 %, that is, PBT being 10–50 % more effective per month in delaying biochemical failure. Figure 1.5 graphs the incremental (or "marginal") dollars per life year gained with PBT, as the assumption of

efficacy is varied. If PBT is only 10–20 % more efficacious in delaying biochemical failure than IMRT, the cost per life year gained exceeds $80,000. At 30 % the value is close to $50,000 per life year, a common threshold for acceptability in cost-effectiveness studies.

Figure 1.6 shows a family of cost-effectiveness curves. Each curve corresponds to a different 5-year probability of FFBF for IMRT, from a low of 74 % to a high of 94 %. For any value of FFBF probability for IMRT, greater efficacy of PBT leads to fewer dollars per life-year gained. The better IMRT is, however, the higher the marginal cost per life year is with PBT. At the highest value of FFBF for IMRT, PBT does not reach the level of $50,000 per life-year over its analyzed range.

As mentioned above, we could push the boundaries of parameter variation beyond their clinically plausible ranges. Figure 1.6 shows the cost-effectiveness curves rising steeply as the efficacy of PBT over IMRT drops. The model is constructed so that if that efficacy were zero, the life expectancy on both models would be equivalent, and thus the cost-effectiveness would be infinite. On the other hand, if the efficacy were

Fig. 1.5 Incremental (or "marginal") dollars per life year gained with PBT (color figure online)

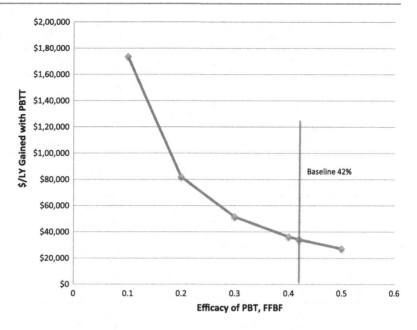

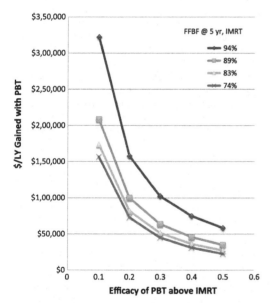

Fig. 1.6 Family of cost-effectiveness curves (color figure online)

Conclusions

Formal medical decision models, which began appearing in the clinical literature in the early 1970s as decision trees, are now almost exclusively represented as STMs. While they would never be considered uncomplicated, STMs can be constructed with modern software at varying levels of complexity. Approaches such as microsimulation and DES enable analysis of uncertainty and variability in decision models, and allow the study of complex problems with heterogeneity and dependencies. Adherence to best practices in model development, parameter estimation and analysis will enhance the validity as well as the transparency of STMs, and thus contribute to their value in health science decision-making.

100 %, the cost on the PBT model would fall to $76,500 (i.e., no additional treatment costs would ever be incurred). The marginal cost-effectiveness of PBT would be under $11,000 per life year—a floor for the value of PBT over IMRT.

References

Briggs, A. H., Weinstein, M. C., Fenwick, E. A. L., Karnon, J., Sculpher, M. J., & Paltiel, A. D. (2012). Model parameter estimation and uncertainty analysis: A report of the ISPOR-SMDM modeling good research practices task force—6. *Medical Decision Making, 32*, 722–732.

Caro, J. J., Briggs, A. H., Siebert, U., & Kuntz, K. M. (2012). Modeling good research practices—Overview: A report of the ISPOR-SMDM modeling good research practices task force—1. *Medical Decision Making, 32*, 667–677.

Howard, R. A., & Matheson, J. (Eds.). (1983). *The principles and applications of decision analysis. General collection* (Vol. 1), *Professional collection* (Vol. 2). Menlo Park, CA: Strategic Decisions Group.

Ingelfinger, F. J. (1975). Decision in medicine. *New England Journal of Medicine, 293*, 254–255.

Konski, A., Speier, W., Hanlon, A., Beck, J. R., & Pollack, A. (2007). Is proton beam therapy cost-effective in the treatment of adenocarcinoma of the prostate? *Journal of Clinical Oncology, 25*, 3603–3608.

Ledley, R. S., & Lusted, L. B. (1959). Reasoning foundations of medical diagnosis. *Science, 130*, 9–21.

Mendenhall, N. P., Hoppe, B. S., Nichols, R. C., Mendenhall, W. M., Morris, C. G., Li, Z., et al. (2014). Five-year outcomes from 3 prospective trials of image-guided proton therapy for prostate cancer. *International Journal of Radiation Oncology, Biology and Physics, 88*, 596–602.

Miller, D. K., & Homan, S. M. (1994). Determining transition probabilities: Confusion and suggestions. *Medical Decision Making, 14*, 52–58.

Owens, D. K., Lohr, K. N., Atkins, D., Treadwell, J. R., Reston, J. T., Bass, E. B., et al. (2010). AHRQ Series Paper 5: Grading the strength of a body of evidence when comparing medical interventions—Agency for Healthcare Research and Quality and the Effective Health-Care Program. *Journal of Clinical Epidemiology, 63*, 513–523.

Owens, D. K., Shachter, R. D., & Nease, R. F, Jr. (1997). Representation and analysis of medical decision problems with influence diagrams. *Medical Decision Making, 17*, 241–262.

Parthan, A., Pruttivarasin, N., Davies, D., Taylor, D. C. A., Pawar, V., Bijlani, A., et al. (2012). Comparative cost-effectiveness of stereotactic body radiation therapy versus intensity-modulated and proton radiation therapy for localized prostate cancer. *Frontiers in Oncology, 2*, 1–8.

Raiffa, H. (1968). *Decision analysis: Introductory lectures on choices under uncertainty.* Reading, MA: Addison Wesley.

Roberts, M., Russell, L. B., Paltiel, A. D., Chambers, M., McEwan, P., & Krahn, M. (2012). Conceptualizing a model: A report of the ISPOR-SMDM modeling good research practices task force—2. *Medical Decision Making, 32*, 678–689.

Ruiz-Primo, M. A., & Shavelson, R. J. (1996). Problems and issues in the use of concept maps in science assessment. *Journal of Research and Science in Teaching, 33*, 569–600.

Siebert, U., Alagoz, O., Bayoumi, A. M., Jahn, B., Owens, D. K., Cohen, D. J., et al. (2012). State-transition modeling: A report of the ISPOR-SMDM modeling good research practices task force—3. *Medical Decision Making, 32*, 690–700.

Sonnenberg, F. A., & Beck, J. R. (1993). Markov models in medical decision making: A practical guide. *Medical Decision Making, 13*, 322–338.

Von Neumann, J., & Morgenstern, O. (1947). *Theory of games and economic behavior* (2nd Ed.). Princeton, NJ: Princeton University Press.

Weinstein, M. C., O'Brien, B., Hornberger, J., Jackson, J., Johannesson, M., McCabe, C., et al. (2003). Principles of good practice for decision analytic modeling in health-care evaluation: Report of the ISPOR task force on good research practices-modeling studies. *Value in Health, 6*, 9–17.

From Laboratory to Clinic and Back: Connecting Neuroeconomic and Clinical Measures of Decision-Making Dysfunctions

4

Ming Hsu and Winston Chiong

Introduction

Impairments in financial and social decision-making capacities are a common symptom in a number of neurological and psychiatric disorders. Such impairments have significant impact on quality of life and overall health outcomes. The NIH estimates that nearly 40 % of the risk of early preventable death in the U.S. is caused by human behavior (Office of Behavioral and Social Sciences Research 2010). However, unlike memory and motor impairments, which are readily recognized as symptoms of more serious underlying neurological conditions, we still largely lack measures to characterize decision-making deficits in clinically meaningful ways.

In the past, the lack of clinical knowledge to tackle to complexity of behavior was compounded by the lack of scientific knowledge on the biological basis of decision-making, at both neural and molecular levels. In the past decade, however, rapid progress has been made in our understanding of neural circuits and neuromodulatory systems that underlie economic decision-making. Moreover, this collaborative effort, from researchers from neuroscience, economics, and psychology, has produced a set of experimental tools that are of great potential value for clinical use (Maia and Frank 2011; Montague 2012). There is now substantial neuroimaging and neuropsychological evidence characterizing the set of brain regions that underlie decision-making, and the computations that are carried out in these regions (Schultz et al. 1997; Hsu et al. 2005; Kable and Glimcher 2007). Second, the experimental paradigms developed have now been used successfully in a number of neuropsychiatric and focal lesion patients, albeit still largely confined to research settings (Frank et al. 2004; Denburg et al. 2007; King-Casas et al. 2008).

Moreover, these applications go beyond relatively simple forms of risk-reward tradeoffs and toward decision-making in the social and interpersonal domains (King-Casas et al. 2005; Fehr and Camerer 2007), which represent some of the most poorly measured forms of dysfunction in clinical settings. The ability to make good decisions in has potentially vast real-world implications. First, we spend much of our lives devoted to the accumulation of financial and social prosperity, and often with much success. To take just one measure, the median net worth of a 65-year-old American in 2007 is more than

M. Hsu (✉)
Haas School of Business, University of California, Berkeley, USA
e-mail: mhsu@haas.berkeley.edu

M. Hsu · W. Chiong
Helen Wills Neuroscience Institute, University of California, Berkeley, USA
e-mail: Winston.Chiong@ucsf.edu

W. Chiong
Memory and Aging Center, University of California, San Francisco, USA

© Springer Science+Business Media New York 2016
M.A. Diefenbach et al. (eds.), *Handbook of Health Decision Science*,
DOI 10.1007/978-1-4939-3486-7_4

double that of a 40-year old (Bucks et al. 2009). For many, however, such wealth comes at a vulnerable time when the cognitive and neurological apparatus that made this possible is beginning to break down (Plassman et al. 2008). It is well known that the elderly are disproportionate targets of fraud across the world, and constitute a conservatively estimated 30 % of all fraud victims in the United States (Templeton and Kirkman 2007; Bucks et al. 2009).

> Impairments in financial and social decision-making capacities have significant impact on quality of life and overall health outcomes, but clinical measures of dysfunction are largely missing. Recent neuroeconomic measures promises to provide such measures, but lack direct evidence that these measures capture clinically relevant behavior, in terms of abnormalities or deficits.

Despite the aforementioned advances, major gaps must be bridged before our newly acquired scientific understanding of decision-making can be applied in clinical settings, to directly improve the care of patients. In particular, much work remains in order to map behavioral and neural measures derived from these paradigms to clinically relevant characteristics. Without this sort of convincing evidence of clinical utility, it is not apparent why neuroeconomic tasks deserve a place in the clinician's toolkit. Here we attempt to shed light on this gap and discuss current challenges in using neuroeconomic measures to: (1) map clinical descriptions of decision-making impairments to laboratory measures and (2) refine and quantify these descriptions. Next, we will focus on a largely untapped source of clinical data in medical charts, which constitute a rich source of primary data, and have been largely untapped in translational research.

The organization of the paper is as follows: Sect. "Neuroeconomic Framework" will provide a selective review of current models and evidence on neural systems underlying decision-making. We will also discuss current approaches to translation research, and the challenges that face them. In Sect. "Medical Charts and Patient Data," we discuss ways to leverage clinical information contained in medical charts, and how neuroeconomic measures can be used to organize these information, and how the two can be combined to generate novel insights that cannot be using either method alone. In Sect. "Conclusion," we conclude by discussing scientific and ethical challenges to a fuller integration of these sources of experimental and clinical data.

Neuroeconomic Framework

Neuroeconomics Is an Old Idea

The conscious application of economic models to understand the inner workings of the brain is largely a new endeavor, dating back only a decade or so (McCabe et al. 2001; Glimcher 2002). However, the study of the biological basis of economic behavior has been with us dating back to the founding of ethology by Lorenz and Tinbergen. Classic works by Tinbergen (1951, 1953), for example, studied bird behavior in the context of what an animal gains by making a decision, including foraging and prey–predator interactions. Economic decision-making, in the sense of acquiring rewards and avoiding punishments, can be clearly seen to fall under the broad umbrella of this scientific tradition.

What changed with the introduction of experimental and behavioral economics ideas into the neuroscientific study of value-based decision-making is twofold. First, experimental economics has provided a broad set of experimental paradigms that have proven to be highly amenable to neuroimaging and neuropsychological studies of behavior in humans. In contrast, previous animal behavior and ethological studies are often naturalistic and difficult to implement in humans due to logistic and ethical constraints. Second, economic theory has provided a set of rigorous and quantitative models of behavior, spanning from relatively simple individual costs-benefit decision-making (e.g., portfolio choice) to complex social and strategic interactions between multiple individuals and groups (e.g., bargaining).

For example, risk taking has been a prominent area of research in neuroscience prior to the introduction of formal economic models (Miller 1992; Bechara et al. 1997). However, there was considerable ambiguity in interpreting subjective attitudes toward risk, which often do not specify the fundamental variables that underlie risk perception and risk taking. Borrowing conceptualizations of risk in economics and finance, neuroeconomic studies model the risk people face in the environment as probability distributions of rewards (Fig. 4.1a). For example, a simple binary outcome lottery is defined by the probability p of winning a larger prize x and the complement $1 - p$ of winning the alternative, smaller, prize y. The risk *preference* or *attitude* of the person is defined by whether they prefer this lottery to its expected value of $p \cdot x + (1 - p) \cdot y$. A person who prefers the lottery to its expected value is said to be risk *seeking*. In contrast, a person who prefers the expected value is said to be risk *averse*. Finally, a person who is indifferent is risk *neutral*. More importantly, the neural correlates of risk processing can now be isolated by systematically manipulating the probability and reward magnitude of the gambles (Kuhnen and Knutson 2005; Preuschoff et al. 2008; Hsu et al. 2009).

Such a quantitative framework has been applied with equal, if not more success, in social behavior. In interpersonal interactions, outcomes are often determined by joint actions of multiple individuals. Here, in addition to learning about rewards and punishments available in the environment, people also need to anticipate and respond to actions of others cooperating or competing for the same rewards. In evolutionary biology and economics, these interactions are described formally using the language of game theory (Fudenberg and Levine 1998; Hofbauer and Sigmund 1998). Specifically, in addition to representing feasible set of rewards and actions available in the environment, people need to also form and update expectations about the actions and consequences of other individuals in the social environment (Fig. 4.1a). Similarly to risk, by manipulating these actions and consequences, the neural correlates of social decision-making can be characterized by manipulating the expectation and consequences of the actions of others (King-Casas et al. 2005; Zhu et al. 2012).

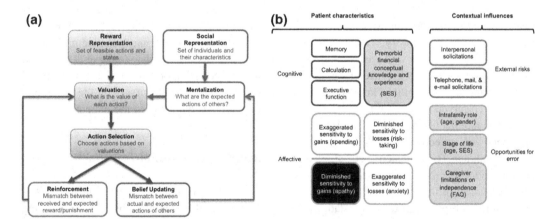

Fig. 4.1 a Economic decision-making in both individual and social (i.e., interpersonal) domains can be described as a series of processes that allows organisms to assign appropriate values to different actions and learning to optimize these action over the course of time. In the social domain, addition to representing feasible set of rewards and actions available in the environment, people need to also (i) represent the set of individuals and their characteristics in the social environment—e.g., whether the situation is a cooperative or competitive one, (ii) form expectation about the likely actions of these individuals, and (iii) detect and correct errors in these expectations, e.g., whether a prosocial action has been reciprocated or betrayed. **b** Applying this framework to patient settings, however, require clinicians and researchers to include a host of characteristics that go beyond this framework, including (i) patient characteristics in other cognitive factors such as memory and affect, and (ii) contextual influences such as familial circumstances and wider social influences

Neuroeconomics in Clinical Context

Beyond isolating specific computational variables that directly influence behavior, however, applications of neuroeconomic models to clinical populations must appreciate the fact that the variation encountered in the clinical context far outstrips those in the lab, or even in typical translational studies. For example, in typical laboratory experiments, participants are screened for memory and language impairments, as well as psychotropic medication. In contrast, these experimentally excluded variables account for much of the decision-making impairments encountered in clinical settings. In the real world, furthermore, economic decision-making is a multidimensional activity that depend upon myriad cognitive and affective resources (Marson et al. 2000), and is strongly influenced by one's social milieu and life circumstances. In addition to decision-making processes themselves, clinical characterizations must also be informed by alterations in cognitive and affective function in different syndromes, as well as account for contextual influences and premorbid individual patient characteristics (Fig. 4.1b). Individual patient cognitive characteristics include disease-related impairment in domains of "fluid" intelligence such as memory, calculation, and executive function, as well as premorbidly acquired "crystallized" intelligence in the form of stored financial conceptual knowledge and experience (Agarwal et al. 2008).

Neuroeconomic research also highlights the importance of affective factors in financial decision-making (Loewenstein et al. 2001; Knutson and Greer 2008); these may have particular relevance in the clinical setting given the recognized neuropsychiatric manifestations of different neuropsychiatric syndromes (Cummings et al. 1994; Levy et al. 1996). For example, applying prospect theory, the most established empirical account of decision-making under risk (Kahneman and Tversky 1979; Tversky and Kahneman 1992), we can distinguish between the disease-related alterations in affective responses to anticipated gains and to anticipated losses. Exaggerated affective responses to gains and blunted responses to losses (or other negative consequences) would predispose patients to errors such as overspending, risky investments, and criminality; while diminished responses to gains and exaggerated responses to losses would predispose patients to conservative decisions (which may or may not be appropriate), and also to anxiety and paranoia about financial matters.

Individual patient's cognitive and affective characteristics interact with contextual influences (Fig. 4.1b). For instance, patients with dementia are less able to critically evaluate telemarketing, e-mail, and personal solicitations. At the same time, if fraud perpetrators target the cognitively impaired, then patients may be at increased risk for receiving such solicitations in the first place (Templeton and Kirkman 2007). Meanwhile, other demographic characteristics may determine whether the opportunity arises for a patient to make a certain kind of error. Some patients, such as wives in some patriarchal cultures, have never have had responsibility for investments or checking, and so would be at less risk for errors in these tasks. Other errors arise in the context of financial issues specific to a stage of life (Nielsen and Mather 2011); for instance, middle-aged patients may be more likely than elderly patients to make errors in purchasing real estate. Finally, some patients' families may act preemptively to limit patients' financial independence and diminish the likelihood of subsequent financial errors, but this depends greatly on the social and family support available to the patient.

Current Translational Approaches

The scientific benefits of a mechanistic understanding of the neural substrates underlying decision-making include: (1) understanding subtypes of decision-making deficits or (2) inferring different causes of these deficits. Most existing measures of financial management in neuropsychiatric illness are primarily designed to identify patients who no longer have the capacity to manage their financial affairs independently. Such tests, however, do not address the many patients present for evaluation at an earlier stage, when they have concerns about their financial management or have made one or two financial errors, yet still manage their finances independently. Also, if risks for different types of error in different syndromes can be established, clinicians will be better-equipped to counsel patients and families to avoid situations that place them at greatest risk (Widera et al. 2011).

In order to justify their clinical application, neuroeconomic tools need to show either diagnostic or prognostic utility. On one hand, potential *diagnostic* applications may identify specific deficits that allow clinicians to recognize the presence of a previously undiagnosed disorder. For example, if certain diseases or injuries to specific systems with the brain are associated with distinctly aberrant profiles in (e.g.,) risk tolerance or temporal discounting, identifying impaired decisions consistent with these traits may allow clinicians to make earlier clinical diagnoses, allowing for earlier treatment and behavioral interventions. On the other hand, *prognostic* applications may be helpful, particularly for patients who have been diagnosed with a disease, in predicting what decision-making errors they might be at greater risk for in the future. This could be used to improve counseling for patients to help them to avoid fraud and other financial harms, and could also be useful for risk stratification to identify high-risk patients for targeted interventions and further study.

Here, by far the most common types of translational studies are those that extend laboratory measures of behavior to clinical populations. For example, Hsu et al. (2005) was able to find behavioral differences in patients with focal lesions to different regions using predictions derived from a neuroimaging study on normal healthy young subjects. Specifically, subjects were asked to choose gambles where the probability distribution was known versus where the probability distribution was unknown. There is substantial evidence that people are averse to the latter, even when normative decision theory suggests they should be valued equivalently (Camerer and Weber 1992). Using fMRI, the authors found a set of regions, in particular the lateral orbitofrontal cortex (LOFC) that showed greater activity under ambiguity compared to risk, whereas the reverse contrast showed greater activity in the striatum (Fig. 4.2a). This result is consistent with existing notions that expected reward differences due to ambiguity aversion is reflected in the striatum, and that LOFC signals uncertainty or salience about the environment. This latter hypothesis was then tested using focal lesion patients with damage to the LOFC. Compared to the control lesion group consisted primarily of temporal pole patients, LOFC patients exhibited less sensitivity to uncertainty in the gambles per se, and were nearly risk and ambiguity neutral (Fig. 4.2b). These results thus were able to shed light on the role of OFC in processing of uncertainty in general, and advance our understanding of the complex affective and behavioral deficits found in neurological patients with damage to the OFC (Bechara et al. 2000).

In the social domain, these paradigms have been successfully applied even in psychiatric disorders, where the etiology is much less clear and diagnostic categories remain controversial (Insel and Fernald 2004). Using an economic exchange task called the Trust game, King-Casas et al. (2008) scanned healthy and borderline personality disorder (BPD) patients during game play (Fig. 4.3a). BPD is a poorly understood mental health condition characterized by long-term patterns of unstable or turbulent emotions. These inner experiences often result in impulsive actions and chaotic relationships with other people (First and Gibbon 1997). The rules of the game are that an investor (always a healthy subject) can invest an amount x between $0 and 20 in the trustee. The amount is tripled to $3x$ by the experimenter, and the trustee can decide to give back to the investor anywhere between $0 and $3x$. The game is then repeated 10 times during the course of the experiment. Behaviorally, whereas the healthy-healthy pairs were able to sustain cooperation through the course of the 10 rounds, the health-BPD pairs experienced significant breakdown in trust, such that investment levels were much lower in the latter portions of the experiment. Neurally, the BPD trustees exhibited diminished responsivity in the insula to inequity signals that were present in the

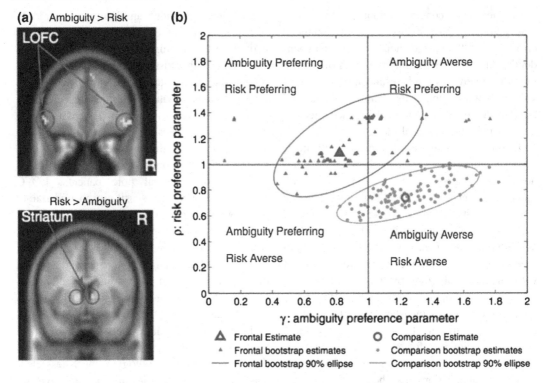

(a) Ambiguity > Risk **(b)**

Fig. 4.2 **a** When participants did not know probability distribution of the gambles (ambiguity), areas of activation included the lateral orbitofrontal cortex (LOFC). In contrast, when the probability distribution is known (risk), the dorsal striatum was significantly activated relative to the ambiguity condition. **b** Using focal lesion patients with LOFC damage, it was found that patients with LOFC damage was significant less ambiguity and risk seeking compared to control patients with lesions in the temporal pole (adapted from Hsu et al. 2005)

investors (Fig. 4.3b). These results provide suggestive evidence that this response might serve as a possible neural marker for BPD.

Medical Charts and Patient Data

Despite these successes in applying neuroeconomic measures of behavior to clinical populations, to date there has been little direct evidence that these measures capture *clinically relevant* behavior, in terms of abnormalities or deficits. That is, does increase risk seeking behavior as assessed in an economic task, or abnormal reward-related neural response as measured in fMRI, predict increased financial risk taking in day-to-day life? One approach to evaluation would insist that such tests undergo clinical trials, in the same manner as medical diagnostic

procedures and treatments (Fig. 4.4a). Such an approach may well be amenable to a select set of tools that tackle the most urgent (or particularly well-understood) problems. It goes without saying, however, that this route is inaccessible for the vast majority of basic science researchers, and puts significant barriers to researchers considering pursuing these questions.

Here we suggest that medical charts are a unique and largely untapped data source that can provide a partial answer to this problem, and may serve as a resource to connect basic and clinical researchers. Moreover, integrating neuroeconomic measures into medical charts would allow for a low-cost and continuous inflow of clinically relevant information that can be scientifically and clinically valuable (Fig. 4.4b). Medical charts offer a focused and unparalleled collection of clinically relevant descriptions of symptoms and

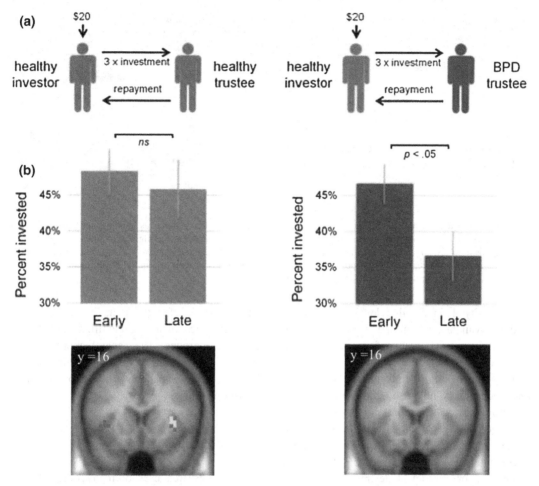

Fig. 4.3 a Healthy and borderline personality disorder (BPD) patients played an economic exchange task called the trust game. The rules of the game are that an investor (always a healthy subject) can invest an amount x between $0 and 20 in the trustee. The amount is tripled to $3x$ by the experimenter, and the trustee can decide to give back to the investor anywhere between $0 and $3x$. The game is then repeated 10 times during the course of the experiment. **b** Behaviorally, whereas the healthy-healthy pairs were able to sustain cooperation through the course of the 10 rounds, the health-BPD pairs experienced significant breakdown in trust, such that investment levels were much lower in the latter portions of the experiment. Neurally, the BPD trustees exhibited diminished responsivity in the insula to inequity signals that were present in the investors (adapted from King-Casas et al. 2008)

deficits. There is already a substantial agreement that patient's health records themselves constitute a valuable resource from a research perspective, and include "a computable collection of fine-grained longitudinal phenotypic profiles" (Jensen et al. 2012). While the data in these records have previously been scattered in paper charts across different physicians' offices (and therefore either inaccessible or only nonsystematically accessible for research), the ongoing adoption of electronic health records and shared protocols for transmitting data between medical practices is hoped to consolidate these data. These changes are expected to improve patient care, while controlling costs (Wu et al. 2006; although see Himmelstein et al. 2010) by limiting the unnecessary repetition of diagnostic tests and procedures, avoiding drug–drug interactions and other harms that may occur when providers are unaware of what other interventions have been prescribed by other providers for the same patient, and improving physicians' diagnostic

(a) Clinical Trials

(b) Integrated Approach

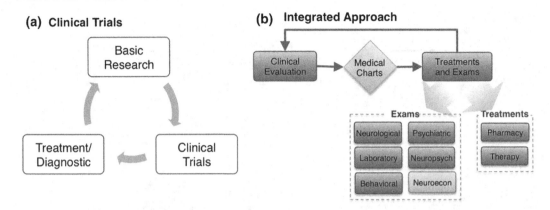

Fig. 4.4 **a** Typical translational approach using clinical trials. This is often most appropriate for novel treatment and diagnostic tools. **b** In contrast, in cases of the heterogenous set of neuroeconomic tools, it is more appropriate to incorporate measures directly in the clinician's toolkit, much as existing neuropsychological exams such as those for language and memory. These can then be refined and improved from scientific study of the relationship between test and clinical outcome

accuracy by having all relevant information readily available when the patient is seen. There is increasing interest from both the academicians and policy makers in connecting this rich domain of clinical information to scientific knowledge. This holds the promise of revolutionizing our classification, diagnosis, and prediction of diseases. Clinical texts in the form of written summaries are a cornerstone of clinical documentation. In the absence of standard behavioral or biological testing of decision-making deficits, these clinical narratives can be a key source of information regarding clinically relevant decision-making deficits.

> Medical charts offer a focused and unparalleled collection of clinically relevant descriptions of symptoms and deficits. These materials can be a unique and largely untapped data source to connect basic and clinical researchers.

Here we consider two broad approaches that could be pursued by researchers in utilizing data from these records; the choice of methods will depend in part on the nature of the records available to researchers, whether other forms of contact with patients are feasible, and on how research groups are able to manage the ethical and practical difficulties associated with research uses of clinical material. The first approach, which has been more extensively discussed in genetics and other domains of research using patient records (Jensen et al. 2012), is a "big data" approach using de-identified patient data from large groups. The second approach is a finer-grained approach correlating clinical data from identifiable patients with experimentally derived measures.

Big Data Approach

Proposed research uses of many other clinical records, as in genetics (Jensen et al. 2012) often involves a "big data" approach, where researchers gather the real-world data from community medical charts, and rely upon large numbers to compensate for the statistical noise of variations in individual physicians' documentation practices. Existing ethical and legal guidelines (discussed in greater detail in the following section) require, with some stringent exceptions, that these data be de-identified unless specific consent for use of these data is obtained. Since it would be impracticable for most research groups to obtain specific consent for such uses from (potentially) thousands of patients with whom they have no preexisting relationship, and since the validity of such "big data" approaches could be vitiated by selection effects (e.g., if the behaviors of patients who refuse to consent to the use of their data are different from those of patients who consent), a uniform approach utilizing de-identified data is most likely to succeed. After potentially identifying information is removed from patients' records, correlations could be sought between data points (such as between financial behaviors, or from financial behaviors to diagnoses).

There are limitations to this "big data" approach as applied to behavioral deficits in neurological and psychiatric diseases. Many of these hurdles reflect the complex cognitive, affective, and behavioral effects of these disorders, which are often far more difficult to quantify than those outside of the CNS. First, the vast majority of medical records are poorly suited for understanding complex behavioral deficits such as economic decision-making. For example, a typical primary care doctor's visit is 15 min, where some part is taken up by paperwork. The type of information documented, especially about behavioral issues like decision-making, will be relatively sparse—e.g. "forgetting to pay bills," and "making mistakes with money". The quantity of information, furthermore, will depend on the features that the physician views as lending support for a particular diagnosis and treatment decisions. It is likely, however, that many of the patients most likely to be of interest in research (i.e., those with behavioral disorders involving decision-making) will also have records from medical specialists in behaviorally oriented fields such as psychiatry and cognitive neurology, and that these records will be of greater potential value.

Second, while correlative approaches between data points in de-identified records have proven useful in other medical domains, there may be limitations to these approaches in the context of decision-making. In domains such as genetics or pharmacology, there is a broad spectrum of potentially informative associations with variables such as allergies to medication, family medical history, or rare adverse outcomes, which may yield previously unsuspected connections. In the case of decision-making, however, many of these parts of the de-identified medical record have little to do with decision-making and are therefore likely to be of low yield. Because there

will be fewer data points in each patient's chart that are directly relevant to existing hypotheses about decision-making, the potential space for revealing correlations between data points in de-identified individual charts will be reduced.

How Medical Charts Can Inform Neuroeconomic Theories and Vice Versa

In contrast, a finer-grained approach would utilize records from patients who have given specific consent for the use of their data in research. The relevant records could either be accessed from existing records, or generated in the course of research evaluations. (For instance, the research visit summaries generated by our group are often sent to a patient's physician at the patient's request, becoming a part of the medical record.) This approach would typically require the research group to have a relationship with the patient, making large numbers logistically difficult. Instead, the value of this approach would be in the opportunity to correlate clinical descriptions of decision-making impairments with other measures, including experimental measures, collected from those patients.

Despite formidable challenges, researchers are now beginning to apply a neuroeconomic framework to medical data. One path to realizing clinical value is for neuroeconomic measures to be integrated into current medical practices (Fig. 4.4b). To do so, however, requires researchers to demonstrate that medical descriptions contain the raw information needed to assess potentially subtle changes in behavior, and that these are robust to confounding factors such as prevalence of comorbidities, diverse socioeconomic status, and presence of general cognitive declines.

To this end, Chiong et al. (In Press) studied susceptibility to financial errors in dementia due to Alzheimer's disease (AD) and behavioral variant frontotemporal dementia (FTD), and assessed whether they differed given the known neuroanatomical targets and behavioral consequences of these syndromes. The authors drew

Table 4.1 Selected patient chart documentation of financial errors (quotes are verbatim)

Alzheimer's disease	Behavioral variant frontotemporal dementia
Increasing obsessive behavior about jewelry and money, suspicious about it being money, constantly asking to see it, count it, and be assured that it is around. She often becomes quite anxious and tearful thinking it is missing or someone has taken it. She has begun hiding it	At baseline, she was quite thrifty and was a successful small business owner. In 2002, she began to be compulsively shopping and she spent a great amount of money on a motor home, two new cars, and in remodeling of the backyard area of her home
In 2006 they received a check back from New York state for $1189 in reimbursement from taxes… he could not figure out how much they owed in taxes that year and simply sent a check	He began giving money out to strangers and was lured into a bogus gambling scheme conceived by his barber. The two of them traveled to Las Vegas at considerable expense on two occasions
[The patient's wife] stated he would forget to pay bills or pay bills twice	He became more aggressive with his investment decisions, and several of his investments lost value in the range of hundreds of thousands of dollars
[S]he started putting her checks and bills in the wrong envelopes	[The patient] started investing massively in lottery tickets, wiring money abroad and falling for scams found in her junk mail or magazines. She reached the credit limit on most of her credit cards and apparently lost tens of thousands of dollars this way

upon both existing neuroeconomic knowledge on neural and cognitive components of financial decision-making and management, as well as clinical experience in evaluating financial errors made by patients with dementia (Table 4.1).

AD is characterized by early memory and executive impairments, reflecting early involvement of the medial temporal lobe and the medial and lateral parietal lobes; whereas FTD is characterized by early alterations in a social and emotional function, reflecting early involvement of the insula and the medial and orbital frontal lobes. While financial errors are observed in both diseases, the authors hypothesized that details recovered from chart data could be used to distinguish between types of financial error that are characteristic of the specific cognitive and affective profiles of each disease.

Using a retrospective chart review approach, Chiong et al. (In Press) found that financial errors are common in AD and bvFTD. 72 % of AD ($N = 100$) and 84 % of bvFTD ($N = 50$) charts included some report of financial impairment. Strikingly, in 16 % of AD cases and 30 % of bvFTD cases, the financial impairment was either the first indicator of cognitive decline or was observed concurrently with the first indicator of decline; and in 34 % of AD cases and 48 % of bvFTD cases, the financial impairment was an early indicator of disease (noted within the first 2 years of illness). While the trend toward greater impairment in FTD in these comparisons was not statistically significant, there were significant between group differences in susceptibility to specific financial errors in AD and bvFTD.

Amnestic financial errors were significantly more common in AD patients (26 %) than bvFTD patients (4 %). In contrast, bvFTD patients were more likely to spend excessively (6 % in AD vs. 34 % in bvFTD) and to otherwise exhibit diminished sensitivity to losses (0 % in AD vs. 36 % in bvFTD) . In some cases, however, the description in the chart was too sparse for more detailed analysis—e.g., one patient who "has made a number of bad decisions with respect to finances." In other cases, the nature of the errors was not recoverable because the patients' decisions had not been monitored by family members, and the patients could not explain what they had done.

In general, financial errors in AD reflected a cognitive vulnerability factor, while financial errors in bvFTD reflected a social and affective vulnerability factor. Social/affective rather than cognitive deficits conferred greater risk for financial errors. This was further supported by factor analysis showing that clinical descriptions of behavior dysfunction can be characterized by two latent factors, with Factor 1 representing social/affective vulnerability and Factor 2 representing cognitive vulnerability to errors. Errors reflecting Factor 1 were less common in AD than in bvFTD (12 % vs. 58 %, $p < 0.001$), while errors reflecting Factor 2 were more common in AD than in bvFTD (29 % vs. 6 %, $p < 0.001$).

Although preliminary, this study presents the first direct evidence to our knowledge that medical charts of dementia patients contain sufficient details about decision-making impairments for a retrospective review (Table 4.1). Due to the inherent limitations of retrospective chart reviews, however, it is impossible to determine whether alterations in neuroeconomic measures precede other cognitive and affective symptoms, whether it correlates with disease progression, nor how they change as a function of treatments. However, these questions can in principle be addressed using the approach we outlined, likely in collaboration with clinical researchers (Fig. 4.4b).

Ethical/Privacy Concerns

Ethical concerns over appropriate respect for patient privacy will be front and center in every discussion of incorporating EHRs in research (Bakalar 2013; Jaret 2013). As observed by one commentator, "In the past, health information privacy has been protected mainly by chaos" (Rothstein 2009). Traditionally, patients' health information has been scattered across paper charts located in dozens of doctors' offices and hospitals, with no centralized resource for sharing or aggregating the information. Thus, the privacy of patients' medical information was protected not only by norms of confidentiality, but also by the practical obscurity conferred by its distribution across multiple incomplete sources. As we have discussed, the comprehensiveness and organization provided by electronic health records opens new possibilities for research; however, because patients are unaccustomed to the prospect of having their records

available for these new purposes, they may also raise concerns.

Existing U.S. regulations, most notably the Health Insurance Portability and Accountability Act (HIPAA) Privacy Rule, limit access to patients' confidential health records. An exemption is allowed for research on materials from which potentially identifying information is removed; one way of satisfying this standard requires expert statistical/scientific consultation to ensure that the risk of reidentification is very small, and another is to remove all data from a list of 18 potential identifiers including names, date of birth, social security and license numbers, and biometric parameters. Some authors have questioned whether de-identification is sufficient to justify the use of health records in the absence of specific consent (Rothstein 2010); among other things, these authors point out that the process of de-identification (and who, if this is done manually, would have access to the raw data in order to perform de-identification) is underspecified, and that patients may have non-privacy interests in asserting control over the use of their records (including religious or ethical objections to the research, or claims to any commercial benefits that ensue). A general problem for all research using de-identified health records is to develop protocols that are flexible enough to address a range of potential individual concerns, and to focus their use on applications in which the potential societal benefit can provide a reasonable rationale for pursuing research given these barriers and questions. These considerations may favor the second, more fine-grained approach described above.

Whether identified records are used with specific consent, or de-identified records are used in the absence of consent, the sensitive nature of psychiatric illnesses and cognitive disorders like dementia also demands special care. The use of these methods to identify people making impaired decisions will specifically identify patients at risk for fraud and exploitation, so data security will be much more important in order to avoid breaches of data by bad actors who might have an interest in identifying targets for criminal activity. More generally, these disorders remain highly stigmatized and have many potential ramifications for employability and insurability. Patients therefore will be especially reluctant to have this information shared without very high confidence in investigators' good faith and commitment to confidentiality.

Conclusion

We now have a reasonable understanding of neural circuits that mediate economic behavior. The behavioral paradigms used in this field have been successfully applied to a variety of clinical populations. Neuroeconomics, therefore, would appear to be well-placed to provide clinical insights into decision-making deficits. However, to extend this scientific success to practical clinical use, there needs to be a sustained effort to ensconce neuroeconomic paradigms in the standard battery of clinical toolkit of cognitive and behavioral functioning, alongside tests of memory, executive function, language, etc.

We present preliminary evidence that medical charts of dementia patients contain sufficient details about decision-making impairments for a retrospective review. Comparing financial errors in AD and bvFTD patients, we found that errors in AD reflected a cognitive vulnerability factor, while financial errors in bvFTD reflected a social and affective vulnerability factor. This account of real-world financial impairment is largely consistent with current neuroeconomic characterization of behavioral deficits in AD and bvFTD patients.

As an initial step to establishing the diagnostic and prognostic usefulness of neuroeconomic measures, research groups can use existing knowledge of what brain systems are involved in different value-based decisions, as well as of what brain systems are impaired in different diseases, to identify behavioral neuroeconomic tasks suited to identify these impairments. This project can further be advanced by the use of information from medical records to systematically assess real-world failures of decision-making in patients. As a later step, establishing the reliability and validity of these measures in a variety of patient groups and settings would encourage the broader adoption of these measures in clinical practice, potentially in a way analogous to existing established measures of neuropsychological domains such as language and executive function. Finally, although data security and ethical concerns are especially pressing given the sensitive nature of these diagnoses and behaviors, this research is also of great clinical importance given the potentially devastating consequences of disordered decision-making for patients and also for their families. Behavioral researchers therefore must be able to communicate to both clinicians and patients on applications where the potential societal benefit can provide a reasonable rationale for pursuing research despite these potential barriers, and to partner with clinical researchers when possible to refine measures that combine clinical applicability with scientific rigor.

References

Agarwal, S., Driscoll, J., et al. (2008). The age of reason: Financial decisions over the lifecycle. *American Economic Association Annual Meeting*.

Bakalar, N. (2013). Sharing psychiatric records helps care. *New York Times*.

Bechara, A., Damasio, H., et al. (1997). Deciding advantageously before knowing the advantageous strategy. *Science, 275*(5304), 1293–1295.

Bechara, A., Tranel, D., et al. (2000). Characterization of the decision-making deficit of patients with ventromedial prefrontal cortex lesions. *Brain, 123*(11), 2189–2202.

Bucks, B. K., Kennickell, A. B., et al. (2009). *Changes in U.S. family finances from 2004 to 2007: Evidence from the survey of consumer finances. D. o. R. a. Statistics*. Washington: Board of Governors of the Federal Reserve System.

Camerer, C. F., & Weber, M. (1992). Recent developments in modeling preferences—uncertainty and ambiguity. *Journal of Risk and Uncertainty, 5*(4), 325–370.

Chiong, W., Hsu, M., et al. Financial errors in dementia: Testing a neuroeconomic conceptual framework. *NeuroCase* (in press).

Cummings, J. L., Mega, M., et al. (1994). The neuropsychiatric inventory comprehensive assessment of psychopathology in dementia. *Neurology, 44*(12), 2308.

Denburg, N., Cole, C., et al. (2007). The orbitofrontal cortex, real-world decision making, and normal aging.

Annals of the New York Academy of Sciences, 1121 (1), 480–498.

Fehr, E., & Camerer, C. F. (2007). Social neuroeconomics: the neural circuitry of social preferences. *Trends in Cognitive Sciences, 11*(10), 419–427.

First, M. B., & Gibbon, M. (1997). *User's guide for the structured clinical interview for DSM-IV axis I disorders SCID-I: Clinician version.* Amer Psychiatric Pub Incorporated.

Frank, M. J., Seeberger, L. C., et al. (2004). By carrot or by stick: Cognitive reinforcement learning in parkinsonism. *Science, 306*(5703), 1940–1943.

Fudenberg, D., & Levine, D. K. (1998). *The theory of learning in games.* Cambridge: MIT press.

Glimcher, P. (2002). Decisions, decisions, decisions: Choosing a biological science of choice. *Neuron, 36* (2), 323–332.

Himmelstein, D. U., Wright, A., et al. (2010). Hospital computing and the costs and quality of care: A national study. *The American Journal of Medicine, 123*(1), 40–46.

Hofbauer, J., & Sigmund, K. (1998). *Evolutionary games and population dynamics.* Cambridge: Cambridge Univ Press.

Hsu, M., Bhatt, M., et al. (2005). Neural systems responding to degrees of uncertainty in human decision-making. *Science, 310*(5754), 1680–1683.

Hsu, M., Krajbich, I., et al. (2009). Neural response to reward anticipation under risk is nonlinear in probabilities. *The Journal of Neuroscience, 29*(7), 2231–2237.

Insel, T. R., & Fernald, R. D. (2004). How the brain processes social information: Searching for the social brain. *Annual Review of Neuroscience, 27*, 697–722.

Jaret, P. (2013). Mining electronic records for revealing health data. *New York Times*: D1.

Jensen, P. B., Jensen, L. J., et al. (2012). Mining electronic health records: Towards better research applications and clinical care. *Nature Reviews Genetics.*

Kable, J. W., & Glimcher, P. W. (2007). The neural correlates of subjective value during intertemporal choice. *Nature Neuroscience, 10*(12), 1625–1633.

Kahneman, D., & Tversky, A. (1979). Prospect theory: An analysis of decision under risk. *Econometrica: Journal of the Econometric Society*, 263–291.

King-Casas, B., Sharp, C., et al. (2008). The rupture and repair of cooperation in borderline personality disorder. *Science, 321*(5890), 806.

King-Casas, B., Tomlin, D., et al. (2005). Getting to know you: Reputation and trust in a two-person economic exchange. *Science, 308*(5718), 78–83.

Knutson, B., & Greer, S. M. (2008). Anticipatory affect: Neural correlates and consequences for choice. *Philosophical Transactions of the Royal Society B: Biological Sciences, 363*(1511), 3771–3786.

Kuhnen, C., & Knutson, B. (2005). The neural basis of financial risk taking. *Neuron, 47*(5), 763–770.

Levy, M. L., Miller, B. L., et al. (1996). Alzheimer disease and frontotemporal dementias: Behavioral distinctions. *Archives of Neurology, 53*(7), 687.

Loewenstein, G. F., Weber, E. U., et al. (2001). Risk as feelings. *Psychological Bulletin, 127*(2), 267.

Maia, T. V., & Frank, M. J. (2011). From reinforcement learning models to psychiatric and neurological disorders. *Nature Neuroscience, 14*(2), 154.

Marson, D. C., Sawrie, S. M., et al. (2000). Assessing financial capacity in patients with Alzheimer disease: A conceptual model and prototype instrument. *Archives of Neurology, 57*(6), 877.

McCabe, K., Houser, D., et al. (2001). A functional imaging study of cooperation in two-person reciprocal exchange. *PNAS, 98*(20), 11832–11835.

Miller, L. A. (1992). Impulsivity, risk-taking, and the ability to synthesize fragmented information after frontal lobectomy. *Neuropsychologia, 30*(1), 69–79.

Montague, P. R. (2012). The scylla and charybdis of neuroeconomic approaches to psychopathology. *Biological Psychiatry, 72*(2), 80–81.

Nielsen, L., & Mather, M. (2011). Emerging perspectives in social neuroscience and neuroeconomics of aging. *Social Cognitive and Affective Neuroscience, 6*(2), 149–164.

Office of Behavioral and Social Sciences Research. (2010). *Better living through behavioral and social sciences.* National Institutes of Health.

Plassman, B. L., Langa, K. M., et al. (2008). Prevalence of cognitive impairment without dementia in the United States. *Annals of Internal Medicine, 148*(6), 427–434.

Preuschoff, K., Quartz, S. R., et al. (2008). Human insula activation reflects risk prediction errors as well as risk. *The Journal of Neuroscience, 28*(11), 2745–2752.

Rothstein, M. A. (2009). Currents in contemporary ethics. *The Journal of Law, Medicine and Ethics, 37*(3), 507–512.

Rothstein, M. A. (2010). Is deidentification sufficient to protect health privacy in research? *The American Journal of Bioethics, 10*(9), 3–11.

Schultz, W., Dayan, P., et al. (1997). A neural substrate of prediction and reward. *Science, 275*(5306), 1593–1599.

Templeton, V. H. M., & Kirkman, D. N. J. (2007). Fraud, vulnerability, and aging: Case studies. *Alzheime's Care Today, 8*(3).

Tinbergen, N. (1951). *The study of instinct.*

Tinbergen, N. (1953). *Social behaviour in animals: With special reference to vertebrates.* Taylor & Francis.

Tversky, A., & Kahneman, D. (1992). Advances in prospect theory: Cumulative representation of uncertainty. *Journal of Risk and uncertainty, 5*(4), 297–323.

Widera, E., Steenpass, V., et al. (2011). Finances in the older patient with cognitive impairment "He Didn't Want Me to Take Over". *JAMA, the Journal of the American Medical Association, 305*(7), 698–706.

Wu, S., Chaudhry, B., et al. (2006). Systematic review: Impact of health information technology on quality, efficiency, and costs of medical care. *Annals of Internal Medicine, 144*(10), 742–752.

Zhu, L., Mathewson, K. E., et al. (2012). Dissociable neural representations of reinforcement and belief prediction errors underlying strategic learning. *PNAS, 109*(5), 1419–1424.

Research Methods for Health Decision Making

Marc T. Kiviniemi and Erin M. Ellis

- Theories of health decision-making and our ability to improve the health of both individuals and populations through decision-making interventions are only as good as the scientific evidence on which those theories and interventions are based.
- Methodology for decision-making research is important both for basic scientific understanding of health decision-making processes and for clinical and public health applications to address decision-making.
- The role of evidence-based practice is as important for interventions related to decision-making as for any other treatment domain.

- Empirical research on health-related preferences helps clarify individual differences in decision-making, and fosters patient-centered interventions, clinical care, and health policy.
- Developing effective interventions to address decision-making issues requires that we understand how decision-making works, and the quality of that understanding will be heavily dependent on the methodology that is used in basic science studies.
- Health decision-making theories seek to describe the *causal* patterns that connect constructs or events. Factors such as attitudes and risk perceptions are proposed to causally influence decision-making concerning health behaviors. Comprehensive knowledge of such causal relations is essential when seeking to understand, predict, or change a health behavior.
- Measurement models must be validated as corresponding to the underlying theoretical construct that it is intended to measure (construct validity) and should also produce consistent and replicable results (reliability) as well as be free from cultural biases that may compromise their reliability or validity for specific demographic or social groups.

M.T. Kiviniemi (✉)
Department of Community Health and Health Behavior, University at Buffalo, SUNY, 314 Kimball Tower, 3435 Main Street, Buffalo, NY 14222, USA
e-mail: mtk8@buffalo.edu

E.M. Ellis
Behavioral Research Program, Cancer Prevention Fellowship Program, National Cancer Institute, 9609 Medical Center Dr., Bethesda, MD 20892-9712, USA
e-mail: erin.ellis@nih.gov

E.M. Ellis
University at Buffalo, Buffalo, USA

© Springer Science+Business Media New York 2016
M.A. Diefenbach et al. (eds.), *Handbook of Health Decision Science*,
DOI 10.1007/978-1-4939-3486-7_5

- Conceptual understanding of decision-making requires a focus on three main types of constructs: inputs to decision-making, decision-making processes, and outcomes of decision-making.
- Explicit measures, such as self-report questionnaires are the most commonly used method of assessing behavior, intentions, risk perceptions, attitudes, and other decision-making constructs. Implicit measures offer a complement to explicit measures of attitudes.
- Decision-making operationalization should reflect the study's theoretical framework and goals, and the factors that influence preferences for the treatment of behavior of interest.

Understanding health, health behaviors, and health care outcomes has always required a focus on decision-making, as the individual person's choices and preferences concerning lifestyle behaviors, preventive measures, and health care options are central to many health-related outcomes. However, the need to understand and address decision-making processes is increasingly critical as health-related issues become more complex. The growing multitude of treatment options for serious illnesses, availability of personalized genetically-based risk information, and the frequently shifting landscape of screening and treatment recommendations all require individuals to play an active role in making decisions about their health and health care. This, in turn, requires scientists and interventionists to understand and address issues of health decision-making in their research and clinical practice.

The other chapters in this volume provide overviews of various content areas important to the field of health decision-making. In this chapter we focus not on a particular content area but on the research methods that are used to develop knowledge of health decision-making inputs, processes, and outputs. We begin by addressing several conceptual issues that are relevant to conducting research on health decision-making. Next, we turn to a discussion of key research design issues, followed by an examination of important points to consider in conceptualizing and measuring constructs that are inputs to or outcomes of health decision-making. Finally, we will discuss methodological issues related to examining decision-making processes themselves.

Why is this notion of health decision-making as an empirical or scientific field important? First, the role of evidence-based practice is as important for interventions related to decision-making as for any other treatment domain. When we are assisting individuals in making decisions, developing treatment protocols accounting for the need for individuals to decide whether to comply with them, or creating public health messages to encourage decision-making on a health issue, our practices should be based on empirical evidence of effectiveness (Glasgow and Emmons 2007). Gathering quality evidence to enable evidence-based practice requires strong research methodology skills. A second important point is that our individual intuitions about how we make decisions and the intuitions of health professionals about how other people make decisions are not always correct (Nisbett and Wilson 1977; Wilson and Schooler 1991). This makes using empirical evidence to guide our understanding of how decisions are made and what influences decisions all the more important.

Methodology for decision-making research has importance both for basic scientific understanding of health decision-making processes and for clinical and public health applications to address decision-making. From the basic scientific perspective, the quality of the research methodology determines the quality of the collected data and thereby the conclusions drawn from that data. Therefore, advancement of the science and development of better theoretical models of decision-making relies on a base of strong research methodology. Research methodology is equally important for practical applications. Developing effective interventions to address decision-making issues requires that we understand how decision-making works, and the quality of that understanding will be heavily dependent on the methodology that is used in basic science studies.

This chapter addresses key topics for understanding research methods in health decision-making. There are many excellent introductions to general issues of research methodology for the social, behavioral, and decision-making sciences (some good starting points include Creswell 2009; Reis and Judd 2000; Shadish et al. 2002). Our focus here is specifically on issues that deal directly with health decision-making applications.

What Are the Causes of Decision-Making Outcomes? Types of Research Studies and Inferences About Causality

Like most scientific theories, health decision-making theories seek to describe the *causal* patterns that connect constructs or events. Factors such as attitudes and risk perceptions are proposed to causally influence decision-making concerning health behaviors. Comprehensive knowledge of such causal relations is essential when seeking to understand, predict, or change a health behavior.

From a methodological perspective, the ability to make causal inferences is importantly dependent on the nature of the *research design*. Research design is a large and complex topic and there are many excellent sources for individuals interested in a deeper knowledge (Maxwell and Delaney 2004; Shadish et al. 2002; Smith et al. 2000). Here we will confine ourselves to two key design considerations that have implications for both causal inferences and for other methodological issues discussed later in the chapter.

First, one must distinguish between observational studies and experimental studies (Shadish et al. 2002). In an observational study, a researcher measures or otherwise observes the variables of interest and then uses statistical tests to examine the interrelations of the different variables (Mark and Reichardt 2004). For example, Liang et al. (2002) were interested in how the number of different treatment options

presented to a patient recently diagnosed with breast cancer related to how satisfied that patient was with her chosen treatment. The researchers conducted a survey of recent patients, asking each patient whether her doctor provided her with treatment options and asking how satisfied she was with the treatment selected. The researchers then looked to see if there was an association between the number of treatment options provided and the degree of satisfaction with treatment (Liang et al. 2002). Note that the key feature here is that the "naturally occurring" state of each variable is simply measured as they occur in the real world, without the researcher making any overt changes to the natural course of the phenomena being observed.

By contrast, in an experimental study the researcher manipulates one variable and ascertains how changes in that manipulated variable influence an outcome variable of interest; the outcome variable is subsequently measured or observed (Smith et al. 2000). When a change in the level of a predictor variable is associated with a sequential change in the outcome variable, this provides evidence that the predictor is *causing* the outcome. In fact, because experimental designs control for extraneous variables and measure an outcome prospectively, they can provide the primary criteria for causal inferences and are considered the gold standard for demonstrating causality (Weinstein et al. 1998). In this way, they differ from observational studies, which can test correlations between variables, but not causal associations.

In our example, a researcher might instead manipulate number of treatment options provided, offering some patients one option, others two options, and others three or more (hopefully in hypothetical scenarios, for ethics sake!) and then measure their satisfaction. If there were a significant difference in satisfaction levels across the different conditions the researcher would conclude that number of options influences satisfaction. Similarly, causal associations can be assessed in the context of public health and clinical interventions by measuring the change from baseline in an outcome variable following the intervention (Weinstein et al. 1998). Such research not only advances decision-making theory, it also helps evaluate the effectiveness of interventions and the pathways through which they engender behavior change.

A second important distinction exists between cross-sectional studies, in which all of the variables are observed at a single time point, and longitudinal studies, in which variables are measured at multiple points over time (Cook and Ware 1983; Weinstein et al. 1998; West et al. 2004). This distinction is most meaningful with respect to the conclusions one draws from observational studies (which will be discussed in more detail in later points in the paper). Although intuitively appealing, cross-sectional research designs that rely on post hoc reports and explanations of past behavior do not provide compelling evidence for causality because they cannot capture the temporal sequences of events. Instead, longitudinal (prospective) and/or experimental designs are preferred because they are specifically aimed at capturing event sequence, thus allowing researchers to draw causal conclusions. For example, to examine the interrelation of changes in behavior and changes in risk perceptions, Gibbons et al. (1997) surveyed smokers at the beginning of a smoking cessation clinic and again at 6 and 12 months following the clinic. Measuring risk perception and smoking behavior at each of these time points allowed the researchers to explore how *changes* in behavior related to *changes* in risk perception.

Once an appropriate study design is selected, the next step is to determine which constructs one is interested in measuring, and the ways in which they will be assessed. When studying psychological constructs, a number of factors should be considered when making these decisions.

Measuring What Cannot Be Seen: Assessing Psychological Constructs

The study of health decision-making often relies on our ability to capture characteristics of individuals that cannot be seen or readily observed by others. Since most psychological constructs, such as feelings, beliefs, and personality traits are not observable, decision-making researchers rely on questionnaires and other instruments to capture these underlying constructs (for a brief discussion of this issue see Brewer 2000). For instance, the Health Belief Model posits that individuals' *expected utility*, or their perceived costs and benefits of a health behavior, will influence their decision to engage in it (Rosenstock 1974). Since researchers cannot directly observe participants' expected utility, this construct is often measured with a decisional balance scale that asks them to rate the extent to which a variety of potential costs and benefits of a behavior are important in their decision of whether or not to engage in it. Consider the striking difference between this methodology and the traditional laboratory tests and direct observations that assess biological risk factors for disease, such as viruses and high cholesterol.

A reliance on psychological constructs has important methodological implications for decision-making research. In order to utilize and test decision-making theories, a measurement model must be specified in which each construct relevant to the theory is defined in a way such that it can be measured, and the associations between each construct are hypothesized and mapped out. Further, each measure or questionnaire must be validated as corresponding to the underlying theoretical construct that it is intended to measure (construct validity). The measure should also produce consistent and replicable results (reliability). Further, measures ought to be free from cultural biases that may compromise their reliability or validity for specific demographic or social groups.

Traditionally, psychological constructs have been assessed with questionnaires; however, to overcome inherent biases and limitations of such measures, technological advances have contributed to an increasingly diverse arsenal of alternative techniques, including implicit measures of attitudes and the use of FMRIs to capture images of brain activity during the decision-making process. These techniques are discussed further in the following sections.

Conducting Research in Health Decision-Making: Measuring Inputs and Outputs of Decision Processes

We now turn to a focus on factors to consider when conducting research on health decision-making. We argue that a conceptual understanding of decision-making requires a focus on three main types of constructs: inputs to decision-making (factors which determine the decisions people make), decision-making processes (the ways in which those inputs are thought of, processed, manipulated to lead to a decision outcome), and outcomes of decision-making (a firm decision, a behavioral intention, an actual behavior). In this section, we describe some of the key methodological considerations relating to each of these constructs.

We consider inputs to decision-making to be any construct which is used by the individual as an information processing factor when making a decision. The specific inputs involved in a particular research project are a conceptual decision on the part of the researcher, and the variety of factors involved in making that decision is beyond the scope of this chapter. Here we consider methodological issues common regardless of the specific constructs or theoretical model underlying a particular research study.

Operationalizing Constructs

One key decision is how one will take the conceptual construct (e.g., perceived benefits) and operationalize it (an operationalization is an observable, measurable definition of the construct). This question about operationalization is relevant for both observational and for experimental studies. First, let us consider observational studies. For example, to conduct research on the role of expected utility on decision-making concerning colorectal cancer screening, one needs to assess perceived benefits of screening. This construct could be operationalized in a number of different ways. First, one might operationalize it as the score obtained on a measure in which participants use a scale to rate how strongly a set of listed perceived benefits influences their behavior. Alternatively, one might operationalize it as the count of the number of benefits a participant lists when asked to verbalize screening benefits. As yet another alternative, one might assess an overall rating of whether a participant perceives very few or many benefits to screening.

Each of these definitions captures something about the idea of perceived benefits, but not necessarily the same thing. If the conceptual definition of perceived benefits focuses mainly on their quantity, the second measure is a useful operationalization. However, if one believes that the strength of the perceived benefit is important, the second measure will not match the operational definition and the first would be preferable. Finally, if one believes that perceived benefits is a gestalt sense on the part of the person rather than a set of individual possible benefits, then the third measure is appropriate. None of them are inherently right or wrong, but each is only a valid measure of decision-making under the terms of a particular conceptual definition of the construct. Thus, if a researcher is to draw conclusions about the role of her/his conceptualization of perceived benefits in decision-making, the operational measure of benefits used must match that conceptual definition.

Explicit Measures

Explicit measures, such as self-report questionnaires, are the most commonly used method of assessing behavior, intentions, risk perceptions, attitudes , and other decision-making constructs. Participants respond to a series of questions with either open-ended responses or by selecting from a series of alternatives. Examples include semantic differentials (ratings of basic evaluative dimensions toward a given construct), feeling thermometers (thermometer-like scales designed to measure a respondent's general feelings toward an object or behavior), and single-item measures (Goddard and Villanova 1996). Such measures can be administered retrospectively in a laboratory or clinical setting, or contemporaneously in natural settings. For instance, daily diaries and other ecological momentary assessment (EMA) techniques seek to study decision-making and behavior over time in real-world settings as subjects go about their daily lives. Such an approach has been shown to reduce recall bias and maximize external validity by prompting participants to report on relevant constructs temporally and contextually much closer to the natural decision-making process (for further discussion of EMA, see: Shiffman et al. 2008; Stone et al. 2007).

A primary advantage of explicit measures of attitudes and other psychological constructs is the straightforward interpretation and statistical analysis that they allow. Compared to implicit measures in particular, there is greater consensus as to what constructs are being measured and how explicit measures assess the constructs (DeCoster et al. 2006). However, explicit measures of health decision-making constructs also have a number of weaknesses, including vulnerability to biases and logistical challenges. They are prone to response bias or social desirability (demand characteristics), in which individuals provide potentially inaccurate information about their beliefs and behaviors in an effort to present themselves in a favorable light or conform to social norms (Couch and Keniston 1960; Eysenck and Eysenck 1963; Phillips 1979). While such risks can be minimized using well-validated published measures, these biases may induce systematic errors that confound results and lead to erroneous conclusions (Podsakoff et al. 2003; Schwarz 1999).

Retrospective self-report questionnaires are also constrained by limitations to participants' own introspection, self-awareness, and memory (LeBel and Paunonen 2011). Further, responses can be influenced by features of the measures themselves, including introductory statements, question wording, and response options (Schwarz 1999; Shiffman et al. 2008). Similarly, the decision-making surrounding some health behaviors, such as risky sexual behavior, is logistically and ethically challenging to study, given their private nature (Schroder et al. 2003).

Closed-ended versus open-ended items. One aspect of operationalization for observational studies concerns whether one will used a closed-ended measure or an open-ended measure. In a closed-ended measure, a set of response options is provided to the participant and the participant uses some sort of rating scale to indicate his/her response. There are several strengths to this approach. First, it provides an easily quantifiable response for each participant, thus enabling use of quantitative statistical tools to analyze data and test hypotheses. Second, it is an approach that can easily be compared across individuals (e.g., seeing which individuals have higher versus lower benefits) and across populations (with some of the caveats noted in weaknesses below). Third, the data management burden on the researcher is reduced relative to open-ended items.

On the other hand, closed-ended items have some inherent weaknesses. Returning to our example of the perceived benefits of colorectal screening, if a "laundry list" approach is used, the measure is really only a valid assessment of perceived benefits if the individual's own perceived benefits are represented by the items on the list; if an individual has a set of perceived benefits that are not captured by the measure, the measure will not accurately capture the "true" value of the individual's perceived benefits. An important task in the design of closed-ended measurement tools is to conduct pretesting to determine specific beliefs and perceptions relevant to the particular study population (Ajzen 2006; Rawl et al. 2001).

Second, most people do not naturally think about their world in terms of seven-point Likert scales, so while it makes the researchers' job easier, using a closed-ended measure makes the participant's job more difficult. To answer a given perceived benefit item, the person must read and comprehend the item, retrieve from memory his/her own thoughts relevant to the item, translate the thoughts in her head into a response that fits somewhere on the seven-point scale, and so on (Tourangeau et al. 2000).

Open-ended items consist of asking a question but *not* providing a closed-ended scale or mechanism for response. For example, one might ask "What do you see as the benefits of cancer screening?" and then have participants respond verbally (with responses recorded by a researcher) or by writing. Such open-ended items can overcome some of the limitations of closed-ended items. First, because no "laundry list" is provided, a participant can (at least theoretically) provide their own self-tailored list of benefits and barriers. Second, because there is not a response scale involved, some of the "translational burden" is removed. Although the person still has to comprehend the question, because the "response options" are whatever the participant chooses to share, there is not the cognitive burden of having to determine how to provide one's thoughts using the response options provided. Third, the open-ended format reduces some possible methodological problems with closed-ended questions (e.g., the problem of response sets discussed above).

The weaknesses of open-ended responses, on the other hand, mirror some of the strengths of other approaches. Because open-ended responses are essentially a raw transcript of a person's thoughts, converting them to a form that is meaningful for comparison and analysis requires active translation on the part of the researcher. There is an involved coding process in which items are categorized into particular categories, extraneous responses are removed, and so on (Marshall and Rossman 1999; Weber 1990). In addition to being time intensive, this process shifts interpretation burden to the researcher and therefore sets up the possibility that the results could be clouded by mistakes and misinterpretations. Second, because the response is free form, the richness of the data is contingent on participants' motivation and ability to fully articulate all their perceived benefits of the health behavior (e.g., Does someone who lists 2 benefits relative to a person who lists 7 really see fewer benefits, or is the person simply tired, lazy, or cognitively taxed?).

Ultimately, the decision of whether to use closed-ended or open-ended items depends on the goals of the researcher, the state of existing measures in the field (e.g., if there is no established closed-ended measure for the construct, one might have to collect open-ended items as a step toward scale development), and the goals of the research.

Implicit Measures

The development of techniques to implicitly measure attitudes began in the 1960s as an effort to avoid the demand characteristics and other biases of explicit measures (DeCoster et al. 2006). Rather than explicitly asking participants to provide an account of their thoughts, feelings, and behavior, implicit measures infer such constructs indirectly from participants' performance on experimental paradigms. Such measures are based on the assumption that people's attitudes exert systematic and predictable influence on their behavior (Greenwald et al. 1998). Therefore, attitudes can be inferred from small differences in performance on a variety of experimental tasks. For instance, many implicit assessments of attitudes rely on response latencies, or the average length of time required to classify objects into one of two categories, with faster speeds thought to reflect stronger associations in memory between the object and its assigned category (De Houwer 2003; Gawronski and Payne 2010; Greenwald et al. 1998). For instance, participants' attitudes about fruits would be deemed negative if the speed with which they are categorized as part of a negatively valenced category (e.g., insects) is faster than the speed required to match them with a positively valenced category (e.g., flowers).

Because participants are not aware of the true purpose of these tasks, implicit measures theoretically overcome the biases associated with explicit measures, thereby providing a more objective measure of people's true thoughts and feelings surrounding health behaviors (DeCoster et al. 2006). Evidence suggests that implicit measures reliably predict a number of health-related attitudes and behaviors, including food preferences (Hollands et al. 2011; Perugini 2005; Richetin et al. 2007), exercise (Bluemke et al. 2010), risky sexual behavior (Czopp et al. 2004), cigarette smoking (Payne et al. 2007), and alcohol use (Houben et al. 2010; Payne et al. 2008). For instance, an implicit measure of attitudes about alcohol was even more predictive of drinking behavior and alcohol-related problems than explicitly measured attitudes about alcohol. The researchers also found that implicit measures were less vulnerable to social desirability bias than explicit measures (Payne et al. 2008).

The interpretation of results from implicit measures is not as straightforward as the interpretation of responses on explicit measure, though. While many studies have reliably predicted health behaviors with implicit measures, implicit and explicit measures of attitudes do not always correlate with each other, and they often differentially correlate with actual behavior (Conner et al. 2007; Fazio and Olson 2003; Gawronski and Payne 2010; Hofmann et al. 2005). Even within the same behavior, such as fruit and vegetable consumption, interventions and experimental studies have produced conflicting results regarding the associations between implicit and explicit measures and their relative power to predict snack selection and food consumption (Hollands et al. 2011; Karpinski and Hilton 2001; Perugini 2005; Spruyt et al. 2007).

Debate remains as to the structure of attitudes themselves and the way in which implicit and explicit measures capture both attitudes and cognitive processing more broadly. Studies that have examined the predictive validity of implicit compared to explicit measures suggest that explicit measures may be particularly valuable predictors of deliberate and volitional behaviors, while implicit measures show greater predictive validity for impulsive or spontaneous behaviors (Friese et al. 2008). Further complicating interpretation is the tendency for different implicit measures to produce conflicting results for identical constructs, suggesting that the mechanisms underlying the measures, rather than genuine differences in attitudes, may be influencing

results (Gawronski 2009; Spruyt et al. 2007). Given these findings, implicit measures seem to offer a promising alternative or complement to explicit measures of attitudes; however, additional research is needed to elucidate their underlying mechanisms and to aid in the interpretation of their findings.

Measuring and Illustrating Causal Pathways

How Do Inputs Lead to Decisions?

Once the factors that influence decision-making are identified, the next step is to describe the relationships between these constructs. Since most theoretical models make assumptions about the ways that predictor variables are associated with each other and behavior, the theory/model that is guiding the research or intervention has implications for the operationalization, measurement, and analysis of *relations between the constructs,* in addition to its implications for operationalization of the constructs themselves. For instance, while a number of health decision-making models contain an affective (emotional) component, the way in which this construct is defined, measured, and situated in relation to other variables varies considerably across theories. Some models, such as the behavioral affective associations model, posit that affect serves as a mediator or intervening variable (types of relationships are discussed further in the next section) between cognitive factors and decision-making (Kiviniemi et al. 2007). Conversely, other models suggest that the influence of affective factors is mediated by cognitive variables (Slovic et al. 2004), while others still argue that both cognitive and affective factors are subcomponents of attitudes, with neither having a direct and independent effect on decision-making (Ajzen and Driver 1992). The way in which affect is conceptualized in relation to other variables has important implications for

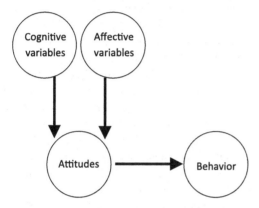

Affective variables as a mediator

Cognitive variables as a mediator

Cognitive and affective variables as subcomponents of attitudes

Fig. 5.1 Illustrates possible alternative ways in which decision-making inputs may lead to behavior

statistical analyses and interpretation. Figure 5.1 illustrates possible alternative ways in which affective inputs may lead to decisions.

Types of Relationships Between Variables

Health decision-making is often more complex than a simple association between one predictor and one outcome variable. Other factors often interact with, confound, and serve as intermediaries between the predictor and outcome of interest (for an expanded discussion on different types of variables and their role in understanding decision-making see Bauman et al. 2002). Therefore, many decision-making theories include *mediator* and *moderator* models that further explicate how, why, and under which

conditions the causal relation exists. Mediators or intervening variables are third variables that explain the process or mechanisms underlying the associations between predictors, such as psychosocial constructs, and health or other outcome variables. For mediation to exist the predictor must temporally precede the mediator and there must be a causal association between the two variables. There must also be a causal association between the mediator and outcome variable after statistically accounting for the mediator (Baron and Kenny 1986; MacKinnon et al. 2002).

It is important to identify mediators in the health decision-making process for two reasons. First, they help researchers understand why and how certain risk factors and behaviors influence health. For instance, low socioeconomic status has been associated with lower cancer screening rates (Coughlin et al. 2006). However, a number of variables may be mediating this association. Low socioeconomic status increases the likelihood of having limited access to transportation and inadequate health insurance coverage, and these variables may be the proximal risk factors explaining the low screening rates (Link and Phelan 1995).

Second, by understanding the mechanisms underlying an intervention's success (or failure), it allows researchers to strengthen, remove, or modify specific components based on their relative influence. Also, once the mechanisms are understood, the interventions or tools can be generalized to a range of health care decisions, diseases, and settings (Chmura Kraemer et al. 2008; Reyna 2008). For instance, a support group for patients newly diagnosed with HIV may achieve its goal of reducing patient stress and anxiety by increasing feelings of social support and reducing feelings of isolation (Beals et al. 2009; Uchino 2006). In this case, the increase in social support serves as the mediator or mechanism through which the intervention achieves its success.

Moderators are conditions that magnify, attenuate, cancel, or reverse an association between two other variables. While mediators tend to be process-level variables, moderators are usually a fixed characteristic, such as gender, age, or a feature of a situation. The association between a predictor and outcome variable will differ in strength or direction at different levels of this fixed characteristic. For instance, we may be interested in identifying whether a treatment or intervention is equally effective across various subpopulations. A weight loss intervention that seeks to increase social support and emotional well-being of participants may be highly effective for women, but ineffective for men, in which case gender would moderate the association between the intervention and the amount of weight lost. Statistically, moderation is demonstrated with a significant interaction term, calculated as the product of the moderator and predictor variables, which suggests that the association between predictor and outcome is different at different levels of the moderator.

There are two other types of variables worth mentioning: covariates and confounders. Covariates are variables that are associated with the outcome of interest. Although technically speaking any variable related to the outcome is a covariate, in common usage we usually use the term to refer to variables that are not directly relevant to one's research question or theoretical framework (Bauman et al. 2002; Last 2007). For instance, when studying the way in which psychological factors, such as attitudes and risk perceptions, influence health outcomes, age and education level are often included as covariates in order to explain additional variability in the outcome of interest. Alternatively, confounding variables are those that are associated with the predictor and outcome, and do change the nature of the relationship between the predictor and outcome (Bauman et al. 2002; Cohen et al. 1983). These four types of relationships between variables are important to understand and account for when developing and testing decision-making models, as they have both statistical and clinical implications.

It is often useful to graphically depict a decision-making model by mapping the relevant variables and the associations between them (see Fig. 5.1) (Earp and Ennett 1991). Such illustrated depictions are referred to as path diagrams, and they not only illustrate underlying theoretical assumptions, but can also help guide complex statistical analyses. Variables are identified as manifest (measured constructs) or latent (theoretical variables that are inferred from manifest variables) using squares and circles respectively, and the associations between variables are identified as causal (depicted by straight arrowed lines) or correlational (using curved lines with double arrows). While path models do not specify a certain statistical analysis in and of themselves, they often are associated with a class of analysis techniques called structural equation modeling (SEM) (Loehlin, 2004). Unlike traditional regression analyses, SEM allows for the simultaneous examination of all the associations between variables in the model, including direct and indirect effects, associations between latent and manifest variables, and unexplained error terms (Kline 2011). These strengths make SEM a powerful tool in health decision-making research.

Outcomes

We now turn to a consideration of the outcomes of health decision-making. In much work in health decision-making, the outcome is some form of behavioral choice—a person decides to be screened for colorectal cancer, an individual elects to change her exercise behavior, a person decides to pursue a particular course of treatment. We will consider two key issues related to behavioral outcomes below. In addition to behavioral outcomes, a growing area of research within decision-making examines preferences among different outcome options (e.g., among different treatment plans for prostate cancer, or between different available screening tests for colorectal cancer). Following the discussion of behavioral outcomes, we will consider some key features of measurement of preferences.

Self-report Versus Observed Behavior

One key methodological choice concerns whether one actually observes the behavioral outcome in question or relies on the individual to self-report her/his behavioral practices. There are tradeoffs to consider here. Because our interest is in actual behavior, assessing actual behavior most closely matches the conceptual outcome of interest. It is the "gold standard" of behavioral measures.

However, there are some downsides to observed behavior. First, in many decision-making research topics, directly observing behavior may not be feasible (e.g., home-based dietary behavior for large samples) or desirable for ethical or other reasons (e.g., condom use during intercourse). Second, direct observation is time, money, and personnel intensive and may not be logistically feasible even if desirable. Third, of necessity, direct observation of behavior involves a narrow time slice of behavior and

therefore may not capture patterns of behavior over time.

On the other hand, self-report measures of behavior are subject to a number of biases. First, individuals must be able to remember their behaviors. This may not be a valid assumption, especially for historical reports or for behaviors which are repeated frequently over time (e.g., what did you eat for lunch last Thursday?) Second, behavioral reports are subject to social desirability biases (e.g., people may be unwilling to report drug use).

Direct Behavior Versus "Behavioroid" Measures

One strategy for overcoming issues with direct measurement of behavior is to utilize a "behavioroid" measure. One might measure a behavior that is not the final outcome of interest but is a necessary step along the way to that outcome. For example, a study of sexual decision-making might examine people's behavior of taking or purchasing condoms as a proxy for condom use during sex (Stone et al. 1994). Similarly, a dietary behavior study might examine food purchasing decisions as a proxy for actual dietary choices (Epstein et al. 2010).

Behavioral Intentions Versus Actual Behavior

A final conceptual distinction to consider is whether to measure behavioral intentions versus actual behavior. Behavioral intentions can be a desirable measure, because forming an intention to engage in a behavior is a key construct in its own right in several decision-making models (e.g., the theories of reasoned action/planned behavior and the transtheoretical model; Ajzen 1985, 1991; Prochaska et al. 1992). However, from a methodological perspective there are two key issues of concern. First, behavioral intentions measures are subject to the social desirability biases described above for other types of behavioral measures. Second, there is a body of work demonstrating that behavioral intentions do not always lead do behavior—in fact, the correspondence is often less than 50 % (Orbell and Sheeran 1998). This is an interesting conceptual research area in its own right. From a methodological perspective, this lack of correspondence is an issue when behavioral intentions measures are being used where actual behavior is the true conceptual variable.

Conclusion

The domain of health decision-making is broad, as the other chapters in this volume will illustrate. Both the range of decision-making principles addressable in research and the multitude of health domains in which decision-making processes are applicable makes for a wide ranging, diverse discipline. However, regardless of the specific topic area or health domain, the core set of research design principles discussed here apply. Careful consideration of the conceptual constructs and research questions, how to best select a study design and operationalize variables in light of those questions, and how to examine the relevant inputs to, processes in, and outputs of decision-making is necessary across specific research topics. Ultimately, our theories of health decision-making and, more importantly, our ability to improve the health of both individuals and populations through decision-making interventions are only as good as the scientific evidence on which those theories and interventions are based. Although high quality health decision-making research is an effortful process, the benefits of that research for both science and society are significant.

SIDEBAR: **Health preferences**

Increasing attention is being given to the empirical assessment of the *preferences* of individuals and society. Originating in economic theory, a preference is a psychological construct that reflects one's attitudes, experiences, motives, and subjective value of alternative outcomes (McDowell 2006). Empirical research on health-related preferences helps clarify individual differences in decision-making, and fosters

patient-centered interventions, clinical care, and health policy (Lauver et al. 2008). The research methods that are used to develop knowledge of health preferences are not unique, and will therefore serve as an illustration of the key points discussed in this chapter.

Operationalizing and Measuring Preferences

Researchers have defined and measured preferences in a number of ways. As with other decision-making constructs, their operationalization should reflect the study's theoretical framework and goals, and the factors that influence preferences for the treatment or behavior of interest (e.g., the accuracy and cost of diagnostic tests; privacy and invasiveness of treatment). Preferences can be measured with closed-ended or open-ended assessments. Commonly used closed-ended assessments include standard gambles and rating scales, which ask individuals to evaluate their health preferences in the face of various risk scenarios, or to rate health states or treatments in relative or absolute terms (Bennett and Torrance 1996; McDonough and Tosteson 2007). Preferences can also be assessed with more traditional measures of attitudes, in which participants use Likert or visual analogue scales to indicate their level of agreement with items. Open-ended questionnaires can also be useful in assessing health goals and preferences, particularly how individuals define a decision and what factors affect their preference (Davey et al. 2004).

Both open- and closed-ended methods of assessing preferences are accompanied by the weaknesses discussed earlier in this chapter. With closed-ended assessments, the nature of the measure itself often influences responses, and preferences tend to vary considerably based on the method of assessment (Johnson et al. 2005). For instance, the response options may imply a normative or standard course of treatment, which people tend to view as safest and use as their default preference, regardless of the other treatment options listed (Johnson et al. 2005). In the case of infrequent medical decisions, people tend to lack preexisting preferences, and the process of completing a measure that assesses their preferences may actually be instrumental in forming them. Therefore, it is particularly important to consider these methodological issues (Johnson et al. 2005; McDowell 2006). Open-ended assessments of preferences also are accompanied by the weaknesses discussed earlier in this chapter, especially the added burden they pose to the research following data collection.

Relationships Between Variables

As with any decision-making model, it is important to consider the many factors influencing the process as well as the associations between them. For instance, in the association between risk perceptions and health behaviors, preferences may be theorized as moderating or mediating the relationship, with implications for both the operationalization of preferences as well as statistical analyses. Further, many researchers argue that patient preferences are most accurately understood when they are based on multiple characteristics of each decision and contextualized within real-world circumstances (Johnson et al. 2005). For instance, by assessing participants' preferences for life-prolonging medical treatments within different real-life scenarios and contextual circumstances, researchers made more accurate predictions of participants' real-life medical decision-making (Winter et al. 2007). Regardless of whether patient preferences are assessed as an *input* in the decision-making process or as an outcome in itself, they should be operationalized and measured appropriately and contextualized within the larger decision-making process.

References

Ajzen, I. (1985). From intentions to actions: A theory of planned behavior. In J. Kuhl & J. Beckmann (Eds.), *Action control: From cognition to behavior* (pp. 11–40). Berlin, Germany: Springer.

Ajzen, I. (1991). The theory of planned behavior. *Organizational Behavior and Human Decision Processes, 50*, 179–211.

Ajzen, I. (2006). Constructing a TPB questionnaire: Conceptual and methodological considerations. Retrieved October 30, 2008 from http://www.people.umass.edu/aizen/pdf/tpb.measurement.pdf

Ajzen, I., & Driver, B. L. (1992). Application of the theory of planned behavior to leisure choice. *Journal of Leisure Research, 24*, 207–224.

Baron, R. M., & Kenny, D. A. (1986). The moderator-mediator variable distinction in social psychological research: Conceptual, strategic, and statistical considerations. *Journal of Personality and Social Psychology, 51*, 1173–1182.

Bauman, A. E., Sallis, J. F., Dzewaltowski, D. A., & Owen, N. (2002). Toward a better understanding of the influences on physical activity: The role of determinants, correlates, causal variables, mediators, moderators, and confounders. *American Journal of Preventive Medicine, 23*, 5–14.

Beals, K. P., Peplau, L. A., & Gable, S. L. (2009). Stigma management and well-being: The role of perceived social support, emotional processing, and suppression. *Personality and Social Psychology Bulletin, 35*, 867–879.

Bennett, K., & Torrance, G. (1996). Measuring health state preferences and utilities: Rating scale, time trade-off, and standard gamble techniques. *Quality of life and pharmacoeconomics in clinical trials, 2*, 253–265.

Bluemke, M., Brand, R., Schweizer, G., & Kahlert, D. (2010). Exercise might be good for me, but I don't feel good about it: Do automatic associations predict exercise behavior? *Journal of Sport and Exercise Psychology, 32*, 137–153.

Brewer, M. B. (2000). Research design and issues of validity. In *Handbook of research methods in social and personality psychology* (pp. 3–16). New York: Cambridge University Press.

Chmura Kraemer, H., Kiernan, M., Essex, M., & Kupfer, D. J. (2008). How and why criteria defining moderators and mediators differ between the Baron & Kenny and MacArthur approaches. *Health Psychology, 27*, S101–S108.

Cohen, S., Kamarck, T., & Mermelstein, R. (1983). A global measure of perceived stress. *Journal of Health and Social Behavior, 24*, 385–396.

Conner, M. T., Perugini, M., O'Gorman, R., Ayres, K., & Prestwich, A. (2007). Relations between implicit and explicit measures of attitudes and measures of behavior: Evidence of moderation by individual difference variables. *Personality and Social Psychology Bulletin, 33*, 1727.

Cook, N. R., & Ware, J. H. (1983). Design and analysis methods for longitudinal research. *Annual Review of Public Health, 4*, 1–23. doi:10.1146/annurev.pu.04.050183.000245.

Couch, A., & Keniston, K. (1960). Yeasayers and naysayers: Agreeing response set as a personality variable. *The Journal of Abnormal and Social Psychology, 60*, 151–174. doi:10.1037/h0040372.

Coughlin, S. S., King, J., Richards, T. B., & Ekwueme, D. U. (2006). Cervical cancer screening among women in metropolitan areas of the United States by individual-level and area-based measures of socioeconomic status, 2000 to 2002. *Cancer Epidemiology, Biomarkers and Prevention, 15*, 2154–2159. doi:10. 1158/1055-9965.epi-05-0914.

Creswell, J. W. (2009). *Research design: Qualitative, quantitative, and mixed methods approaches* (3rd ed.). Thousand Oaks, CA US: Sage Publications Inc.

Czopp, A. M., Monteith, M. J., Zimmerman, R. S., & Lynam, D. R. (2004). Implicit attitudes as potential protection From risky sex: Predicting condom use with the IAT. *Basic and Applied Social Psychology, 26*, 227–236.

Davey, H. M., Lim, J., Butow, P. N., Barratt, A. L., & Redman, S. (2004). Women's preferences for and views on decision-making for diagnostic tests. *Social Science and Medicine, 58*, 1699–1707. doi:10.1016/s0277-9536(03)00339-3.

De Houwer, J. (2003). The extrinsic affective Simon task. *Experimental Psychology, 50*, 77–85. doi:10.1026//1618-3169.50.2.77.

DeCoster, J., Banner, M. J., Smith, E. R., & Semin, G. R. (2006). On the inexplicability of the implicit: Differences in the information provided by implicit and explicit tests. *Social Cognition, 24*, 5–21.

Earp, J. A., & Ennett, S. T. (1991). Conceptual models for health education research and practice. *Health Education Research, 6*, 163–171. doi:10.1093/her/6.2.163.

Epstein, L. H., Dearing, K. K., Roba, L. G., & Finkelstein, E. (2010). The influence of taxes and subsidies on energy purchased in an experimental purchasing study. *Psychological Science, 21*, 406–414. doi:10.1177/0956797610361446.

Eysenck, S. B. G., & Eysenck, H. J. (1963). Acquiescent response set in personality questionnaires. *Life Sciences, 2*, 144–147. doi:10.1016/0024-3205(63)90026-2.

Fazio, R. H., & Olson, M. A. (2003). Implicit measures in social cognition research: Their meaning and use. *Annual Review of Psychology, 54*, 297–327.

Friese, M., Hofmann, W., & Wänke, M. (2008). When impulses take over: Moderated predictive validity of explicit and implicit attitude measures in predicting food choice and consumption behaviour. *British Journal of Social Psychology, 47*, 397–419.

Gawronski, B. (2009). Ten frequently asked questions about implicit measures and their frequently supposed, but not entirely correct answers. *Canadian Psychology/Psychologie Canadienne, 50*, 141.

Gawronski, B., & Payne, B. K. (2010). *Handbook of implicit social cognition: Measurement, theory, and applications*. New York: Guilford Press.

Gibbons, F. X., Eggleston, T. J., & Benthin, A. C. (1997). Cognitive reactions to smoking relapse: The reciprocal relation between dissonance and self-esteem. *Journal of Personality and Social Psychology, 72*, 184–195.

Glasgow, R. E., & Emmons, K. M. (2007). How can we increase translation of research into practice? Types of evidence needed. *Annual Review of Public Health, 28*, 413–433. doi:10.1146/annurev.publhealth.28.021406. 144145.

Goddard, R. D, I. I. I., & Villanova, P. (1996). Designing surveys and questionnaires for research. In F. T. L. Leong & J. T. Austin (Eds.), *The psychology research handbook: A guide for graduate students and research assistants* (pp. 85–97). Thousand Oaks, CA US: Sage Publications Inc.

Greenwald, A. G., McGhee, D. E., & Schwartz, J. L. K. (1998). Measuring individual differences in implicit cognition: The implicit association test. *Journal of Personality and Social Psychology, 74*, 1464–1480. doi:10.1037/0022-3514.74.6.1464.

Hofmann, W., Gawronski, B., Gschwendner, T., Le, H., & Schmitt, M. (2005). A meta-analysis on the correlation between the Implicit association test and explicit self-report measures. *Personality and Social Psychology Bulletin, 31*, 1369–1385.

Hollands, G. J., Prestwich, A., & Marteau, T. M. (2011). Using aversive images to enhance healthy food choices and implicit attitudes: An experimental test of evaluative conditioning. *Health Psychology, 30*, 195.

Houben, K., Havermans, R. C., & Wiers, R. W. (2010). Learning to dislike alcohol: Conditioning negative implicit attitudes toward alcohol and its effect on drinking behavior. *Psychopharmacology (Berl), 211*, 79–86. doi:10.1007/s00213-010-1872-1.

Johnson, E. J., Steffel, M., & Goldstein, D. G. (2005). Making better decisions: From measuring to constructing preferences. *Health Psychology, 24*, S17–S22. doi:10.1037/0278-6133.24.4.s17.

Karpinski, A., & Hilton, J. L. (2001). Attitudes and the implicit association test. *Journal of Personality and Social Psychology, 81*, 774–788. doi:10.1037/0022-3514.81.5.774.

Kiviniemi, M. T., Voss-Humke, A. M., & Seifert, A. L. (2007). How do I feel about the behavior? The interplay of affective associations with behaviors and cognitive beliefs as influences on physical activity behavior. *Health Psychology, 26*, 152.

Kline, R. B. (2011). *Principles and practice of structural equation modeling*. New York: Guilford press.

Last, J. M. (2007). *Dictionary of public health*. New York: Oxford University Press.

Lauver, D. R., Worawong, C., & Olsen, C. (2008). Health goals among primary care patients. *Journal of the American Academy of Nurse Practitioners, 20*, 144–154. doi:10.1111/j.1745-7599.2007.00296.x.

LeBel, E. P., & Paunonen, S. V. (2011). Sexy but often unreliable: The impact of unreliability on the replicability of experimental findings with implicit measures. *Personality and Social Psychology Bulletin, 37*, 570–583. doi:10.1177/0146167211400619.

Liang, W., Burnett, C. B., Rowland, J. H., Meropol, N. J., Eggert, L., Hwang, Y.-T., et al. (2002). Communication between physicians and older women with localized breast cancer: Implications for treatment and patient satisfaction. *Journal of Clinical Oncology, 20*, 1008–1016. doi:10.1200/jco.20.4.1008.

Link, B. G., & Phelan, J. (1995). Social conditions as fundamental causes of disease. *Journal of health and social behavior*, pp. 80–94.

Loehlin, J. C. (2004). *Latent variable models: An introduction to factor, path, and structural equation analysis* (4th ed.). Mahwah, NJ US: Lawrence Erlbaum Associates Publishers.

MacKinnon, D. P., Lockwood, C. M., Hoffman, J. M., West, S. G., & Sheets, V. (2002). A comparison of methods to test mediation and other intervening variable effects. *Psychological Methods, 7*, 83.

Mark, M. M., & Reichardt, C. S. (2004). Quasi-experimental and correlational designs: Methods for the real world when random assignment isn't feasible. In C. Sansone, C. C. Morf & A. T. Panter (Eds.), *The Sage handbook of methods in social psychology* (pp. 265–286). Sage Publications, Inc.

Marshall, C., & Rossman, G. B. (1999). *Designing qualitative research* (3rd ed.). Thousand Oaks, CA US: Sage Publications Inc.

Maxwell, S. E., & Delaney, H. D. (2004). *Designing experiments and analyzing data: A model comparison perspective* (2nd ed.). Mahwah, NJ US: Lawrence Erlbaum Associates Publishers.

McDonough, C. M., & Tosteson, A. N. A. (2007). Measuring preferences for cost-utility analysis: How choice of method may influence decision-making. *Pharmacoeconomics, 25*, 93–106.

McDowell, I. (2006). *Measuring health: A guide to rating scales and questionnaires*. USA: Oxford University Press.

Nisbett, R. E., & Wilson, T. D. (1977). Telling more than we can know: Verbal reports on mental processes. *Psychological Review, 84*, 231–259.

Orbell, S., & Sheeran, P. (1998). 'Inclined abstainers': A problem for predicting health-related behaviour. *British Journal of Social Psychology, 37*, 151–165.

Payne, B. K., Govorun, O., & Arbuckle, N. L. (2008). Automatic attitudes and alcohol: Does implicit liking predict drinking? *Cognition and Emotion, 22*, 238–271.

Payne, B. K., McClernon, F. J., & Dobbins, I. G. (2007). Automatic affective responses to smoking cues. *Experimental and Clinical Psychopharmacology, 15*, 400.

Perugini, M. (2005). Predictive models of implicit and explicit attitudes. *British Journal of Social Psychology, 44*, 29–45. doi:10.1348/014466604x23491.

Phillips, J. P. (1979). A method for the investigation of irrelevant response set in ordered metric and original questionnaires. *British Journal of Mathematical and Statistical Psychology, 32*, 252–268. doi:10.1111/j.2044-8317.1979.tb00597.x.

Podsakoff, P. M., MacKenzie, S. B., Lee, J.-Y., & Podsakoff, N. P. (2003). Common method biases in behavioral research: A critical review of the literature and recommended remedies. *Journal of Applied Psychology, 88*, 879–903.

Prochaska, J. O., DiClemente, C. C., & Norcross, J. C. (1992). In search of how people change: Applications to addictive behaviors. *American Psychologist, 47*, 1102–1114.

Rawl, S. M., Champion, V., Menon, U., Loehrer, P. J., Vance, G. H., & Skinner, C. S. (2001). Validation of scales to measure benefits of and barriers to colorectal cancer screening. *Journal of Psychosocial Oncology, 19*, 47–63.

Reis, H. T., & Judd, C. M. (2000). *Handbook of research methods in social and personality psychology*. New York, NY US: Cambridge University Press.

Reyna, V. F. (2008). Theories of medical decision making and health: An evidence-based approach. *Medical Decision Making, 28*, 829–833. doi:10.1177/0272989x08327069.

Richetin, J., Perugini, M., Prestwich, A., & O'Gorman, R. (2007). The IAT as a predictor of food choice: The case of fruits versus snacks. *International Journal of Psychology, 42*, 166–173.

Rosenstock, I. M. (1974). Historical origins of the health belief model. *Health Education Monographs, 2*, 1–8.

Schroder, K., Carey, M., & Vanable, P. (2003). Methodological challenges in research on sexual risk behavior. II. Accuracy of self reports. *Annals of Behavioral Medicine, 26*, 104–123.

Schwarz, N. (1999). Self-reports: How the questions shape the answers. *American Psychologist, 54*, 93–105.

Shadish, W. R., Cook, T. D., & Campbell, D. T. (2002). *Experimental and quasi-experimental designs for generalized causal inference*. Boston, MA: Houghton Mifflin.

Shiffman, S., Stone, A. A., & Hufford, M. R. (2008). Ecological momentary assessment. *Annual Review of Clinical Psychology, 4*, 1–32. doi:10.1146/annurev.clinpsy.3.022806.091415.

Slovic, P., Finucane, M. L., Peters, E., & MacGregor, D. G. (2004). Risk as analysis and risk as feelings: Some thoughts about affect, reason, risk, and rationality. *Risk Analysis, 24*, 311–322.

Smith, E. R., Reis, H. T., & Judd, C. M. (2000). Research design. In *Handbook of research methods in social and personality psychology* (pp. 17–39). Cambridge: Cambridge University Press.

Spruyt, A., Hermans, D., De Houwer, J., Vandekerckhove, J., & Eelen, P. (2007). On the predictive validity of indirect attitude measures: Prediction of consumer choice behavior on the basis of affective priming in the picture–picture naming task. *Journal of Experimental Social Psychology, 43*, 599–610. doi:10.1016/j.jesp.2006.06.009.

Stone, A. A., Shiffman, S., Atienza, A., & Nebeling, L. (2007). *The Science of real-time data capture: Self-reports in health research*. Oxford: Oxford University Press.

Stone, J., Aronson, E., Crain, A. L., Winslow, M. P., & Fried, C. B. (1994). Inducing hypocrisy as a means of encouraging young adults to use condoms. *Personality and Social Psychology Bulletin, 20*, 116–128. doi:10.1177/0146167294201012.

Tourangeau, R., Rips, L. J., & Rasinski, K. (2000). *The psychology of survey response*. New York, NY US: Cambridge University Press.

Uchino, B. N. (2006). Social support and health: A review of physiological processes potentially underlying links to disease outcomes. *Journal of Behavioral Medicine, 29*, 377–387. doi:10.1007/s10865-006-9056-5.

Weber, R. P. (1990). *Basic content analysis* (2nd ed.). Thousand Oaks, CA US: Sage Publications Inc.

Weinstein, N. D., Rothman, A. J., & Sutton, S. R. (1998). Stage theories of health behavior: Conceptual and methodological issues. *Health Psychology, 17*, 290–299. doi:10.1037/0278-6133.17.3.290.

West, S. G., Biesanz, J. C., & Kwok, O.-M. (2004). Within-subject and longitudinal experiments: Design and analysis issues. In C. Sansone, C. C. Morf & A. T. Panter (Eds.), *The sage handbook of methods in social psychology* (pp. 287–312). Sage Publications, Inc.

Wilson, T. D., & Schooler, J. W. (1991). Thinking too much: Introspection can reduce the quality of preferences and decisions. *Journal of Personality and Social Psychology, 60*, 181–192. doi:10.1037/0022-3514.60.2.181.

Winter, L., Dennis, M. P., & Parker, B. (2007). Religiosity and preferences for life-prolonging medical treatments in African–American and white elders: A mediation study. *Omega: Journal of Death and Dying, 56*, 273–288. doi:10.2190/OM.56.3.d

Part II
Decision Making on the Individual Level

A Fuzzy-Trace Theory of Judgment and Decision-Making in Health Care: Explanation, Prediction, and Application

6

Priscila G. Brust-Renck, Valerie F. Reyna,
Evan A. Wilhelms and Andrew N. Lazar

In this chapter, we discuss how an evidence-based theory of human behavior and decision-making—Fuzzy-Trace Theory (FTT)—can be used to better understand and improve public health and medicine. Initially, we present an overview of the theory, describing its core principles as well as illustrative evidence. The evidence includes research prior to FTT as well as current research from independent laboratories. Applications are discussed in the areas of risk perception, prevention, detection, and diagnosis of disease, as well as decision-making regarding treatment. We then present findings from interventions designed to improve health judgments and medical decision-making. FTT provides guidelines for the development of such interventions because it predicts reactions to health messages and explains the causal mechanisms of judgment and decision-making. Specifically, FTT has been applied to designing public health programs and patient education tools that effectively communicate risks and benefits, and to tools for health care providers. By focusing on theoretically motivated mechanisms of judgment and decision-making, old interventions can be enhanced and new ones can be designed. Examples of interventions are given from HIV-AIDS prevention, genetic risk of breast cancer, biologic therapy for arthritis, and cardiovascular disease. Finally, we present implications and recommendations for future research.

Preparation of this manuscript was supported in part by the National Institutes of Health National Cancer Institute Award Number R21CA149796 and National Institute of Nursing Research R01NR014368-01 to the second author.

P.G. Brust-Renck · E.A. Wilhelms
Department of Human Development, Cornell University, Ithaca, USA

V.F. Reyna (✉)
Departments of Human Development and Psychology, Center for Behavioral Economics and Decision Research and Cornell Magnetic Resonance Imaging Facility, Cornell University, 331 Martha van Rensselaer Hall, Ithaca, NY 14853, USA
e-mail: vr53@cornell.edu

A.N. Lazar
Weill Cornell Medical College, Cornell University, Ithaca, USA

Background: Fuzzy-Trace Theory

FTT is a theory of memory, reasoning, judgment, and decision-making that also describes how these develop across the lifespan (Reyna 2012a b). Central to the theory are five components of social cognition that are relevant to the medical decisions of patients and providers: (a) background knowledge; (b) mental representations of new inputs; (c) retrieval of principles and social values; (d) application of principles and values to representations (which can elicit processing interference, as in probability judgments), and (e) individual differences, notably, the ability to inhibit interference (Reyna and Brainerd 1995, 2011). Background knowledge refers to

© Springer Science+Business Media New York 2016
M.A. Diefenbach et al. (eds.), *Handbook of Health Decision Science*,
DOI 10.1007/978-1-4939-3486-7_6

information stored in long-term memory that affects how a person processes incoming stimuli such as health messages. This knowledge could be understanding of numbers, other educational knowledge, or personal experience (Reyna 2012b; Reyna et al. 2009).

Stimuli, such as auditory and visual inputs, are encoded in two kinds of mental representations in parallel: verbatim and gist (Reyna 2011). A verbatim representation is a memory of the precise surface form (e.g., exact words, numbers, or pictures), whereas a gist representation is a qualitative understanding of the deeper or bottom-line meaning of an event or stimulus (Reyna 2008, 2012b). The verbatim representation reflects the objective facts, whereas the gist reflects a subjective and impressionistic interpretation. In addition, retrieval cues differ in their tendency to elicit verbatim versus gist representations, which means that judgments about the same event can vary depending on the cues in questions (e.g., Mills et al. 2008). In fact, FTT is the only theory that can predict these specific variations in health judgments within individuals.

Knowledge helps shape gist representations, and these representations are also influenced by personal characteristics such as culture, prejudices, beliefs, and worldview, among other factors that affect understanding (Mills et al. 2008; Reyna and Adam 2003). People typically extract multiple gist representations of the same input (Reyna and Brainerd 1995). For example, consider a 55-year-old female who is trying to determine her risk for breast cancer by using the Breast Cancer Risk Estimation Tool from the National Cancer Institute website (http://www.cancer.gov/bcrisktool/). Suppose further that the online estimation tool determines that her lifetime risk is 20 %. From this information, the woman encodes a verbatim representation of "20 %." She also typically extracts multiple gist interpretations of what that percentage *means*.

When considering breast cancer risk estimates derived from the online tool, two women may view a risk of 20 % differently. One may see 20 % as a "high risk" relative to an average woman's risk of 12.2 %, whereas a second woman may not know the average woman's risk and view 20 % as a "low risk" because it is substantially lower than 50 % (i.e., it probably would not happen; Brewer et al. 2009). Background knowledge—knowledge of the average risk—influences how the gist of the risk estimate of 20 % is interpreted, as high or low (Fagerlin et al. 2005). Although gist representations are subjective, and thus differ across individuals, they are not arbitrary. Usually, a small number of gist representations encompass most people's interpretations of risks for the same information —especially if those people share background knowledge.

Gist representations are encoded at multiple levels in a hierarchy that roughly correspond to levels of measurement, from the most crude to the most fine-grained level of precision (Reyna 2004, 2008, 2012b; Reyna et al. 2003). Thus, a crude level of gist for quantities (e.g., number of patients who survived whose cancer was detected early; numerical probability of developing breast cancer) corresponds to the simplest distinctions about quantities, namely, nominal or categorical level (e.g., "All of the early-detection patients survived" or "I am at risk for developing breast cancer"). In parallel, a person might also encode a representation of the same information at an ordinal level of precision (e.g., "My risk of breast cancer is higher than average"), and then again at yet more precise levels, such as interval or ratio levels (e.g., "My risk is 1 in 5").

Note that "1 in 5" is technically not a representation of the verbatim stimulus, which was 20 % in our example, but is, rather, verbatim *based* because it involves a computation performed on the exact number presented (Reyna and Brainerd 2008). People who are higher in numeracy (the ability to understand and use numbers) are more likely to spontaneously perform such computations (e.g., Reyna et al. 2009). These computations do not necessarily bring decision-makers closer to the right decision, which hinges instead on distilling the essential qualitative gist of the options (Reyna 2008).

Once information is encoded in gist and verbatim representations, decision-makers retrieve principles and personal values that are applied to these representations (Reyna 2004, 2008; Reyna and Brainerd 2011). Consider the example of a woman deciding whether to have a lumpectomy or a mastectomy after being diagnosed with early-stage breast cancer. Studies have shown that long-term survival for lumpectomy (plus radiation therapy) is similar to that for mastectomy, but recurrence rates are slightly higher for lumpectomy (American Cancer Society 2012). For many patients, values relevant to this decision include survival, recurrence, and cosmetics in that order of priority. However, there are two main ways to interpret the gist of the risks depending on whether a small increase in recurrence is understood as "same" or "higher": One gist interpretation is that survival is the same, recurrence is the same, and therefore the decision hinges on cosmetics, which favors lumpectomy. Another gist interpretation is that survival is the same, but recurrence rates are higher with lumpectomy, which favors mastectomy. Cosmetics do not figure in the latter decision because they would be considered only if the preceding dimensions were equivalent. This example shows that the representation of options helps determine which values are retrieved and applied.

Retrieving moral and social values is a cue-dependent process. Thus, according to FTT, value clarification methods can help patients by prompting retrieval (Fagerlin et al. 2013). As our example with lumpectomy illustrated, a primary value that is retrieved concerns survival (life is better than death) and a cancer diagnosis can be initially equated with death. A patient retrieving only this value would likely choose surgery (e.g., to "remove" the cancer and avoid death; see Reyna 2008). However, decision aids often elicit additional values, such as quality of life that are not easily retrieved, despite their relevance. The accessibility of values in memory is a result of overall priority for that individual as well as contextual cues (Reyna 2008), which together determine which values are applied to decisions.

Applying retrieved principles to representations is a distinct phase of information processing (Reyna 2012a). According to FTT, this processing can be interfered with by confusion caused by

overlapping classes, such as the class of women with breast cancer and the class of women with genetic mutations (e.g., BRCA 1 or 2) that increase the probability of breast cancer (Reyna 1991; Reyna and Brainerd 1994; Reyna and Mills 2007a). For example, people confuse the probability that a woman might develop breast cancer given that she has a genetic mutation with the probability that a woman has a genetic mutation given that she has breast cancer (Reyna et al. 2001). Research has shown that such confusion, which produces errors in probability judgment, is a result of overlapping and nested classes rather than lack of understanding of ratios and probabilities (Reyna 2004; Reyna et al. 2003, 2009). This class-inclusion effect will be further explored under detection and diagnostic tests. The ability to inhibit interference, for example from overlapping classes, increases from childhood to adulthood, but, nonetheless, varies across adults. This ability to inhibit helps people think coherently about combining different probability (and risk) judgments relevant to health (e.g., cancer risk and genetic risk; Reyna et al. 2009).

An Explanatory Approach to Health Decisions

FTT originated from extensive evidence in psychology, both basic and applied science. The upshot of this work is that bottom-line meaning (i.e., gist) is key for how people encode information and decide about health promoting choices (Reyna 2008, 2012b). In the next section, we review some of the applications of FTT in providing a bridge between health information—which has limited effects on judgments and decisions when expressed in highly precise form—and effective communications that influence medical decision-making (Reyna 2008). We first address the preexisting knowledge patients and health providers bring to decisions (e.g., numeracy). We then discuss how risks and benefits of health information are perceived, including lifestyle risks in the sexual health domain (e.g., in HIV-AIDS prevention) and vaccination risks, and how these perceptions are related to healthy choices. In the final sections, we discuss how the results of diagnostic tests are commonly mis-judged (due to interference in processing), how gist representations determine treatment deci-sions, and whether patients truly understand and consent to risks of medication or surgery.

Background Knowledge and Health Decisions

As our earlier discussion about knowledge illustrated, the role of knowledge in FTT goes beyond arbitrary associations, recitation of facts, or mindless computational skills (e.g., Reyna et al. 2012). According to FTT, knowledge allows decision-makers to understand causal mechanisms that underlie health messages, and, thus, extract appropriate representations. For example, the knowledge of laypeople is limited with respect to transmission of sexually trans-mitted infections (STIs; Adam and Reyna 2005; Reyna and Adam 2003). Most laypeople assume that sexual transmission of infections occurs only through exchange of bodily fluids; hence, meth-ods such as condoms must be effective because they provide a mechanical barrier that blocks this exchange. Therefore, people overestimate the effectiveness of condoms in preventing skin-to-skin transmission of STIs such as herpes simplex virus (HSV) and human papillomavirus (HPV). Reyna and Adam (2003), for example, found that students overestimated effectiveness of condoms significantly more than physicians and public health experts.

Similarly, few people have sufficient knowl-edge to understand public health messages about the rationale for vaccination, including such concepts as herd immunity (Reyna 2012b). Even worse, vaccinations occur in the context of meaning threats—mysterious illnesses (whose cause is unknown, e.g., autism or narcolepsy) that co-occur with vaccinations. Meaning threats produce a greater impetus for people to "connect the dots" to understand their world and the mysterious adverse events that are happening in it (Betsch et al. 2012). FTT offers an explanatory

framework to understand how anti-vaccination messages can be more effective in this context than official information sources, such as gov-ernment Web sites.

Consistent with this framework, Downs et al. (2008) have demonstrated that, to those with little background knowledge, health communications from official sources are cryptic, whereas anti-vaccination messages tell a compelling and plausible story. Such web sites that produce more coherent and meaningful gist will be more influential in decision-making, which can be an obstacle for public health (Betsch et al. 2012; Reyna 2012b). To take one example among many, anti-vaccination messages have associated the measles, mumps, rubella (MMR) vaccine with the development of autism as a result of alleged mercury in the vaccine. Autism develops around the same age that the MMR vaccine is adminis-tered. Little is known about the causes of autism and the number of children with the disease is increasing; autism constitutes a "meaning threat" because of its mysterious origin. However, if an individual has the background knowledge that the MMR vaccine is a live vaccine and the presence of mercury in a live vaccine would kill it, the anti-vaccine explanation becomes implausible. Therefore, if people *understand* how vaccines work, there should be less reason to avoid the MMR vaccine (Reyna 2012b).

Lack of knowledge is also exemplified with respect to innumeracy, associated with serious errors of probability and risk estimation in medicine and public health (Reyna and Brainerd 2008; Reyna et al. 2009). Despite the surfeit of resources containing health information, many people still lack basic numerical understanding, in particular, ratios and probabilities, that is required to process this information to maintain health (consistent with FTT's predictions; see Detection and Diagnosis).

Much of the health information available to patients is expressed as numerical risks, such as risk of neurologic disorders from measles vaccine being 1 out of 3333 doses (Stratton et al. 2012). The ability to extract the gist from this numerical information—that 1 person out of 3333 is a small frequency of neurologic disorder *relative to* how common measles was before the vaccine—is associated with training in public health and medicine, as this knowledge introduces meaning to numbers (Reyna 2012b; Reyna and Lloyd 2006). However, FTT's conception of numeracy builds on prior theories of judgment and decision-making (e.g., Kahneman 2003, 2011), but it goes beyond traditional theories of numeracy, which focus on analytical, quantitative ability, to emphasize qualitative understanding of the meaning (gist) of numerical information (Reyna and Brainerd 2008). As an example, Peters et al. 2008, emphasize affective meaning, but their theory relies on traditional dualism between low-level intuition and high-level analysis, the latter subsuming numeracy.

In summary, differences in background knowledge have an effect on how information is understood, influencing the gist representations that are encoded in decision-making. Research has shown that people rely on simple gist in decision-making even when they can recall exact information (Kühberger and Tanner 2010; Reyna 2012a; Reyna and Brainerd 1995). Gist representations incorporate meaning; they reflect inferences or connecting the dots among inputs. Background knowledge supplies some of the missing dots that allow people to go beyond the literal language of health facts. In the presence of meaning threats (mysterious adverse events), stories that seem to explain adverse events fill the vacuum of inadequate knowledge.

Risk Perceptions and Judgments: Effects of Retrieval Cues

In the previous section, an overview of errors of knowledge was presented, in which education played an important role in understanding risks. Risk estimation, however, is not only dependent on knowledge. Evidence suggests that different retrieval cues have varied (and sometimes paradoxical) effects on how individuals estimate risks, even those with advanced training.

Reyna and Adam (2003) investigated this point by asking the same question about the risk of a young woman to contract STIs in two different ways: the first question asked about risk of STIs, (including HPV) and the second question was identical except that it "unpacked" the concept of STIs by enumerating examples, such as HIV-AIDS, chlamydia, genital herpes, syphilis, or gonorrhea. The 174 physicians, other health care professionals, and medical students surveyed were aware of what STIs were; knowledge did not change when different STIs were specified. Nevertheless, across all groups, there was a small but significant within-subject effect of "unpacking" the question. Subjects raised their risk estimates (closer to the correct estimate) for the "unpacked" version (although estimates were still lower than the factual answer of approximately 50 %). However, the "unpacking" provided more specific retrieval cues that improved accuracy of risk estimates. This unpacking effect for health risk judgments was replicated in a sample of 120 health education professionals (Adam and Reyna 2005).

In addition to changes in risk judgment, retrieval cues have also been shown to change personal risk perception estimates when knowledge remains the same (Mills et al. 2008; Reyna et al. 2011). Mills et al. (2008) have called these effects on risk perception *paradoxical* because perception of risk is sometimes positively correlated, and sometimes negatively correlated, with risk taking for the same individual (see also Brewer et al. 2004). FTT predicts that verbatim cues to risk perceptions (e.g., estimation of exact personal risk of unprotected sex using a 0–100 % scale) will have positive correlations with risk taking, whereas gist cues to risk perception (e.g., estimation of personal risk of unprotected sex using global categories, such as "low," "medium," or "high") will have negative correlations with risk taking. This reversal occurs because, on the one hand, risk takers tend to estimate lower vulnerability when asked global questions (retrieving their gist representations, which reflect limited understanding of their risk), but they acknowledge higher risk when cued for specific behaviors. On the other hand, those who avoid risk tend not to have risky behaviors available to retrieve, yielding lower specific estimates of risk (e.g., on 0–100 % scales). Nevertheless, risk avoiders perceive high risk when asked for their global judgments (e.g., associated with sexual behavior).

This paradoxical prediction was borne out in a study with 596 adolescents that used various measures of risk perception to investigate risky sexual behavior (Mills et al. 2008). The measures of risk perception included scales with verbatim cues versus gist cues (see Reyna 2008; Reyna and Brainerd 1995, for details of predictions). In addition to the 0–100 % scale, the verbatim scales included a measure of specific risk, containing items that mentioned concrete consequences of risky sex (e.g., pregnancy/STIs in the next 6 months), and asked for personal estimates of those risks. The global gist scales included measures of categorical thinking (e.g., "Even low risks happen to someone"), gist values/principles (e.g., "Avoid risk,"), and global risk categories of "low," "medium," or "high." Behavioral measures of risk taking (outcomes) included intentions to have sex, whether the subject had initiated sex, and number of sexual partners. As predicted, each of the verbatim measures correlated positively with risk taking outcomes, and each of the global gist measures correlated negatively with those outcomes. Reyna et al. (2011) replicated these reversals with 153 adolescents and young adults, and showed that the verbatim and gist scales loaded on orthogonal dimensions in a principal components analysis.

In summary, judgment and perception of risk are associated with the retrieval cues used to measure them, and the simple shift in cue from verbatim to gist produces changes in reported perception of risk and reversals in responses to public health questions (Mills et al. 2008; Reyna et al. 2011). This effect of retrieval cues for verbatim versus gist representations can affect both patients and health care professionals, because it does not depend on training or knowledge (what is stored in memory), but rather on the nature of the cue that retrieves what is stored (Adam and Reyna 2005; Reyna and Adam 2003; Reyna and Lloyd 1997).

Gist and Preventive Health in Light of Representation and Retrieval

As noted in the section on risk perception, which gist or verbatim representations are endorsed and retrieved is associated with how much risk a person takes in their lifestyle choices (e.g., number of sexual partners). More can be predicted, however, by considering which gist principles are endorsed. Mills et al. (2008) made an additional distinction separating those who endorse the categorical avoidance of risk, "No risk is better than some risk" and those who endorse the ordinal gist principle, "Less risk is better than more risk." The FTT prediction (consistent with the negative correlations discussed in the previous section between gist representations of risk and risk taking) is that endorsement of simplest, categorical principles should be associated with less (unhealthy) risk taking and endorsement of relative, ordinal principles should be associated with more (unhealthy) risk taking.

The FTT rationale for this prediction is as follows: Although both principles express the view that risk is bad, the relative principle makes finer distinctions than the categorical principle. In contrast to other theories, a core principle of FTT is that *advanced* cognition is gist based. Development progresses from reliance on more precise verbatim-based analysis to simpler gist-based intuition, a result supported by studies comparing children to adults and novices to experts, including medical experts (e.g., Reyna et al. 2014; Reyna and Farley 2006; Reyna and Lloyd 2006). Therefore, adolescents are more likely to think more precisely about risks than adults, and those who think more precisely are more likely to take unhealthy risks.

Results were consistent with these predictions. Adolescents who only endorsed the relative principle were more than twice as likely to have initiated sex (61 % compared to 30 %) than if they endorsed only the categorical principle. Endorsement of both or neither principle resulted in intermediate level of being sexually active (44 and 46 %, respectively). Although both categorical and relative principles are based on gist (categorical and ordinal levels of gist), the less precise principle (i.e., categorical) was associated with endorsement of protective health behaviors (Mills et al. 2008). More generally, decision processes that rely on less precise mental representations are often more developmentally advanced than those that rely on more precise representations.

In summary, as predicted by FTT, endorsement of categorical gist principles (e.g., "No risk is better than some risk") was associated with risk prevention in public health (compared to endorsement of more precise principles). This tenet of FTT that associates reliance on simple (categorical) gist representations regarding sexual behavior with protective effects, instead of the trade offs of risks and benefits, has been used to explain the decrease in risk taking that occurs from adolescence to adulthood (see Reyna et al.'s 2011 study comparing adolescents to young adults, as well as Reyna and Farley's 2006 literature review in multiple domains of public health). Overall, these studies suggest that emphasis on gist-based thinking about risk avoidance has a protective effect on health behaviors.

Detection and Diagnosis: Base Rates and Combining Probabilities

In the preceding sections, we discussed how gist-based decision processes support advanced cognition. In particular, categorical gist is often used to cut to the essential bottom line of important decisions, and to avoid tradeoffs between risks and rewards when those tradeoffs obscure what is most important (e.g., not acquiring an incurable, deadly disease, HIV-AIDS). Studies of medical experts making diagnostic decisions further support this hypothesis: Physicians who were the most accurate according to evidence-based guidelines used the simplest, categorical distinctions to

make decisions about patients (Reyna and Lloyd 2006). Gist-based processing also has the advantage of being less vulnerable to interference. In this section, we show how such interference can compromise the way physicians and patients process information about the results of diagnostic tests.

In a classic study, Eddy (1982) asked physicians to estimate the probability that a woman had breast cancer given a positive diagnostic test result. The base rate of breast cancer (i.e., the probability of breast cancer in the population) was given as 1 % and the test sensitivity (i.e., the probability of a positive result for women with breast cancer) as 80 % (the false-positive rate was 9.6 %). Most physicians estimated the post-test probability of cancer for this woman around 75 %, but the correct answer was much lower than that, around 8 %. This phenomenon has been called base rate neglect because post-test probability judgments display insufficient adjustment for base rates. Although some have claimed that these probability judgments are not "natural" based on speculation about evolution, an early explanation from FTT for the phenomenon (and how to fix it) had to do with confusions about overlapping classes (e.g., Reyna 1991, 2004; Reyna and Brainerd 1994, 2008). This explanation has been tested in many experiments and accounts for data from multiple laboratories (e.g., Barbey and Sloman 2007; Reyna and Mills 2007a).

The explanation leads to a number of important predictions that are relevant to decision-making about health. As expected by FTT, confusion of conditional probabilities in clinical judgment of post-test probability (base rate errors) occurs for most people, including both patients and physicians (Reyna et al. 2001). That is, processing errors in probability estimation do not reflect lack of reasoning competence or low levels of knowledge or experience in health care (Reyna et al. 2003). To assess processing errors independently of disease knowledge, Reyna and Adam (2003) asked physicians and other health care professionals to make post-test probability judgments about an *unknown* disease with a base rate of 10 % in the general population. They were informed that the patient tested positive and that the diagnostic test had 80 % sensitivity and 80 % specificity (i.e., the proportion of patients without the disease who tested negative; both sensitivity and specificity were defined for subjects). To minimize computational burden, subjects were asked whether the correct post-test probability was either around 30 or 70 %.

Only 31 % of physicians selected the correct option, which is significantly below chance (the only group to respond around chance at 55 % correct were experts in public health, for whom base rate neglect is a common topic). Other health care professionals scored below 30 % correct and different groups of undergraduates who were not health care professionals ranged from 36 to 45 % correct (Adam and Reyna 2005; Reyna and Adam 2003). High school students scored 33 % correct, similar to trained physicians (Reyna 2004). The fact that the effect was obtained for both untrained high school students and trained physicians supports the FTT prediction that processing interference is not related to knowledge or expertise, but instead is a judgment error that is present in advanced reasoners as a result of class-inclusion confusion (Reyna 1991; Reyna et al. 2003). Individual differences in the ability to inhibit interference—an "executive" function in the brain—mitigate susceptibility to class-confusion errors (Reyna and Mills 2007b).

Specifically, people confuse sensitivity with post-test probability, which are conditional probabilities (analogous to confusing breast cancer risk given a BRCA mutation with mutation risk given breast cancer). Focal classes are in the numerators, and people tend to forget about denominators in their confusion about overlapping classes (Reyna and Brainerd 1994, 2008). Ergo, they think of sensitivity as though it were post-test probability (and vice versa) because the numerators are the same (the joint probability of both having disease and testing positive); only the denominators (which are momentarily forgotten about) differ. Naturally, neglecting base rates (or pre-test probabilities) can produce large errors in diagnostic judgments (Eddy 1982; Lloyd and Reyna 2001; Reyna et al. 2001; Reyna and Lloyd 2006).

In summary, accurate detection and diagnosis of diseases involve combining probability estimates about overlapping classes, such as the classes of patients with disease and of patients with positive test results. These combined judgments are subject to errors that occur as a result of confusion about overlapping classes, producing denominator neglect and base rate neglect. Experts as well as laypeople are vulnerable to these errors, as predicted by FTT. As we discuss in the next section, interventions that reduce these errors have been developed and tested for experts and laypeople.

Interventions Based on Evidence: Theory and Data

Specific interventions for health and medical decision-making are suggested by the principles of FTT and have been evaluated in research (e.g., Brewer et al. 2012; Fraenkel et al. 2012; Lloyd and Reyna 2001; Reyna et al. 2008). Although the focus of other interventions has been on increasing how much people know about health facts, interventions based on FTT also take into consideration how health knowledge is mentally represented, retrieved, and processed coherently in decision-making, as well as how interference is inhibited. The goal is to transmit knowledge while encouraging people to extract the appropriate gist for the decision (e.g., "My risk is high" so I should get screening for breast cancer), retrieve relevant values and principles (e.g., "Avoid recurrence"), and implement such values so as to reduce interference from class-inclusion confusion (Reyna 2008; Reyna and Brainerd 2011). In this section, we review some of the public health and medical interventions that are motivated by FTT and discuss how they accomplished these goals.

Interventions Targeting Representation and Retrieval of Values

Unlike other approaches, FTT implies that health communication and decision support should begin with the message in mind (Reyna 2008). In other words, the first step in designing an intervention is to identify the gist that is to be communicated, the functionally significant "bottom line" of the information in as integrated a form as possible. As we have discussed, there can be more than one such bottom line generated from different perspectives. Experienced patients and providers can provide iterative drafts of proposed gist representations, which naturally should be informed by the most rigorous scientific evidence. In addition to developing new materials, it is also possible to transform existing communications or interventions—to "gistify" them—by translating arbitrary facts into meaningful messages (e.g., deciding which facts are essential to decision-making, explaining the reasons behind the essential facts, integrating facts, and deleting irrelevant details) in order to improve efficacy. Despite the simplicity of this approach of focusing on simple meaning and on causal understanding of that meaning, initial results from a variety of interventions have been surprisingly successful.

For example, the effectiveness of representation-targeted risk communication techniques was investigated in Brewer et al.'s (2012) study about breast cancer recurrence risk. One hundred thirty-three patients were interviewed who were eligible for the Oncotype DX genomic test. This genomic test estimates 10-year risk of distant recurrence of early-stage estrogen receptor-positive breast cancer. The results help patients decide whether to add adjuvant chemotherapy to endocrine therapy to prevent recurrence. Risk of recurrence varies along a continuum, but there are values that can be roughly categorized as low, intermediate, and high. Subjects were randomly assigned to different descriptions of risk of recurrence, which varied in complexity, and included a detailed standard report from a commercial assay with (1) a simple explanation of risk, (2) the explanation followed by a simple graphic presenting recurrence risk information on a continuum (gist), (3) both explanation and graphic accompanied by a description of the graphic and confidence interval reports, or (4) an additional format that involved an icon array. Subjects were asked to estimate risk of 10-year

recurrence as well as to rate their understanding and easiness of understanding of the material.

The standard detailed report generated a greater number of errors in estimating level of risk (low, intermediate, or high) compared to simpler formats, whereas the newly developed gist-based risk continuum format generated the fewest errors in risk estimation (Brewer et al. 2012). Moreover, the standard report format was rated as least understandable and the least liked format, whereas the gist-based risk continuum graphical format was rated among the most understandable and most liked formats. Consistent with FTT, simple but meaningful presentation of risk (e.g., as a continuum with qualitative categories), not merely numbers, enhanced understanding (Reyna 2008, 2012b; Brust-Renck et al. 2013). Simple line graphs readily convey relative ordering or trends across time, but other graphical displays highlight different relationships among numbers. According to FTT, the use of the correct type of graphic facilitates the process of extracting the relevant gist (see also Fraenkel et al. 2012, 2015).

Interventions aimed at representation and retrieval have also been implemented in an FTT-based intervention in a randomized control trial of 734 adolescents focusing on reducing the risk of pregnancy and STIs from unprotected sex (Reyna 2008; Reyna et al. 2008). The gist-based intervention was compared to (1) a standard multicomponent intervention ("Reducing the Risk"; Reyna et al. 2005) and (2) an unrelated control group. The experimental intervention was based on FTT and included the same content as the standard intervention but emphasized gist representations of risk (e.g., "Even low risks happen to someone"), as well as identification and automatic retrieval of gist values (e.g., "Avoid risk"; "Better to not put my partner at risk"). All three interventions consisted of 14-h classes in small groups of high school students either in school settings or after school programs. Effectiveness of the interventions was assessed via testing that occurred prior to the intervention, immediately after, and 3, 6, and 12 months later.

Overall, the goal of the gist-based intervention was to reduce (or avoid) pregnancy and STIs from unprotected sex. High school students were encouraged to understand the gist of information about risky behaviors (gist lasts longer in memory compared to memorization of verbatim details), recognize risky situations rapidly, retrieve relevant values, and engage in automatic gist-based thinking (that is faster than verbatim and deliberative analysis of risk (Reyna 2008; Reyna et al. 2008). Such gist-based intuitive and automatic thinking should provide additional benefits in emotional situations; gist is more resistant to interference from emotion and stress (Rivers et al. 2008). Results comparing the three interventions (i.e., gist-enhanced, standard, and control) demonstrated that the enhanced curriculum produced significant improvements (relative to controls) for 17 out of 26 outcomes, and was more effective than the others across a range of outcomes (e.g., knowledge, attitudes, and behaviors), lasting as long as 12 months after program delivery (Reyna et al. 2008; also Reyna and Farley 2006, Table 4).

Interventions Targeting Processing Interference Due to Class-Inclusion Confusion

In 1991, Reyna extended the analysis of class-inclusion confusions to the conjunction fallacy, logical reasoning biases (e.g., syllogisms), and other errors of probability judgment. As FTT explained, such confusions "can be diminished by, for example, providing a notational scheme such as Venn diagrams … or superordinate-set tags" (p. 319) (Reyna and Brainerd 2008). The thrust of those interventions is to keep the classes discrete—to separate, for example, the class of people who had breast cancer and a positive test result from other classes, such as the people without breast cancer who also had a positive test result. Once classes can be considered separately, they can be more easily recombined (assembled from the separate judgments) in different ways to yield conjunction

judgments, conditional probabilities, and other combinatorial judgments (e.g., Wolfe et al. 2013, 2015; Wolfe and Reyna 2010). For example, when classes are separated, it is possible to "flip the denominators" more easily, to consider *among those who had a positive test result*, how many had cancer versus did not have cancer.

This hypothesis has been tested in a variety of populations, ranging from expert physicians to the general population, using diagrams, 2×2 tables (and asking for separate estimates for each of the four classes in each cell of the table), and icon arrays that label classes distinctively so that denominators can be easily flipped visually. Even children's probability judgments are improved with such interventions (e.g., Reyna and Brainerd 1994). Although presenting probabilities (e.g., 0.01) in terms of frequencies (e.g., 1 in 100) often accomplishes this same separation of classes, frequencies are not inherently easier to manipulate than probabilities. For example, Cuite et al. (2008) studied 16,133 people's performance on multiple computational tasks involving health risks and found that performance was very similar for frequency (55 % accurate) and probability (57 % accurate) versions.

Many scholars have assumed that emphasizing numbers and providing calculators should improve health-related judgments and decisions (see Reyna et al. 2009). Lloyd and Reyna (2001) compared the use of a Bayesian online clinical calculator to an icon array that visually represented base rates, sensitivity, and specificity using the principles of FTT. Residents and medical students estimated the post-test probability of disease given a positive or negative test result. Results showed that subjects would often miss the question using the Bayesian calculator (despite being taught Bayes' theorem), for example, when estimating the probability of a test being negative rather than the probability of the patient having a disease given a negative test result (a class-inclusion confusion).

Rather than focusing on precise calculation, the goal of the FTT intervention was to increase gist-based thinking and decrease interference from overlapping classes. The intervention therefore focused on teaching subjects to visually estimate relative magnitude on a 10-by-10 grid with 100 squares (each square represented a woman with potential ischemic heart disease). Once the grid was constructed, squares were completed with pre-test information regarding the chances of ischemic heart attack and of coronary heart disease; then sensitivity and specificity were added by writing in + or − signs above each square. The grid accounted for all relevant classes, making it possible to visually estimate positive and negative predictive value (the probability of disease given a positive test result and the probability of no disease given a negative test result, respectively). The key to the intervention was to represent each class discretely (patients with the disease and either a positive or a negative result, and patients without the disease and either a positive or a negative result). Because classes were represented discretely, diagnostic errors were reduced, as predicted by FTT (Lloyd et al. 2001; Lloyd and Reyna 2001).

Conclusions and Future Directions: Gist in Public Health and Medical Decision-Making

Remarkably often, experts in public health are at a loss when asked what the point of information on a public Web page is other than to "provide information"—but toward what end? Similarly, experts in medical decision-making frequently disavow helping patients make any particular decision, and restrict decision-making support to situations in which there is no right or wrong choice, variously referred to as "equipoise" or "preference-sensitive" decisions (Elwyn et al. 2009).

Although it is certainly important to help people face tough choices when there is no right answer, according to FTT, the mental representations that are encoded, the values that are retrieved, and the application of values to representations all hinge on the functional significance of information—the meaning that matters (i.e., gist). Human information processing suppresses details to arrive at an essential bottom line: which option provides life rather than death, relief rather than suffering, mobility rather than disability. When people lack background information, they become lost in details; it is difficult for them to summarize the main point of information and to demonstrate an appreciation of the gist of key facts that should inform their decision-making. People encode both verbatim and multiple gist representations of information into memory independently, but tend to rely on the gist in judgment and decision-making (Reyna 2008; Reyna et al. 2015). Hence, people can get the verbatim facts right, and still not derive the proper meaning, which is necessary for informed consent (Reyna and Hamilton 2001).

This theoretical approach implies that judgment and decision-making cannot be stripped of meaningful content. Instead, the work of extracting the essential gist of options for different prevention, diagnosis, and treatment situations must be performed using systematic techniques for surveying patients and providers (e.g., Fraenkel et al. 2012; Table 6.1). A number of valid and reliable scales have been developed that have been successfully transferred across health situations (e.g., categorical thinking scales; Mills et al. 2008; Reyna 2008). Although progress has been made in research on meaning in multiple disciplines, humans remain far better at extracting gist than artificial systems.

In contrast to other theoretical approaches, the goal in FTT is not numerical precision or trading off precise numerical outcomes (e.g., the number treated who survived) against precise degrees of risk (e.g., the number of adverse events in the treatment group)—although in some difficult decisions the devil is in the details. Rather, the goal is to integrate the facts into a bottom line that captures the qualitatively important distinctions, not the quantitative minutia. Implementing this FTT approach would represent a significant change in current approaches to decision analysis and decision support for patients, and in education for health care providers (Lloyd and Reyna 2009).

FTT does not claim that numbers are unimportant, but that numbers lack meaning out of context and that the meaning that matters is

Table 1 Empirically supported applications of a fuzzy-trace theory of judgment and decision-making

Processing problem	Intervention	Theoretical framework	Results
Failure to retrieve knowledge in context (i.e., misinterpretations of messages) generates biases in risk assessment, even when explicit, specific cues relevant to mode of transmission are mentioned	Asking a patient in the emergency room whether he is "taking anything for pain" instead of asking whether he is taking ibuprofen (Reyna and Lloyd 1997)	Relevant gist-based retrieval cues can help patients remember health information	When cued with the gist of "medication for pain," the patient accurately recalled the name of the medication, however the verbatim drug name "ibuprofen" failed to elicit the accurate response with same patient the first time he was asked
Communication of a precise estimate of risk tailored for the patient does not necessarily mean that the patient extracts the essential gist of whether the risk is low or high (ordinal gist distinction)	Presenting two bar graphs, positioned side-by-side, to demonstrate the benefit of adding a specific medication to a traditional disease-modifying anti-rheumatic treatment [clear language such as "higher bar is better" was also used (Fraenkel et al. 2012)]	Presentation of meaningful graphical formats affects the ease with which people extract the gist of those inputs (e.g., meaning of the numerical relations)	Using this gist-based tool to promote accurate gist representations increased knowledge and patient willingness to escalate care in a pre- and post-test comparison
Failure to endorse the appropriate values about risk that elicits global meaning of risk-relevant behaviors results in compensatory decision-making (i.e., risk vs. benefit trade off) and less risk avoidance	Presenting values that arthritis patients could endorse (e.g., "it is important to reduce my chances of becoming disabled, even if it means taking medications with a risk of serious side effects") followed by feedback about options to better control their arthritis (Fraenkel et al. 2012)	Relying on meaning and endorsing simple, categorical (gist) principles are associated with less (unhealthy) risk taking	The tool substantially increased the proportion of patients making an informed value-concordant choice (i.e., those who favored medication use to minimize disease activity were more likely to show interest in changing their medication to better control their arthritis)
Failure to inhibit a salient and compelling gist (e.g., the meaning or essence of the target category that seems to fit the query) pulls reasoning toward the class-inclusion error	Illustrating relations between classes using analogies (e.g., the relation between AIDs and immune disorders are "like the relation between roses and flowers;" Wolfe and Reyna 2010)	Semantic manipulations make the gist of the classes more evident and more resistant to interference from class-inclusion	Analogies that highlighted set relations increased semantic coherence by helping people to accurately constrain their gist-based probability judgments to fit the appropriate set relations
Interference from nested class-inclusion relations (e.g., basal cell carcinoma and nonmelanoma) pushes reasoning away from the correct path	Making nested relations discrete and transparent through the presentation of 2 × 2 tables (subjects made separate probability judgments for each cell; Wolfe and Reyna 2010)	Separating nested classes reduces denominator neglect by making class-inclusion relations transparent	Teaching the use of optimal strategies reduced denominator neglect (i.e., 2 × 2 tables) reduced reasoning fallacies about meaningful information

usually simple (Reyna 2013). It is not informed consent to know that one's risk of death from surgery is exactly 0.02 and to be able to precisely differentiate that quantity and easily transform it into decimals and fractions without having a clue about whether that number is low or high (and whether to feel worried or relieved). To be sure, understanding that a risk of 0.02 is higher than

0.002 is helpful for patients and providers, especially given a rising tide of research knowledge; this ability is assessed in current measures of numeracy (Reyna et al. 2009). However, research needs to be conducted on how to measure *gist numeracy*, the ability to extract the qualitative essence of numbers—what numbers mean in context, including the relevant qualitative relations among numbers.

Although we emphasize the significance of content and context, unlike some theorists, we do not argue that conjunction fallacies, base rate neglect, and other biases are not errors. On the contrary, the interventions summarized in this chapter were designed to curb such errors by applying evidence-based understanding of the mechanisms that generate them. In this connection, FTT has been used to design effective public health programs and patient education tools, ranging from adolescents' HIV-AIDS prevention, to patients' arthritis medication choices, to physicians' judgments of cardiac risk (e.g., Reyna and Lloyd 2006).

One of the implications of this work for future research is to better understand how developmental differences in judgment and decision-making play out on in health and medicine. Lifestyle choices, such as diet and exercise, begin to take root in adolescence as young people gain more independence, and these choices have long-term impact on major killers, such as cancer and heart disease. For the first time in history, increases in heart disease are now being predicted because of poor diet and exercise in adolescence (Shay et al. 2011). However, FTT predicts that decision-making in adolescence about health will differ from mature decision-making in adults (e.g., Reyna et al. 2011). As we have discussed, reliance on gist processing increases with age and expertise (Reyna et al. 2003, 2014; Reyna and Brainerd 2011). The implications of these differences for obesity prevention and lifestyle choices (and for public health programs) have not been investigated.

Recommendations for Practice

1. **Do not stop at the numbers**.
   - Provide qualitative representations that capture the meaning (gist) of information to achieve understanding of risk; the gist is the essential element in informed consent.
   - Just because patients can repeat an exact probably (e.g., 20 %) does not mean that they comprehend what that specific probability means (e.g., whether risk is low or high).

2. **Give meaningful reasons for facts**.
   - Provide a more coherent and meaningful gist by explaining *the reasons behind* the directives to effectively communicate health information to those with little background knowledge.
   - For example, explain that the reason that HIV, HPV, and herpes simplex are incurable and not treatable with antibiotics is because they are viruses.

3. **Begin with a bottom-line message in mind**.
   - Identify the gist that is meant to be communicated, the bottom-line, relevant meaning of information, by distilling its simplest qualitative essence.
   - You cannot communicate a message if you do not know what it is.

4. **Find the qualitative pivot points**.
   - Find the qualitative pivot points in a decision (i.e., the consequences that are categorically different from other consequences); focus on the bottom line of messages that represent the simplest distinction between options.
   - Make distinctions between life versus death, being unable to work versus being able to work, irre-

versible permanent damage versus reversible damage (e.g., joint damage in rheumatoid arthritis), or bearable pain versus an unbearable peak of pain (e.g., colonoscopy).

5. **Encourage the endorsement of simple healthy principles and values**.
   - Lifestyle gist principles represent patients' own personal values (e.g., survival, quality of life) and can be practiced sufficiently to be automatically retrieved in the context of risky choices.
   - Endorsing categorical avoidance of risk, such as "Avoid risk" and "No risk is better than some risk," has been associated with protective effects regarding risky behavior.

6. **Use graphs that facilitate extracting a salient gist**.
   - Provide meaningful graphical representations that facilitate perceptual estimation of the gist relation; the picture should match the concept.
   - People can intuitively grasp gross differences in heights in visual displays (e.g., simple bar graphs and risk ladders) to signify the gist of relative magnitude (e.g., which treatment has "higher" and which was "lower" risk).

7. **Keep classes of events separately**.
   - Explain the probabilities separately of overlapping classes to reduce confusion about probability judgment: for example, probability of getting cancer without the cancer gene; of having the gene without the cancer; of getting cancer with the cancer gene; and of having the gene with cancer.
   - Use a 2 × 2 table to separate each class of events and to make clear the

different probabilities of false positives, false negatives, true positives, and true negatives.

References

Adam, M. B., & Reyna, V. F. (2005). Coherence and correspondence criteria for rationality: Experts' estimation of risks of sexually transmitted infections. *Journal of Behavioral Decision Making, 18*(3), 169–186. doi:10.1002/bdm.493.

American Cancer Society. (2012). *Cancer facts & figures 2012*. Atlanta: American Cancer Society.

Barbey, A. K., & Sloman, S. A. (2007). Base-rate respect: From statistical formats to cognitive structures. *Behavioral and Brain Sciences, 30*, 287–297.

Betsch, C., Brewer, N. T., Brocard, P., Davies, P., Gaissmaier, W., Haase, N., et al. (2012). Opportunities and challenges of web 2.0 for vaccination decisions. *Vaccine, 28*(30), 3727–3733. doi:10.1016/j.vaccine.2012.02.025

Brewer, N. T., Richman, A. R., DeFrank, J. T., Reyna, V. F., & Carey, L. A. (2012). Improving communication of breast cancer recurrence risk. *Breast Cancer Research and Treatment, 133*, 553–561. doi:10.1007/s10549-011-1791-9.

Brewer, N. T., Tzeng, J. P., Lillie, S. E., Edwards, A. S., Peppercorn, J. M., & Rimer, B. K. (2009). Health literacy and cancer risk perception: Implications for genomic risk communication. *Medical Decision Making, 29*, 157–166. doi:10.1177/0272989X08327111.

Brewer, N. T., Weinstein, N. D., Cuite, C. L., & Herrington, J. (2004). Risk perceptions and their relation to risk behavior. *Annals of Behavioral Medicine, 27*, 125–130.

Brust-Renck, P. G., Royer, C. E., & Reyna, V. F. (2013). Communicating numerical risk: Human factors that aid understanding in health care. *Reviews of Human Factors and Ergonomics, 8*, 235–276. doi:10.1177/1557234X13492980.

Cuite, C. L., Weinstein, N. D., Emmons, K., & Colditz, G. (2008). A test of numeric formats for communicating risk probabilities. *Medical Decision Making, 28*(3), 377–384. doi:10.1177/0272989X08315246.

Downs, J. S., Bruin de Bruine, W. D., & Fischhoff, B. (2008). Parents' vaccination comprehension and decisions. *Vaccine, 26*, 1595–1607. doi:10.1016/j.vaccine.2008.01.011.

Eddy, D. M. (1982). Probabilistic reasoning in clinical medicine: Problems and opportunities. In D. Kahneman,

P. Slovic, & A. Tversky (Eds.), *Judgment under uncertainty: Heuristics and biases* (pp. 249–267). Cambridge, UK: Cambridge University.

Elwyn, G., Frosch, D., & Rollnick, S. (2009). Dual equipoise shared decision making: Definitions for decision and behaviour support interventions. *Implementation Science, 4*, 75. doi:10.1186/1748-5908-4-75.

Fagerlin, A., Pignone, M., Abhyankar, P., Col, N., Feldman-Stewart, D., Gavaruzzi, T., et al. (2013). Clarifying values: An updated review. *BMC Medical Informatics and Decision Making, 13*(Suppl 2), S8. doi:10.1186/1472-6947-13-S2-S8.

Fagerlin, A., Zikmund-Fisher, B. J., & Ubel, P. (2005). How making a risk estimate can change the feel of that risk: Shifting attitudes toward breast cancer risk in a general public survey. *Patient Education and Counseling, 57*(3), 294–299.

Fraenkel, L., Matzko, C. K., Webb, D. E., Oppermann, B., Charpentier, P., Peters, E., Reyna, V. F., & Newman, E. D. (2015). Use of decision support for improved knowledge, values clarification, and informed choice in patients with rheumatoid arthritis. *Arthritis Care and Research, 67*(11), 1496–1502. doi:10.1002/acr.22659.

Fraenkel, L., Peters, E., Charpentier, P., Olsen, B., Errante, L., Schoen, R. T., et al. (2012). A decision tool to improve the quality of care in rheumatoid arthritis. *Arthritis Care & Research, 64*(7), 977–985. doi:10.1002/acr.21657.

Kahneman, D. (2003). A perspective on judgment and choice: Mapping bounded rationality. *American Psychologist, 58*(9), 697–720. doi:10.1037/0003-066X.58.9.697.

Kahneman, D. (2011). *Thinking fast and slow*. New York: Farrar, Strauss, Giroux.

Kühberger, A., & Tanner, C. (2010). Risky choice framing: Task versions and a comparison of prospect theory and fuzzy-trace theory. *Journal of Behavioral Decision Making, 23*(3), 314–329. doi:10.1002/bdm.656.

Lloyd, A., Hayes, P., Bell, P. R. F., & Naylor, A. R. (2001). The role of risk and benefit perception in informed consent for surgery. *Medical Decision Making, 21*(2), 141–149. doi:10.1177/0272989X0102100207.

Lloyd, F. J., & Reyna, V. F. (2001). A web exercise in evidence-based medicine using cognitive theory. *Journal of General Internal Medicine, 16*(2), 94–99. doi:10.1111/j.1525-1497.2001.00214.x.

Lloyd, F. J., & Reyna, V. F. (2009). Clinical gist and medical education: Connecting the dots. *Journal of the American Medical Association, 302*(12), 1332–1333. doi:10.1001/jama.2009.1383.

Mills, B., Reyna, V. F., & Estrada, S. (2008). Explaining contradictory relations between risk perception and risk taking. *Psychological Science, 19*, 429–433. doi:10.1111/j.1467-9280.2008.02104.x.

Peters, E., Slovic, P., Västfjäll, D., & Mertz, C. K. (2008). Intuitive numbers guide decisions. *Judgment and Decision Making, 3*, 619–635. Retrieved from journal.sjdm.org/8827/jdm8827.html

Reyna, V. F. (1991). Class inclusion, the conjunction fallacy, and other cognitive illusions. *Developmental Review, 11*, 317–336. doi:10.1016/0273-2297(91)90017-I.

Reyna, V. F. (2004). How people make decisions that involve risk: A dual process approach. *Current Directions in Psychological Science, 13*, 60–66. doi:10.1111/j.0963-7214.2004.00275.x.

Reyna, V. F. (2008). A theory of medical decision making and health: Fuzzy trace theory. *Medical Decision Making, 28*(6), 850–865. doi:10.1177/0272989X08327066.

Reyna, V. F. (2011). Across the lifespan. In B. Fischhoff, N. T. Brewer, & J. S. Downs (Eds.), *Communicating risks and benefits: An evidence-based user's guide* (pp. 111–119). USA: U.S. Department of Health and Human Services, Food and Drug Administration. Retrieved from http://www.fda.gov/ScienceResearch/SpecialTopics/RiskCommunication/default.htm

Reyna, V. F. (2012a). A new intuitionism: Meaning, memory, and development in fuzzy-trace theory. *Judgment and Decision Making, 7*(3), 332–359. Retrieved from journal.sjdm.org/11/111031/jdm111031.html

Reyna, V. Г. (2012b). Risk perception and communication in vaccination decisions: A fuzzy-trace theory approach. *Vaccine, 30*(25), 3790–3797. doi:10.1016/j.vaccine.2011.11.070

Reyna, V. F. (2013). Intuition, reasoning, and development: A fuzzy-trace theory approach. In P. Barrouillet & C. Gauffroy (Eds.), *The development of thinking and reasoning* (pp. 193–220). Hove, UK: Psychology Press.

Reyna, V. F., & Adam, M. B. (2003). Fuzzy-trace theory, risk communication, and product labeling in sexually transmitted diseases. *Risk Analysis, 23*, 325–342. doi:10.1111/1539-6924.00332.

Reyna, V. F., Adam, M. B., Poirier, K., LeCroy, C. W., & Brainerd, C. J. (2005). Risky decision-making in childhood and adolescence: A fuzzy-trace theory approach. In J. Jacobs & P. Klaczynski (Eds.), *The development of children's and adolescents' judgment and decision-making* (pp. 77–106). Mahwah, NJ: Erlbaum.

Reyna, V. F., & Brainerd, C. J. (1994). The origins of probability judgment: A review of data and theories. In G. Wright & P. Ayton (Eds.), *Subjective probability* (pp. 239–272). New York: Wiley.

Reyna, V. F., & Brainerd, C. J. (1995). Fuzzy-trace theory: An interim synthesis. *Learning and Individual Differences, 7*, 1–75. doi:10.1016/1041-6080(95)90031-4.

Reyna, V. F., & Brainerd, C. J. (2008). Numeracy, ratio bias, and denominator neglect in judgments of risk and probability. *Learning and Individual Differences, 18*(1), 89–107. doi:10.1016/j.lindif.2007.03.011.

Reyna, V. F., & Brainerd, C. J. (2011). Dual processes in decision making and developmental neuroscience: A fuzzy-trace model. *Developmental Review, 31*, 180–206. doi:10.1016/j.dr.2011.07.004.

Reyna, V. F., Chapman, S., Dougherty, M., & Confrey, J. (2012). *The adolescent brain: Learning, reasoning, and decision making*. Washington, DC: American Psychological Association.

Reyna, V. F., Chick, C. F., Corbin, J. C., & Hsia, A. N. (2014). Developmental reversals in risky decision-making: Intelligence agents show larger decision biases than college students. *Psychological Science, 25*(1), 76–84. doi:10.1177/0956797613497022.

Reyna, V. F., Estrada, S. M., DeMarinis, J. A., Myers, R. M., Stanisz, J. M., & Mills, B. A. (2011). Neurobiological and memory models of risky decision making in adolescents versus young adults. *Journal of Experimental Psychology. Learning, Memory, and Cognition, 37*(5), 1125–1142. doi:10.1037/a0023943.

Reyna, V. F., & Farley, F. (2006). Risk and rationality in adolescent decision-making: Implications for theory, practice, and public policy. *Psychological Science in the Public Interest, 7*(1), 1–44. doi:10.111/j.1529-1006.2006.00026.x.

Reyna, V. F., & Hamilton, A. J. (2001). The importance of memory in informed consent for surgical risk. *Medical Decision Making, 21*, 152–155. doi:10.1177/0272989X0102100209.

Reyna, V. F., & Lloyd, F. J. (1997). Theories of false memory in children and adults. *Learning and Individual Differences, 9*(2), 95–123. doi:10.1016/S1041-6080(97)90002-9.

Reyna, V. F., & Lloyd, F. J. (2006). Physician decision making and cardiac risk: Effects of knowledge, risk perception, risk tolerance, and fuzzy processing. *Journal of Experimental Psychology, 12*(3), 179–195. doi:10.1037/1076-898X.12.3.179.

Reyna, V. F., Lloyd, F. J., & Brainerd, C. J. (2003). Memory, development, and rationality: An integrative theory of judgment and decision-making. *Emerging Perspectives on Judgment and Decision research* (pp. 201–245). New York: Cambridge University Press.

Reyna, V. F., Lloyd, F., & Whalen, P. (2001). Genetic testing and medical decision making. *Archives of Internal Medicine, 161*(20), 2406–2408. doi:10.1001/archinte.161.20.2406.

Reyna, V. F., & Mills, B. A. (2007a). Converging evidence supports fuzzy-trace theory's nested sets hypothesis (but not the frequency hypothesis). *Behavioral and Brain Sciences, 30*(3), 278–280. doi:10.1017/S0140525X07001872.

Reyna, V. F., & Mills, B. A. (2007b). Interference processes in fuzzy-trace theory: Aging, Alzheimer's disease, and development. In D. Gorfein & C. MacLeod (Eds.), *Inhibition in cognition* (pp. 185–210). Washington: APA Press.

Reyna, V. F., Mills, B. A., & Estrada, S. M. (2008, October). Reducing risk taking in adolescence: Effectiveness of a gist-based curriculum. In *Paper presented at the 30th Annual Meeting of the Society of Medical Decision Making*, Philadelphia, PA.

Reyna, V. F., Weldon, R. B., & McCormick, M. J. (2015). Educating intuition: Reducing risky decisions using fuzzy-trace theory. *Current Directions in Psychological Science, 24*(4), 392–398. doi: 10.1177/0963721415588081.

Rivers, S. E., Reyna, V. F., & Mills, B. (2008). Risk taking under the influence: A fuzzy-trace theory of emotion in adolescence. *Developmental Review, 28* (1), 107–144. doi: 10.1016/j.dr.2007.11.002.

Reyna, V. F., Nelson, W., Han, P., & Dieckmann, N. F. (2009). How numeracy influences risk comprehension and medical decision making. *Psychological Bulletin, 135*, 943–973. doi:10.1037/a0017327.

Shay, C. M., Ning, H., Daniels, S. R., & Lloyd-Jones, D. M. (2011). Prevalence of ideal cardiovascular health in U. S. children and adolescents: Findings from the national health and nutrition examination survey (2003–2008). In *Paper presented at the Annual Meeting of the American Heart Association*, Orlando, Florida.

Stratton, K., Ford, A., Rusch, E., & Clayton, E. W. (2012). Measles, mumps, and rubella vaccine. Report of the committee to review adverse effects of vaccines, Institute of Medicine. In *Adverse Effects of Vaccines: Evidence and Causality* (pp. 103–237). Washington, DC: National Academy of Sciences.

Wolfe, C. R., Fisher, C. R., & Reyna, V. R. (2013). Semantic coherence and inconsistency in estimating conditional probabilities. *Journal of Behavioral Decision Making, 26*(3), 237–246. doi:10.1002/bdm.1756.

Wolfe, C. R., & Reyna, V. F. (2010). Semantic coherence and fallacies in estimating joint probabilities. *Journal of Behavioral Decision Making, 23*(2), 203–223. doi:10.1002/bdm.650.

Wolfe, C. R., Reyna, V. F., Widmer, C. L., Cedillos, E. M., Fisher, C. R., Brust-Renck, P. G., & Weil, A. M. (2015). Efficacy of a web-based intelligent tutoring system for communicating genetic risk of breast cancer: A fuzzy-trace theory approach. *Medical Decision Making, 35*(1), 46–59. doi: 10.1177/0272989X14535983.

Cognitive Mechanisms and Common-Sense Management of Cancer Risk: Do Patients Make Decisions?

7

Howard Leventhal, Jessica S. Yu, Elaine A. Leventhal and Susan M. Bodnar-Deren

Our chapter has two primary goals. The first is to describe a model of the mechanisms underlying the "common-sense processes" involved in everyday management of health risks. The second, intertwined with the first, is to apply the model to decisions and management of cancers in three areas: screening, care seeking, and end-of-life planning. We first spell out two themes underlying how the model represents the processes involved in people's everyday approach to "decision" making for managing threats of cancers. The first theme concerns the role of words and conscious deliberation in health decisions. Academics value words, spoken and written, and greatly overestimate their importance in decision-making in everyday life (for a similar view, see Beach 2009). Everyday life, however, unfolds rapidly: We awaken, brush teeth, dress, toilet, take meds, down a quick breakfast, and head to work. Conscious, verbally marked concepts collaborate in the ongoing, automatic behavioral flow, but it is not always easy to detect when and how it directs specific actions. For example, internal or public speech may be engaged when comparing the color of a shirt or blouse to pants or skirt when dressing, but most behaviors in the sequence of events in the dressing script are automatic. *In short, the bulk of daily behaviors, which include actions such as reaching, lifting, walking, eating, and taking a prescribed medication, are automatically generated behaviors that are embedded in behavioral sequences, or "scripts"* (Abelson 1976, 1981). Post-action doubts such as "Did I take my meds? Lock the door?" attest to the fact that most scripts are performed at a moment with little involvement of conscious deliberation and/or choosing among alternatives.

The interaction between deliberative-executive and automatic systems is a central focus of the common-sense model (CSM), consistent with the distinction between central and peripheral processing of messages in communication theories (Petty and Cacioppo 1984) and slow versus quick decisions in cognitive science (Kahneman 2013). CSM pays particular attention to the interaction of automatic and more

H. Leventhal (✉)
Department of Psychology and Institute for Health, Rutgers University, 112 Paterson St., New Brunswick, NJ 08901, USA
e-mail: hleventhal@ifh.rutgers.edu

J.S. Yu
VA Palo Alto Health Care System, Palo Alto, CA, USA
e-mail: jessica.yu@rutgers.edu

E.A. Leventhal
Department of Medicine and Institute for Health, Rutgers, RWJ Medical School, Rutgers University, 2 Beekman Place, 7C., New York, NY 10022, USA

S.M. Bodnar-Deren
Department Sociology, Virginia Commonwealth University, 827 West Franklin Street, Richmond, VA 23226, USA
e-mail: smbodnar@vcu.edu

© Springer Science+Business Media New York 2016
M.A. Diefenbach et al. (eds.), *Handbook of Health Decision Science*,
DOI 10.1007/978-1-4939-3486-7_7

conscious, executive processes, postulating that the executive needs to slow and carefully review both the environmental context and automatic actions to find "slots," i.e., pauses between automatic sequences in which to insert new responses to manage illness threats (Gobet 1998; Leventhal et al. 2016; Posner and Rothbart 1998; Leventhal et al. 2012). Mental rehearsal of the response allows subsequent, automatic performance (Phillips et al. 2013). Example of automatic response sequences are reported by patients skillful in self-management of chronic conditions; for example, patients with asthma link use of an inhaler by placing it in the bathroom and using as part of their morning routines, a strategy that generated nearly a fourfold increase in treatment adherence in comparison to that for patients who rely on memory (Brooks et al. 2014). Moreover, the odds ratio was reduced little if at all by moderating factors such as education, ethnicity, or literacy. Conscious "action planning" to identifying locations for inserting action can be difficult if daily behavioral sequences are over learned, complex, and not amenable to self-examination, and if the new action is complex or infrequent. The process is also difficult to complete in chaotic environments, e.g., where multiple individuals arise simultaneously and use the same facilities. Although we believe it critical to create automatic action sequences that can generate beneficial health outcomes, it is clear that it is difficult to alter many automatic, health damaging behavioral sequences; smoking and excessive consumption of alcohol are but two examples.

The second theme underlying our analysis involves two developmental sequences. The first is the lengthy, developmental history of chronic conditions such as coronary diseases, Type 2 diabetes, and many cancers. The second is the individual's developmental history. From the intrauterine environment (Finch 1994, 1995), through childhood, adolescence, adulthood, and older age, multiple factors interact in the complex ecology of the socio-bio-behavioral systems involved in the development of life. Much of the history is silent, buried in interactions among our genetic makeup and the environments that generate our epigenetic history. The interaction among the two sequences is affected by how and when a cancer intrudes in the life cycle, and how it alters the context for both automatic action and deliberative decision-making. The interplay will be influenced by an individual's life history and the context formed by her or his culture and family as well as by the individual's perceptions and beliefs about cancer and how the cancer is detected, e.g., symptomatically and experienced as an existent threat, testing that reveals presymptomatic disease or genetic testing that augurs future vulnerability. It is easy to forget however, that common sense, e.g., awareness of the history and presence of cancer in family members played a similar role well before modern technology came on the scene. For cancers unlike many other conditions, the threat combines the images of a lingering, painful existence, with disfiguring treatments and unavoidable death.

"Stages" in Cancer History

Studies examining patient decisions and adaptation to cancer typically focus on a specific stage such as: (1) *preclinical*; research focused on prevention and screening; (2) *diagnosis or discovery*; factors associated with response to detection; (3) *choice and initiation of treatment*, e.g., surgery, radiation, etc.; (4) *transition between treatments*, e.g., from surgery to adjuvant therapies, (5) *living with cancer*, and (6) *end-of-life*, e.g., planning and treatment preferences when terminally ill (see Kreuter et al. 2007). Although convenient for empirical work, these divisions underplay the contributions of two sets of moderating factors previously mentioned: (1) The stage of the patient's life cycle in which the cancer occurs, e.g., breast cancer has quite different ramifications for a 45–year-old mother of two versus an 80-year-old grandmother; and (2) The continuity of personal histories particularly with regard to highly automatic, everyday behaviors. Both issues require the examination as to how events at earlier stages of life and prior experience with cancer impact decisions and adaptation at later points in time.

Individuals face multiple challenges trying to generate new behaviors and reorganize daily, largely automatic behavioral sequences as they confront the uncertainties and demands of the diagnosis of cancer and the transitioning from treatment to treatment and the termination of treatment following treatment failure or presumed cure. Each transition involves readjustments in one's view of cancer, its treatments, and the new vulnerabilities acquired from treatments described as "lifesaving". End-of-life planning and confrontation with immanent death requires addressing existential issues that may or may not have been considered at earlier stages. CSM provides a reasonably detailed though still incomplete analysis of the mental models of cancer(s), the processes by which experience with disease, treatment, and social communication update and elaborate these models, and opens the door to the analysis as to how these processes affect ongoing decisions regarding continuing treatment and changes in daily life. Modeling these processes suggests hypotheses respecting effects within and across stages, e.g., from prediagnosis through diagnosis and treatment. It is also open to more detailed conceptualization of survivorship and ultimate death.

The Common-Sense Framework

The CSM specifies the content and operation of the cognitive, affective, and behavioral system shaping people's daily perception and personal and interpersonal responses to illness. The model posits a multilevel system with feed-forward and feedback controls that generate perceptions and interpretations of signs of present illness risks, projects future risks, and generates goals and plans for goal-directed actions and expectations regarding outcomes. The system evaluates outcomes and updates both the representations and "skills" for managing the evolving threats of the disease as the individual transitions through the "stages" from detection and treatment to survivorship and/or terminal illness and death. The

variables that are updated are embedded in four prototypes: (1) the *SELF*, healthy, and sick; (2) *illness prototypes*, e.g., cancer(s); (3) *procedures for prevention, detection, and treatment* ranging from diet and physical activity through tests (mammography; PSA; surgeries; radiation; chemotherapy), and (4) *action plans*, the strategies and skills for performance, *and action planning*, the strategies for creating plans for implementing and sustaining action. The parameters of these four sets of prototypes or schemata generate the "priors" or expectations that are updated as new information is generated by the outcomes from actions and communications from family, friends, practitioners, and media. CSM is Bayesian at its core.

By defining specific cognitive, affective, and behavioral variables and the dynamics of their operation, CSM provides insights into the generation of frameworks within which individual's perceive, set goals and plan, act, and interpret outcomes for disease management. Two executive functions are of critical importance in this planning process: (1) *anticipating and/or projecting future states of self and environment, and* (2) *monitoring behavior in context to identify behavioral sequences in which to insert action for implementing disease management*. The first, projecting futures, generates motivation to deal with both immediate and, depending upon disease stage, the existential threat of cancer. A critical product of the second is creating largely automatic, efficient action sequences ("action plans") that can be performed with little or no conscious deliberation. Finally, CSM links the memory structures and interpersonal processes that give meaning to the experience of symptoms, function, and treatment in different social and institutional contexts. Comparisons of one's symptoms, perceived causal experience, treatment, and outcomes to observation of another individual with cancer, can enhance or undermine the credibility of the other's comments and advice. In addition, comparison of one's present with prior experience and expectations respecting treatment induced disease changes can affect trust in a clinician's recommendations if communicated expectations are not confirmed by experience.

Our first task is to sketch how CSM represents the content and operation of the factors involved in disease management. We then examine how these factors operate at two points in time; detection of cancer and end-of-life decisions. As our approach is dynamic and focused on process rather than "static," we give little attention to individual difference moderators, e.g., traits such as optimism, except where CSM can describe the mechanisms underlying how an important moderating factor such as self-efficacy is expressed in action.

Content in CSM

Self schema: Interactions among the SELF SCHEMA, its physical, cognitive, affective, and social parameters, and ILLNESS schemata of cancers, generate active mental representations of what it means to be ill rather than well. A cursory examination of any neuroanatomy text makes clear that the SELF schema has shape and location; the prototype is grounded in the anatomy and function of the brain and body. Feedback (somatic; functional; social; etc.) generated by an individual's actions update and expand the physical, cognitive, and social parameters of the neuroanatomical template; "What I am and what I can do physically, cognitively and socially." Updating the SELF however, occurs slowly over much of the life span though it can be far more rapid during developmental transitions, e.g., adolescence, and in following major insults such as severe injury, The rate of change in the parameters of the self, are also likely to vary by system, e.g., representations of the environment or a specific cancer may be rapid whereas skilled motor responses may require intensive practice.

In CSM as other models, the self-prototype integrates experiences across domains, e.g., somatic, functional (cognitive and physical), and social events. Although people generally rely upon words to communicate about the Self, nonverbal routines, e.g., pointing, exposing a body part or performing a movement, are used in many settings, e.g., medical office, on the playing field, to share the underlying referents of words, e.g., "Is this lump my cancer?" As the experiential background underlying an individual is often invisible to an observer, or visible only with technology, an observer with limited access to these data may not accurately reflect who that individual is biologically, and "what s/he should or can and cannot do." Apart from their importance for social sharing, both concepts and their concrete referents play a crucial role in the executive control of automatic action and deliberative thoughts that generate expectations about the future self. Thus, the executive can imagine the SELF as social-emotionally isolated if cancer threatens culturally valued physical features and functions, e.g., mastectomy and loss of breast, prostatectomy and loss of sexual function, and these expectations can provoke emotional distress and searches for untested and often harmful treatments. The search for "miracle" cures is often activated when an individual envisages a death from cancer that is painful and prolonged, for example, Steve Jobs' decision to rely on a combination of complementary alternative medical treatments instead of surgery when he was first diagnosed with pancreatic cancer (Isaacson 2011). This will be addressed in the section on end-of-life planning.

Illness schemata: Illness schemata can be generic and vague or highly specific with detailed referents. For example, the prototype for *acute illnesses* includes symptoms and a label, the *identity* of the illness, relatively brief *timelines* (days), limited *consequences* and an array of *causes* and expectations for *control*. Although the general acute prototype is readily articulated and socially shared (Robbins et al. 2015), its parameters will vary for specific conditions; a stomachache and a head or chest cold will differ markedly with respect to symptom pattern and means of control but may overlap respecting cause (e.g., stress) and timelines. Each condition's concrete features, symptoms, time frame, causes and means of control are linked to verbally labeled concepts, e.g., "I have a stomach ache" or "I have a chest cold," and the activation of the concept defined by one or more experienced factors integrates an array of prior experiences in addition to the immediate concrete referents that gave rise to the labels (Andrews et al. 2009; Meyer et al. 1985; Halm et al. 2006).

Although cancer is our focus, it is critical to include a detailed description of the general prototype for acute conditions, as it is the *default* for the interpretation of somatic and functional deviations. The acute prototype is omnipresent, a generator of priors or expectations regarding the causes, durations, and actions for eliminating and controlling somatic and functional deviations whether the condition underlying these experiences is acute or chronic. The acute schemata is always "in the background," seeding doubts and raising hopes about the meaning of symptoms and expected outcomes of treatment (race for the cure), biasing the longer term picture of treatment outcomes for virtually all chronic conditions and plays a critical role in how patients interpret and respond during several transitions in the diagnosis and treatment of cancer.

Unlike schemata for acute conditions, schemata for specific chronic conditions frequently lack clear referents, leaving patients uncertain and failing to act to manage the condition. To manage the uncertainty associated with a chronic condition, patients may automatically enact behavioral sequences for controlling acute conditions, such as the everyday cold, creating actions and expectations to reach at short-term goals that may interfere with effective management for the long term. Examples can be seen in patients with chronic hypertension (Meyer et al. 1985), asthma (Halm et al. 2006), and heart failure (Albert 2013). For example, valid referents for the concepts heart failure will include chronic fatigue, swollen legs, and bouts of breathlessness in the absence of arm and chest pain, symptoms typically attributed to acute myocardial infarction (Horowitz et al. 2004). Patients with heart failure who expect chest or arm pain for all diseases of the heart, and attribute breathlessness and chronic fatigue to aging, may fail to seek help when decompensating.

Linking the heart to chest pain and not swollen legs is consistent with common sense, as we feel heart beats in the chest, not in the lungs and legs. It is also likely that such misconceptions will be reinforced by social contacts.

In the absence of direct experience with cancer in early life, the concept and concrete referents of the prototype will be based on information ranging from observations of family members and friends managing cancers, media stories, public health campaigns, and cultural beliefs. The absence of personal somatic and functional content can open a door to imagery rich in affective content that overlaps partially at best, with the experience of cancer. In addition, the cancer schemata held by many people may fail to differentiate between treatable cancers, e.g., basal cell carcinoma, and death-dealing melanoma. As a consequence, media and social messages about cancer may be assimilated and interpreted by a prototype in which all cancers are invasive and painful and lead to suffering from futile treatments on a doorway to death (Henry 1999). Representations based on a prototype representing cancer as a "dismal" death-dealing entity can activate defensive reactions that create barriers to deliberative, decision-making, and the avoidance of screening and adoption of preventive behaviors. They may also affect responses and expectations during diagnosis and treatment, influencing behavior and emotional reactions posttreatment that disrupt the planning needed to deal with management of a terminal illness. It is important to remember however, that illness schemata are less stable than SELF schemata; they are changeable with personal experience and public education campaigns. For example, the Australian skin cancer awareness campaign led to marked changes in the public's representation of cancer 1980–2001 (Montague et al. 2001). Other research indicates that between 1964 and 2001, skin cancer screening rates in Australia increased from 18 % in 1964 to 77 % in 2001; a change which appears to be associated with increased information from television and family members (MacTiernan et al. 2014; Donovan et al. 2004). There is also some evidence that media campaigns about colorectal (Cram et al. 2003), oral (Jedele and Ismail 2010) and breast (Yanovitzky and Blitz 2000) cancers were associated with an increase in screenings in the U.S.

Treatment schemata: Schemata of management and treatment procedures (surgery, medication, healthy nutrition, various physical activities) also integrate abstract concepts and verbal labels with imagined and/or actual concrete experiences. Cancer patients are often provided a wealth of treatment options complicating decision-making as patients must understand their alternatives, conceptually and experientially. As many patients diagnosed with cancer lack both the array of abstract concepts and concrete experience to make comparative decisions, they may neither know nor be able to imagine and anticipate how a treatment will feel, let alone understand how it works. For example, in deciding between surgery and chemotherapy, a surgeon may state that cancer is controlled and possibly cured by complete removal of the tumor whereas a radiologist may state that the tumor is destroyed by burning. As burning does not literally remove dead tumor cells, patients may have, but fail to express, doubts about its efficacy. Although complete removal of a breast lump may seem like a cure, removal of breast tissue may affect sexual attractiveness producing an unanticipated discrepancy with self-appearance and posttreatment regrets. Thus, different treatments for the same disorder may differ in perceived efficacy; removing tumor with surgery may seem closer to a cure, radiation as temporary control, and also differ in expectations of posttreatment outcomes and everyday experiences given treatment induced changes in appearance and function (Mukherjee 2010).

Two important issues need to be kept in mind; first, verbally communicated expectations about treatment experience may fail to match reality. Given a practitioner's limited knowledge of a patients' social and cultural environment, practitioner predictions of ease of posttreatment recovery may fail to match patient expectations and posttreatment experience physically and socially. Second, laypersons misperceptions and misinterpretations are not necessarily a sign of

illiteracy or innumeracy; they may reflect fears and motives similar in some respects to some surgical practitioner's blind commitments to radical mastectomy; such is the history of cancer (Mukherjee 2010).

Treatment procedures also have complex time frames including their duration and time until one experiences beneficial outcomes during and after treatment ends. For example, the severity and duration of pain (McAndrew et al. 2008), are affected by the emotional reactions accompanying patient's prototypes of disease and treatment as well as the biology of recovery. Current assessment of patients' perceptions of treatment are focused on a respondent's reports of the "necessity" and "concerns" respecting their own treatment regimens and "necessities" and "concerns" about treatments in general (Horne and Weinman 1999). A patient's endorsement of items on these scales provides a useful, overview of his or her preferences for specific treatments and are consistent predictors of adherence (Horne et al. 1999). Knowing a patient's responses to these scales can inform practitioner–patient exchanges and improve shared decision-making. As the scales do not however, assess perceptions or expectations respecting time frames for outcomes, posttreatment somatic experience or life disruptions, or the specific experiences and objective tests that a patient uses to judge treatment efficacy, the practitioners likely need to more fully explore the patient's representations of disease and treatment. These details will be touched upon when we address aspects of shared decision-making.

Representations Dynamics: The Matching Process

The representations of illness threats, the active, mental models that create the framework for decisions, are often products of the interaction or interpretation of somatic and functional changes with one or more illness schemata. Mental representations can also be activated by observation of illness and media messages. Activated representation generates motives for action along with expectations respecting action outcomes, an ongoing process that shapes behaviors and interprets feedback from actions to control a perceived threat. CSM provides a reasonably detailed picture of four of the steps involved in the activation of mental models: (1) the observation of somatic and functional stimuli in one's self or others that deviate from "normal, healthy SELF"; (2) the creation of meaning when observed deviations are matched to illness schemata, e.g., cancer(s); (3) the automatic and deliberative responding elicited by the representations; and (4) the role of interpersonal communication in the matching process. Each of these steps is moderated and mediated by the mental representations active at that time and each have significant implications for screening, detection and treatment pf cancer, survivorship and end-of-life planning.

1. *Detection*: The SELF is a prototype defined by a broad set of parameters that generate expectations for the evaluation of somatic sensations and physical and mental function (i.e., this is how I am physically, behaviorally, and cognitively). Similar processes also are involved when observing other individuals. Appraisals occur both deliberatively, i.e., a conscious sense of self as "normal" and healthy versus ill or likely to become ill, and automatically, the latter involving an array of control systems "appraising" and regulating the interior milieu, posture, and movement. Deviations from self are often detected subliminally, below the threshold for conscious deliberative decisions and action, and individuals are often unaware of their automatic responses to these cues; for example, scratching to alleviate an itch, or rubbing a sore arm can occur with minimal or no conscious awareness. When a stimulus is highly salient however, a severe pain or major change in function, both automatic and conscious processes will be jointly involved in matching an experienced somatic or functional change to an illness schemata (see Fig. 7.1).

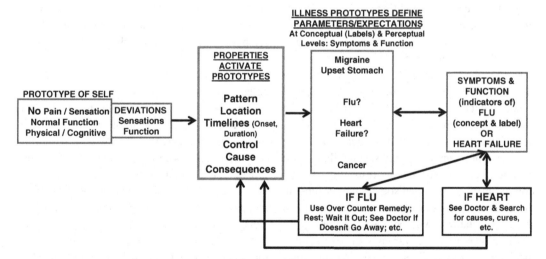

Fig. 7.1 Matching deviations from self to illness prototypes: prototypes are averages of a history of experiences with SELF and specific illnesses. Prototype for FLU and prototype for HEART FAILURE can share expected pattern and location of some symptoms (obstructed breathing; fatigue), though they differ markedly in timelines, control, and outcomes. The process is computational as each prototype assigns different weights to each deviation. Repetition forms modules (stomach problem; migraine; etc.) that generate higher order, declarative structure, e.g., ACUTE and CHRONIC models. As the number of conditions increase with age and properties fit two or more prototypes there is increasing uncertainty in the construction of representations. Representations based on histories of repeated construction are activated rapidly and can interfere with the construction of new, biologically valid representations, a problem with many chronic, asymptomatic conditions onset in the later years of life

2. *Matching and meaning*: Active representations have substantive content in one or more of five categories, and the variables in each category are involved in the matching process. (1) The *identity* of a condition involves a match of concrete experience with diagnostic labels. The concrete features include the **pattern and location** of symptoms and the type of functional changes. Thus, a lump in the breast forms a ready match with the illness schemata for breast cancer, urinary or rectal bleeding and difficulty with urination or defecation, can match, respectively, the schema for prostate and colon cancer. However, the connection between concrete experience and illness concepts is often ambiguous, and lack of clarity may open a window for fantasy and emotional distress, an outcome that seems likely when individuals are asymptomatic prior to being diagnosed with cancer. (2) *Timelines*. Both objective (clock) and felt time with respect to the rate of onset, total duration and time to respond to treatment are critical for matching a somatic event to a label. Both clock and experienced time are key differentiators of acute from chronic conditions. The clarity of time frames, particularly rate of onset and freedom from symptom posttreatment, vary by disease and treatment and may be vague for many cancers and an individual's experience for many chronic conditions can be inconsistent with prior temporal expectations and the time frames of the biological system both prior to and post diagnosis and treatment. (3) *Consequences*. The activation of schemata for any specific illness and treatment, create expectations respecting disruption of function, work and social relationships. In the absence of direct experience with an illness, these expectations will be based primarily on observation of family and friends and exposure to media. (4) *Causes*. Illness and treatment representations of the cause of cancer will reflect personal experience (exposures to radiation; atmospheric pollution; smoking) and abstract knowledge (family history of risk) often backed with direct observation, e.g., looking like an aunt who had breast cancer. (5) *Control*. Many though not all disease schemata have implications for action ranging from screening to detect risk, seeing the doctor for advice and diagnosis, and using family or culturally available alternative products for prevention and treatment. Choice of action will be affected by the identity of the disease, e.g., cancer (breast, uterine, colon, or prostate) or cardiac, and perceptions and beliefs about cause. Treatment schemata can also influence choices in potentially beneficial and harmful ways (Polacek et al. 2007; Bickell et al. 2009; Neugut et al. 2012); for example, patients may decide against chemotherapy because it is perceived as extremely distressing and unnecessary given that their tumor was excised, or avoid surgery if they believe surgery lets cancer cells spread. Although the processes involved in matching illness and treatment concepts and experiences are similar for acute and chronic conditions, coherence among the representations of illness and treatment are typically simpler and more easily achieved for acute conditions, e.g., disease present when symptomatic, rapid onset with limited duration, treatment terminates illness, etc. Prototypes and representations of cancer will differ from both the mental models of acute conditions as well as from the mental models for other chronic conditions. These differences require detailed discussion in shared decision-making,

3. *Responding*: When deviations among variables in one or more of the categories match two prototypes, e.g., one for a chronic the other for an acute condition, the probability for action on the more common, less threatening acute condition may outweigh accepting the risk of the chronic threat. The consequences can be serious if the less threatening, acute match leads to delay, inappropriate care seeking and disease progression. Mismatching to an incorrect prototype has been studied in detail for patients with myocardial infarction (MI) and patients with heart failure. The study by Bunde and Martin (2006) mentioned earlier, reported more rapid care seeking for patients with MI when the pattern and location of their symptoms were consistent with MI. The data showed that both the abstract concept (having a prior history) and specific features (pain in chest; novelty of the pain; pain in arm) made small, positive contributions to

rapid care seeking. Although the contribution of each factor was small, they were independent of one another and added up to a sizeable effect. In addition, care seeking was slowed if symptoms were perceived as gastric in origin.

Overlap need not be between two or more illness schemata to lead to delay and ineffective self-management; it can be with an illness schemata and the prototype of self. For example, patients may perceive symptoms of heart failure such as chronic system-wide fatigue, swollen legs, and frequent breathlessness, as signs of aging or pulmonary problems. Misperception is especially likely when chest or arm pain are believed to be necessary signs of cardiovascular disease, and chronic fatigue and breathlessness are unlikely to motivate use of cardiac medication or lead to calls for assistance, when attributed to aging.

4. *Communication and sharing*: Although numerous studies have examined the intrapersonal process and confirmed that the match of somatic and functional deviations with illness prototypes affects care seeking, fewer have examined how the process is moderated by interpersonal comparisons (Vollmann et al. 2010; Leventhal et al. 1992). This is a major gap as interpersonal sharing of symptoms and treatments is common, particularly among elderly respondents (Stoller 1998). Cameron et al. (1993) present a good example of the importance of interpersonal communication in care seeking in the responses of 111 patients interviewed while waiting to see an internist at a medical clinic; their responses were compared to those of matched controls interviewed by phone. Symptoms were critical for care seeking; 100 % of care seekers reported new symptoms in comparison to 30 % of the 111, matched controls. Most strikingly, 92 % of the care seekers discussed their symptoms with a family member or friend and 50 % were urged to seek care. In contrast, only 61 % of the non-care seeking controls spoke to someone and only 9 % were advised to seek care. The care seekers also reported a greater number of symptoms, longer times since onset, and having labeled and acted to control them.

The process of searching for and matching symptoms to schemata (location and pattern; time frames; etc.) is often reinforced in visits to the doctor. After the usual social niceties, "getting down to business" likely includes a sequence of questions such as, "What's bothering you?" "Where is it?" "What does it feel like?" "How long has it been going on?" "Did anything happen or did you do anything that may have brought it on?" "What if anything did you do to take care of it?", and "What happened?" These questions strongly imply that this form of self-appraisal is an essential part of preparing for your medical visits. Patient and practitioner however, may map the observed features to different illness prototypes—the patient's based upon common-sense views and fears, respectively, activated by self and family history. Unfortunately, patients may not communicate these "subjective cognitive and affective additions" to practitioners.

Action and Outcome Appraisal

The vast majority of symptomatic and functional deviations elicit well learned responses, e.g., take an OTC for headache, antiacid for stomach upset, rest for signs of cold, that terminate the event in an expected time frame. Coherence between illness and treatment models, i.e., matching of expected time frames for illness and treatment with observed outcomes, is typical for most acute conditions. Achieving coherence is far more complex for chronic conditions and while many of the challenges are common to all chronic conditions, differences exist often among conditions bearing similar names, e.g., type 1 and type 2 diabetes, and cancers of different types in different sites. Matches between treatment expectations and outcomes may also vary over the life history of the same condition. Managing the variation across and within conditions over the life span, requires executive function, *action planning to create, implement and sustained action for chronic conditions*. The process requires observing, organizing, and reorganizing ongoing behavior and updating expectations and methods of evaluating outcomes.

Action plans and action planning. Early studies on the effects of fear communication on attitudes, intentions, and behavior, set the stage for the development of the CSM by providing a window into the process of planning (Leventhal 1970; Leventhal et al. 1965). Action planning involves three sets of executive function: (1) examining the everyday environment (equivalent to providing a map of the university campus to taking a tetanus shot—Leventhal et al. 1965); (2) identifying specific behavioral sequences in that environment (reviewing class changes); (3) linking the response to an action sequence to insure adherence; get a tetanus shot when walking past the health service, i.e., from building X to Y. In the fear studies, steps such as these were presented by the research team; they were not self-generated by the participant. As actions for management of chronic conditions are conducted in each patient's unique environment, self-generated action plans are critical for successful control. In addition, self-generated plans are critical, as the environments in which daily, behavioral sequences occur, differ across individuals and within individuals over time. It is important to note that the strategies for performing an action are not identical to the skills and strategies for generating a strategy and the plan for a one-time intervention can differ in many respects from that for a chronic, life-long action.

Given the variance in individuals and environments, stimulating self-generated planning may seem an impossible task. We do not doubt it challenging but believe that a common set of principles underlies all planning. These include: (a) Environmental and behavioral monitoring; (b) Identifying behavioral sequences that appear in daily life; (c) comparison of sequences to identify the one best suited for including a new action, e.g., using an inhaler to control the inflammation underlying asthmatic attacks, or self-examination to detect cancer; (d) Rehearsal and refinement of the behaviors and clarification of outcome expectations. In the language of the CSM framework, searching for units, i.e., well-structured behavioral units that are repeated daily; involves chunking the behavioral stream (a above); assessing the compatibility or fit of specific features of the units to the responses to be implemented, e.g., if a medication needs to be taken with water, is the behavioral sequence performed where water and glasses are present and can the medication be stored and visible in that location, and rehearsal, or imagining one's self in context and mimicking the action required in that context, e.g., to alter food buying in the super market, imagine or look and point at the items needed for effective management. Rehearsal is observed in the arm and hand movements of ballet dancers who use such gestures to memorize movement sequences (Kirsh 2010). The process is designed to establish automatic response programs for consistent adherence.

Outcome appraisal. In many behavioral models, reinforcement is defined as receipt of an expected outcome at the termination of action. Outcomes for managing illnesses are rarely immediately contingent with performance; even relieving headache with aspiring or acetaminophen takes time, though often aided by the more immediate "placebo" benefit of swallowing the pill. With chronic conditions, benefits are not only often remote in time, they may be perceptually invisible. Beliefs to the contrary, people cannot "feel" when blood pressure is elevated or controlled (Meyer et al. 1985), cannot tell when A1c is lowered by medication or appropriate diet and exercise, nor can most patients with asthma feel the immediate benefit of using daily anti-inflammatory medication to moderate chronic, pulmonary inflammation, though the effects of medication for managing flares are visible immediately (Halm et al. 2006). The gap between action and feedback and the absence of palpable feedback are critical issues for the initiation of management, both to preventive and control the progression of disease, and perhaps most importantly for maintaining behavior over the long term. Deficits in maintenance are visible not only in asthma, hypertension, and diabetes management, but in the maintenance of treatment to prevent catastrophic disease recurrence; for example, the high levels of nonadherence to ACE inhibitors and beta blocker to prevent recurrence of heart attack (Akincigil et al. 2008).

Management of a Developing Disorder: Cancer

The Bayesian core of the Common-Sense Model clarifies how we conceptualize prototypes and active mental representations, and reveals how much we have yet to understand about the content and processes involved in updating prototypes during the history of cancer. The updating process is critical for understanding how representations of cancer and treatments and planning change as a patient transitions from well to at risk, diagnosed, treated, and "cured" or terminal, creating at times unexpected variability in decisions. The parameters, means and variances, of the prototypes involved in this process are anchored in history. For the self, that includes abstract sense of one's vulnerability to cancer based on family history or cultural and community beliefs and global perceptions of health (SAH). Global, self-assessments of health (SAH) are anchored in the history of one's physical function and the pattern, location and salience of somatic sensations (Mora et al. 2008). Each of these specific variables has its history, its average and variability, implicit time frames for change, perceptions of causes, methods of control (rest or exercise to enhance function), and consequences associated with its values. Changes of these values during transitions introduces uncertainty and unexpected decisions and does so at all levels, i.e., how one conceives of the self and how one experiences function and symptoms. It is worth noting that self-assessment of health are powerful predictors of mortality both in community samples (Idler and Benyamini 1997; Benyamini and Idler 1999) and in some studies, better predict mortality than medical markers for patients with advanced cancer (Shadbolt et al. 2002).

Parameters of the prototypes of cancer(s), and treatments, interact with the values of the self, amplifying or minimizing the cancer threat. If cancer has been diagnosed, does sense of self and family history suggest the cancer will by symptomatic and disrupt function, progress rapidly, and perceived to be controllable, or untreatable and death dealing? Is the cancer expected to lead to different treatments? Are the treatments perceived to be effective? Do they have negative consequences for oneself such as damaging one's physical image, e.g., mastectomy destroying femininity and disrupting or embarrassing oneself in daily life, e.g., the need for an external bag following removal of the bladder or colon? The common-sense representations affect updating and decisions, though it is unclear how expectations generated by prototypes of self, cancer and treatment, interact with one another and with information from practitioners, family, friends, and media, in updating a patient's representations, decisions, and actions. Uncertainty associated with high levels of distress may lead to rigidity with decisions fixed on the necessity or avoidance of specific treatments. The picture is further complicated when the symptoms attributed to the cancer may be only partially related to the underlying condition, and inconsistencies exist between the temporal trajectory of the cancer, the benefits of treatment, and the time courses of the individual's experience of somatic, functional, and emotional responses. Examples of the consequences of discrepancies between the biology and experience of illness have been recorded for infectious conditions, the clearing of symptoms resulting in cessation of use of antibiotics before pathogens are eradicated (Hawkings et al. 2007), and potentially life threatening conditions, prevention of recurrence of MI, in which 50 % of patients stop beta blockers and ACE inhibitors after 2 years, asymptomatic period (Akincigil et al. 2008). Given the absence of symptoms these patients updated their cardiovascular status from seriously ill to one as cured rather than from seriously ill to at risk. Their cardiologists may not have informed them of this inconsistency and the new, life-long status of their self. Similar issues arises for patients at the termination of successful treatment for cancer, i.e., what does it mean to conceptualize oneself as "a cancer survivor". The question for each of these examples, is what conditions lead to updating of self, disease and treatment that provides a valid representation, one that minimizes threat to life.

Creating Representations: Transitions in the Development of Cancer

Ditto and Hawkins (2005) emphasize that many, unexpected negative or positive experiences with cancer and its treatment add to the complexity faced by patients, clinicians, and researchers for understanding and optimizing the planning process and decisions during the disease history. The interplay among the patient and family members further complicate the decisional process; a task such as appointing durable power of attorney to a specific family member or an outsider can be difficult if not close to impossible, when long term animosities and jealousies exist among family members. The difficulty of resolving complex family issues can be present even for seemingly trivial issues, such as changes in food preferences, as well as more significant factors, such as changes in a patient's employment and the financial demands of treatment. The decisional processes are visible from screening to end-of-life planning and moderated by cultural, community and economic factors and the participants' ability to discuss and engage in shared decision-making.

Decisions to screen. Multiple studies have examined the moderating effects of factors such as cultural beliefs, ethnicity, age, and gender on decisions to screen. Barriers to screening and delays in early detection of cancer, such as mistrust of the medical care system, are often associated with cultural and ethnic variables (Consedine et al. 2004). For example, lung cancer is often first detected at an advanced stage among individuals from ethnic minorities who both express fatalistic views of cancer and mistrust of the care system (Bergamo et al. 2013). Data on delay and failure to screen for colon cancer (colonoscopy) reveal a similar array of beliefs acting as barriers to screening, e.g.,

perceiving oneself as vulnerable and believing that colon cancer can be prevented (Bromley et al. 2015; Codori et al. 2001). Specific comments such as, "surgery spread the cancer" (when discussing the death of a friend soon after hospitalization and surgery), and the perceived risks of colonoscopy, e.g., fear that the scope will perforate the colon, indicate that treatment representations can also affect decisions to avoid screening (Bergamo et al. 2013). These statements represent expectations of negative outcomes from screening that are based on underlying prototypes, and are barriers to screening and early detection. Beliefs such as these are at the more detailed, i.e., "lower" level of the hierarchy of cognitive factors involved in the decision process and given their variety and number, are unlikely to appear as significant variables in multiple regression models. They are critical however, for development and testing of interventions and for clinical practice. The impact of such detailed beliefs, generated by social chatter and flawed interpretations of concrete observation, is amplified by cancers that occur with no prior symptoms and apparent cause in individuals with no known family history. Cancer can be both a threat and mystery, given its incongruity with the acute, default model that defines much of the life-long experience with illness for many if not most individuals.

Treatment decisions. Once diagnosed, patients can face multiple treatment options depending upon the location and type of tumor (Diefenbach et al. 2002). Genomic testing has and will continue to increase the oncologists understanding and ability to select targeted, nonsurgical therapies for stopping the multiplication and spread of some but not all types of cancer (Schilsky 2010). For example, genetic tests for breast cancer have not yielded significant guidance for treatment as it is unclear which of the detected mutations promotes cell proliferation, nor are gene specific therapies available if known (Kolata 2016). At this point in time, little is known as to how patients perceive and understand what they are told about targeted therapies and how the information will affect treatment decisions. Studies have shown that patients choose active cancer therapy for seemingly small benefits, regardless of potential side effects and toxicities in comparison to the choices that would be made by oncologists considering similar situations; discrepancies also occur in patients with COPD (Balmer et al. 2001; Hirose et al. 2005). It has also been observed that patients transitioning through cancer and treatment may come to accept and adapt to the functional changes associated with treatments they had previously rejected (Saraiya et al. 2008). Both choices for aggressive treatment and tolerance of treatment impact can reflect perceived threats to life; treat of die, a common representation of cancer for many patients. Tolerance of treatment can also reflect adaptation; increasing familiarity with aversive stimuli can remove the affective component that drives avoidance altering the representation of treatment and is anticipated consequences (Johnson 1973). Changes in preferences are common, they have been recorded from before to after hospitalization (Ditto et al. 2005), and are expressed in less vivid detail among older than younger patients (Lowenstein 2005); reduced detail may minimize anticipated affective distress.

Studies of failure to accept and undergo adjuvant therapy are at variance however, with the conclusion that patients are overly eager for treatment. Adjuvant therapy involves months of multiple cycles of chemotherapy to destroy cancer cells that may have migrated from the tumor site and avoided the surgical knife; it is recommended following surgery for breast and colon cancers. National data indicate that approximately 30 % of women do not transition to recommended, adjuvant treatment post breast surgery as per the Surveillance, Epidemiology, and End Results (SEER) program. These figures are not stable, however, as a recent randomized trial found unexpectedly high levels of acceptance of adjuvant treatment, approximately 98 % doing so in both intervention and control arms, among women many of whom were members of ethnic minorities (Bickell et al. 2014). The high rates in the trial relative to those reported by SEER and by descriptive data collected a few years earlier in the very same community, highlight the malleability of treatment representations and the possibility of changes in their coherence with the representation of the disease; for these breast cancer patients it made sense to transition to chemotherapy to minimize the threat of recurrence. There are a number of "myths" respecting patients' response to chemotherapy, two related to expectations of the differences in responses of anxious and nonanxious women to chemotherapy treatments. The major myth is that anxiety increases awareness and increased reporting of treatment induced somatic symptoms and amplifies distress during treatment. A study by Rabin et al. (2001), that interviewed women before and after chemotherapy cycles, illustrates one aspect of the myth; anxious patients reported more symptoms of anxiety both during and between treatment cycles. Anxious patients reports of chemotherapy symptoms were no different in number and duration from those reported by nonanxious women. It was critical therefore, to examine the two types of symptoms separately. One might conclude that the women "knew" the difference between chemotherapy and their anxious selves and investigators need to make the same differentiation. The second example is from an early stage 2, randomized trial assessing the toxicity and tolerance for tamoxifen in women previously treated for breast cancer (Cameron et al. 1998). The trait "anxious" women reported more concrete symptoms (indicators of tamoxifen, not anxiety), than their nontrait anxious peers. These symptoms were however, related to objectively monitored differences, the anxious women showing less bone loss over the year long period. Although the outcome, and others, were not anticipated, they were predictable consequence of the interaction between the enzyme that metabolizes both tamoxifen and cortisol; it "prefers" cortisol and the anxious women likely offered it a more desirable target leaving more tamoxifen in place to prevent bone loss.

The findings for symptom reporting by patients in treatment have a special importance for treatment; noxious symptoms can encourage nonadherence. Nonadherence however, is not solely a function of the presence of noxious symptoms: how these symptoms are represented, i.e., are they perceive as signs of damage to the body or signs that treatment is working, killing cancer cells and protecting the body. How treatment is perceived and interpreted will vary as hoped for outcomes change over time. This difference in the representation of cancer and treatments is nontrivial as it will have major impact on decisions to continue and transition from one form of treatment to another, e.g., surgery to adjuvant therapy, or to terminate treatment assuming one is cured or that the cancer is uncontrollable and deadly.

Survivorship: Self posttreatment. Following termination of successful treatment, many patients appear to consider themselves "cured," a theme in patient testimonials in televised ads from major cancer centers. What however, is the meaning of "I'm cancer free; cured"? Does the patient regard his or her Self as the physical and psychological being he or she was prior to the onset of cancer, or is this a new, changed self? If it is changed, how has it changed? Many patients point to major changes wrought by cancer and treatment in their values and perception of everyday life. The question less frequently addressed, is how "survivors" represent their physical selves; their vulnerabilities to recurrence of cancer(s) and to other chronic, life threatening conditions. The treatments that succeeded in removing a virulent tumor and the chemotherapies that controlled the spread of cancer cells, have also created vulnerabilities absent in the pre-cancer self. These vulnerabilities not only include risk of recurrence of the cancer, and cancer in other sites, but the increased risk of cardiomyopathy and eventual heart failure (Slamon and Pegram 2001), the extent of this latter risk varies by chemotherapy regimen (Gianni et al. 2010; El-Jawahri et al. 2010; American Society of Clinical Oncology 2016). Multisite randomized trials are currently underway to improve the transition to survivorship. In these trials are assessing whether the medical realities inherent in survivorship have been integrated into the prototype and representations of the self, engaged in daily activities, (yet aware of old and new vulnerabilities), and combined with an action plan for self-monitoring for early detection of risk. Keeping self-monitoring in "a box" with a well-structured action plan is designed to random if not constant somatic monitoring from intruding on daily activities, i.e., a way of avoiding a ruminative, self-monitoring system and associated, pervasive worry that disrupts a return to life.

An individual's ability to return to normal, everyday life, to live as a cancer survivor, is affected by multiple factors, some intrapsychic, e.g., presence of a self-monitoring plan, others contextual, both interpersonal (e.g., do family members stimulate worry or adopt helping roles as sentinels), and systemic (e.g., ability to reengage with work). One might expect that successful entry to daily life among patients entering survivorship would be easier for those who were previously employed in professions and high end technical positions; in either case, their skills are desired and return facilitated by institutional norms. On the other hand, those employed in construction, manufacturing, or sales may have been forced to resign when entering treatment and given little or no opportunity to reengage posttreatment. The door to daily life is opened or shut by others; decisions are made by the system not the individual. Support programs can play an important role in helping patients return to a normal daily life; for women treated for breast cancer joining has been found related to common-sense beliefs about cause and likelihood of control (Cameron et al. 2005). Efforts are also underway to develop programs for training oncologists to assist patients with survivorship and to and assess their efficacys. Qualitative data suggests that the efficacy of these programs will depend on whether they can activate patients to engage in communication and self-management in addition to increase their overall knowledge of causes of and means of controlling cancer risk (Hudson et al. 2012).

End-of-Life Planning

Federal (U.S.) law requires health care facilities receiving Medicare and Medicaid funds, to notify patients of their treatment options in writing; the options include the right to die, and the need to create an advance directive (AD). The law encourages discussion prior to completion of an AD, assuming that the discussions and AD that is generated will reflect the individual's wishes at the time s/he is severely ill. Although unstated, the rules assume patients can project themselves into a partially or completely unknown future, anticipate the treatments they would want, and make decisions regardless of their current age and distance from death, and for all possible diseases. Though these expectations may be unachievable, advanced planning is an important step for considering the alternatives one may face when incapacitated and leaving loved ones the burden of making decisions without their input (Singer et al. 1999). Despite the legal requirement, only 1/3 to 1/2 of US adults have an AD (Moorman 2011; U.S. Department of Health and Human Services 2008; Later and King 2007), and fewer than 50 % of terminally ill American adults have a formal AD in their medical record (Kass-Bartelmas and Hughes 2003). Evidence respecting discussion and sharing end-of-life wishes is relatively scarce. We do not know for example, how many adults have discussed AD with family members and physicians though studies find that many individuals who have completed an AD have neither shared this with someone nor know where they have stored it post completion (Perkins 2007). Even if an individual has discussed end-of-life wishes, completed and stored an AD and shared with family member assigned durable power of attorney to another person, there is less than 100 % assurance that these wishes will be enacted by medical practitioners at critical moments (IOM 2015). Discrepancy between patients and health care providers should not be surprising given the discrepancy between patients and practitioners as to what is important when terminally ill. In comparison to the lengthy, abstract lists created by experts, patients' focus on five issues; 1. Pain and symptom management; 2. Avoidance of inappropriate prolongation of dying; 3. Sense of control; 4. Relieving burden on others; and 5. Strengthening bonds with loved ones (Institute of Medicine Committee (Field and Cassel 1997); Statement by American Geriatric Society (1997); Singer et al. 1999, Table 1).

Advocates for advanced planning assume that general instructions are adequate to encourage young and physically healthy individual's to create meaningful plans, whereas detailed statements are best used to prompt individuals who are in the midst of dealing with life threatening cancer and treatment (Butler et al. 2014). Thus, instructions to plan and the plans generated by well and the very ill, vary from "general statements (e.g., no heroic measures) to careful delineations of specific medical treatments to be used or withheld in specific medical conditions". Ditto and Hawkins (2005) have cautioned however, that the details used to stimulate advanced planning by very ill patients should vary substantially over the course of treatment, and that use of the same prompts for individuals at different places with cancer and treatment can create plans that are discrepant with experience. They also note that treatment experiences that are unanticipated can amplify uncertainty and emotional distress, disrupting further planning and optimal decisions. Discrepancies between expectations and experience should not be surprising as expectations are influenced by a lifetime of experience with acute conditions and exposure to mass media; the expectations based on the acute model are likely greatly at odds with the disease and its aversive treatments. Given the variation in disease and treatment over time, it may be unrealistic to expect discussions and an AD formed when one is well and decades or years from death, to accurately reflect the expectations and desires an individual will express when terminally ill (Hawkins et al. 2005; Saraiya et al. 2008). A patient's representation of end-stage prostate cancer and/or colon cancer may fail to reflect important differences in the demands of living with each during the final months of life. Thus, forecasting how one will prefer to respond to future pain, disruption of function, and treatments involves a great deal of uncertainty and need for constant updating at an experiential level. The updating process also need to consider that a patient's prototypes of cancer and treatments are unlikely to address his or her experience for cancers varying in aggressiveness, stage and type. Whether the uncertainty is primarily from deficits in the content or the resistance to change of the self-prototype, or is due to the prototypes of the cancer and/or treatment, or whether uncertainty arises from the interaction of the three, may require development of interventions that allow patients to adapt to anticipate and seek continual discussions with their oncologists to update expectations associated with changes in the course of the disease and treatment. These are complex but researchable questions.

Uncertainty and self-assessments. Projecting a valid picture of future preferences depends to some degree upon the accuracy of the representation of the self as it is now and how it is evolving. Many studies have shown that people typically fail to predict their future preferences, decisions, and affective states (Dunning et al. 2004). We might anticipate therefore, that current SAH, a critical baseline for prediction of future health, would also be inaccurate. Data suggest however, that SAH are generally accurate. In more than 200 studies, SAH made on simple, five point scales (excellent, very good, good, fare, and poor), have proven to be valid predictors of mortality from representative samples drawn in multiple nations (Idler and Benyamini 1997; Jyhla 2009). These judgments have also proven to be valid predictor of mortality among terminal cancer patients, often superior to "objective" medical measures (Shadbolt et al. 2002; Saraiya et al. 2008). Given that SAH are valid predictors of the future course of terminal cancer, one might expect that focusing patients on the basis of these judgments, physical and cognitive function and symptoms (Gonzalez et al. 2002; Mora et al. 2008), might improve the utility of their planning, treatment decisions and successful transitions through the end of life. Planning would addresses the expected experience of physical and cognitive function and symptoms,

the pattern (identity), time frames, impact on daily life (consequences), means of control, and factors increasing symptoms and dysfunction (causal factors). There is evidence that accurate expectations respecting the sensory feel of stressful treatments and action plans can both minimize emotional distress and improve outcomes in clinical settings, though these settings are far less threatening than treatments for terminal cancer (child birth: Leventhal et al. 1989; cast removal: Johnson et al. 1975; endoscopy: Johnson and Leventhal 1974). We do not know whether procedures such as these would both minimize distress and allow patients to generate effective realistic frameworks for deciding to opt for or against aggressive treatments and/or hospice. The reality however, is that there may be no way of predicting the course of cancer at the end of life. Projecting this trajectory calls for constant recurring and updating discussions between the doctor and patient, as changes over time will require shifts in treatment strategies. As an example, most patients with end-stage pancreatic cancer have severe pain, and wasting, but one of us (EAL) had a patient with pancreatic cancer who had no abdominal pain, and knew she was terminal. Pain relief was not central for this patient; relieving abdominal pressure from ascites was, as was being surrounded by family at home and assured that pain relieve was available if needed.

By focusing patients on the variable and unpredictable aspects of the factors in each of the five areas of illness and treatment representations, i.e., time frames and symptoms in particular, they may be better prepared to make reasoned comparisons between current and anticipated futures and to anticipate and accept changes in their preferences and treatment decisions. It is not unusual to observe seemingly contradictory shifts in treatment decision. As mentioned before, a patient may ask for aggressive care at time of crisis even though their AD had specified conservative care, and return the AD to conservative care after the crisis is averted (Saraiya et al. 2008). One might hypothesize that this shift is a product of an array of strategies, some automatic others conscious and deliberative, designed to defend the integrity of the Self system. Equally frequent however, are shifts from an AD that specified use of advanced life support, to conservative management after experiencing life support treatment, accompanied by statements such as "... never again on the respirator". Unfortunately, there is a paucity of evidence both on how to assess the variability of the prototype of the self and little evidence on the processes or conditions useful for generating reasoned comparisons between the prototype of self now and possible future selves. The comparison process could be better understood by studies asking: (1) Are the treatment choices by patients facing the possibility of death different than the treatment choices of patients who are not? Will individuals make the same treatment choices when in good health versus when receiving treatment for cancer (Saraiya et al. 2008)? Clinical examples may suggest hypotheses respecting the mechanisms involved in these decisional shifts, but data are essential; anecdotes are not enough.

Moderators of planning. It has been shown that planning is moderated by contextual factors such as religious affiliation, the level of instrumental and emotional support from family and friends and age related changes in cognitive function and emotional responding (Carstensen and Hartel 2006). Active planning, for example, is precluded by religious commitments among African Americans (Carr 2011) and fundamental Protestants (Garrido et al. 2013); leaving death "in God's hands" rules out discussions of preferences for aggressive treatments versus hospice and palliative care. It can also preclude assigning durable power of attorney in the event that one is unable to make decisions or assert what is perceived as "God's" preferences. Leaving death in God's hands may address existential questions surrounding death and minimize the fear of death but it can also close the door to self and family engagement in decision-making, leaving decisions in the hands of oncologists and hospital procedures.

Age related changes introduce yet another set of moderators to end-of-life planning. Data show that in comparison to older subjects (over 65), younger subjects (less than 30) include more situation-specific details in narratives depicting both past and future, everyday events; the total number of situation-specific and "abstract" nonsituation-specific comments are similar as elderly respondents include more "abstract" elements (Addis et al. 2007, 2008). Our unpublished data replicated Addis et al. (2007, 2008) for everyday events and showed similar age effects for familiar acute conditions, young subjects (M age = 21) generating more event-specific details in narratives than did older participants (M age = 84). The age difference shrank, however, as younger participants used fewer specific, disease and treatment details in narratives for complex, less well understood chronic conditions. From the perspective of CSM, both age and cultural commitments that leave death in God's hands, remove the individual from the experiential details of planning; abstract formulations both minimize the specifics of planning and lower the fear and emotional distress elicited by detailed imagery of the extremely ill, aggressively treated, dying self (Leventhal and Scherer 1987). How practitioners can share the patient's perspective, allowing patient and family to understand and see the implications of alternative treatments versus hospice, is an open question. CSM suggests it will much more than "being emotionally supportive" to bridge this divide (Phillips et al. 2013).

Moderators: details and abstractions. Given the uncertainties surrounding individual differences in physical health and the presence of multiple chronic conditions among the elderly (over 65 and free of chronic diseases a rarity) planning for future health calamities might be better served by the initial adoption of a broad conceptual framework focused on the goals of planning and shared decision, prior to focusing on the details of alternative treatments for the current status of the life threatening cancer. The advantage of viewing the future through a nonsituation-specific framework rather than an array of situation-specific details, allows executive processes to attend to and evaluate a variety of behavioral scripts appropriate for treatment of different chronic conditions as well as cancers.

This approach is consistent with the role of higher order, executive processes in creating and generalizing skills and well learned scripts across settings.

It is clear that we need to better understand when and how the broad abstract concepts hidden in cultural factors such as ethnicity, religious spirituality in contrast to secular commitments and focus on family, affect the generation of event-specific detail in thinking about treatments when terminally ill. Second, it also is important to examine the similarities and differences between abstract, nonspecific constructions of future health and end-of-life events across different illness threats. Although all may be non-situation specific, some may be better frameworks for addressing the uncertainties in planning for a diversity of conditions and treatments at the end of life and among these, some may be better for generalizing from specific past illness events to the future, others perhaps for facing the open ended realities of terminal illness. Finally, it will be important to understand how the threat of death itself affects projecting future planning. Does conscious absorption with this existential threat disrupt projecting the details needed for realistic coping? By contrast, does this threat motivate social exchanges, discussion for valid end-of-life planning when "implicit", i.e., external to consciousness and out of working memory. Research is needed to address these questions and translate the findings to clinical settings coupled with ongoing quality assessment.

Generating Futures: Planning and Decisions

Our brief examination of some of the processes underlying how an individual may perceive and respond as s/he transitions from wellness to detection of risk, diagnosis, treatment, survivorship, and planning and deciding at the end of life, has opened more questions than it has answered. The opportunities for research are vast. It is also clear that the complexity of the processes involved at the individual, social and system levels calls for

multiple methods and models. Although we have focused on cognitive and behavioral processes at the individual patient levels, models are needed at the social and system levels. It is extremely important that these models "speak to one another," that their content and conceptual structure allow for integration of processes and findings across levels. For example, it is not sufficient to suggest that trust is essential for communication and shared decisions making between patients, family members, and practitioners, and to point out that it is more difficult to establish trust among ethnic minorities and non-ethnic oncologists. The details of previous experiences with practitioners that undermined trust, and the communication among group members that supported distrust, need to be modeled at both the social level and the individual, common-sense level. Once we describe and link the processes operating on both sides of the chasm of mistrust, we will be prepared to develop and test effective and efficient ways of restoring trust and enhance quality of life and where possible, health outcomes. This will require developing and testing interventions whose content, structure (e.g., face-to-face communication; electronic reminders; etc.), and underlying processes are based on developed and developing theoretical models. Much of the testing will be experimental, using randomized designs with patients categorized on theoretically relevant characteristics as well as traditional moderators such as ethnicity, income, and education. As interventions modules contain multiple components, their complexity calls for methods to identify critical elements, the specific message components that shape the representations of cancer and treatments and activate the planning for action in each of the several identified patient subgroups. It will also be important to identify components that establish the framework for successful reception of the elements that shape the details of behavior. For example, though patients at all levels of education and literacy may respond similarly to common intervention components to initiating planning and encourage self-examination for decision-making, different intervention components may be important to set the framework for attending to and processing information among different educational levels. Qualitative methods will also be needed to guide the process from its initiation and development of intervention components through the assessment as to how they are perceived and responded to, and to the examination of the methods used by patients to implement action and overcome barriers for implementing action in their home environments. As the processes underlying perception and action to confront illness threats range from abstract/conceptual to the detailed experiential, and behavioral, each of which is regulated by partially conscious and largely automatic processes, the task of understanding and creating effective and efficient programs for improving patient decisions and health outcomes is formidable. It is challenging, engaging, and merits our best efforts.

References

Abelson, R. P. (1976). Script processing in attitude formation and decision making. In J. S. Carroll & J. W. Payne (Eds.), *Cognition and social behavior.* Oxford, England: Lawrence Erlbaum.

Abelson, R. P. (1981). Psychological status of the script concept. *American Psychologist, 36*(7), 715–729.

Addis, D., Wong, A., & Schacter, D. (2007). Remembering the past and imagining the future: Common and distant neural substrates during event construction and elaboration. *Neuropsychologia, 45,* 1363–1377.

Addis, D., Wong, A., & Schacter, D. (2008). Age-related changes in the episodic simulation of future events. *Psychological Science, 19*(1), 33–41.

Akincigil, A., Bowblis, J. R., Levin, C., Jan, S., Patel, M., & Crystal, S. (2008). Long-term adherence to evidence based secondary prevention therapies after acute myocardial infarction. *Journal of General Internal Medicine, 23,* 115–121.

Albert, N. M. (2013). Parallel paths to improve heart failure outcomes: Evidence matters. *American Journal of Critical Care, 22,* 289–297.

American Geriatric Society. (1997). Measuring quality of care at the end of life: A statement of principles. *Journal of the American Geriatric Society, 45,* 526–527.

American Society of Clinical Oncology. (2016). *Cancer. Net: ASCO's patient information website.* Retrieved on March 18, 2016 from: http://www.cancer.net/about-us/asco-answers-patient-education-materials

Andrews, M., Vigliocco, G., & Vinson, D. (2009). Integrating experiential and distributional data to learn semantic representations. *Psychological Review, 116,* 463–498.

Balmer, C. E., Thomas, P., & Osborne, R. J. (2001). Who wants second-line, palliative chemotherapy? *Psycho-Oncology, 10*(5), 410–418.

Beach, L. R. (2009). *Narrative thinking and decision making: How the stories we tell ourselves shape our decisions, and vice versa.* Online publication retrieved from: www.leeroybeach.com

Benyamini, Y., & Idler, E. L. (1999). Community studies reporting associations between self-rated health and mortality: Additional studies, 1995–1998. *Research on Aging, 21*(3), 392–401.

Bergamo, C., Lin, J. J., Smith, C., Lurslurchachai, L., Halm, E. A., Powell, C. A., et al. (2013). Evaluating beliefs associated with late-stage lung cancer presentation in minorities. *Journal of Thoracic Oncology, 8* (1), 12–18.

Bickell, N. A., Weimann, J., Fei, K., Lin, J. J., & Leventhal, H. (2009). Underuse of breast cancer adjuvant treatment: Patient knowledge, beliefs and medical mistrust. *Journal of Clinical Oncology, 27,* 5160–5167.

Bickell, N. A., Geduld, A. N., Joseph, K. A., Sparano, J. A., Kemeny, M. M., Oluwole, S., et al. (2014). *Journal of Oncology Practice, 10*(1), 48–56

Bromley, E. G., May, F. P., Federerf, M. L., Spiegela, B. M. R., & van Oijenb, M. G. H. (2015). Explaining persistent under-use of colonoscopic cancer screening in African Americans: A systematic review. *Preventive Medicine, 7,* 40–48.

Brooks, T. L., Leventhal, H., Wolf, M. S., O'Conor, R., Morillo, J., Martynenko, M., et al. (2014). Strategies used by older asthmatics for adherence. *Journal of General Internal Medicine, 29*(11), 1506–1512.

Bunde, J., & Martin, R. (2006). Depression and prehospital delay in the context of myocardial infarction. *Psychosomatic Medicine, 68*(1), 51–57.

Butler, M., Ratner, E., McCreedy, E., Shippee, N., & Kane, R. L. (2014). Decision aids for advance care planning: an overview of the state of the science. *Annals of Internal Medicine, 161*(6), 408–418.

Cameron, L. D., Leventhal, E. A., & Leventhal, H. (1993). Symptom representations and affects as determinants of care seeking in a community-dwelling, adult sample population. *Health Psychology, 12,* 171–179.

Cameron, L. D., Leventhal, H., & Love, R. R. (1998). Trait anxiety, symptom perceptions, and illness-related responses among women with breast cancer in remission during a tamoxifen clinical trial. *Health Psychology, 17*(5), 459.

Cameron, L. D., Booth, R. J., Schlattre, M., Ziginskas, D., Harman, J. E., & Benson, S. R. C. (2005). Cognitive and affective determinants of decisions to attend a group psychosocial support program for women with breast cancer. *Psychosomatic Medicine, 67,* 584–589.

Carr, D. (2011). Racial differences in end-of-life planning: Why don't Blacks and Latinos prepare for the inevitable? *OMEGA-Journal of Death and Dying, 63* (1), 1–20.

Carstensen, L. L., & Hartel, C. R. (2006). *Socioemotional influences on decision making: The challenge of choice. When I'm 64.* Washington (DC): National Academies Press (US) National Research Council (US) Committee on Aging Frontiers in Social Psychology, Personality, and Adult Developmental Psychology. Retrieved on March 16, 2016 from: http://www.ncbi.nlm.nih.gov/books/NBK83777/

Codori, A. M., Petersen, G. M., Mighoretti, D. L., & Boyd, P. (2001). Health beliefs and endoscopic screening for colorectal cancer: Potential for cancer prevention. *Preventive Medicine, 33*(2), 128–136.

Consedine, N. S., Magai, C., Krivoshekova, Y. S., Ryzewicz, L., & Neugut, A. I. (2004). Fear, anxiety, worry, and breast cancer screening behavior: A critical review. *Cancer Epidemiology, Biomarkers and Prevention, 13*(4), 501–510.

Cram, P., Fendrick, A. M., Inadomi, J., Cowen, M. E., Carpenter, D., & Vijan, S. (2003). The impact of a celebrity promotional campaign of the use of colon cancer screening. *Archives of Internal Medicine, 163* (13), 1601–1605.

Diefenbach, M. A., Uzzo, R. G., Hanks, G. E., Greenbert, R. E., Horwitz, E., Newton, F., et al. (2002). Decision-making strategies for patients with localized prostate cancer. *Seminars in Urologic Oncology, 20* (1), 55–62.

Ditto, P. H., & Hawkins, N. A. (2005). Advance directives and cancer decision making near the end of life. *Health Psychology, 24*(4), S63–S70.

Ditto, P. H., Hawkins, N., & Pizzaro, D. A. (2005). Imagining the end of life: On the psychology of advanced medical decision making. *Motivation and Emotion, 29*(4), 475–496.

Donovan, R., Carter, O. B. J., Jalleh, G., & Hones, S. C. (2004). Changes in beliefs about cancer in Western Australia, 1964–2001. *Medical Journal of Australia, 181*(1), 23–25.

Dunning, D., Heath, C., & Suls, J. M. (2004). Flawed self-assessment. *Psychological Science in the Public Interest, 5*(3), 69–106.

El-Jawahri, A., Pdogurski, L. M., Eichler, A. F., Plotkin, S. R., Temel, J. S., Mitchell, S. L., et al. (2010). Use of video to facilitate end-of-life discussions with patients with cancer: A randomized control trial. *Journal of Clinical Oncology, 28*(2), 305–311.

Field, M. J., & Cassel, C. K. (1997). The Institute of Medicine. In *Approaching death: Improving care at the end of life.* Washington, DC: National Academy Press.

Finch, C. E. (1994). The evolution of ovarian oocyte decline with aging and possible relationships to Down syndrome and Alzheimer disease. *Experimental Gerontology, 29*(3–4), 299–304.

Finch, C. E. (1995). Non-genetic factors in the individuality of brain aging: Cell numbers, developmental environment, and disease. *Brain and Memory: Modulation and Mediation of Neuroplasticity: Modulation and Mediation of Neuroplasticity,* 183.

Garrido, M. M., Idler, E. L., Leventhal, H., & Carr, D. (2013). Pathways from religion to advance care planning: Beliefs about control over length of life and end-of-life values. *The Gerontologist, 53*(5), 801–816.

Gianni, L., Eiermann, W., Semiglazov, V., Manikhas, A., Lluch, A., Tjulandin, S., et al. (2010). Neoadjuvant chemotherapy with trastuzumab followed by adjuvant trastuzumab versus neoadjuvant chemotherapy alone, in patients with HER2-positive locally advanced breast cancer (the NOAH trial): A randomised controlled superiority trial with a parallel HER2-negative cohort. *The Lancet, 375*(9712), 377–384.

Gobet, F. (1998). Expert memory: A comparison of four theories. *Cognition, 66,* 115–152.

Gonzalez, J. S., Chapman, G. B., & Leventhal, H. (2002). Gender differences in the factors that affect self-assessments of health. *Journal of Applied Biobehavioral Research, 7,* 133–156.

Halm, E. A., Mora, P., & Leventhal, H. (2006). No symptoms, no asthma: The acute episodic disease belief is associated with poor self-management among inner-city adults with persistent asthma. *Chest, 129,* 573–580.

Hawkings, N. J., Butler, C. C., & Wood, F. (2007). Antibiotics in the community: A typology of user behaviours. *Patient Education and Counseling, 73,* 146–152.

Hawkins, N. A., Ditto, P. H., Danks, J. H., & Smucker, W. D. (2005). Micromanaging death: Process preferences, values, and goals in end-of-life medical decision making. *The Gerontologist, 45*(1), 107–117.

Henry, D. P. (1999). Coping with cancer. A personal odyssey. *Patient Education and Counseling, 37*(3), 293–297.

Hirose, T., Horichi, N., Ohmori, T., Kusmoto, S., Sugiyama, T., Shirai, T., et al. (2005). Patients' preferences in chemotherapy for advanced non-small-cell lung cancer. *Internal Medicine, 44*(2), 107–113.

Horne, R., & Weinman, J. (1999). Patients' beliefs about prescribed medicines and their role in adherence to treatment in chronic physical illness. *Psychosomatic Research, 47*(6), 555–567.

Horne, R., Weinman, J., & Hankins, M. (1999). The beliefs about medicines questionnaire: The development and evaluation of a new method for assessing the cognitive representation of medication. *Psychology and Health, 14*(1), 1–24.

Horowitz, C. R., Rein, S. B., & Leventhal, H. (2004). A story of maladies, misconceptions and mishaps: Effective management of heart failure. *Social Science and Medicine, 58,* 631–643.

Hudson, S. V., Miller, S. M., Hemler, J., Ferrante, J. M., Lyle, J., Oeffinger, K. C., et al. (2012). Adult cancer survivors discuss follow-up in primary care: 'Not what i want, but maybe what i need'. *The Annals of Family Medicine, 10*(5), 418–427.

Idler, E. L., & Benyamini, Y. (1997). Self-rated health and mortality: A review of twenty-seven community studies. *Journal of Health and Social Behavior, 38*(1), 21–37.

IOM (Institute of Medicine). (2015). *Dying in America: Improving quality and honoring preferences near the end of life*. Washington, DC: The National Academies Press.

Isaacson, W. (2011). *Steve jobs*. New York: Simon & Schuster.

Jedele, J. M., & Ismail, A. I. (2010). Evaluation of a multifaceted social marketing campaign to increase awareness of and screening for oral cancer in African Americans. *Community Dental Oral Epidemiology, 38*, 371–382.

Johnson, J. E. (1973). Effects of accurate expectations about sensations on the sensory and distress components of pain. *Journal of Personality and Social Psychology, 27*(2), 261–275.

Johnson, J. E., & Leventhal, H. (1974). Effects of accurate expectations and behavioral instructions on reactions during a noxious medical examination. *Journal of Personality and Social Psychology, 29*(5), 710–718.

Johnson, J. E., Kirchoff, K. T., & Endress, M. P. (1975). Altering children's distress behavior during orthopedic cast removal. *Nursing Research, 24*(6), 404–410.

Jyhla, M. (2009). What is self-rated health and why does it predict mortality? Towards a unified conceptual model. *Social Science and Medicine, 69*, 307–316.

Kahneman, D. (2013). *Thinking, fast and slow*. New York, NY: Farrar, Straus, and Giroux.

Kass-Bartelmas, B. L., & Hughes, R. (2003). Advance care planning: Preferences for care at the end of life. *Research in Action*, (12). Retrieved from the Agency for Healthcare Research and Quality website: http://www.ahrq.gov/research/endliferia/endria.pdf

Kirsh, D. (2010). Thinking with the body. In S. Ohlsson & R. Caatrambone (Eds.), *Proceedings of the 32nd Annual Conference of the Cognitive Science Society* (pp. 2864–2869). Austin, TX: Cognitive Science Society.

Kolata, G. (2016). When gene tests for breast cancer reveal grim data but no guidance. *The New York Times*. March 11, 2016. Retrieved from: http://www.nytimes.com/2016/03/12/health/breast-cancer-brca-genetic-testing.html?_r=0

Kreuter, M. W., Green, M. C., Cappella, J. N., Slater, M. D., Wise, M. E., Storey, D., et al. (2007). Narrative communication in cancer prevention and control: A framework to guide research and application. *Annals of Behavioral Medicine, 33*(3), 221–235.

Later, E. B., & King, D. (2007). Advance directives: results of a community education symposium. *Critical care nurse, 27*(6), 31–35.

Leventhal, H. (1970). Findings and theory in the study of fear communications. *Advances in Experimental Social Psychology, 5*, 119–186.

Leventhal, H., Singer, R., & Jones, S. (1965). Effects of fear and specificity of recommendation upon attitudes and behavior. *Journal of Personality and Social Psychology, 2*(1), 20.

Leventhal, H., & Scherer, K. (1987). The relationship of emotion to cognition: A functional approach to a semantic controversy. *Cognition and emotion, 1*(1), 3–28.

Leventhal, E. A., Leventhal, H., Schacham, S., & Easterling, D. V. (1989). Active coping reduces reports of pain from childbirth. *Journal of Consulting and Clinical Psychology, 57*(3), 365–371.

Leventhal, H., Diefenbach, M. A., & Leventhal, E. A. (1992). Illness cognition: Using common sense to understand treatment adherence and affect cognition interactions. *Cognitive Therapy and Research, 16*(2), 143–163.

Leventhal, H., Leventhal, E. A., Cameron, L., Bodnar-Deren, S., Breland, J. Y., Hash-Converse, J., et al. (2012). Modeling health and illness behavior: The approach of the common sense model (CSM). In A. Baum & T. A. Revenson (Eds.), *Handbook of health psychology* (2nd ed.).

Leventhal, H., Phillips, L. A., & Burns, E. A. (2016). Modeling management of chronic illness in everyday life: A common-sense approach. *Psychological Topics; Health Psychology: Current research and trends*, 187.

Lowenstein, G. (2005). Projection bias in medical decision making. *Medical Decision Making, 25*(1), 96–105.

MacTiernan, A., Fritschi, L., Sleven, Tl, Jalleh, G., Donovan, R., & Heyworth, J. (2014). Public perceptions of cancer risk factors: A Western Australian study. *Health Promotion Journal of Australia, 25*, 90–96.

McAndrew, L. M., Musumeci-Szabo, T. J., Mora, P. A., Vileikyte, L., Burns, E., Halm, E. A., et al. (2008). Using the common sense model to design interventions for prevention and management of chronic illness threats: From description to process. *British Journal of Health Psychology, 13*(2), 195–204.

Meyer, D., Leventhal, H., & Gutmann, M. (1985). Common-sense models of illness: The example of hypertension. *Health Psychology, 4*, 115–135.

Montague, M., Borland, R., & Sinclair, C. (2001). Slip! Slop! Slap! and SunSmart, 1980–2000: Skin cancer control and 20 years of population-based campaigning. *Health Education and Behavior, 28*(3), 290–305.

Moorman, S. M. (2011). Older adults' preferences for independent or delegated end-of-life medical decision-making. *Journal of Aging and Health, 23*(1), 135–157.

Mora, P. A., DiBonaventura, M. D., Idler, E., Leventhal, E. A., & Leventhal, H. (2008). Psychological factors influencing self-assessment of health: Toward an understanding of the mechanisms underlying how people rate their own health. *Annals of Behavioral Medicine, 36*, 292–303.

Mukherjee, S. (2010). *The emperor of all maladies: A biography of cancer*. New York, NY: Scribner.

Neugut, A. I., Clarke Hillyer, G., Kushi, L. H., Lamerato, L., Leoce, N., Nathanson, D., et al. (2012). Noninitiation of adjuvant chemotherapy in women with localized breast cancer: The breast cancer quality of care study. *Journal of Clinical Oncology, 31*, 3800–3809.

Perkins, H. S. (2007). Controlling death: The false promise of advance directives. *Annals of Internal Medicine, 147*(1), 51–57.

Petty, R. E., & Cacioppo, J. T. (1984). The effects of involvement on responses to argument quantity and quality: Central and peripheral routes to persuasion. *Journal of Personality and Social Psychology, 46*, 69–81.

Phillips, L. A., Leventhal, H., & Leventhal, E. A. (2013). Assessing theoretical predictors of long-term medication adherence: Patients' treatment-related beliefs, experiential feedback, and habit development. *Psychology and Health,*. doi:10.1080/08870446.2013.793798.

Polacek, G. N. L. J., Ramos, M. C., & Ferrer, R. L. (2007). Breast cancer disparities and decision-making among U.S. women. *Patient Education and Counseling, 65*, 158–165.

Posner, M. I., & Rothbart, M. K. (1998). Attention, self-regulation and consciousness. *Philosophical Transactions Royal Society B. Biological Sciences, 353*, 1915–1927.

Rabin, C., Ward, S., Leventhal, H., & Schmitz, M. (2001). Explaining retrospective reports of symptoms in patients undergoing chemotherapy: Anxiety, initial symptom experience, and posttreatment symptoms. *Health Psychology, 20*(2), 91.

Robbins, T., Hemmer, P., Leyble, K., & Robbins, S. (2015). Assessing Prior Beliefs and Memory for Symptom and Illness Relationships. In Poster presented at the Annual Meeting of the Psychonomic Society, Chicago, Il.

Saraiya, B., Bodnar-Deren, S., Leventhal, E., & Leventhal, H. (2008). End-of-life planning and its relevance for patients' and oncologists' decisions in choosing cancer therapy. *Cancer, 113*(S12), 3540–3547.

Schacter, D. L., & Addis, D. R. (2007). The cognitive neuroscience of constructive memory: Remembering the past and imagining the future. *Philosophical Transactions Royal Society B. Biological Sciences, 362*, 773–786.

Schilsky, R. L. (2010). Personalized medicine in oncology: The future is now. *Nature Reviews Drug Discovery, 9*, 363–366.

Shadbolt, B., Barresi, J., & Craft, P. (2002). Self-rated health as a predictor of survival among patients with advanced cancer. *Journal of Clinical Oncology, 20*(10), 2514–2519.

Singer, P. A., Martin, D. K., & Kelner, M. (1999). Quality end-of-life care: Patients' perspectives. *JAMA, 281*, 163–168.

Slamon, D., & Pegram, M. (2001). Rationale for trastuzumab (Herceptin) in adjuvant breast cancer trials. In *Seminars in oncology* (Vol. 28, pp. 13–19). WB Saunders.

Stoller, E. P. (1998). Medical self-care: Lay management of symptoms by elderly people. In M. Ory & G. DeFreis (Eds.), *Self-care in later life: Research, programs, and policy perspectives* (pp. 24–61). New York: Springer.

U.S. Department of Health and Human Services. (2008). *Advance directives and advance care planning: Report to congress.* Retrieved on March 17, 2016 from https://aspe.hhs.gov/basic-report/advance-directives-and-advance-care-planning-report-congress

Vollmann, M., Scharloo, M., Salewski, C., Dienst, A., Schonauer, K., & Renner, B. (2010). Illness representations of depression and perceptions of the helpfulness of social support: Comparing depressed and never-depressed persons. *Journal of Affective Disorders, 125*, 213–220.

Yanovitzky, I., & Blitz, C. L. (2000). Effect of media coverage and physician advice on utilization of breast cancer screening by women 40 years and older. *Journal of Health Communication, 5*, 117–134.

The Influence of Affect on Health Decisions

8

Ellen Peters and Louise Meilleur

Recommendations for health decision-making

Instead of a focus on providing complete and accurate information, the emphasis in supporting decision-making needs to shift to providing usable, meaningful, and accurate information that will support better choices. This shift brings with it a new level of responsibility for health practitioners and communicators who will need to know how to present information to patients in ways that ethically support good decision-making. It also requires a delicate balance between informing patients (about information and its meaning) and telling them what to do (this option is excellent whereas that one is only fair). The provision of more subjective interpretations may be difficult and health professionals who prefer to provide only "objective facts" may resist this change. Nonetheless, patients need more than mere exposure to information; they also need to be able to understand and use that information. Providing information in formats that allow them to draw affective meaning from the information may help patients understand and use important information more in health and health-related decisions.

Applications: Using Affect to Facilitate Better Health Decisions

Understanding how affect influences judgment and choice is important because it is often a better predictor than thoughts. In addition, affect manipulations can facilitate judgment and choice. By making the affective meaning of important information easier to access, complex information can be processed more effectively, allowing for comparison between different options and influencing choices. Affect, of course, also can hinder decision-making. When emotions are high, health care providers should ensure that patients have time to stop and think; otherwise, perceptions of the disease and treatment options may be biased when dealing with the immediate emotion of a new diagnosis. Understanding how to maximize the beneficial effects of affect while minimizing any harms will assist patients in making better, more reasoned choices about their health.

E. Peters (✉) · L. Meilleur
Department of Psychology, The Ohio State University, 1835 Neil Ave., Columbus, OH 43210, USA
e-mail: Peters.498@osu.edu

L. Meilleur
e-mail: Meilleur.1@osu.edu

The Influence of Affect on Health Decisions

When deciding whether or not to vaccinate, what cancer treatment to choose, or whether to exercise and eat well, it is often assumed that people "make" choices; they deliberately evaluate information about treatments and screening options, represent the information appropriately, carefully weigh risks and benefits, and then choose the "best" option that is concordant with their individual values. Increasingly though, evidence suggests that preferences are often constructed instead. They are developed "on-the-spot" and influenced by cues in the situation (Lichtenstein and Slovic 2006).

This construction appears to be driven by two different modes of thinking—an affective, experiential mode and a deliberative one (Epstein 1994; Kahneman 2003). Processing in the deliberative mode is conscious, analytical, reason-based, verbal, and relatively slow. It is the deliberative mode that policy makers tend to consider in attempts to inform choices (e.g., provide more information for better choices). Decision makers, however, often want to reduce the amount of effort exerted. As a result, a decision maker choosing among six diets might identify the most important attribute (e.g., quickest way to drop the pounds) and choose the diet that maximizes it, ignoring all other attributes.

More recent research, however, has developed and tested theories of judgment and decision-making that incorporate the affect of the experiential system as a key component in the process of constructing values and preferences. One of the primary functions of affect is to highlight information important enough to warrant further consideration. Within these theories, integral affect (positive and negative feelings about a stimulus) and incidental affect (positive and negative feelings such as mood states that are independent of a stimulus but can be misattributed to it) are used to predict and explain a wide variety of judgments and decisions (Slovic et al. 2002; Schwarz and Clore 2003). In this chapter, we review these theories and their evidence base and suggest future avenues for

research concerning the role of affect in health decision-making.

Health-related decisions require an accurate understanding of provided information so that decision makers can choose options that meet their health care needs. This understanding is generally thought to emerge from the deliberative mode (e.g., understanding *what* a number is). Affect provides a different kind of understanding. As shown in a number of studies, affect provides meaning and motivation to choice processes (Damasio 1994), and it is critical to facilitating informed choice (affect is a part of the gist understanding of Fuzzy Trace Theory; Reyna 2008). Thus, affect is intrinsic to the process of communicating health information and facilitating patient choices. It can be used to persuade (e.g., fear appeals) but can also hinder a person's ability to make the best decision (e.g., by exacerbating perceived risk or overwhelming the patient). In this chapter, we focus on the multiple roles of affect in medical decisions and outline four key functions that affect plays in health judgments and decisions.

Four Functions of Affect in Constructing Judgments and Decisions

Mild incidental affect and integral affect are ubiquitous in everyday life. Imagine finding a dollar lying on the sidewalk (a mild positive mood state is induced) or considering whether you will have a bowl of oatmeal or a chocolate croissant for breakfast (mild negative and positive integral affective feelings are experienced). These feelings can influence the processing of information and, thus, what is judged or decided. For example, a 35-year-old woman who is being counseled about amniocentesis may evaluate its risks differently depending on whether she just learned that her best friend was in a car accident or that her husband won a long-earned promotion at work. The absolute risk of the procedure is the same, but its risks and benefits will be perceived in light of the emotions she is experiencing. In particular, she is likely to perceive less risk and more benefit when elated about her husband's success and the opposite when she is fearful about her friend's prognosis. As reviewed below, research in this area has begun to delineate some of the various ways that affect alters how we process information, form judgments, and make decisions.

When studying the influence of affect in decision-making, researchers have focused on two key approaches. The first examines the effects of valenced affect (good or bad feelings) such as in the Affect-Heuristic (Finucane et al. 2000; Slovic et al. 2002) and Risk-As-Feelings (Loewenstein et al. 2001) hypotheses. In both, affect is used intuitively to inform judgments based on an experienced feeling of goodness or badness towards information or an option. The second approach examines the effect of discrete emotions (e.g., anger versus fear) based on cognitive appraisals and motivations underlying a specific emotion. This research demonstrates that two discrete emotions with the same valence can have very different effects on judgments such as risk perceptions (Lerner and Keltner 2001). It suggests that emotional appraisals other than valence (e.g., certainty) can also exert influence on judgment and decision processes. In this chapter, we focus primarily on the influence of valenced affect because emotions are often mixed (Peters et al. 2004) and occur naturally only for brief periods of time. Health decisions, in particular, often involve complex mixtures of emotion over time.

We argue that affect plays four separable roles in health decisions. We describe them briefly here and then expand on each role below. First, affect can act as *information*. Most recent research in affect has considered this informational value. That is, at the moment of judgment or choice, decision makers consult their feelings about a target or option and ask "how do I feel about this?" (Schwarz and Clore 2003; Slovic et al. 2002). These feelings then act as information in a heuristic process to guide the formation of judgments and decisions. Second, affect can act as a *spotlight* focusing us on different information—numerical cues, for example—depending on the extent of our affect. Third, it can *motivate* us to take action or do extra work. Finally, affect, when present, acts as a *common*

currency allowing us to compare and integrate very different attributes more effectively than when it is absent.

Affect as Information

One of the most comprehensive theoretical accounts of the role of affect and emotion in decision-making was presented by the neurologist, Antonio Damasio (1994). In seeking to determine "what in the brain allows humans to behave rationally," Damasio argued that a lifetime of learning leads decision options and attributes to become "marked" by positive and negative feelings linked directly or indirectly to somatic (bodily) states. When a negative somatic marker is linked to an outcome, it acts as information by sounding an alarm warning us away from that choice. When a positive marker is associated with the outcome, it becomes a beacon of incentive drawing us towards that option. Affect developed through experience thus provides information about what to choose and avoid. Damasio claims that we make better quality, more efficient decisions by consulting and being guided by these feelings. Without these feelings, information in a decision lacks meaning, does not get used, and the resulting choice suffers.

The Affect Heuristic is based, in part, on this earlier research. Affective reactions occur faster than cognitive appraisals (Zajonc 1980) and appear to be used in addition to or instead of cognitive thoughts to influence judgments. For example, positive affect about an option (such as a medication or an exercise routine) appears to lead to perceptions of more benefits and less risk; the opposite is true for negative affect (i.e., reduced perceptions of benefits and increased risk perceptions; Finucane et al. 2000; Slovic et al. 2007).

Affect appears to act as information in the construction of risk perceptions (Loewenstein et al. 2001; Peters and Slovic 1996). For example, Johnson and Tversky (1983) induced negative affect in participants and found that it led to a generalized increase in perceived risk across many adverse events, rather than simply increasing risk perceptions for cognitively similar events. These findings are important because they illustrate affect's causal impact on risk perceptions. Peters et al. (2006) also linked affect to the adjustment process in fatality estimates. Specifically, they found that decision makers asked to estimate the number of annual US fatalities from various causes of death anchored on a provided number (the actual number of deaths from a different disease) and then appeared to adjust away from the anchor based on the extent of their worry about the disease under consideration. Thus, affect is a possible mechanism underlying the adjustment process.

Much of the research on the use of affect as information has focused on the valence of affect (good or bad) as opposed to discrete emotions. Although the positive or negative valence of emotion does act as information, two discrete emotions that are similarly valenced (e.g., anger and fear) also can influence risk perceptions differently (Lerner and Keltner 2001). For example, DeSteno et al. (2000) induced either a sad or angry mood in participants and found that, when participants were induced to anger, they later rated events that caused angry reactions as more likely than sad events. Conversely, participants induced to sadness rated sad events as more likely than angering events. These differences between same-valence emotions are presumably due to other appraisals (e.g., certainty) or behavioral predispositions that are inherent components of the emotion (by this latter explanation, these results could perhaps be more fruitfully categorized under the function of affect as a direct motivator of behavior).

Decision makers appear to consult their affective feelings and use them as information in judgment and decision processes. Affect as information thus acts as a substitute for the assessment of more normatively-relevant information such as probabilities and outcomes (Kahneman 2003). Without affect, information appears to lack meaning and to be weighed less in judgment and choice processes. As a result, affect tends to be beneficial although it sometimes causes detrimental effects. For example, women tend to greatly overestimate their risk of breast cancer. When they learn the correct risk

numbers, the relief experienced in comparison with their overestimation can lead to decreased risk perceptions (Fagerlin et al. 2005). Thus, counseling for breast cancer screening may sometimes result in lower risk perceptions, which in turn lead to reduced mammography rates.

Frequently, when making health decisions, people face unfamiliar situations that require the evaluation of many pieces of new information. Peters et al. (2009) were interested in the processes by which decision makers bring meaning to dry, cold facts and whether affect may be used to facilitate the valuation of different options and new information. In particular, they attempted to influence the interpretation of health-plan attributes by providing numeric information along with affective cues that could be used to evaluate the overall goodness or badness of a health plan. In two separate studies, older-adult and younger-adult participants were presented with attribute information (quality of care and member satisfaction) about two health plans. The information was presented in bar chart format with the actual score displayed to the right of the bar chart (see Fig. 8.1). The information for half of the subjects in each group was supplemented by the addition of evaluative categories (i.e., the category lines plus affective labels that placed the health plans into categories of poor, fair, good, or excellent). The attribute information was designed such that Plan A was good on both attributes while Plan B was good on quality of care but fair on member satisfaction. The specific scores for quality of care and member satisfaction were counterbalanced across subjects such that, for half of the subjects, the average quality of care scores were higher; for the other half, average member satisfaction scores were higher. They predicted and found that evaluative categories influenced choices. Specifically, individuals (older and younger) preferred health plan A more, often when the categories were present (plan A was in the better affective category when the categories were present). Further tests of the manipulation supported its affective basis. These findings suggest that information about treatment and other options can be communicated in ways that convey affective meaning to facilitate information use.

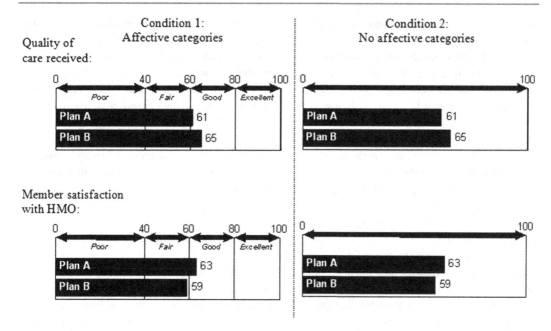

Fig. 8.1 Example of evaluative (affective) categories

Affect as Common Currency

Considerably less work has been done on the other three proposed functions of affect in the construction of preferences. Several theorists have suggested that affect plays a role as a common currency, allowing decision makers to compare apples to oranges (Cabanac 1992; Peters 2006). This role may be due to affect being simpler in some ways than thoughts. It comes in simple "flavors," (e.g., positive and negative) whereas thoughts include more and more complex, cost-benefit and other tradeoffs. By translating more complex thoughts into simpler affective evaluations, decision makers can compare and integrate good and bad feelings rather than attempting to make sense out of a multitude of conflicting logical reasons.

In the health-plan choice studies of Peters et al. (2009), evaluative categories were hypothesized to act as overt markers of affective meaning in choices. If true, then these overt markers should help participants to consider relevant information (that is not considered when evaluative categories are not present) such that they can apply that information to a complex judgment. Thus, evaluative categories should influence not just the choice of a health plan, as shown in previous studies, but it should help decision makers to take into account more information and be more sensitive to variation in information. Peters et al. (2009) conducted a test of this hypothesis. Participants were asked to judge the attractiveness of a hospital. They received information about three quality attributes presented with one of three numerical scores (e.g., hospital A scored 78 out of 100 points when patients rated its quality of care). The hospitals evaluated thus represented a $3 \times 3 \times 3$ design of low, medium, and high scores on each of the three attributes; 27 versions were constructed.

They found that judgments of less numerate adults (those who scored lower on a test of probabilistic understanding) were influenced more than the highly numerate by the presence versus absence of evaluative categories. In particular, less numerate adults did not significantly use any provided numeric information when evaluative categories were not provided; they relied instead on current mood states, whether good or bad, to judge the quality of a hospital.

When evaluative categories were present, however, they used the provided information instead and judged a hospital as more attractive when told that it provided greater quality of care based on numeric indicators compared to worse quality of care. In other words, with evaluative categories, the less numerate became sensitive to the different levels of numeric information. More numerate adults were more successful in their information use even in the absence of evaluative categories, but providing information in a more affective format also helped more and less numerate judges to integrate more information into their judgments.

In situations where patients are faced with the stress of a new diagnosis and must evaluate a large quantity of unfamiliar information in a short period of time, it is possible that the situation causes enough cognitive overload that all patients "act like" less numerate adults. As a result, the use of evaluative categories may allow them to evaluate options more accurately and take into consideration more information when choosing between different treatment options. Future research should examine the benefits and any unintended drawbacks of such an approach in settings where stress and time pressure can be experimentally varied and then (if the approach looks promising) in patient populations.

The power of affect thus can be harnessed and used as an intervention to improve decisions and the decision-making process. The use of methods such as evaluative categories does call, however, for a different emphasis in health and other communications. Instead of a focus on providing complete and accurate information, the emphasis shifts to providing usable, meaningful, and accurate information that will support better choices. It brings with it a new level of responsibility for health practitioners and communicators who would need to know how patients currently respond to information, and would need to bring their expertise to bear not only on what information to provide, but also on how to present that information in ways that ethically support good decision-making. It also requires a delicate balance between informing patients (about information and its meaning) and being

paternalistic (this option is excellent whereas that one is only fair). The provision of more subjective interpretations may be difficult and be resisted by health professionals who prefer to provide only "objective facts," but it is important to help patients understand and use provided information rather than simply exposing patients to data. Providing information in a more affective format may help patients understand and use important information more when making their choices.

Affect as a Spotlight

In a third function for affect, Peters et al. (2003) proposed that affect plays a role as a lens or spotlight in a two-stage process. First, the quality of affective feelings (e.g., weak versus strong or positive versus negative) focuses the decision maker on different information. Then, that information (rather than the feelings themselves) is used to guide the judgment or decision. Although the impact of incidental feelings has been shown to function as a spotlight in memory and judgment (e.g., mood-congruent biases on memory; Bower 1981), little research has examined how feelings about a target might alter what information becomes salient.

In one relevant example, strong affect associated with outcomes seems to desensitize people to numeric information such as the probability or magnitude of an outcome. Hsee and Rottenstreich (2004), for example, demonstrated that strong affect desensitized people to the magnitude or scope of a stimulus in judgments of its subjective value. In their studies, participants, faced with affect-rich objects (e.g., a picture of a cute animal in need of help), seemed to base their valuation on the presence or absence of at least one object while being relatively insensitive to greater numbers of the object (e.g., whether one or four pictured cute animals were in need). In contrast, when the object was affect-poor (the same animal depicted with a number of dots), value was closer to a linear function, and decision makers were willing to pay more for larger numbers of the object. Watson et al. (1999) showed what may be a similar effect with genetic counseling in women with a family history of breast cancer. In particular, women who were quite worried demonstrated probability neglect; less worried women were more sensitive to probability levels. As a result, when patients are highly emotional about a disease or treatment, it may be particularly difficult to accurately convey important information such as the objective risk of a disease.

More recently, Peters et al. (2012) found that decision makers neglected time in affect-rich and not affect-poor settings. These findings may be important in health decisions involving time such as the decision to vaccinate against hepatitis when traveling to Mexico for either a week's vacation or a 6 months stay for business. Travelers should be more inclined to vaccinate for the longer stay, but if the prospect is affect-rich (the pleasure of vacation or discomfort of disease), they may ignore time and choose to vaccinate for the shorter trip as well. A potentially more troublesome effect is that, for the longer trip, they may be more likely to vaccinate if it is affect-poor (and they are sensitive to time) than affect-rich (and they weigh only affect but future affect is less salient than immediate). Many negative health behaviors (tobacco use, high caloric consumption, sedentary lifestyles) do not pose an immediate threat to health, but their effects accumulate over time. As such, it is difficult to motivate patients to make behavioral changes to avoid a consequence that may not come for years. Future research concerning the interaction of affect and time could explore the repeated decisions necessary to improve and maintain good health.

In another example relevant to health decisions, Alhakami and Slovic (1994) demonstrated that the negative correlation between perceptions of risk and benefit is mediated by affect. In other words, decision makers with positive affect towards a treatment tend to perceive it as high in benefit and low in risk; the reverse happens if decision makers have a negative affect about it. Although this effect has been interpreted in terms of the role of affect as information, it may be related to affect's role as a spotlight. The affect-as-spotlight hypothesis predicts that

decision makers who have positive feelings about a treatment will spend more time looking at its benefits and will remember them better while they spend less time looking at its risks and will remember them less well. It predicts the reverse for treatments that they do not like.

In a recent study, Ferrer et al. (2012) tested the influence of an "affective booster" on framing effects. Participants were provided information about colon cancer screening in either a gain frame (e.g., testing can find precancerous polyps before they become cancerous), or a loss frame (e.g., without screening, precancerous polyps will not be found before they turn to cancer). Because losses loom larger than gains, the loss frame resulted in greater intentions to screen for cancer. However, when participants were asked to vividly imagine that they received (or did not receive) the screening and how they would feel to find out that they did not have colon cancer (or developed cancer if they did not receive the screening), participants in the gain condition who received this vivid affective booster showed a marked increase in their intentions to screen (the affective booster had no effect on participants in the loss condition, perhaps due to ceiling effects or defensive response). They also measured self-efficacy and found that the affective booster was effective in increasing self-efficacy only in the gain condition. The affective booster in the gain frame appeared to act as a spotlight highlighting the participant's ability to avoid colon cancer, thus resulting in greater intentions to screen.

Affect as a Motivator of Behavior

In a fourth role for affect, it functions as a motivator of behavior. Classical theories of emotion include, as the core of an emotion, a readiness to act and the prompting of plans (Frijda 1986). Although affect is a much milder experience compared to a full-blown emotion state, recent research has demonstrated that we tend to automatically classify stimuli around us as good or bad and that this tendency is linked to behavioral tendencies (Chen and Bargh 1999). In multiple studies, for example, research has demonstrated that negative affect is a better predictor of health behaviors such as getting vaccinated or screened than more cognitive predictors such as perceived vulnerability or risk (Chapman and Coups 2006; Diefenbach et al. 1999; McCaul et al. 1996). Negative affect may also motivate improved daily health choices such as the decision to eat more fruit to reduce cancer risk (Ferrer et al. 2013).

Although one-time decisions about health care treatments or options are critical to the well-being of patients, these daily health-related decisions are likely to have a broader and more significant impact. Historically, the majority of deaths were caused by communicable diseases and accidental injury, but, in the past century, behavior-related disease has become a major cause of mortality. Mortality rates are generally presented by the disease that caused the death (e.g., cancer, stroke), but in actuality, health behaviors like tobacco use and excessive caloric intake/lack of physical exercise are the true cause of death (Mokdad et al. 2004) as they lead to the specific disease that causes death. Affect also plays a role in these decisions. Kwan and Bryan (2010), for example, measured integral affect towards exercising and found that increased positive affect and decreased negative affect, experienced during exercise, were associated with greater motivation to exercise three months later. Thus, affect plays an important role, not just in one-time decisions (e.g., choosing a treatment), but in the repeated decisions necessary to maintain many healthy behaviors.

Affect also appears to be linked with the extent of deliberative effort decision makers are willing to put forth to make the best decision (Peters et al. 2003). For example, people who experience strong affect regarding a health decision may work harder to find and process information about treatments and other options and may take on more positive health behaviors (e.g., Hovick et al. 2011).

Decision makers' motivation to maintain or attain positive moods also might lead those in a positive mood to make better decisions among treatment, screening, and other options. Research

has already begun to examine whether mild positive mood interventions may lead to improved health behaviors (Ogedegbe et al. 2012). Alternatively, patients may delay a decision if they do not believe the outcome will sufficiently maintain or improve their mood. Expectations of what an outcome will do to one's mood therefore may influence decisions in unexpected ways. For example, when considering genetic testing, a patient may perceive screening for breast cancer as helping her to avoid cancer risk (and protect her mood), thus leading to increased screening rates. However, in cases where patients dread the disease or treatment, that negative affect may create an expectation of a negative mood state and the patient may decide not to be screened in order to avoid the knowledge and dread of increased risk. For example, a patient with a family history of early colon cancer may have such negative feelings about treatments (e.g., need for colostomy) that they may choose not to be screened in order to avoid the negative emotions that accompany knowledge of increased disease risk (Croyle and Lerman 1999). Future research could consider communication or other interventions that take advantage of the human tendency to want to be in positive mood states and avoid negative mood states.

Factors that Influence the Balance Between Affect and Deliberation

Many factors are involved in determining what sources of affective and non-affective information are used in making a decision and how they are used (e.g., affect as information vs. as a spotlight). Decision importance is one obvious factor in health decisions where outcomes can mean life or death. It is likely that, for simple, unimportant decisions, we rely more heavily on affect rather than deliberating at length (Kahneman 2003; Slovic et al. 2002). High-impact decisions, on the other hand, are likely to be deliberated more thoroughly, with the best decisions involving an interaction of affect and deliberation (Damasio 1994). Prior experience may increase reliance on affect as decision makers rely on memories of past feelings rather than on memories of the situational details.

Factors that influence the ease (or difficulty) of processing such as familiarity, cognitive load, time pressure, or decision complexity can also influence the reliance on affect over deliberation. For example, Shiv and Fedorikhin (1999) found that, when asked to remember a long string of numbers at the same time (a high-cognitive load), people were more likely to choose chocolate cake (the affect-rich option), whereas people in a low-load situation tended to choose fruit salad. In another study, Finucane et al. (2000) found that placing participants under time pressure increased the inverse relationship between risks and benefits. With little time for deliberation, participants were thought to rely more on affect to infer benefits and risks, thus causing perceptions of them to align even more negatively. Considering how common increased cognitive load and time pressure are in our daily lives, the potential impact on decision-making is far reaching. In medical decisions about treatment options, it may be possible to assist the decision maker by reducing cognitive load and time pressure and allowing patients more time in a comfortable setting with new and unfamiliar information (Peters et al. 2013).

Future Research Directions in Affect

Throughout this chapter, we have presented possible future research directions when they were relevant to a particular function of affect. Overall, however, further research is needed to understand the process mechanisms that underlie the influence of affect and emotions in health decisions. Affect, for example, does appear to play a role in what information becomes salient in a decision or disappears outside of the spotlight. This role has barely been described at this point, and additional studies are needed to understand the characteristics of the affective reaction (and in interaction with the situation) that causes affect to function in this way. Through a more clear descriptive understanding

of the process, researchers may also be able to identify ways in which affect can be used prescriptively to cause more important health information to loom in affect's spotlight while less important information fades into the background.

Important research is also needed to understand the impact of mixed discrete emotions (e.g., he is angry about and fearful of her cancer) on the emerging mixed appraisals and decisions. What little research exists suggests that, with mixed emotions, appraisals that differ in direction across the mixed emotions (e.g., appraisals of certainty are greater with anger and lower with fear) cancel one another out. The mixed appraisals drop out in terms of their predictive value in the mixed emotions that guide risk perceptions and other judgments. The valence appraisal, however, appears to increase in predictive power relative to other appraisals (Peters et al. 2003).

Affect is often discussed as being comprised of two dimensions—valence (good or bad) and arousal (intensity). Little is known, however, about the differential effects of valence and arousal in health decision-making. The well-known negativity effect—negative losses and emotions have a bigger impact on decisions and judgments than positive gains and emotions—is likely due, in part, to valence but could also be due to arousal and the confound of negative things generally being higher in arousal. Research in the area of eating behaviors indicates a complex relationship between arousal, valence, and individual differences, with the effect on behavior dependent on their interaction (Macht 2008). For example, high arousal emotions tend to reduce consumption regardless of valence, whereas moderate arousal emotions increase consumption differently depending on the valence of emotion and individual differences in consumption motivation (whether people are dieters, emotional eaters, or normal eaters).

Further research, of course, is needed. In what situations do high/low arousal and positive/negative valence best facilitate healthy behaviors? We can see, for example, the effectiveness of high arousal, negative valence messages in tobacco warning labels used outside of the US (e.g., Hammond 2011), but could they be more effective if either the valence or level of arousal were varied and what level of each dimension results in the greatest impact to smokers intentions to quit? Or perhaps specific emotions should be used (e.g., fear appeals)?

Recent research has also questioned how well explicit, reportable thoughts predict health behaviors as opposed to more implicit reactions that exist beneath the level of awareness. Using fMRI data, Falk et al. (2012) collected the neural responses of participants viewing anti-smoking advertisements from three different media campaigns. After the fMRI session, participants completed a survey about the advertisements, ranking their projected effectiveness, their favorite advertisements, and each advertisement's individual effectiveness. A priori, the researchers had identified the ventral subregion of the medial prefrontal cortex (MPFC) as a region of interest due to its association with behavioral change (Falk et al. 2010). This area has been associated with affect's influence on decisions in past studies (Damasio 1996). Falk et al. then used the extent of the neural activity in this area and self-reported judgments to predict which of the three advertisement campaigns was most effective, using the number of calls placed to quit smoking phone lines as the dependent measure. MPFC activation was a significantly better predictor of the advertisement campaign that elicited the most quit-line calls than the explicit judgments participants made after watching the advertisements. Falk et al. suggested that an unconscious mechanism is involved in determining the influence of different ads on smokers. Given the link with Damasio's research, it seems likely that this mechanism would concern the function of affect as information. Of course, because the researchers did not assess self-reported affect and emotions to the advertisements, it is unclear whether self-report measures might predict as well as the more expensive neuroimaging technique. After all, a history of studies exists illustrating the greater predictive power of self-reported affect over more cognitive assessments in health behaviors (e.g., Diefenbach et al. 1999).

Is Affect Rational?

Affect's influence in health decisions can be overwhelming. Patients may suffer undue anxiety or fear, vastly overestimate risks (e.g., with breast cancer patients), or avoid choices among treatment options. Affect can also be a distraction when it provides information or motivation to attend to or act on emotional information at the expense of other more important message content. Often times, when people consider the impact of emotion on health decisions, these negative impacts are most salient, but they neglect the critical importance of affect. Damasio (1994) and others argue that integral affect increases the accuracy and efficiency of the decision process, and its absence (e.g., in patients with damage to the ventral MPFC) degrades decision performance. Decision researchers have expanded on this view of affect in health and other decisions. Affect is rational in the sense that some level of integral affect is necessary for information to have meaning so that decisions can be made. This "affective rationality" is a key for health communications that have normally focused less on the role of affect and more on deliberative means (Hibbard and Peters 2003). Previous warning labels on cigarette packages in the United States exemplify this deliberative approach, providing only factual information about the related risks of tobacco use. Based on evidence of the greater effectiveness of affective and graphic warning labels (Hammond 2011), the FDA proposed new labels to take effect in 2012.

Affect's role in health decisions is also likely to be nuanced; it therefore deserves careful empirical study. Affect sometimes will help and other times hurt decision processes. Which occurs will depend on the affect elicited by the stimulus (including how information is presented), how affect influences the information processing that takes place in the construction of preferences, and how that particular influence matches whatever processing will produce the best decision for the individual in a given situation. In other words, the presence of affect does not guarantee good or bad decisions; it does guarantee that communicated information will be processed in ways that are different from when it is not present. Understanding these processes presents important challenges in health decision-making research.

Acknowledgments This paper is based in part on the chapter "The functions of affect in the construction of preferences" by E. Peters, which appears in S. Lichtenstein and P. Slovic (Eds.), 2006, The construction of preference. New York: Cambridge University Press. Preparation of this paper was supported in part by the National Science Foundation (SES-1047757 and -1155924).

References

Alhakami, A. S., & Slovic, P. (1994). A psychological study of the inverse relationship between perceived risk and perceived benefit. *Risk Analysis, 14*(6), 1085–1096.

Bower, G. (1981). Mood and memory. *American Psychologist, 36*(2), 129–148.

Cabanac, M. (1992). Pleasure: The common currency. *Journal of Theoretical Biology, 155*, 173–200.

Chapman, G. B., & Coups, E. J. (2006). Emotions and preventive health behavior: Worry, regret, and influenza vaccination. *Health Psychology: Official Journal of the Division of Health Psychology, American Psychological Association, 25*(1), 82–90.

Chen, M., & Bargh, J. A. (1999). Consequences of automatic evaluation: Immediate behavioral predispositions to approach or avoid the stimulus. *Personality and Social Psychology Bulletin, 25*(2), 215–224.

Croyle, R. T., & Lerman, C. (1999). Risk communication in genetic testing for cancer susceptibility. *Journal of the National Cancer Institute, 25*, 59–66.

Damasio, A. R. (1994). *Descartes' error: Emotion, reason, and the human brain*. New York: Avon.

Damasio, A. R. (1996). The somatic marker hypothesis and the possible functions of the prefrontal cortex. *Biological Sciences, 351*(1346), 1413–1420.

DeSteno, D., Petty, R. E., Wegener, D. T., & Rucker, D. D. (2000). Beyond valence in the perception of likelihood: The role of emotion specificity. *Journal of Personality and Social Psychology, 78*(3), 397–416.

Diefenbach, M. A., Miller, S. M., & Daly, M. B. (1999). Specific worry about breast cancer predicts mammography use in women at risk for breast and ovarian cancer. *Health Psychology, 18*(5), 532–536.

Epstein, S. (1994). Integration of the cognitive and the psychodynamic unconscious. *American Psychologist, 49*(8), 709–724. doi:10.1037//0003-066X.49.8.709.

Fagerlin, A., Zikmund-Fisher, B. J., & Ubel, P. A. (2005). How making a risk estimate can change the feel of that risk: Shifting attitudes toward breast cancer risk in a general public survey. *Patient Education and Counseling, 57*(3), 294–299.

Falk, E. B., Berkman, E. T., Harrison, B., Lieberman, M. D., & Mann, T. (2010). Predicting persuasion-induced behavior change from the brain. *Journal of Neuroscience, 30*(25), 8421–8424.

Falk, E. B., Berkman, E. T., & Lieberman, M. D. (2012). From neural responses to population behavior: Neural focus group predicts population-level media effects. *Psychological Science, 23*(5), 439–445.

Ferrer, R., Bergman, H., & Klein, W. M. P. (2013). Worry as a predictor of nutrition behaviors: Results from a nationally representative survey. *Health Education and Behavior, 40*(1), 88–96.

Ferrer, R. A., Klein, W. M. P., Zajac, L. E., Land, S. R., & Ling, B. S. (2012). An affective booster moderates the effect of gain- and loss-framed messages on behavioral intentions for colorectal cancer screening. *Journal of Behavioral Medicine, 35*(4), 452–461.

Finucane, M. L., Alhakami, A., Slovic, P., & Johnson, S. M. (2000). The affect heuristic in judgments of risks and benefits. *Journal of Behavioral Decision Making, 13*, 1–18.

Frijda, N. H. (1986). *The emotions: Studies in emotion and social interaction*. New York: Cambridge University Press.

Hammond, D. (2011). Health warning messages on tobacco products: A review. *Tobacco Control, 20*(5), 327–337.

Hibbard, J. H., & Peters, E. (2003). Supporting informed consumer health care decisions: Data presentation approaches that facilitate the use of information in choice. *Annual Review of Public Health, 24*, 413–433. doi:10.1146/annurev.publhealth.24.100901.141005.

Hovick, S. R., Freimuth, V. S., Johnson-Turbes, A., & Chervin, D. D. (2011). Multiple health risk perception and information processing among African Americans and Whites living in poverty. *Risk Analysis, 31*(11), 1789–1799. doi:10.1111/j.1539-6924.2011.01621.x.

Hsee, C. K., & Rottenstreich, Y. (2004). Music, pandas, and muggers: On the affective psychology of value. *Journal of Experimental Psychology: General, 133*(1), 23–30.

Johnson, E. J., & Tversky, A. (1983). Affect, generalization, and the perception of risk. *Journal of Personality and Social Psychology, 45*, 20–31.

Kahneman, D. (2003). A perspective on judgment and choice: Mapping bounded rationality. *American Psychologist, 58*(9), 697–720.

Kwan, B. M., & Bryan, A. D. (2010). Affective response to exercise as a component of exercise motivation: Attitudes, norms, self-efficacy, and temporal stability of intentions. *Psychology of Sport and Exercise, 11*(1), 71–79.

Lerner, J. S., & Keltner, D. (2001). Fear, anger, and risk. *Journal of Personality and Social Psychology, 81*(1), 146–159.

Lichtenstein, S., & Slovic, P. (2006). *The construction of preference*. Cambridge, New York: Cambridge University Press.

Loewenstein, G. F., Weber, E. U., Hsee, C. K., & Welch, E. S. (2001). Risk as feelings. *Psychological Bulletin, 127*(2), 267–286.

Macht, M. (2008). How emotions affect eating: A five-way model. *Appetite, 50*(1), 1–11.

McCaul, K. D., Reid, P. A., Rathge, R. W., & Martinson, B. (1996). Does concern about breast cancer inhibit or promote breast cancer screening? *Basic and Applied Social Psychology, 18*(2), 183–194.

Mokdad, A. H., Marks, J. S., Stroup, D. F., & Gerberding, J. L. (2004). Actual causes of death in the united states, 2000. *JAMA: The Journal of the American Medical Association, 291*(10), 1238–1245.

Ogedegbe, G. O., Boutin-Foster, C., Wells, M. T., Allegrante, J. P., Isen, A. M., Jobe, J. B., et al. (2012). A randomized controlled trial of positive-affect intervention and medication adherence in hypertensive African Americans. *Archives of Internal Medicine, 172*(4), 322–326. doi:10.1001/archinternmed.2011.1307.

Peters, E. (2006). The functions of affect in the construction of preferences. In S. Lichtenstein & P. Slovic (Eds.), *the construction of preference* (pp. 454–463). New York: Cambridge University Press.

Peters, E. M., Burraston, B., & Mertz, C. K. (2004). An emotion-based model of risk perception and stigma susceptibility: Cognitive appraisals of emotion, affective reactivity, worldviews, and risk perceptions in the generation of technological stigma. *Risk Analysis, 24*(5), 1349–1367.

Peters, E., Dieckmann, N. F., Vastfjall, D., Mertz, C. K., Slovic, P., & Hibbard, J. H. (2009). Bringing meaning to numbers: The impact of evaluative categories on decisions. *Journal of Experimental Psychology: Applied, 15*(3), 213–227.

Peters, E., Klein, W. M. P., Kauffman, A., & Meilleur, L. (2013). More is not always better: Intuitions about effective public policy can lead to unintended consequences. *Social Issues and Policy Review, 7*(1), 114–148.

Peters, E., Kunreuther, H., Sagara, N., Slovic, P., & Shley, D. R. (2012). Protective measures, personal experience, and the affective psychology of time. *Risk Analysis, 32*(12), 2084–2097.

Peters, E., & Slovic, P. (1996). The role of affect and worldviews as orienting dispositions in the perception and acceptance of nuclear power. *Journal of Applied Social Psychology, 26*, 1427–1453.

Peters, E., Slovic, P., & Gregory, R. (2003). The role of affect in the WTA/WTP disparity. *Journal of Behavioral Decision Making, 16*, 309–330.

Peters, E., Slovic, P., Hibbard, J. H., & Tusler, M. (2006). Why worry? Worry, risk perceptions, and willingness to act to reduce medical errors. *Health Psychology, 25*(2), 144–152.

Reyna, V. F. (2008). A theory of medical decision making and health: Fuzzy trace theory. *Medical Decision Making, 28*(6), 850–865.

Schwarz, N., & Clore, G. L. (2003). Mood as information: 20 years later. *Psychological Inquiry, 14*, 294–301.

Shiv, B., & Fedorikhin, A. (1999). Heart and mind in conflict: Interplay of affect and cognition in consumer decision making. *Journal of Consumer Research, 26*, 278–282.

Slovic, P., Finucane, M. L., Peters, E., & MacGregor, D. G. (2002). The affect heuristic. In T. Gilovich, D. Griffin, & D. Kahneman (Eds.), *Heuristics and biases: The psychology of intuitive judgment* (pp. 397–420). New York: Cambridge University Press.

Slovic, P., Peters, E., Grana, J., Berger, S., & Dieck, G. S. (2007). Risk perception of prescription drugs: Results of a national survey. *Drug Information Journal Drug Information Journal, 41*(1), 81–100.

Watson, M., Lloyd, S., Davidson, J., Meyer, L., Eeles, R., Ebbs, S., et al. (1999). The impact of genetic counselling on risk perception and mental health in women with a family history of breast cancer. *British Journal of Cancer, 79*(5–6), 5–6.

Zajonc, R. B. (1980). Feeling and thinking: Preferences need no inferences. *American Psychologist American Psychologist, 35*(2), 151–175.

Strategies to Promote the Maintenance of Behavior Change: Moving from Theoretical Principles to Practice

9

Alexander J. Rothman, Austin S. Baldwin, Rachel J. Burns and Paul T. Fuglestad

There is strong consensus that efforts to promote and improve people's health will depend, at least in part, on people's behavioral decisions; decisions that cross a broad range of domains (Roberts and Barnard 2005; U.S. Department of Health and Human Services 2011). Some decisions involve behaviors that occur frequently (e.g., food intake; physical activity; the use of substances such as tobacco and alcohol), whereas other decisions involve behaviors that occur regularly, but infrequently (e.g., yearly check-up; flu vaccination) or that emerge at specific times in one's life (e.g., cancer screening). Regardless of the domain, strategies are needed to help people make behavioral decisions that increase the likelihood that they will live healthy, productive lives. To this end, some investigators have relied on strategies that shape the beliefs and skills that guide people's behavioral decisions (e.g., increasing awareness of the benefits or costs posed by different behaviors), whereas other investigators have relied on strategies that constrain or shape people's behavioral options (e.g., policies that place limits on where people can smoke).

In this chapter, we focus on intervention strategies that have been developed to shape the thoughts, feelings, and skills that guide people's health behaviors (Conner and Norman 2005; Rothman and Salovey 2007). However, we examine these approaches through a particular perspective—their ability to promote the maintenance of behavior change. The benefits that emerge if people make healthier behavioral choices in domains such as diet, physical activity, and substance use require that people not only initiate a healthy pattern of behavior (e.g., increase their physical activity), but also sustain that pattern of behavior over time. Thus, interventions that are able to elicit a new, healthy pattern of behavior are necessary, but not sufficient. Research has consistently revealed that people who are able to make significant changes in their behavior are not necessarily able to maintain those changes over time and, thus, attention needs to be directed toward specifying the factors that facilitate and inhibit sustained behavior change (Rothman et al. 2004, 2009).

Looking across the strategies that investigators have developed to promote sustained behavior change, we have identified three intervention approaches. One approach rests on the premise that to promote successful maintenance the psychological factors and behavioral skills

A.J. Rothman (✉)
Department of Psychology, University of Minnesota, 75 East River Road, Minneapolis, MN 55455, USA
e-mail: rothm001@umn.edu

A.S. Baldwin
Southern Methodist University, Dallas, TX, USA

R.J. Burns
University of Minnesota, Minneapolis, MN 55455, USA

P.T. Fuglestad
University of North Florida, Jacksonville, FL, USA

© Springer Science+Business Media New York 2016
M.A. Diefenbach et al. (eds.), *Handbook of Health Decision Science*,
DOI 10.1007/978-1-4939-3486-7_9

that led to the initial change in behavior need to be reinforced continually. The second approach rests on the premise that people will maintain a new pattern of behavior if they are provided with the appropriate set of motivation, beliefs, and behavioral skills at the outset of the behavior change process. The third approach rests on the premise that the set of psychological factors and behavioral skills that facilitate the initiation of behavior change are distinct from those that facilitate behavioral maintenance and, thus, different intervention strategies are needed at each phase of the behavior change process. In the sections to follow, we consider each of the three intervention approaches; first describing the theoretical rationale that underlies the approach and then the evidence available from interventions designed to promote behavioral maintenance. Although the majority of interventions conducted to date have focused on the maintenance of weight loss, interventions in other behavioral domains, when available, are considered. Following our review of these three approaches, we turn to two promising intervention techniques that offer opportunities for innovation—using financial incentives to promote behavior change and tailoring intervention strategies to address an individual's particular needs or psychological dispositions.

Intervention Strategy I: Continually Reinforcing the Determinants of Initial Behavior Change

The first strategy proposes that the psychological factors and behavioral skills individuals possess or develop that guide initial changes in behavior (e.g., self-monitoring, stimulus control, cognitive restructuring; Wadden et al. 2005) must be reinforced continually. To date, most of the work that has evaluated this intervention approach has targeted behaviors that underlie weight loss (but see Joseph et al. 2011). This approach has been referred to as a "continued care" intervention model (Perri and Corsica 2002; Svetkey et al. 2008; Wadden et al. 2005) and the rationale

for using this approach in the domain of weight loss rests on the recognition of obesity as a chronic disorder that requires long-term care (National Institutes of Health 1998).

Evidence from randomized controlled trials (RCTs) indicates that this intervention approach can be effective for long-term weight loss maintenance (Perri et al. 2008; Svetkey et al. 2008; Wing et al. 2006). In this area, investigators have been particularly interested in the relative effectiveness of different modes of delivering continued care [e.g., face-to-face contact vs. web-based contact (Svetkey et al. 2008; Wing et al. 2006) or telephone contact (Perri et al. 2008)], the duration of continued care during the maintenance period [e.g., 12 months (Perri et al. 2008) to 30 months (Svetkey et al. 2008)], and the frequency of contacts with the intervention staff [e.g., biweekly (Perri et al. 2008) or monthly (Svetkey et al. 2008; Wing et al. 2006)].

Findings from these RCTs indicate that some forms of continued care result in slower weight regain compared to minimal contact during the maintenance period and that some forms of contact between intervention staff and participants are more effective. For example, face-to-face contact was found to afford the slowest rate of weight regain (Perri et al. 2008; Svetkey et al. 2008; Wing et al. 2006), whereas web-based contact was found to be no better than control (Svetkey et al. 2008; Wing et al. 2006). However, Perri et al. (2008) found that continued care provided via telephone had similar effects to face-to-face contact and both were more effective than a minimal contact control condition. The findings suggest that some form of personal contact, whether face to face or over the telephone, may be a necessary component for a continued care approach to be effective. Consistent with the premise underlying this approach, individuals who received continued care were more likely to continue to self-monitor their dietary behavior, and self-monitoring mediated the intervention effect on weight regain (Perri et al. 2008). However, findings from these trials also suggest that while a continued care approach can delay or slow the rate of relapse, it does not completely prevent it (Kiernan et al. 2013; Perri and Corsica 2002; Wadden et al. 2005).

Intervention Strategy II: Instantiating the Appropriate Set of Motivations and Skills at the Outset of Treatment

The second class of intervention strategies to promote the maintenance of behavior change is grounded on the premise that people are more likely to maintain changes in their behavior if, at the outset, they are motivated to initiate the change for the right reasons and have appropriate expectations for what the change in their behavioral practices will entail. Most of the intervention work in this area is based on Self-Determination Theory (SDT; Ryan and Deci 2000). SDT is a general theory of human motivation that has provided valuable insights into the decision processes that underlie the maintenance of health behavior change.

According to SDT, maintenance is more likely when motivation for the change and the skills needed to make it are internalized by the individual. Three factors—autonomy, competence, and relatedness—facilitate the internalization of the motivation and skills. Autonomy occurs when the individual personally endorses or identifies with the importance of the behavior, in contrast to engaging in the behavior change due to external pressure. Competence occurs when the individual has the skills and confidence to make the change. Relatedness occurs when the individual feels a connection to and trusts those promoting and supporting the change. Observational data across different behavioral domains [e.g., weight loss (Williams et al. 1996), glycemic control among Type 2 diabetics (Williams et al. 2004), and medication adherence among chronically ill patients (Williams et al. 1998)] have provided empirical support that autonomy and perceived competence are associated with long-term maintenance. Moreover, a recent meta-analysis observed that autonomy, competence, and relatedness are all reliably related to internalized motivation and skills, and that

internalized motivation and skills are reliably related to better physical health (Ng et al. 2012).

Trials that have evaluated interventions targeting autonomy and competence have similarly supported the efficacy of an SDT approach to promoting the maintenance of behavior change. For example, an intervention to support autonomy and competence in smoking cessation was designed to allow participants to make their own decisions about cessation, including whether and when they were ready to quit smoking (as opposed to an intervention-imposed quit date; Williams et al. 2002). The autonomy-supportive intervention led to higher rates of smoking abstinence after two years compared to an education-based control intervention, and changes in autonomous motivation and perceived competence for smoking cessation mediated the effect of intervention on abstinence (for similar findings see Silva et al. 2011; Williams et al. 2009).

The premise that successful maintenance is predicated on how people are trained at the outset of behavior change can also be seen in a recent weight loss intervention in which individuals learned and practiced maintenance-specific skills prior to their initial weight loss efforts in order to capitalize on their initial motivation and to provide opportunities to experience success with weight maintenance before being faced with the challenge of maintaining actual weight loss (Kiernan et al. 2013). To test this premise, participants were randomized to either a weight loss first condition (20 week weight loss program followed by 8 weeks of continued care) or a maintenance first condition (8 weeks of maintenance skills followed by the 20 week program). Both conditions provided the same period of active intervention, but participants in the maintenance first condition spent the initial 8 weeks learning and practicing maintenance skills (e.g., daily weighing to collect data about weight fluctuations, practicing a 1-week disruption in new dietary habits). Findings revealed that there was no difference in weight loss across intervention conditions at the end of the active intervention period, but participants in the maintenance first intervention regained less weight over the subsequent 12 months (3.2 vs. 7.3 lb). Although this is the only intervention of this type reported to date, these findings suggest that this may be a promising approach to health behavior change maintenance.

Intervention Strategy III: Targeting the Specific Sets of Motivations and Skills that Facilitate the Initiation and Maintenance of Behavior Change

The third class of intervention strategies to promote the maintenance of behavior change is grounded on the premise that initiation and maintenance are each different phases of the behavior change process and the criteria that shape decisions to initiate and decisions to maintain a change in behavior are distinct (Rothman et al. 2011; Schwarzer et al. 2007).

Two theoretical frameworks have guided research in this area. First, Rothman (2000) and Rothman et al. (2011) proposed that the decision to initiate a new pattern of behavior is guided by people's favorable expectations for the behavior change and confidence in their ability to successfully change behavior (i.e., self-efficacy), whereas the decision to maintain that pattern of behavior is guided by an assessment of whether the experiences and outcomes associated with the new behavior are worth the effort required (i.e., perceived satisfaction). In addition, initiation is conceptualized as an approach-based self-regulatory process (i.e., progress toward one's goals is indicated by a reduction in the discrepancy between one's current state and a desired reference state), whereas maintenance is conceptualized as an avoidance-based self-regulatory process (i.e., progress toward one's goals is indicated by maintaining the discrepancy between one's current state and an undesired reference state). In the domain of smoking cessation, there is evidence to support the theoretical premise that beliefs about one's ability to change behavior (i.e., self-efficacy) are more important when initiating a change, whereas perceptions of satisfaction are more important when people are faced with the decision

to maintain the change (Baldwin et al. 2006). In addition, evidence across both smoking cessation and weight loss interventions suggests that people's self-regulatory mindset differentially predicts their ability to initiate and maintain a new pattern of behavior and is consistent with the conceptualization of initiation and maintenance as approach- and avoidance-based regulatory processes, respectively (Fuglestad et al. 2008, 2013).

Second, the Health Action Process Approach model (HAPA; Schwarzer et al. 2007) also emphasizes different phases of the behavior change process: non-intentional, intentional, and action. The non-intentional phase is when a person has not formed an intention to act. The intentional phase is when a person has already formed an intention but has not changed her or his behavior (or is acting below a recommended level). The action phase is when a person is acting at the recommended level (Lippke et al. 2005; Schwarzer et al. 2007). The intentional and action phases could be considered analogous to the initiation and maintenance phases described by Rothman et al. (2011). Different psychological factors are believed to be more important at different phases of the behavior change process. Specifically, risk perceptions, outcome expectancies, and motivational self-efficacy predict forming intentions for people in the non-intentional phase, whereas action planning and recovery self-efficacy predict behavior for people in the intentional and action phases (Lippke et al. 2005; Schwarzer et al. 2007; Sniehotta et al. 2005).

Evidence from RCTs provides some support for the efficacy of this approach to behavior change maintenance. Guided by the Rothman framework (Rothman 2000; Rothman et al. 2011) and Self-Determination Theory (Ryan and Deci 2000), West et al. (2011) conducted a RCT in which all participants enrolled in a standard weight loss program for 6 months. Following this initial weight loss period, participants were randomized to a satisfaction- and motivation-focused condition (the novel intervention), a continued care condition (reinforcement of weight loss skills), or a control condition. The novel intervention was designed to strengthen participants' satisfaction with their progress and elicit personal motivations for engaging in long-term behavior changes. The results indicated that both maintenance conditions resulted in smaller weight regains compared to the control condition, but they did not differ from one another. However, the extent to which people focused on the progress they made (a form of satisfaction) predicted lower rates of weight regain in both maintenance conditions. Moreover, among people who received the novel intervention, the extent to which they focused on the progress they made was a stronger predictor of maintained weight loss than other factors. Although this was a single RCT, these findings suggest that having people focus on different factors and skills when faced with maintenance may be effective.

Several HAPA-based randomized interventions have examined the efficacy of planning at different phases of behavior change. For example, orthopedic rehabilitation patients were randomized to an interviewer-assisted planning intervention or one that was self-directed (Ziegelmann et al. 2006), and reported different types of planning: action planning (predicted to be more important initially) and coping planning (predicted to be more important for maintenance). Consistent with predictions, coping planning accounted for physical activity minutes, above and beyond action planning, at both 4 weeks and 6 months after the intervention but not 2 weeks after. This pattern of findings suggests that coping planning is relevant only when people are faced with the decision to maintain the change they have made. Taken together, there is an emerging body of evidence that interventions can be more effective if they target the specific factors that underlie successful initiation and maintenance of behavior change, respectively.

Emerging Intervention Technique: The Impact of Financial Incentives on Maintenance of Behavior Change

Each of the three classes of intervention approaches to promote behavioral maintenance has a distinct objective; however, there are numerous techniques that can be used to meet these objectives. We now turn to a discussion of two emerging intervention techniques that may be useful means through which the goal of a specific approach to interventions is achieved.

The premise that the provision of financial incentives will motivate behavior change is a principle that has reemerged as an intriguing intervention technique. Typically, this approach involves awarding or reimbursing an incentive (i.e., money, prizes, coupons) if a person achieves a specified criterion within a predetermined time period. The incentivized criterion can be the performance of a behavior (e.g., taking medication daily) or the downstream consequence of a behavior (e.g., losing 2 lb in 2 weeks).

Providing financial incentives to elicit behavior change is based on the premise that people's behavioral choices reflect a weighing of benefits and costs and that the failure to take action (e.g., be more physically active) reflects a determination that the costs outweigh the benefits. The provision of a financial incentive that is contingent upon meeting a particular criterion is designed to alter the cost-benefit analysis, such that the benefits of taking action to meet the criterion outweigh the costs of not acting. The use of financial incentives to promote behavior change is also rooted in operant conditioning theory (Skinner 1953)—the provision of an incentive in response to a behavior affords the opportunity to develop an association between a behavior and its consequences, which, in turn, can increase or decrease of the frequency of the behavior. Furthermore, the structure of an incentive program can vary along two theoretically meaningful, orthogonal dimensions that may have implications for its influence on people's health behavior (Burns et al. 2012).

First, incentives can differ in reinforcement procedure. With positive reinforcement, a behavior is performed more frequently because it is associated with the provision of a pleasant stimulus, whereas negative reinforcement increases the frequency of the target behavior by associating it with the removal of an unpleasant stimulus (Skinner 1953). For example, in weight loss interventions, incentives that are structured as positive reinforcement takes the form of cash rewards or lotteries (e.g., Francisco et al. 1994; Volpp et al. 2009), whereas incentives that are structured as negative reinforcement involve deposit contracts or payroll deductions (e.g., meeting a criterion removes the threat of not getting one's money returned; Jeffery et al. 1993; Volpp et al. 2008). Because people perceive the costs of losing a particular amount of money to be greater than the perceived benefit associated with gaining the same amount of money (Tversky and Kahneman 1991), one would expect an incentive program structured as negative reinforcement to be more effective than an incentive program structured as positive reinforcement.

Second, incentives can differ in the frequency at which the target behavior is reinforced (i.e., reinforcement schedule). With fixed ratio scheduling, a target behavior is consistently reinforced after every nth behavior, whereas with variable ratio scheduling, a target behavior is reinforced at an unpredictable rate (but at an average of every nth behavior; Skinner 1953). A fixed ratio schedule provides a greater degree of certainty and predictability. Research with nonhuman animals suggests that incentives provided on a fixed ratio schedule are more effective at eliciting an initial change in behavior, but incentives provided on a variable ratio schedule are more effective at sustaining behavior over time (see McSweeney 2004).

The efficacy of financial incentives to elicit initial changes in behavior change has been tested in a range of health domains, including weight loss (Volpp et al. 2008), smoking cessation (Volpp et al. 2009), vaccination (Moran et al. 1996), and screening (Slater et al. 2005). The predominant finding is that incentives increase the likelihood that people will perform the incentivized behavior or achieve the incentivized outcome, but once the financial incentive is removed the initiated behavior or outcome is not sustained (Burns et al. 2012; Kane et al. 2004).

Only a few studies have examined the efficacy of financial incentives on maintaining health behavior change directly. In the domain of weight loss maintenance, one study used deposit contracts in which reimbursement was contingent upon maintaining body weight or meeting physical activity and diet goals; weight regain amongst participants in the deposit contract conditions did not differ from that of participants in a control condition after one year (Kramer et al. 1986). In the domain of smoking cessation, two studies have demonstrated that participants who are offered a cash reward for maintaining a specified period of abstinence were more likely to be abstinent that participants who were assigned to a control condition (Donatelle et al. 2000; Volpp et al. 2009). However, in both studies, the incentive condition included intervention components that were not offered to other participants (e.g., strategies for increasing social support; incentives to attend a smoking cessation program), so it is unclear if the differences in sustained abstinence between the groups reflect the effectiveness of the incentive or other differences between the groups.

To date, the use of incentives as an intervention technique has not been strongly grounded in theoretical perspectives that might offer insights into how or when they may be most effective (Burns et al. 2012). What has emerged is a tremendous heterogeneity in how incentive programs have been structured, which has precluded any systematic test of whether specific combinations of reinforcement procedure and reinforcement schedule might be particularly effective in eliciting favorable rates of behavioral maintenance. The three classes of intervention strategies we have identified provide a productive frame for thinking through how and when to use incentives to promote sustained behavior change. The continued care model of intervention strategies would suggest that the provision of incentives needs to be sustained if people are going to successfully maintain an initial change in their behavior. As has been done for weight loss treatment and smoking cessation treatment, there would be value in systematically examining the effect of incentive programs of different, extended durations; though the repeated provision of the same incentive may result in habituation to the incentive, diminishing its value.

The premise that successful maintenance depends on people initiating a change in behavior under the right conditions would suggest that how the incentive program is designed to elicit initial changes in behavior is critical. SDT would suggest that any provision of incentives would need to be done thoughtfully and in a manner that still enables people to develop a sense of autonomy and competence. Moreover, building on the perspective underlying the intervention conducted by Kiernan et al. (2013), there might be value in providing people with a set of skills and expectations that would complement the strengths of an incentive-based program and enable them to manage the transition that comes with the end of the incentive program.

Finally, incentive programs could be structured around the premise that the initiation and maintenance of behavior change are responsive to different strategies. For example, there might be value in shifting the schedule and structure of the reinforcement as people transition from initiation to maintenance. In the domain of weight loss treatment, Burns et al. (2012) observed that an incentive program that provided positive reinforcement on a fixed schedule might be effective at eliciting initial changes in behavior, but to support the maintenance of those changes it would be beneficial if it shifted to providing negative reinforcement on a variable schedule.

Emerging Intervention Technique: Leveraging Psychological Dispositions to Enhance the Effect of Intervention Strategies to Promote the Maintenance of Behavior Change

A second promising approach to enhancing the effectiveness of intervention strategies designed to support maintenance is to consider whether differences in stable psychological dispositions modify how these strategies facilitate or inhibit the behavior change process. Across the three broad classes of intervention approaches discussed earlier, strategies designed to promote the maintenance of behavior change depend on their ability to support or mitigate factors that guide

people's behavioral decisions. To date, limited attention has been paid to whether specific strategies might be more effective for certain groups of individuals. Across a number of research programs, investigators have observed that because people's dispositional tendencies affect how information is processed and how the pursuit of personal goals is managed, people's psychological dispositions can modify the effectiveness of strategies designed to promote behavior change (Rothman and Baldwin 2012). What have emerged from this body of research are two broad approaches: strategies that are particularly effective because they compensate for people's weaknesses and strategies that are particularly effective because they capitalize on people's strengths.

Compensating for people's weaknesses. Across an array of behavioral domains (e.g., smoking, exercise), investigators have observed that people high in conscientiousness are more likely to act on their intentions than are people who are low in conscientiousness (e.g., Conner et al. 2009; Rhodes et al. 2005). This is particularly true when the behavior is performed under nonoptimal conditions such as unusual circumstances with additional barriers (Conner et al. 2007) or high stress (Schwartz et al. 1999). Conscientiousness may prove to be beneficial because it represents people's tendency to be thorough and deliberate in their actions. People who are trying to change their behavior and are lower in conscientiousness may benefit from additional support or training, especially when having to deal with unexpected or stressful circumstances.

Consistent with research on conscientiousness, Fuglestad et al. (2008) found that people who score low on prevention focus—which indicates that they are *not* dispositionally inclined to be vigilant or careful as they regulate their behavior—were less successful at maintaining cessation in a smoking cessation trial or at maintaining weight lost during a weight loss trial. However, people's level of prevention focus was not related to their ability to successfully *initiate* a change in their behavior in either of these domains. It may be that the optimal delivery of an intervention strategy will depend on directing it toward a specific group of people at a particular point of time in the behavior change process. For example, efforts to promote the maintenance of behavior change (e.g., more frequent intervention contacts or the provision of additional intervention techniques) might be directed toward people who not only score low on prevention focus, but also are working to maintain an initial change in their behavior.

Capitalizing on people's strengths. An alternative strategy is to develop intervention procedures that leverage an individual's strengths. Higgins' (2005) theory of regulatory fit provides a useful conceptual model of the process by which matching strategies to people's psychological dispositions can augment their effectiveness. According to the theory, people feel a sense of "fit" when the strategies they use to pursue an outcome match their psychological dispositions; this sense of fit increases people's motivation, which, in turn, leads to increased performance. A number of studies have utilized this approach to promote healthful behavior change (e.g., Latimer et al. 2008a, b; Tam et al. 2010; Williams-Piehota et al. 2006, 2009), and those that have explicitly examined the mechanisms that underlie this approach have found that when intervention strategies match a person's disposition they express greater motivation to perform and satisfaction with the behavior in question (e.g., Latimer et al. 2008b; Tam et al. 2010).

However, only a few studies have examined the effectiveness of this approach on relatively longer term outcomes. For example, several studies have utilized the National Cancer Institute's Cancer Information Service to deliver intervention messages to promote changes in diet or physical activity that either matched or mismatched people's coping styles (Williams-Piehota et al. 2009), need for cognition (Williams-Piehota et al. 2006), or regulatory focus (Latimer et al. 2008a, b). Across these studies, when messages were designed to match people's psychological dispositions, they elicited a more pronounced improvement in initial outcomes (e.g., 2 weeks or 2 months), but the observed difference between matched and mismatched messages did not hold for longer term outcomes (e.g., 4 months; but see Latimer et al. 2008a). Yet, it should be noted that none of these studies focused on intervention approaches that were designed specifically to promote sustained behavior change.

The premise that matching intervention strategies to dispositions will heighten their effectiveness has implications for efforts to advance all three classes of intervention strategies identified earlier. In the context of a continued care approach to promoting maintenance, it may be that different groups of people would benefit from the continued provision of different facets of an intervention. For example, people who score low on conscientiousness might benefit from the continued provision of a tool that facilitates planning or self-monitoring, whereas those who score high on conscientiousness might benefit from a tool that helps people recognize the favorable outcomes that are afforded by their behavior. Alternatively, when investigators are able to triage people, dispositional differences might guide decisions about the frequency or intensity of the intervention—some people might benefit from frequent, in-person contact, whereas others might not need additional support.

To the extent that successful maintenance is predicated on how people initiate the behavior, there could be systematic differences in what people need emphasized at the outset. Even if everyone would benefit from an intervention approach that supports autonomy and competence, people may differ systematically in how they respond to different strategies for providing support. What might prove to be particularly productive is the premise that as people move through the behavior change process they differ in whether or what type of assistance they need. Given the thesis that the initiation and the maintenance of a pattern of behavior are distinct self-regulatory tasks, people may find that they have skills that support one phase of the process but not another. Consistent with this perspective, Fuglestad et al. (2008) found that scoring high on promotion focus was beneficial when people were charged with the task of initiating weight loss, but scoring high on prevention focus was beneficial when people were charged with the task of maintaining weight loss. This type of relationship would suggest that interventionists would want to be able to both leverage people's strengths (e.g., maximizing the match between promotion focus and behavioral initiation) and compensate for people's weaknesses (e.g., addressing the mismatch between promotion focus and behavioral maintenance). An example of the latter strategy would be to restructure the task of behavioral maintenance in a manner that resonates with how people who are promotion focused regulate their behavior. Although the prospect of needing to take into account both psychological dispositions and phases of the behavior change process may be daunting, it has the potential to optimize the delivery of intervention resources to people who are striving to sustain new patterns of behavior.

Final Thoughts and Future Directions

There is a clear need for effective, evidence-based intervention strategies that enable people to not only initiate, but also maintain a new pattern of behavior. As investigators continue to design and test strategies to support the maintenance of behavior change, it is critical that these strategies are grounded on a set of principles that specify what facilitates and/or inhibits maintenance (Rothman 2004). In this chapter, we have identified three classes of intervention strategies that are each grounded on a different set of theoretical principles. Although within each class of strategies an intriguing array of findings have

emerged, more empirical work is needed before any strong recommendations can be made. In particular, there are three lines of inquiry that would benefit from more focused attention. First, within each class of strategy, investigators should specify more explicitly the mechanisms that underlie the hypothesized effect of an intervention approach and make sure the manner in which the strategy is designed, implemented, and evaluated is consistent with the underlying model. Second, little is known regarding the relative effectiveness of the different classes of intervention strategies that have been identified. The study conducted by West et al. (2011) stands as an excellent exemplar of this type of work as it compared the effectiveness of a continued care intervention program and a satisfaction-based intervention program. Third, further consideration needs to be given to the different ways in which maintenance unfolds across behavioral domains. In some domains, behavioral decisions need to be made daily (e.g., diet, physical activity), whereas in other domains decisions need to be made every six months (e.g., dental exam) or every year (e.g., cancer screening). Furthermore, in some cases maintenance involves continually *not* performing a behavior (e.g., smoking cessation), whereas in others maintenance involves continually performing a behavior (e.g., physical activity). To date, very little is known—both empirically and theoretically—as to whether the different facets of behavioral domains would benefit from different intervention strategies. Taken together, the implementation of well-designed studies that are guided by an explicit theoretical framework will enable us to develop the evidence base needed to provide a clear, useful, productive roadmap for practice (Table 1).

Table 1 Take home messages

1. To date, intervention strategies that have been developed to promote sustained behavior change can be organized around three intervention approaches
2. Research on each approach has provided some supporting evidence, but greater clarity is needed regarding underlying mechanisms and the relative effectiveness of each intervention approach
3. Two classes of intervention techniques—providing financial incentives to promote behavior change; matching intervention strategies to people's psychological dispositions—offer promising areas for future research

References

Baldwin, A. S., Rothman, A. J., Hertel, A. W., Linde, J. A., Jeffery, R. W., Finch, E., & Lando, H. (2006). Specifying the determinants of the initiation and maintenance of behavior change: An examination of self-efficacy, satisfaction, and smoking cessation. *Health Psychology, 25*, 626–634.

Burns, R. J., Donovan, A. S., Ackermann, R. T., Finch, E. A., Rothman, A. J., & Jeffery, R. W. (2012). A theoretically grounded systematic review of material incentives for weight loss: Implications for interventions. *Annals of Behavioral Medicine, 44*, 375–388.

Conner, M., Grogan, S., Fry, G., Gough, B., & Higgins, A. R. (2009). Direct, mediated and moderated impacts of personality variables on smoking initiation in adolescents. *Psychology and Health, 24*, 1085–1104.

Conner, M., & Norman, P. (Eds.). (2005). *Predicting health behaviour: Research and practice with social cognition models* (2nd ed.). Buckingham, UK: Open University Press.

Conner, M., Rodgers, W., & Murray, T. (2007). Conscientiousness and the intention-behaviour relationship: Predicting exercise behaviour. *Journal of Sports and Exercise Psychology, 29*, 518–533.

Donatelle, R. J., Prows, S. L., Champeau, D., & Hudson, D. (2000). Randomised controlled trial using social support and financial incentives for high risk pregnant smokers: Significant other supporter (SOS) program. *Tobacco Control, 9*(Suppl. III), 67–69.

Francisco, V. T., Paine, A. L., Fawcett, S. B., Johnston, J., & Banks, D. (1994). An experimental evaluation of an incentive program to reduce serum cholesterol levels among health fair participants. *Archives of Family Medicine, 3*, 246–251.

Fuglestad, P. T., Rothman, A. J., & Jeffery, R. W. (2008). Getting there and hanging on: The effect of regulatory focus on performance in smoking and weight loss interventions. *Health Psychology, 27*, S260–S270.

Fuglestad, P. T., Rothman, A. J., & Jeffery, R. W. (2013). The effects of regulatory focus on responding to and avoiding slips in a longitudinal study of smoking cessation. *Basic and Applied Social Psychology, 35*, 426–435.

Higgins, E. T. (2005). Value from regulatory fit. *Current Directions in Psychological Science, 14*(4), 209–213.

Jeffery, R. W., Forster, J. L., French, S. A., Kelder, S. H., Lando, H. A., McGovern, P. G., et al. (1993). The healthy worker project: A work-site intervention for weight control and smoking cessation. *American Journal of Public Health, 83*, 395–401.

Joseph, A. M., Fu, S. S., Lindgren, B., Rothman, A. J., Kodl, M., Lando, H., et al. (2011). Chronic disease management for tobacco dependence improves long-term abstinence from smoking: A randomized, controlled trial. *Archives of Internal Medicine, 171*, 1894–1900.

Kane, R. L., Johnson, P. E., Town, R. J., & Butler, M. (2004). A structured review of the effect of economic incentives on consumers' preventive behavior. *American Journal of Preventive Medicine, 27*, 327–352.

Kiernan, M., Brown, S. D., Schoffman, D. E., Lee, K., King, A. C., Taylor, C. B., et al. (2013). Promoting healthy weight with "stability skills first": A randomized trial. *Journal of Consulting and Clinical Psychology, 81*, 336–346.

Kramer, F. M., Jeffery, R. W., Snell, M. K., & Forster, J. L. (1986). Maintenance of successful weight loss over 1 year: Effects of financial contracts for weight maintenance or participation in skills training. *Behavior Therapy, 17*, 295–301.

Latimer, A. E., Rivers, S. E., Rench, T. A., Katulak, N. A., Hicks, A., Hodorowski, J. K., & Salovey, P. (2008a). A field experiment testing the utility of regulatory fit messages for promoting physical activity. *Journal of Experimental Social Psychology, 44*, 826–832.

Latimer, A. E., Williams-Piehota, P., Katulak, N. A., Cox, A., Mowad, L., Higgins, E. T., & Salovey, P. (2008b). Promoting fruit and vegetable intake through messages tailored to individual differences in regulatory focus. *Annals of Behavioral Medicine, 35*, 363–369.

Lippke, S., Ziegelmann, J. P., & Schwarzer, R. (2005). Stage-specific adoption and maintenance of physical activity: Testing a three-stage model. *Psychology of Sport and Exercise, 6*, 585–603.

McSweeney, F. K. (2004). Dynamic changes in reinforcer effectiveness: Satiation and habituation have different implications for theory and practice. *The Behavior Analyst, 27*, 171–188.

Moran, W. P., Nelson, K., Wofford, J. L., Velez, R., & Case, L. D. (1996). Increasing influenza immunization among high-risk patients: Education or financial incentive? *American Journal of Medicine, 101*, 612–620.

National Institutes of Health/National Heart, Lung, and Blood Institute. (1998). Clinical guidelines on the identification, evaluation, and treatment of overweight and obesity in adults: The evidence report. *Obesity Research, 6*, 51S–210S.

Ng, J. Y. Y., Ntoumanis, N., Thogersen-Ntoumani, C., Deci, E. L., Ryan, R. M., Duda, J. L., & Williams, G. C. (2012). Self-determination theory applied to health contexts: A meta-analysis. *Perspectives on Psychological Science, 7*, 325–340.

Perri, M. G., & Corsica, J. A. (2002). Improving the maintenance of weight lost in behavioral treatment of obesity. In T. A. Wadden & A. J. Stunkard (Eds.), *Handbook of obesity treatment* (pp. 357–379). New York, NY: Guilford Press.

Perri, M. G., Limacher, M. C., Durning, P. E., Janick, D. M., Lutes, L. D., Bobroff, L. B., et al. (2008). Extended-care programs for weight management in rural communities: The treatment of obesity in underseved rural settings (TOURS) randomized trial. *Archives of Internal Medicine, 168*, 2347–2354.

Rhodes, R. E., Courneya, K. S., & Jones, L. W. (2005). The theory of planned behaviour and lower-order personality traits: Interaction effects in the exercise domain. *Personality and Individual Differences, 38*, 251–265.

Roberts, C. K., & Barnard, R. J. (2005). Effects of exercise and diet on chronic disease. *Journal of Applied Physiology, 98*, 3–30.

Rothman, A. J. (2000). Toward a theory-based analysis of behavioral maintenance. *Health Psychology, 19*, S64–S69.

Rothman, A. J. (2004). Is there nothing more practical than a good theory?: Why Innovations and advances in health behavior change will arise if interventions are more theory-friendly. *International Journal of Behavioral Nutrition and Physical Activity, 1*, 11.

Rothman, A. J., & Baldwin, A. S. (2012). A person X intervention strategy approach to understanding health behavior. In K. Deaux & M. Snyder (Eds.), *Handbook of personality and social psychology* (pp. 729–752). New York, NY: Oxford University Press.

Rothman, A. J., Baldwin, A., & Hertel, A. (2004). Self-regulation and behavior change: Disentangling behavioral initiation and behavioral maintenance. In K. Vohs & R. Baumeister (Eds.), *The handbook of self-regulation* (pp. 130–148). New York, NY: Guilford Press.

Rothman, A. J., Baldwin, A. S., Hertel, A. W., & Fuglestad, P. (2011). Self-regulation and behavior change: Disentangling behavioral initiation and behavioral maintenance. In K. Vohs & R. Baumeister (Eds.), *Handbook of self-regulation: Research, theory, and applications* (2nd ed., pp. 106–122). New York, NY: Guilford Press.

Rothman, A. J., & Salovey, P. (2007). The reciprocal relation between principles and practice: Social psychology and health behavior. In A. Kruglanski & E. T. Higgins (Eds.), *Social psychology: Handbook of basic principles* (2nd ed., pp. 826–849). New York, NY: Guilford Press.

Rothman, A. J., Sheeran, P., & Wood, W. (2009). Reflective and automatic processes in the initiation and maintenance of food choices. *Annals of Behavioral Medicine, 38*, S4–S17.

Ryan, R. M., & Deci, E. L. (2000). Self-determination theory and the facilitation of intrinsic motivation, social development and well-being. *American Psychologist, 55*, 68–78.

Schwartz, M. D., Taylor, K. L., Willard, K. S., Siegel, J. E., Lamdan, R. M., & Moran, K. (1999). Distress, personality, and mammography utilization among women with a family history of breast cancer. *Health Psychology, 18*, 327–332.

Schwarzer, R., Schuz, B., Ziegelmann, J. P., Lippke, S., Luszczynska, A., & Scholz, U. (2007). Adoption and maintenance of four health behaviors: Theory-guided longitudinal studies on dental flossing, seat belt use, dietary behavior, and physical activity. *Annals of Behavioral Medicine, 33*, 156–166.

Silva, M. N., Markland, D., Carraça, E. V., Vieira, P. N., Coutinho, S. R., Minderico, C. S., et al. (2011). Exercise autonomous motivation predicts 3-year weight loss in women. *Medicine and Science in Sports and Exercise, 43*, 728–737.

Skinner, B. F. (1953). *Science and Human Behavior.* Cambridge, MA: B.F. Skinner Foundation.

Slater, J. S., Henly, G. A., Ha, C. N., Malone, M. E., Nyman, J. A., Diaz, S., & McGovern, P. G. (2005). Effect of direct mail as a population-based strategy to increase mammography use among low-income underinsured women ages 40–64 years. *Cancer Epidemiology, Biomarkers and Prevention, 14*, 2346–2352.

Sniehotta, F. F., Scholz, U., & Schwarzer, R. (2005). Bridging the intention–behaviour gap: Planning, self-efficacy, and action control in the adoption and maintenance of physical exercise. *Psychology & Health, 20*, 143–160.

Svetkey, L. P., Stevens, V. J., Brantley, P. J., Appel, L. J., Hollis, J. F., Loria, C. M., et al. (2008). Comparison of strategies for sustaining weight loss: The weight loss maintenance randomized controlled trial. *JAMA, 299*, 1139–1148.

Tam, L., Bagozzi, R. P., & Spanjol, J. (2010). When planning is not enough: The self-regulatory effect of implementation intentions on changing snacking habits. *Health Psychology, 29*, 284–292.

Tversky, A., & Kahneman, D. (1991). Loss aversion in riskless choice: A reference-dependent model. *The Quarterly Journal of Economics, 106*, 1039–1061.

U.S. Department of Health and Human Services. (2011). *Health indicators warehouse.* Retrieved from http://healthindicators.gov

Volpp, K. G., John, L. K., Troxel, A. B., Norton, L., Fassbender, J., & Loewenstein, G. (2008). Financial incentive–based approaches for weight loss. *JAMA, 300*, 2631–2637.

Volpp, K. G., Troxel, A. B., Pauly, M. V., Glick, H. A., Puig, A., Asch, D. A., et al. (2009). A randomized, controlled trial of financial incentives for smoking cessation. *New England Journal of Medicine, 360*, 699–709.

Wadden, T. A., Crerand, C. E., & Brock, J. (2005). Behavioral treatment of obesity. *The Psychiatric clinics of North America, 28*, 151–170.

West, D. S., Gorin, A. A., Subak, L. L., Foster, G., Bragg, C., Hecht, J., et al. (2011). A motivation-focused weight loss maintenance program is an effective alternative to a skill-based approach. *International Journal of Obesity, 35*, 259–269.

Williams, G. C., Gagne, M., Ryan, R. M., & Deci, E. L. (2002). Facilitating autonomous motivation for smoking cessation. *Health Psychology, 21*, 40–50.

Williams, G. C., Grow, V. M., Freedman, Z. R., Ryan, R. M., & Deci, E. L. (1996). Motivational predictors of weight loss and weight-loss maintenance. *Journal of Personality and Social Psychology, 70*, 115–126.

Williams, G. C., Lynch, M., & Glasgow, R. E. (2007). Computer-assisted intervention improves patient-centered diabetes care by increasing autonomy support. *Health Psychology, 26*, 728–734.

Williams, G. C., McGregor, H. A., Zeldman, A., Freedman, Z. R., & Deci, E. L. (2004). Testing a self-determination theory process model for promoting glycemic control through diabetes self-management. *Health Psychology, 23*, 58–66.

Williams, G. C., Niemiec, C. P., Patrick, H., Ryan, R. M., & Deci, E. L. (2009). The importance of supporting autonomy and perceived competence in facilitating long-term tobacco abstinence. *Annals of Behavioral Medicine, 37*, 315–324.

Williams, G. C., Rodin, G. C., Ryan, R. M., Grolnick, W. S., & Deci, E. L. (1998). Autonomous regulation and long-term medication adherence in adult outpatients. *Health Psychology, 17*, 269–276.

Williams-Piehota, P., Latimer, A. E., Katulak, N. A., Cox, A., Silvera, S. A., Mowad, L., & Salovey, P. (2009). Tailoring messages to individual differences in monitoring-blunting styles to increase fruit and vegetable intake. *Journal of Nutrition Education and Behavior, 41*, 398–405.

Williams-Piehota, P., Pizarro, J., Navarro Silvera, S. A., Mowad, L., & Salovey, P. (2006). Need for cognition and message complexity in motivating fruit and vegetable intake among callers to the cancer information service. *Health Communication, 19*, 75–84.

Wing, R. R., Tate, D. F., Gorin, A. A., Raynor, H. A., & Fava, J. L. (2006). A self-regulation program for maintenance of weight loss. *The New England Journal of Medicine, 355*, 1563–1571.

Ziegelmann, J. P., Lippke, S., & Schwarzer, R. (2006). Adoption and maintenance of physical activity: Planning interventions in young, middle-aged, and older adults. *Psychology & Health, 21*, 145–163.

Uncertainty and Ambiguity in Health Decisions

10

Paul K.J. Han

- The evidence-based medicine (EBM) and growing shared decision-making (SDM) movements have increased the amount, visibility, and importance of uncertainty in health care, and make it imperative to understand how uncertainty affects decision-making and other psychological outcomes, and how these outcomes can be optimized.
- The three main sources of uncertainty in health care are: (1) probability—the randomness of future outcomes; (2) ambiguity—lack of reliability, inadequate, or imprecise information; (3) complexity—aspects of decision-relevant information that make it difficult to understand.
- Ambiguity is the most prominent source of uncertainty in health decisions, and attributable to insufficient or conflicting scientific evidence regarding the net benefits and harms of a given intervention for an individual patient. Therefore, ambiguity is the primary rationale for shared decision-making.
- Ambiguous information about health risks leads to heightened perceptions of risks, and ambiguity concerning the outcomes of health-protective measures makes people less willing to adopt them.
- Uncertainty arising from conflicting evidence alone, even without numeric estimates of probability, leads to avoidance of decision-making a phenomenon known as "conflict aversion"
- Ambiguity may diminish perceptions of trust and the credibility of information or its source, affect emotions as well as cognitions, and increase anxiety.
- Moderators of ambiguity aversion include the emotional state of the decision-maker, whether gains or losses are at stake, negative mood states, personality, self-perceptions of competence, and motivational factors.
- The objective is to enable patients and clinicians to effectively manage the ambiguity that increasingly pervades all health decisions due to escalating efforts to promote shared decision-making.

Introduction

Uncertainty is central to health decisions across the entire continuum of medical care—from disease prevention and screening, to disease treatment, to end-of-life care. For numerous decisions in all these domains, uncertainty is not

P.K.J. Han (✉)
Center for Outcomes Research and Evaluation,
Maine Medical Center, 39 Forest Avenue, Portland,
ME 04101, USA
e-mail: hanp@mmc.org

© Springer Science+Business Media New York 2016
M.A. Diefenbach et al. (eds.), *Handbook of Health Decision Science*,
DOI 10.1007/978-1-4939-3486-7_10

only a complicating factor but a precondition for the decisions themselves. Should a 50-year-old man have prostate-specific antigen (PSA) testing to screen for prostate cancer? Should a 60-year-old woman with chronic stable angina undergo coronary artery bypass graft surgery? Should a 70-year-old man with severe chronic obstructive pulmonary disease be referred for hospice care? In cases like this there would be no decision to make if uncertainty did not exist— i.e., if the right course of action was clear. Uncertainty is the omnipresent problem that makes these and many other health decisions both possible and necessary.

The centrality of uncertainty in healthcare decisions raises the need to understand its effects on patients and clinicians, and recent healthcare trends have heightened this need. The evidence-based medicine (EBM) movement has not only expanded the base of scientific knowledge supporting medical decisions, but highlighted substantial limitations in this knowledge. At the same time, an increasing cultural emphasis on patient autonomy and informed patient choice, manifest by the growing shared decision-making (SDM) movement, has created an ethical imperative to communicate these limitations to clinicians and patients. These convergent trends have increased the amount, visibility, and importance of uncertainty in health care, and make it imperative to understand how uncertainty affects decision-making and other psychological outcomes, and how these outcomes can be optimized.

In the current chapter, I will address this task by providing an overview of important theoretical and empirical work on the effects of uncertainty in healthcare decisions. I will first discuss the concept of uncertainty and provide a working definition to guide further analysis and discussion. I will then review theory and evidence on the effects of one important type of uncertainty, known as "ambiguity" or "epistemic uncertainty," on health decisions and patient well-being. I will argue that ambiguity in healthcare decisions has important psychological effects that need to be better understood and accounted for, and I will suggest potentially fruitful directions for future research in this area.

Varieties of Uncertainty in Health Decisions

Any discussion of uncertainty in health decisions must begin by establishing a working definition of the concept, since the term "uncertainty" has multiple meanings. Following Smithson (1989) and recent work on this topic (Han et al. 2011), I define uncertainty as the *subjective consciousness of ignorance*. As such, uncertainty is a metacognition characterized by one's self-awareness of incomplete knowledge about some aspect of the world. In health care as well as all other domains of life, this metacognitive awareness of ignorance arises from multiple sources and pertains to multiple issues. The three main sources are (Fig. 1): (1) probability, (2) ambiguity, and (3) complexity (Han et al. 2011). *Probability* (otherwise known as "risk") refers to the fundamental indeterminacy or randomness of future outcomes, and has also been termed "aleatory" or "first-order" uncertainty; the exemplar in health care is the point estimate of risk (e.g., "20% probability of benefit from treatment") or a clinical practice guideline or recommendation (e.g., "all breast cancer patients with Stage I disease should undergo lumpectomy and radiotherapy"). *Ambiguity* refers to the lack of reliability, credibility, or adequacy of information about probability, and is thus also known as "epistemic" or "second-order" uncertainty (Camerer and Weber 1992). Ambiguity arises in situations in which the risk information needed for decision-making is unavailable, inadequate, or imprecise; the exemplar is the confidence interval around a point estimate (e.g., "10–30 % probability of benefit from treatment"), or formal ratings statements to grade the quality of evidence supporting clinical practice guidelines (e.g., "The available evidence is insufficient to assess effects on health outcomes"). *Complexity* refers to features of decision-relevant information that make it difficult to understand; examples include the presence of conditional probabilities or of multiplicity in risk factors, outcomes, or decisional alternatives, which diminish their comprehensibility or produce information overload.

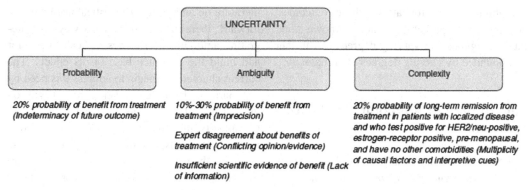

Examples and representations of different sources of uncertainty in the example of response to breast cancer treatment

Fig. 1 Sources of uncertainty in clinical evidence (Han et al. 2011)

These three fundamental *sources* of uncertainty—probability, ambiguity, complexity—are manifest in a variety of concrete, substantive *issues*, which can be usefully conceptualized as falling into three main categories—scientific, practical, and personal (Fig. 2) (Han et al. 2011). Scientific uncertainty in health decisions encompasses uncertainties about diagnosis, prognosis, causal explanations, and treatment recommendations. Practical uncertainty applies to the structures and processes of care; examples include uncertainty about the competence of one's healthcare providers, the quality of care one can expect to receive, or the procedures one must undertake to access care. Personal uncertainty pertains to psychosocial and existential issues including the effects of one's illness or treatment on one's goals or outlook on life, personal relationships, or sense of meaning in life. Scientific uncertainty is disease-centered, whereas practical and personal uncertainties are system- and patient-centered, respectively. Importantly, for all these specific *issues* of uncertainty—scientific, practical, and personal—the underlying cause may be any of the *sources* comprising the first dimension of uncertainty (probability, ambiguity, complexity). Any or all of these sources may engender uncertainty about not only diagnosis, prognosis, causal explanations, and treatment recommendations (scientific uncertainty) but also the expected quality of care and the procedures required to access care (practical uncertainty), as well as the effects of illness or treatment on one's personal relationships and goals in life (personal uncertainty). In theory,

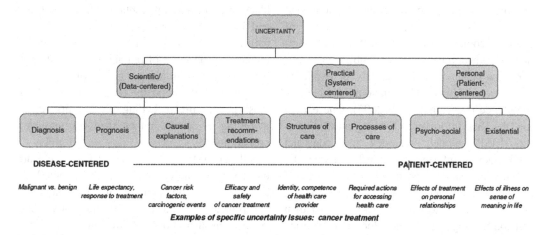

Examples of specific uncertainty issues: cancer treatment

Fig. 2 Issues of uncertainty in clinical evidence (Han et al. 2011)

probabilities exist for all of these outcomes, although these probabilities are unknown—and thus ambiguous—in varying degrees and further compounded by varying degrees of complexity.

The Primacy of Ambiguity in Health Decisions

Although probability, ambiguity, and complexity are each important and pervasive in health decisions, the current chapter focuses on ambiguity because it is the most prominent source of uncertainty in "preference-sensitive" health decisions for which clinical equipoise exists and shared decision-making is thought to be essential. In these situations, the predominant uncertainty is epistemic and attributable to insufficient or conflicting scientific evidence regarding the net benefits and harms of a given intervention for an individual patient. If sufficient evidence did exist, the course of action would be clear and less dependent on patient preferences. Ambiguity is thus the primary driver of shared decision-making.

Yet in spite of significant progress in understanding the nature and effects of ambiguity in decisions making generally, the effects of ambiguity on health decisions have received disproportionately little attention from behavioral researchers and are thus less well characterized than those of probability. For example, a great deal of research has been devoted to describing how risk perceptions affect health decisions, and perceived risk (or "perceived likelihood") of health outcomes is a central construct in several theories of health behavior. In contrast, no major theory of health behavior directly or explicitly integrates ambiguity, although some allude to its importance (Leventhal et al. 2003). One exception, the Risk Information Seeking and Processing (RISP) model, includes the construct "sufficiency of information" (Griffin et al. 1999, 2004), which can be construed as the inverse of ambiguity. However, the RISP model focuses solely on health information seeking rather than decision-making per se, and does not integrate insights from the large behavioral decision theory

literature on ambiguity. The critical need moving forward, therefore, is to develop ways of integrating ambiguity in theories of health behavior and build the evidence base on its effects. The current chapter will begin to address this need by summarizing theoretical and empirical insights on the effects of ambiguity in health decisions. Complexity, the other major source of uncertainty in health decisions, also deserves greater attention although theory and evidence on its effects are even less well developed, and discussion of this topic is beyond the scope of the current analysis.

Effects of Ambiguity in Decision-Making: Ambiguity Aversion

Ambiguity, otherwise known as epistemic or "second order" uncertainty—i.e., uncertainty *about* probability—has been recognized by behavioral scientists as a key source of uncertainty since the classic work of Ellsberg in (1961), who showed that in games of chance, people show a clear preference against choice options involving unknown (ambiguous) versus known probabilities—a phenomenon known as "ambiguity aversion" (Camerer and Weber 1992; Ellsberg 1961). In Ellsberg's original decision-making paradigm, which has subsequently come to be known as the "Ellsberg paradox," subjects were asked their preferences for betting between two events involving equal likelihoods of winning: (1) drawing a red (or black) ball from an urn containing exactly 50 red and 50 black balls, or (2) drawing a red (or black) ball from an urn containing 100 balls in an unknown proportion of red and black. Although the likelihood of drawing a given colored ball in each case is theoretically equivalent ($P = 0.5$), most people prefer betting on the first event involving a certain rather than an uncertain probability.

Ellsberg (1961) thus deduced that "there are uncertainties that are not risks," that people base risky decisions upon judgments about not only the probability and utility of alternative outcomes, but also about a "third dimension"—the "nature of one's information" concerning the likelihood of these outcomes. This phenomenon represents a violation of rational decision-making axioms (specifically, Savage's "sure-thing principle") of subjective expected utility theory. Ambiguity aversion is nonrational from a normative standpoint, furthermore, since probability itself should arguably already encompass uncertainty about the future (Howard 1988; Morgan et al. 2009); nevertheless, from a descriptive standpoint it is a valid account of how people behave. When information is ambiguous, decision-makers behave as though the likelihood associated with the ambiguous option is lower than it really is, and they favor the unambiguous option. Ambiguity aversion thus amounts to a pessimistic bias that Viscusi (1997) has described as an "alarmist response" to risk information, a systematic tendency of decision-makers to "devote excessive attention to the worst case scenarios" contained in ambiguous risk information. This pessimistic bias has been shown to be robust, persisting even when odds favor the ambiguous option (Curley and Yates 1985, 1989; Keren and Gerritsen 1999).

This aversion to unknown versus known probabilities is also observed when ambiguity pertaining to probabilities is operationalized in other ways. For example, when decision-makers are presented with probability estimates in which second-order uncertainty is described by confidence intervals, they form pessimistic judgments of these estimates and avoid decision-making (Han et al. 2011b; Kuhn 1997; Kuhn and Budescu 1996; Viscusi 1997; Viscusi et al. 1999). Evidence from experiments incorporating hypothetical health-related decisions has shown that ambiguous information about health risks leads to heightened perceptions of these risks, and that ambiguity concerning the outcomes of health-protective measures makes people less willing to adopt them (Ritov and Baron 1990; Viscusi 1997; Viscusi et al. 1991). Communicating ambiguity about cancer risk estimates has been shown to increase cancer risk perceptions and worry (Han et al. 2011b). These responses provide further proof that ambiguity is an influential factor in judgment and decision-making—over and above the influence of probability itself—and that its effects generalize not only to different representations of epistemic uncertainty, but to different decision-making domains including health.

Importantly, ambiguity aversion also generalizes to choice situations that do not involve explicit probability estimates. Epistemic uncertainty arising from conflicting evidence alone, even without numeric estimates of probability, also leads to avoidance of decision-making—an effect Smithson has called "conflict aversion" (Smithson 1999). Supporting evidence for this effect in the health domain includes intervention studies that have demonstrated that informing people about uncertainties concerning cancer screening measures decreases their interest in screening (Frosch et al. 2003; Volk et al. 2003). Perceptions of ambiguity regarding expert recommendations for cancer prevention and screening have been shown to be negatively associated with both cancer-protective behaviors and perceptions that may influence these behaviors (Han et al. 2006, 2007a, b).

Ambiguity Aversion: Associated Effects

Most experimental research on ambiguity aversion has been undertaken in the field of behavioral economics, and has consequently focused on the effects of ambiguity on decisions and risk perceptions in hypothetical games of chance. Yet ambiguity may affect other psychological outcomes and be manifest in ways other than the avoidance of decision-making and pessimistic appraisals of risk that classically define ambiguity aversion.

For example, ambiguity may have cognitive effects other than heightened risk perceptions. It stands to reason that ambiguity would diminish perceptions of trust and the credibility of information or its source, given that lack of credibility of risk information is part of the definition of ambiguity itself. These effects have been a great concern of policy analysts although they have not been extensively studied, and evidence for their extent is limited (Frewer 2004; Frewer et al. 2002; Gutscher et al. 2012; Johnson and Slovic 1995).

Other potential cognitive outcomes of ambiguity have been identified in nonexperimental studies in the healthcare domain. In survey-based studies, perceived ambiguity regarding cancer prevention recommendations have been found to be associated with diminished perceptions of the preventability of cancer (Han et al. 2006, 2007b). A longitudinal study showed that perceived ambiguity regarding recommendations for mammography screening was associated with reduced intentions for mammography as well as diminished future uptake of mammography (Han et al. 2007a). Another study showed that the communication of scientific uncertainty (including both probability and ambiguity) to breast cancer patients was associated with reduced satisfaction with decision-making, another important decision-related cognition (Politi et al. 2011).

Finally, ambiguity may affect emotions as well as cognitions. A substantial body of research in clinical psychology has shown that uncertainty more generally (involving various sources aside from ambiguity) is associated with anxiety, and patients with anxiety disorders are thought to exhibit a pathological propensity to appraise uncertain situations in a negative manner (Buhr and Dugas 2002; Ladouceur et al. 1997). It stands to reason that ambiguity is also anxiety provoking, and one experimental study in the healthcare domain showed that exposing ambiguity in cancer risk information (manifest by imprecision in risk estimates, represented using confidence intervals) led to heightened cancer worry (Han et al. 2011b).

Moderators of Ambiguity Aversion

As the foregoing review has shown, ambiguity aversion is a robust effect that generalizes to different operationalizations of ambiguity, types of evidence, and choice domains; however, it is not universal. In experimental manipulations of the Ellsberg paradox, for example, a substantial minority of decision-makers—more than 30 % in some studies—exhibit either ambiguity indifference or ambiguity seeking (Camerer and Weber 1992; Einhorn and Hogarth 1986). Ambiguity aversion is thus clearly a moderated phenomenon, and some of the factors that influence it have begun to be identified.

Aspects of both the decision and the evidence at hand may moderate ambiguity aversion. In choice situations involving probabilities, one influential factor may be the magnitude of the probabilities at hand. When the unambiguous option is associated with very low probabilities, decision-makers become indifferent to ambiguity and may even seek it (Curley and Yates 1989; Einhorn and Hogarth 1985; Lauriola and Levin 2001). There is also some evidence that ambiguity aversion depends on whether gains or losses are at stake (Camerer and Weber 1992; Einhorn and Hogarth 1986; Kahn and Sarin 1988; Viscusi and Chesson 1999). With potential gains (e.g., winning money) people are ambiguity averse, while with potential losses (e.g., losing money) people are ambiguity seeking, although this finding has not been consistently obtained (Keren and Gerritsen 1999). Accumulating evidence also suggests that the source of ambiguity moderates ambiguity aversion; specifically, decision-makers demonstrate greater aversion to ambiguity arising from conflicting than from imprecise risk information (Cabantous 2007; Smithson, 1999).

The emotional state of the decision-maker is another factor that may moderate ambiguity aversion, although evidence supporting this possibility is mostly indirect. For example, research studies examining people's responses to ambiguous information have shown that anxiety leads to cognitive processing biases in the interpretation of ambiguous information (Beck et al. 1986; Lawson and MacLeod 1999; MacLeod and Cohen 1993). These biases are both attentional and interpretive; individuals with both trait and state anxiety attend selectively to threat-related information, while also imposing threatening or pessimistic interpretations on ambiguous stimuli (Calvo and Castillo 1997; Hazlett-Stevens and Borkovec 2004; MacLeod and Cohen 1993; Mathews and MacLeod 1994). Negative mood states also have been shown to bias risk-related perceptions and judgments in situations that are ambiguous with respect to their certainty or controllability; fear leads to pessimistic risk estimates and risk-averse choices, while anger leads to optimistic risk estimates and risk-seeking choices (Calvo and Castillo 1997; Hazlett-Stevens and Borkovec 2004; Lerner and Keltner 2000, 2001; MacLeod and Cohen 1993; Mathews and MacLeod 1994). In the health domain, cancer fear has also been shown to increase people's tendency to interpret ambiguous information about cancer in a negative manner (Miles et al. 2009). Cross-sectional data has also suggested that cancer worry may moderate ambiguity aversion (Han et al. 2006).

Individual personality differences may also moderate ambiguity aversion. Dispositional optimism, perhaps the most well established of these differences, has been shown in several studies to be associated with less aversive responses to ambiguous probabilities (Bier and Connell 1994; Han et al. 2011; Highhouse 1994; Pulford 2009). Ambiguity aversion (or its complement, ambiguity tolerance) itself may be a fundamental, stable personality trait. Aversion ambiguity to as a trait characteristic has been directly measured in one recent study (Han et al. 2009); however, this measure has not been validated. There have been no other attempts to measure aversion to Ellsberg-type ambiguity as a personality trait, although researchers from various psychological disciplines have developed measures of tolerance or intolerance of "uncertainty" as a more general phenomenon, which appears to be phenomenologically related to ambiguity aversion. These include measures of "tolerance of ambiguity" (Budner 1962; Furnham and Ribchester 1995), "need for cognitive closure" (Kruglanski and Webster 1996), "uncertainty orientation" (Sorrentino et al. 1988), and "intolerance of uncertainty" (Buhr and Dugas 2002). In the health domain, related measures include "tolerance for ambiguity" (Geller et al. 1990, 1993), "monitoring and blunting" (Miller 1987), and physicians' reactions to uncertainty (Gerrity et al. 1990). It stands to reason that individual differences in these traits should

moderate ambiguity aversion, although this has yet to be conclusively shown and at least one study failed to demonstrate a relationship between ambiguity aversion and "tolerance of ambiguity" as assessed by a measure developed in the distant past by Budner (1962; Cabantous 2007). However, the Budner measure showed poor reliability in that study ($\alpha = 0.41$), and its content validity for assessing tolerance of "ambiguity" of the Ellsberg variety (epistemic uncertainty) is also debatable.

Causes of Ambiguity Aversion

Although progress has been made in identifying various moderators of ambiguity aversion, the phenomenon's ultimate causes have yet to be determined and alternative theoretical explanations have been proposed. One is the so-called "competence hypothesis" (Heath and Tversky 1991), which postulates that ambiguity aversion is driven primarily by decision-makers' self-perceived level of knowledge and skill in the decision-making task at hand. When decision-makers perceive that they are relatively uniformed or incompetent, they avoid decision-making. Presumably, this is the case in the Ellsberg paradox, an unfamiliar gambling scenario in which subjects lack knowledge that presumably others (e.g., the experimenter) might know. In contrast, ambiguity aversion has been shown to be diminished in circumstances where people possess greater knowledge and competence in decision-making (Heath and Tversky 1991). An extension of this explanation is the "comparative ignorance hypothesis" (Fox and Tversky 1995; Fox and Weber 2002), which postulates that ambiguity aversion results from an implicit comparison with less ambiguous events or with more knowledgeable individuals. According to this hypothesis, it is the process of comparison that is essential to ambiguity aversion; the contrast between an ambiguous and less ambiguous prospect or information source "makes the less familiar bet less attractive or the more familiar bet more attractive" (Fox and Tversky 1995).

Supporting this hypothesis, ambiguity aversion has been shown to disappear in noncomparative contexts involving evaluation of ambiguous prospects in isolation. This effect, however, does not completely account for ambiguity aversion since other studies have demonstrated ambiguity-averse responses even in noncomparative conditions (Arlo-Costa and Helzner 2005; Chow and Sarin 2001).

Nevertheless, available evidence suggests that self-perceptions of competence and comparative judgments of ambiguity in choice circumstances do play a major role in ambiguity aversion (Klein et al. 2010), and that specific motivations underlie this phenomenon. Frisch and Baron (1988) have argued that ambiguity aversion manifests decision-makers' use of a "missing information" heuristic that biases people against making decisions or taking action when information is incomplete, and that use of this heuristic is greater when decision-makers perceive that missing information is knowable by others. The underlying reason postulated by several investigators (Curley et al. 1986; Heath and Tversky 1991) is that people are concerned about how their decisions will be evaluated by others, and desire to justify their decisions and avoid blame for making bad decisions based on insufficient information. This social motivation, characterized more specifically as "fear of negative evaluation" (FNE), has been experimentally shown to be a powerful determinant of ambiguity aversion (Trautman et al. 2008). In the same vein, other experimental data has shown that manipulating the Ellsberg task to make it a cooperative venture undertaken with a partner or friend—rather than a competitive task against a more knowledgeable but potentially hostile opponent—leads people to be ambiguity indifferent or even ambiguity seeking (Kuhberger and Perner 2003). Collectively, these data suggest that social motivations play a key role in ambiguity aversion. An open question for the future, however, is whether social motivations exert the same strong influence in both experimental and real choice tasks other than the Ellsberg paradigm.

Ambiguity Aversion in Health Decisions: Implications and Future Research Needs

Available evidence suggests that ambiguity has predictable and robust effects on judgments and decisions, some of which have begun to be demonstrated in the health domain. These effects have several important clinical implications that will be increasingly important to address as shared decision-making continues to become the new normative standard for health care, increasing the production and consumption of ambiguity in health decisions. These implications, in turn, point to several specific gaps in our knowledge that represent fruitful targets for future research.

First, although ambiguity is ethically necessary to communicate to patients, it is psychologically aversive and may lead to undesired outcomes. In theory, communicating ambiguity maximizes patient autonomy by allowing them to decide for themselves whether the available scientific evidence justifies action. Ambiguity aversion could thus be construed as an adaptive response, promoting appropriate skepticism and conservatism in the face of scientific uncertainty. On the other hand, the outcomes that characterize ambiguity aversion—heightened risk perceptions and worry, pessimistic judgments of the benefits and harms of medical intervention, avoidance of decision-making—may diminish patient well-being and lead to refusal of potentially beneficial interventions. Ambiguity aversion thus presents a major challenge for efforts to promote shared decision-making. It calls for a greater understanding of the circumstances in which the communication of ambiguity is appropriate and necessary, and the optimal methods for both communicating ambiguity and mitigating ambiguity aversion—i.e., improving ambiguity tolerance among patients and clinicians.

Second, both theoretical and empirical work is needed to better understand the phenomenon of ambiguity in health decisions. Conceptual research is needed to specify the circumstances in which the communication of ambiguity is ethically justified, and to incorporate ambiguity in broader explanatory theories of health behavior. Such work could then provide the basis for empirical studies aimed at testing how ambiguity interacts with cognitive and other factors in influencing health judgments and decisions, and elucidating the mechanisms of ambiguity aversion as a more general phenomenon in real-world decision-making. This remains an important need given that existing hypotheses do not fully account for ambiguity aversion. The comparative ignorance hypothesis, for example, is an inadequate causal explanation since ambiguity aversion also occurs in noncomparative choice contexts. It is possible that the validity of the comparative ignorance hypothesis is a function of the experimental paradigm typically used to demonstrate ambiguity aversion (hypothetical gambling scenarios involving an uninformed subject and a potentially knowledgeable but untrustworthy experimenter). In other types of actual choice situations such as healthcare decision-making, comparative ignorance may play a lesser causal role.

More work is also needed to identify what factors moderate ambiguity aversion. A clearer understanding of these factors could help clinicians identify decision and patient characteristics that place people at risk for aversive reactions to the communication of ambiguity. Past research has identified some important moderators of ambiguity aversion, including individual differences such as dispositional optimism. On the other hand, a great deal of work has isolated tolerance or intolerance of uncertainty and ambiguity as a fundamental trait-level moderating factor of its own. The open question is whether tolerance or intolerance of uncertainty and ambiguity can be reduced to other, more fundamental psychological characteristics or processes, as opposed to being conceptualized and measured as an irreducible individual difference in its own right.

From a clinical and health policy perspective, the ultimate goal of research on ambiguity is to develop interventions to mitigate ambiguity aversion—i.e., to enable patients and clinicians to tolerate the ambiguity that increasingly pervades all health decisions due to the burgeoning efforts to promote shared decision-making. This type of work is in its infancy, but at least two potential approaches exist. The first focuses on the cognitive dimension of communication and the development of representational methods that convey ambiguous information in a manner that reduces ambiguity aversion. Evidence from at least one study suggests that visual representations of uncertainty may be effective in reducing aversion to ambiguity regarding individualized disease risk estimates (Han et al. 2011b). The second approach focuses not on the cognitive dimension of communication, but on the provision of psychological support in health decision-making under ambiguity. The essential components remain to be defined, but likely involve factors that are not strictly cognitive—e.g., empathy, relationship building between patients and clinicians, emotional support. These components of "patient-centered communication" (Epstein and Street 2007) may be most important means of improving tolerance of ambiguity; however, they are the least understood and represent a key focus for future research.

References

Arlo-Costa, H., & Helzner, J. (2005). *Comparative ignorance and the Ellsberg phenomenon*. Paper presented at the 4th International Symposium on Imprecise Probabilities and their Applications.

Beck, A. T., Emery, G., & Greenberg, R. C. (1986). *Anxiety disorders and phobias: A cognitive perspective*. New York: Guilford Press.

Bier, V. M., & Connell, B. L. (1994). Ambiguity seeking in multi-attribute decisions: Effects of optimism and message framing. *Journal of Behavioral Decision Making, 7*, 169–182.

Budner, S. (1962). Intolerance of ambiguity as a personality variable. *Journal of Personality, 30*, 29–59.

Buhr, K., & Dugas, M. (2002). Intolerance for uncertainty scale: Psychometric properties of the English version. *Behaviour Research and Therapy, 40*, 931–946.

Cabantous, L. (2007). Ambiguity aversion in the field of insurance: Insurers' attitude to imprecise and conflicting probability estimates. *Theory and Decision, 62*, 219–240.

Calvo, M. G., & Castillo, M. D. (1997). Mood-congruent bias in interpretation of ambiguity: Strategic processes and temporary activation. *Quarterly Journal of Experimental Psychology, 50A*(1), 163–182.

Camerer, C., & Weber, M. (1992). Recent developments in modeling preferences: Uncertainty and ambiguity. *Journal of Risk and Uncertainty, 5*, 325–370.

Chow, C. C., & Sarin, R. K. (2001). Comparative ignorance and the Ellsberg Paradox. *Journal of Risk and Uncertainty, 22*(2), 129–139.

Curley, S. P., & Yates, J. F. (1985). The center and range of the probability interval as factors affecting ambiguity preferences. *Organizational Behavior and Human Decision Processes, 36*, 273–287.

Curley, S. P., & Yates, J. F. (1989). An empirical evaluation of descriptive models of ambiguity reactions in choice situations. *Journal of Mathematical Psychology, 33*, 397–427.

Curley, S. P., Yates, J. F., & Abrams, R. A. (1986). Psychological sources of ambiguity avoidance. *Organizational Behavior and Human Decision Processes, 38*, 230–256.

Einhorn, H. J., & Hogarth, R. M. (1985). Ambiguity and uncertainty in probabilistic inference. *Psychological Review, 92*(4), 433–461.

Einhorn, H. J., & Hogarth, R. M. (1986). Decision making under ambiguity. *Journal of Business, 59*(4), S225–S250.

Ellsberg, D. (1961). Risk, ambiguity, and the savage axioms. *Quarterly Journal of Economics, 75*, 643–669.

Epstein, R. M., & Street, R. L. J. (2007). *Patient-centered communication in cancer care: Promoting healing and reducing suffering* (p. 07-6225). Bethesda, MD: NIH Publication.

Fox, C. R., & Tversky, A. (1995). Ambiguity aversion and comparative ignorance. *Quarterly Journal of Economics, 110*, 585–603.

Fox, C. R., & Weber, M. (2002). Ambiguity aversion, comparative ignorance, and decision context. *Organizational Behavior and Human Decision Processes, 88*, 476–498.

Frewer, L. (2004). The public and effective risk communication. [Review]. *Toxicology Letters, 149*(1–3), 391–397.

Frewer, L. J., Miles, S., Brennan, M., Kuznesof, S., Ness, M., & Ritson, C. (2002). Public preferences for informed choice under conditions of risk uncertainty. *Public Understanding of Science, 11*, 363–372.

Frisch, D., & Baron, J. (1988). Ambiguity and rationality. *Journal of Behavioral Decision Making, 1*, 149–157.

Frosch, D. L., Kaplan, R. M., & Felitti, V. J. (2003). A randomized controlled trial comparing internet and video to facilitate patient education for men considering the prostate specific antigen test. *Journal of General Internal Medicine, 18*(10), 781–787.

Furnham, A., & Ribchester, T. (1995). Tolerance of ambiguity: A review of the concept, its measurement and applications. *Current Psychology, 14*(3), 179–199.

Geller, G., Faden, R. R., & Levine, D. M. (1990). Tolerance for ambiguity among medical students: Implications for their selection, training and practice. *Social Science and Medicine, 31*(5), 619–624.

Geller, G., Tambor, E. S., Chase, G. A., & Holtzman, N. A. (1993). Measuring physicians' tolerance for ambiguity and its relationship to their reported practices regarding genetic testing. *Medical Care, 31*(11), 989–1001.

Gerrity, M. S., DeVellis, R. F., & Earp, J. A. (1990). Physicians' reactions to uncertainty in patient care. A new measure and new insights. *Medical Care, 28*(8), 724–736.

Griffin, R. J., Dunwoody, S., & Neuwirth, K. (1999). Proposed model of the relationship of risk information seeking and processing to the development of preventive behaviors. [Research Support, Non-U.S. Gov't]. *Environmental Research, 80*(2 Pt 2), S230–S245.

Griffin, R. J., Neuwirth, K., Dunwoody, S., & Giese, J. (2004). Information sufficiency and risk communication. *Media Psychology, 6*, 23–61.

Gutscher, H., Earle, T., & Siegrist, M. (Eds.). (2012). *Trust in cooperative risk management: Uncertainty and scepticism in the public mind*. London: Routledge.

Han, P. K., Klein, W. M., & Arora, N. K. (2011a). Varieties of uncertainty in health care: A conceptual taxonomy. *An International Journal of the Society for Medical Decision Making, 31*(6), 828–838.

Han, P. K., Klein, W. M., Lehman, T., Killam, B., Massett, H., & Freedman, A. N. (2011b). Communication of uncertainty regarding individualized cancer risk estimates: Effects and influential factors. [Research Support, N.I.H., Intramural]. *An International Journal of the Society for Medical Decision Making, 31*(2), 354–366.

Han, P. K., Kobrin, S. C., Klein, W. M., Davis, W. W., Stefanek, M., & Taplin, S. H. (2007a). Perceived ambiguity about screening mammography recommendations: Association with future mammography uptake and perceptions. *Cancer Epidemiology Biomarkers and Prevention, 16*(3), 458–466.

Han, P. K., Moser, R. P., & Klein, W. M. (2006). Perceived ambiguity about cancer prevention recommendations: Relationship to perceptions of cancer preventability, risk, and worry. *Journal of Health Communication, 11*(Suppl 1), 51–69.

Han, P. K., Moser, R. P., & Klein, W. M. (2007b). Perceived ambiguity about cancer prevention recommendations: Associations with cancer-related perceptions and behaviours in a US population survey. *Health Expectations, 10*(4), 321–336.

Han, P. K., Reeve, B. B., Moser, R. P., & Klein, W. M. (2009). Aversion to ambiguity regarding medical tests and treatments: Measurement, prevalence, and relationship to sociodemographic factors. *Journal of Health Communication, 14*(6), 556–572.

Hazlett-Stevens, H., & Borkovec, T. D. (2004). Interpretive cues and ambiguity in generalized anxiety disorder. *Behaviour Research and Therapy, 42*(8), 881–892.

Heath, C., & Tversky, A. (1991). Preference and belief: Ambiguity and competence in choice under uncertainty. *Journal of Risk and Uncertainty, 4*, 5–28.

Highhouse, S. (1994). A verbal protocol analysis of choice under ambiguity. *J Economic Psychology, 15*, 621–635.

Howard, R. A. (1988). Uncertainty about probability: A decision analysis perspective. *Risk Analysis, 8*(1), 91–98.

Johnson, B. B., & Slovic, P. (1995). Presenting uncertainty in health risk assessment: Initial studies of its effects on risk perception and trust. *Risk Analysis, 15* (4), 485–494.

Kahn, B. E., & Sarin, R. K. (1988). Modeling ambiguity in decisions under uncertainty. *Journal of Consumer Research, 15*(2), 265–272.

Keren, G., & Gerritsen, L. E. M. (1999). On the robustness and possible accounts of ambiguity aversion. *Acta Psychologica, 103*, 149–172.

Klein, W. M. P., Cerully, J. L., Monin, M. M., & Moore, D. A. (2010). Ability, chance, and ambiguity aversion: Revisiting the competence hypothesis. *Judgment and Decision Making, 5*, 192–199.

Kruglanski, A. W., & Webster, D. M. (1996). Motivated closing of the mind: "Seizing" and "freezing". *Psychological Review, 103*(2), 263–283.

Kuhberger, A., & Perner, J. (2003). The role of competition and knowledge in the Ellsberg task. *Journal of Behavioral Decision Making, 16*, 181–191.

Kuhn, K. M. (1997). Communicating uncertainty: Framing effects on responses to vague probabilities. *Organizational Behavior and Human Decision Processes, 71*(1), 55–83.

Kuhn, K. M., & Budescu, D. V. (1996). The relative importance of probabilities, outcomes, and vagueness in hazard risk decisions. *Organizational Behavior and Human Decision Processes, 68*(3), 301–317.

Ladouceur, R., Talbot, F., & Dugas, M. J. (1997). Behavioral expressions of intolerance of uncertainty in worry. Experimental findings. *Behavior Modification, 21*(3), 355–371.

Lauriola, M., & Levin, I. P. (2001). Relating individual differences in attitude toward ambiguity to risky choices. *Journal of Behavioral Decision Making, 14* (2), 107–122.

Lawson, C., & MacLeod, C. (1999). Depression and the interpretation of ambiguity. *Behaviour Research and Therapy, 37*(5), 463–474.

Lerner, J. S., & Keltner, D. (2000). Beyond valence: Toward a model of emotion-specific influences on judgement and choice. *Cognition and Emotion, 14*(4), 473–493.

Lerner, J. S., & Keltner, D. (2001). Fear, anger, and risk. *Journal of Personality and Social Psychology, 81*(1), 146–159.

Leventhal, H., Brissette, I., & Leventhal, E. A. (2003). The common-sense model of self-regulation of health and illness. In L. D. Cameron & H. Leventhal (Eds.), *The Self-regulation of health and illness behaviour* (pp. 42–65). London: Routledge.

MacLeod, C., & Cohen, I. L. (1993). Anxiety and the interpretation of ambiguity: A text comprehension study. *Journal of Abnormal Psychology, 102*(2), 238–247.

Mathews, A. M., & MacLeod, C. (1994). Cognitive approaches to emotions and emotional disorders. *Annual Review of Psychology, 45*, 25–50.

Miles, A., Voorwinden, S., Mathews, A., Hoppitt, L. C., & Wardle, J. (2009). Cancer fear and the interpretation of ambiguous information related to cancer. *Cognition and Emotion, 23*, 701–713.

Miller, S. M. (1987). Monitoring and blunting: Validation of a questionnaire to assess styles of information seeking under threat. *Journal of Personality and Social Psychology, 52*(2), 345–353.

Morgan, G., Dowlatabadi, H., Henrion, M., Keith, D., Lempert, R., McBride, S., et al. (Eds.). (2009). *Best practice approaches for characterizing, communicating, and incorporating scientific uncertainty in decision making. A Report by the U.S. Climate Change Science Program and the Subcommittee on Global Change Research (Synthesis and Assessment Product 5.2M).* Washington, DC: National Oceanic and Atmospheric Administration, U.S. Climate Change Science Program.

Politi, M. C., Clark, M. A., Ombao, H., Dizon, D., & Elwyn, G. (2011). Communicating uncertainty can lead to less decision satisfaction: A necessary cost of involving patients in shared decision making? *Health Expectations, 14*(1), 84–91.

Pulford, B. D. (2009). Is luck on my side? Optimism, pessimism, and ambiguity aversion. *The Quarterly Journal of Experimental Psychology (Hove), 62*(6), 1079–1087.

Ritov, I., & Baron, J. (1990). Reluctance to vaccinate: Omission bias and ambiguity. *Journal of Behavioral Decision Making, 3*, 263–277.

Smithson, M. (1989). *Ignorance and uncertainty: Emerging paradigms.* New York: Springer.

Smithson, M. (1999). Conflict aversion: Preference for ambiguity versus conflict in sources and evidence. *Organizational Behavior and Human Decision Processes, 79*(3), 179–198.

Sorrentino, R. M., Bobocel, D. R., Gitta, M. Z., Olson, J. M., & Hewitt, E. C. (1988). Uncertainty orientation and persuasion: Individual differences in the effects of personal relevance on social judgments. *Journal of Personality and Social Psychology, 55*(3), 357–371.

Trautman, S. T., Vielder, F. M., & Wakker, P. P. (2008). Causes of ambiguity aversion: Known versus unknown preferences. *Journal of Risk and Uncertainty, 36*, 225–243.

Viscusi, W. K. (1997). Alarmist decisions with divergent risk information. *The Economic Journal, 107*, 1657–1670.

Viscusi, W. K., & Chesson, H. (1999). Hopes and fears: The conflicting effects of risk ambiguity. *Theory and Decision, 47*, 157–184.

Viscusi, W. K., Magat, W. A., & Huber, J. (1991). Communication of ambiguous risk information. *Theory and Decision, 31*, 159–173.

Viscusi, W. K., Magat, W. A., & Huber, J. (1999). Smoking status and public responses to ambiguous scientific risk evidence. *Southern Economic Journal, 66*(2), 250–270.

Volk, R. J., Spann, S. J., Cass, A. R., & Hawley, S. T. (2003). Patient education for informed decision making about prostate cancer screening: A randomized controlled trial with 1-year follow-up. *The Annals of Family Medicine, 1*(1), 22–28.

Adult Age Differences in Health-Related Decision-Making: A Primer

11

Corinna E. Löckenhoff, Chu Hsiao, Julia Kim and Katya Swarts

Across the industrialized world, older adults, especially those in their 80 and 90s, constitute the fastest-growing demographic group (CDC 2007). Compared to younger adults, they are at a disproportionate risk for a variety of acute and chronic conditions and thus more likely to face difficult healthcare choices (CDC 2007). Simultaneously, growing emphasis on informed choice encourages patients to take an active role in decision-making (Wennberg et al. 2007). Thus, there is a historical peak in the number of older patients, and they are more involved in their medical decisions than ever before. Moreover, age-related limitations in physical, interpersonal, and economic resources (Baltes 1997) may make it more difficult for older adults to recover from poor choices. Therefore, while sound decision-making skills are critical at any age, they are particularly important in the later years.

This chapter provides an overview of current research on decision-making in older adults (i.e., those 60 years and over) with particular emphasis on health-related choices. We begin with a review of potential mechanisms including cognitive and emotional aging, age-related motivational shifts, as well as aging stereotypes, and cohort effects. Next, we examine age differences in specific aspects of decision-making. We conclude with directions for future research and implications for practice.

C.E. Löckenhoff (✉)
Department of Human Development, Cornell University, G60B MVR Hall, Ithaca, NY 14853, USA
e-mail: CEL72@cornell.edu

C. Hsiao
College of Medicine, University of Florida, 1682 SW 16th St., Gainesville, FL 32608, USA
e-mail: chujhsiao@gmail.com

J. Kim
Western University of Health Sciences, 309 E. Second St., Pomona, CA 91766, USA
e-mail: juliajskim@gmail.com

K. Swarts
School of Medicine, University of Virginia, 870 Estes St., Charlottesville, VA 22903, USA
e-mail: katyaswarts@gmail.com

Potential Mechanisms of Age Differences in Decision-Making
Cognitive Aging

When considering cognitive aging, it is critical to differentiate between gradual changes found in healthy aging and the steep cognitive decline associated with dementia and other neurological conditions. There is no question that dementia, even in its early stages, severely limits decision-making capability (Frank et al. 1999). The effects of healthy aging, which are the focus of the present chapter, are more subtle (Salthouse and Davis 2006) and differ significantly for resource rich, deliberative processes (cognitive mechanics),

© Springer Science+Business Media New York 2016
M.A. Diefenbach et al. (eds.), *Handbook of Health Decision Science*,
DOI 10.1007/978-1-4939-3486-7_11

and intuitive, and experience-based processes (cognitive pragmatics).

Cognitive Mechanics

Well-documented age decrements in the acquisition and effortful processing of novel information may influence decision-making in a number of ways. Aging is associated with slower *processing speed* as well as limitations in *working memory*, the ability to manipulate small sets of information during ongoing tasks; *executive functioning*, the ability to systematically allocate processing resources (Salthouse and Davis 2006); *inhibitory processing*, the ability to suppress task-irrelevant materials (Kim et al. 2007); and *numeracy,* the ability to reason from numbers (Peters et al. 2007).

In combination, age deficits in deliberate processing may negatively affect older adults' choices, especially in complex decision scenarios that involve large amounts of information and a mix of relevant and irrelevant material. Nevertheless, apparent deficits in effortful cognition may sometimes represent an advantage. For instance, older adults' smaller working memory capacity may make them better at identifying associations (Healey and Hasher 2009), and limitations in the ability to screen out non-essential information may become advantageous if the information is useful in subsequent tasks (Kim et al. 2007).

Cognitive Pragmatics

In contrast to the downward age trajectory in effortful processing, acquired skills, knowledge, and experience remain fairly stable with age. While memory for specific situations and contexts shows marked age decrements, general world knowledge, or *crystallized intelligence* is well preserved (Salthouse and Davis 2006). Thus, older adults can draw on a rich knowledge base and may be able to retrieve preferences from memory instead of having to construct them on the spot. Further, as decision-makers acquire expertise, they shift from analytic decision styles toward *rule-based, heuristic* styles requiring less cognitive resources (Reyna and Brainerd 2011).

Older decision-makers may also engage in strategic resource allocation. According to the *Selective Optimization with Compensation* framework (Baltes 1997), older adults select personally relevant aspects of functioning, optimize them through targeted resource allocation, and use compensatory strategies (e.g., delegation, assistive technology) to address losses in other areas. In social reasoning tasks, for instance, older adults use more effortful strategies when personal relevance is high (Hess et al. 2001).

Overall, a reliance on prior experience and heuristic processing is likely to benefit older adults' choices, but there are some important caveats. First, although world knowledge is well-preserved, age decrements in *source memory* limit recall for the context in which a piece of information was first encountered (Spencer and Raz 1995). This may make it difficult to link choice characteristics to a specific option or result in faulty information being misremembered as accurate (Skurnik et al. 2005). Further, while heuristic decision strategies are low in cognitive effort, they may also give rise to systematic biases (Kahneman 2003).

Emotional Aging

Any meaningful choice involves not only deliberative and experiential reasoning but also emotional factors (Peters et al. 2007) that can be broadly grouped into *integral affect* (i.e., emotional responses to decision options) and *incidental affect* (i.e., decision-irrelevant mood states). Choices that require difficult trade-offs may also elicit *trade-off aversion* (Luce 2005), a negative emotional response that is not associated with specific outcomes but the decision process itself. To optimize choices, decision-makers need to attend to integral affect while simultaneously regulating incidental affect and trade-off aversion (Peters et al. 2007).

Realistic decisions also involve delayed outcomes and joint decisions requiring the accurate prediction of emotional responses in oneself and others (Löckenhoff 2011).

Research on emotional aging suggests that older adults are generally well-prepared for these challenges: *Emotional well-being* and the ability to regulate one's emotions remain fairly stable with age (Scheibe and Carstensen 2010), but age groups differ in preferred *emotion-regulatory strategies*. Compared to younger adults, older adults emphasize antecedent-focused strategies that aim to avoid aversive states over response-focused strategies such as emotional detachment or suppression (Urry and Gross 2010).

Insight into emotional processes is also well preserved with age. *Affective forecasting* of future emotional responses, shows age-related improvements (Nielsen et al. 2008), and older adults are less likely than younger adults to underestimate the intensity of their future emotions (Löckenhoff et al. 2011). Older adults are also high in *empathy* and well-attuned to the emotions of others. Although they have some difficulty discerning emotions from photos and videos (Ruffman et al. 2008), they perform well when material is presented verbally. *Emotional intelligence*, the understanding of others' mental states (Happé et al. 1998), and the ability to infer others' emotions (Richter and Kunzmann 2011) show age-related stability or improvements. Moreover, older adults show higher levels of *sympathy* with others' feelings (Richter and Kunzmann 2011).

Cognitive tasks that draw on *affective processing* are also relatively spared with age. When stimuli are emotionally neutral, working memory, source memory, and long-term recall show significant age-related decrements, but for emotionally salient material, few age differences are found (for a review see Scheibe and Carstensen 2010). In addition to a generalized focus on emotional material, older adults selectively allocate processing resources toward positive and away from negative material (Mather and Carstensen 2005). This *positivity effect* has been replicated across a spectrum of tasks ranging from neural activation (Samanez-Larkin et al. 2007) and attention (Isaacowitz and Choi 2011) to long-term recall (Kennedy et al. 2004).

Although affective processing, emotion regulation, and emotional awareness remain stable or even improve with age, age groups differ in specific strategies and this may affect decision making. On the one hand, high levels of positive emotions and a selective focus on positive material may make older adults less susceptible to aversive trade-offs and encourage creative choices (Isen and Labroo 2003). On the other hand, an exclusive focus on the positive could prevent older adults from processing aversive yet relevant information (Löckenhoff and Carstensen 2007).

To evaluate the implications of emotional aging for decision-making, it is critical to understand the underlying mechanisms. Some have interpreted favorable age trajectories as the result of decrements in neural functioning (Cacioppo et al. 2011) or a compensatory response to age-losses in cognitive mechanics (Labouvie-Vief et al. 2010). Others view emotion-rich reasoning as the hallmarks of a mature, experience-based decision-making style (Reyna and Brainerd 2011). Growing evidence suggests that age-related shifts in motivational priorities may play a role as well.

Motivational Priorities and Time Horizons

Life span theories of motivation have long emphasized the role of maturational processes and age-related losses (Baltes 1997), but recent theoretical developments have cast a spotlight on age-associated shifts in time horizons. According to Socioemotional Selectivity Theory (SST; Carstensen 2006), advancing age is associated with the awareness that future time horizons are shrinking and people adjust their goal priorities accordingly. Specifically, SST predicts that open-ended time horizons in young adulthood lead to a prioritization of goals and activities that benefit the future, such as the acquisition of new information or the establishment of new social contacts. In advanced age, as time horizons are shrinking, priorities are thought to shift toward optimizing immediate well-being via meaningful experiences and close relationships.

SST has been tested across many different contexts ranging from occupational settings to social partner preferences (for a review see Carstensen 2006). With regard to cognitive processing, the theory has informed research on the age-related positivity effect, arguing that older adults preferentially process emotionally salient and positive material because it benefits their emotional well-being (Carstensen 2006). Consistent with a motivational explanation, the positivity effect appears to require active cognitive control (Mather and Knight 2005) and is stronger when emotional goals are activated (Kennedy et al. 2004).

Applying SST to decision contexts, one would expect to find a positivity effect in information acquisition. Moreover, older adults' focus on emotion might make them more sensitive to incidental affect and trade-off aversion during difficult choices. Also, when weighing immediate versus delayed outcomes, older adults' focus on the present could lead them to prioritize current well-being at the expense of the future. Finally, because advanced age and limited time horizons are associated with an emphasis on close and emotionally rewarding relationships (Carstensen 2006), older adults may be more likely than younger adults to consider the opinions of others.

Cohort Effects and Aging Stereotypes

Age differences in decision-making may not only stem from changes in the individual but also reflect age- and history-graded factors at the societal level. *Cohort effects* capture the influence of unique historical environments on different birth cohorts. Life philosophies and values as well as nutrition habits are typically shaped during the late teens and early 20s and remain relatively stable thereafter (Schewe and Meredith 2004). Conceivably, attitudes toward health-related decisions may be acquired in similar ways. In particular, it has been suggested that older cohorts born up to WWII have been socialized to take a passive stance in their healthcare and defer to physicians' authority, whereas the baby boom cohorts and beyond are more likely to value active involvement and individual choice (Laganà and Shanks 2002).

Aging stereotypes, in turn, reflect societally shared beliefs about aging and older adults that may or may not accurately reflect reality (Hummert et al. 1994). Although aging stereotypes incorporate both positive and negative aspects (Hummert et al. 1994), there appears to be wide-spread agreement that physical health, the ability to perform everyday tasks, and new learning decrease with age (Löckenhoff et al. 2009). There are several pathways by which stereotypes of aging may influence health-related choices. First, the implicit activation of negative age stereotypes may inhibit cognitive performance, a phenomenon also referred to as 'stereotype threat' (for a review see Hess 2005). Second, older adults who accept stereotypes of physical aging may have low expectations for the success of medical treatments (Hudak et al. 2002). Finally, stereotypes of aging may bias healthcare providers, inhibit effective communication with older patients, and lead to an undertreatment of preventable health conditions because they are misconstrued as "normal" aging (Laganà and Shanks 2002).

In summary, age differences in decision-making may stem from a variety of factors ranging from cognitive pragmatics to goal priorities and societal influences. Of course, these variables do not operate in isolation but interact with each other as older individuals tackle realistic healthcare choices. While some factors may exacerbate each other, others may cancel each other out and lead to an apparent absence of age effects. In the remainder of this chapter, we discuss evidence for the relative role of these mechanisms in specific aspects of the decision-making process.

Age Differences in Health-Related Choices

Pre-decisional Information Seeking and Preferences for Choice

Across a wide range of decision domains, older adults not only show lower rates of pre-decisional information seeking than their younger counterparts (for a review see Mata and Nunes 2010), but they also make decisions more quickly (e.g., Meyer and Pollard 2004). In addition, older adults prefer to choose among fewer options than their younger counterparts. This pattern is found in hypothetical consumer and healthcare choices (Reed et al. 2008) and extends to clinical settings where older patients are less likely to seek second or third opinions (Meyer and Pollard 2004) or to consider multiple treatment approaches (Beisecker 1988).

At first glance, decrements in information seeking and reduced preferences for choice might be explained by global limitations in information processing capacity (Salthouse and Davis 2006). However, age effects also depend on contextual factors and differ across types of information. In particular, older adults are more likely than younger adults to focus on personally relevant information (Squiers et al. 2005) which may reflect the Selective Optimization with Compensation principle (Baltes 1997) in that limited processing resources are directed toward the most relevant information. Also, even though patients of all ages are increasingly likely to seek information online, older adults are less likely to follow this trend (Bennett et al. 2009)—most likely due to limited experience with computers.

Age differences in other aspects of information seeking are more troubling. When considering their choices, older adults may indeed be wearing the proverbial "rose-colored glasses". In health-related decision scenarios, older adults were found to review a disproportionate amount of positive information (Löckenhoff and Carstensen 2007). Moreover, although older adults may be more deferent to physicians' opinions (Laganà and Shanks 2002), they do not

necessarily turn to them for information: While information seeking from medical providers is negatively associated with age, information seeking from nonmedical sources such as family and friends is relatively spared (Bennett et al. 2009). This focus on positive information from close social partners is consistent with the age-related shifts in motivational priorities proposed by SST. In further support of this notion, older adults who showed a positivity effect in decision-making also reported limited future horizons and more positive emotional responses (Löckenhoff and Carstensen 2007, 2008).

In summary, older as compared to younger decision-makers seek less information and prefer information that is personally relevant, positive in valence, and drawn from sources outside of the medical establishment. Overall, age effects tend to be modest in size, and a recent simulation study suggests that reduced information seeking among older adults has only minor effects on decision quality (Mata and Nunes 2010). Nevertheless, seeking less information may sometimes cause problems. Laboratory research examining decisions about medication adherence found that lower information seeking is linked with higher error rates (Willis et al. 1999). In patient populations, reduced rates of information seeking may also limit access to supportive services (Bennett et al. 2009). Finally, older adults' tendencies to focus on the positive and seek information from social partners as opposed to the medical establishment could make them more susceptible to unproven medical practices or fraud.

Decision Strategies

Age groups also differ in specific decision strategies. When presented with information in a tabular format, older adults generally favor strategies that are less systematic and complex. Specifically, while younger adults are more likely to engage in compensatory strategies where lower scores on some aspects can be compensated by higher scores on others, older adults are more likely to use non-compensatory and satisficing strategies (i.e., picking the first option that meets a minimal standard; Johnson 1990). Older decision-makers are also more likely to review multiple characteristics within a given option instead of comparing characteristics across options (Johnson 1990).

Age differences in decision strategies are generally consistent with limitations in cognitive mechanics, but of course, realistic choices do not occur in a vacuum and decision-makers need to integrate newly acquired information with prior knowledge. Consistent with the favorable age trajectory in cognitive pragmatics, age is associated with greater reliance on existing cognitive frameworks during judgments (Gilinsky and Judd 1994). This pattern extends to health-related choices where older adults rely more on general background knowledge and prior experiences (Gould 1999), whereas younger adults are more likely to engage in an exhaustive review of the available information (Berg et al. 1999).

Although experiential decision styles allow older adults to leverage their knowledge base and well-preserved affective functioning, its implications for decision quality are equivocal. On the one hand, experiential reasoning may help older adults parse the flood of information associated with complex medical choices. For instance, when asked to make hypothetical choices among over-the-counter drugs, older adults were more likely than younger adults to focus on medically relevant characteristics (Stephens and Johnson 2000). However, relying too much on prior experience may limit the encoding of new medical information, especially when it is personally relevant and contradictory to prior beliefs (Okun and Rice 2001). Also, in health-related tasks of daily living, inappropriate use of previous experiences was identified as a significant cause of errors among older adults (Willis et al. 1999).

Distributing Outcomes Over Time

Many healthcare choices not only involve trade-offs among different types of outcomes but also decisions about the temporal distribution of events (e.g., when planning long-term treatment regimens). Among younger adults, there is a wide-spread tendency to devalue delayed outcomes relative to immediate ones, a phenomenon also known as *temporal discounting* (Frederick et al. 2002). For instance, younger adults tend to prefer smaller, immediate monetary gains over larger but delayed payouts. Growing evidence suggests that at least for monetary outcomes, older adults are less likely to devalue the future, and age differences in affective forecasting may contribute to such effects (Löckenhoff 2011).

Age groups also differ in their preferences for sequences of events. Whereas younger adults generally prefer improving sequences where the best is saved for last (Frederick et al. 2002), this tendency is less common among older adults (Löckenhoff et al., in press).

Taken together, these findings suggest that the age-related emphasis on emotion regulatory goals does not necessarily lead older adults to optimize current well-being at all cost. Instead, they appear to prefer a balanced distribution of events, a trend consistent with their well-preserved affective forecasting skills. To date, this line of research has been limited to laboratory settings and further research examining implications for realistic healthcare choices is needed.

Decision Avoidance and Delegation

Perhaps the most striking aspect of age differences in decision-making is the tendency toward choice avoidance, deferral, or delegation (Finucane et al. 2002). In hypothetical tasks, older adults are more likely than younger adults to delegate and to postpone difficult choices (Chen et al. 2011) and these findings extend to patient populations. Older cancer patients are more likely than younger patients to defer decisions to their physician (Pinquart and Duberstein 2004) and desired involvement in medical choices decreases with age (Ende et al. 1989).

In some respects, older adults' tendency to avoid choices may be adaptive. Reasoning from the SOC framework (Baltes 1997), choice delegation could be considered a compensatory strategy that allows older adults to achieve satisfactory decisions without having to invest precious cognitive resources. Avoiding emotionally difficult decisions may also benefit emotional well-being: Older adults who deferred such choices in a laboratory scenario were found to report lower levels of negative emotions (Chen et al. 2011).

Nevertheless, there is a potential for negative outcomes. For one, choice avoidance may limit older adults' willingness to seek out necessary medical treatments (Hudak et al. 2002). Further, although exploring multiple opinions and treatment options increases decision complexity, it can result in better outcomes, especially among older patients who face higher rates of complications and co-morbidities (CDC 2007). Finally, while there may be emotional benefits to delegating choices, joint and surrogate decision-making pose their own challenges.

Joint Decisions

Health-related choices, especially those among the severely ill, involve multiple stakeholders including patients, their close social partners, and medical providers (Posma et al. 2009). Although choice delegation becomes more frequent with age, there is a continuum ranging from a completely passive role to a fully active role. In patient samples, less than half of older patients embrace a fully passive role (Pinquart and Duberstein 2004) and preferences for active decision involvement are even higher among community dwelling older adults (Moorman 2011).

Although most older individuals desire some level of involvement in their healthcare choices, their active participation may be jeopardized by the interpersonal dynamics of joint medical decisions. Medical providers are less likely to encourage active participation among older than among younger adults (Street et al. 1995), and older adults are less assertive in communicating their wishes (Petrisek et al. 1997). Cohort effects

on the side of the patient and aging stereotypes on the side of the provider are likely to contribute to this pattern (Laganà and Shanks 2002) and may lead to a vicious cycle of poor patient–physician communication.

Relatives and confidants also play an important role in treatment decisions (Fried and O'Leary 2008), and older adults' high empathy, combined with the age-related emphasis on close relationships (Carstensen 2006), may make them particularly attuned to the wishes of others. Unfortunately, close confidants are fairly inaccurate in predicting patients' actual preferences. According to a recent review (Shalowitz et al. 2006), surrogates incorrectly predict patients' preferences in at least one-third of the cases with some studies finding agreement at chance level. Research further suggests that surrogates typically err in the direction of overtreatment (Shalowitz et al. 2006) putting older patients at risk of unwanted interventions.

Decision Quality and Satisfaction

Although prior research has found age differences in multiple aspects of decision-making, the evidence for age differences in *objective decision quality* is surprisingly equivocal. In laboratory studies, the direction of age effects strongly depends on task contingencies and specific criteria for assessing decision quality. While older adults perform worse in decisions that involve effortful processing or new learning, tasks that rely on experiential or affective processing are well preserved with age (Peters et al. 2007). In clinical scenarios, objective choice quality is even more difficult to gauge because the 'best' choice may depend not only on the age of the patient but also on their specific health history. However, studies involving hypothetical choices among standardized health scenarios found little evidence for age differences in decision quality (Meyer and Pollard 2004; Zwahr et al. 1999).

In contrast, there is a clear age effect in *choice satisfaction*. Older adults recall their past choices more favorably than younger adults and they report higher levels of satisfaction with their chosen option (e.g., Löckenhoff and Carstensen 2007). In part, these effects may be due to an age-related positivity effect, but they may also reflect older adults' preference for intuitive and experiential decision styles which typically result in higher choice satisfaction (Wilson et al. 1993). Although high satisfaction with past choices has obvious benefits for psychological well-being, it may also prevent learning from suboptimal choices and thus be a cause for concern.

Conclusion

In conclusion, the current literature documents age differences in virtually every aspect of the decision-making process ranging from pre-decisional information seeking and decision strategies to the interpersonal dynamics of joint and delegated choices. Over the past two decades, research on the underlying mechanisms of such effects has shifted from an exclusive focus on cognitive aging to a wider range of explanatory variables including emotional aging, motivational priorities, as well as interpersonal, and societal factors. As discussed above, many of the observed age effects are consistent with more than one of these explanations and systematic research is needed to determine their relative contribution in realistic decision contexts. To achieve this goal, the field has to move beyond the prevalent focus on correlational studies and the practice of focusing on one variable at a time. Instead, researchers should aim to experimentally manipulate variables of interest and explore interactions among multiple factors. Research examining the implications of emotional aging for decision-making has made a promising start in this direction (e.g., Chen et al. 2011; Mather and Knight 2005).

Once such gaps in the literature have been addressed, it may be possible to develop targeted interventions to promote high-quality decisions across the life span. Initial efforts in this direction are promising: Limitations in information seeking and the age-related positivity effect, for example, can be addressed through the experimental elicitation of information-seeking goals (Löckenhoff and Carstensen 2007). Also, training physicians to be more empathic and patients to be more assertive can significantly improve their mutual communication (Berkhof et al. 2011). However, interventions need to be carefully tested to avoid unintentional side effects. For instance, older adults were found to perform worse when asked to adopt the analytic processing style typically seen in younger adults (Mikels et al. 2010).

From a practical point of view, fostering good choices in late life not only benefits the well-being of individual older adults but also society as a whole. Evidence shows that many treatments and procedures are not medically necessary but primarily catered to emotional needs of patients and their relatives (Wennberg et al. 2007). Therefore, optimizing choice among America's aging patient population will not only limit human suffering by tailoring treatment to patients' actual medical needs, but also preserve limited societal resources.

Acknowledgements The preparation of this chapter was supported by funds from the Lois and Mel Tukman Endowment to Corinna E. Löckenhoff. We thank Jingbo Yi and Connie Jung for their help with the review of the literature.

References

Baltes, P. B. (1997). On the incomplete architecture of human ontogeny—selection, optimization, and compensation as foundation of developmental theory. *American Psychologist, 52*(4), 366–380. doi:10.1037/0003-066X.52.4.366.

Beisecker, A. E. (1988). Aging and the desire for information and input in medical decisions. *Gerontologist, 28*(3), 330–335.

Bennett, J. A., Cameron, L. D., Whitehead, L. C., & Porter, D. (2009). Differences between older and younger cancer survivors in seeking cancer information and using complementary/alternative medicine. *Journal of General Internal Medicine, 24*(10), 1089–1094. doi:10.1007/s11606-009-0979-8.

Berg, C. A., Meegan, S. P., & Klaczynski, P. (1999). Age and experiential differences in strategy generation and information requests for solving everyday problems. *International Journal of Behavioral Development, 23* (3), 615–639. doi:10.1080/016502599383720.

Berkhof, M., van Rijssen, H. J., Schellart, A. J. M., Anema, J. R., & van der Beek, A. J. (2011). Effective training strategies for teaching communication skills to physicians: An overview of systematic reviews. *Patient Education and Counseling, 84*(2), 152–162. doi:10.1016/j.pec.2010.06.010.

Cacioppo, J. T., Berntson, G. G., Bechara, A., Tranel, D., & Hawkley, L. C. (2011). Could an aging brain contribute to subjective well-being? The value added by a social neuroscience perspective. In A. Todorov, S. T. Fiske, & D. A. Prentice (Eds.), *Social neuroscience: Toward understanding the underpinnings of the social mind* (pp. 249–262). New York, NY: Oxford University Press.

Carstensen, L. L. (2006). The influence of a sense of time on human development. *Science, 312*(5782), 1913–1915. doi:10.1126/science.1127488.

CDC. (2007). *The state of aging and health in America 2007.* Whitehouse Station, NJ: The Merck Company Foundation.

Chen, Y. W., Ma, X. D., & Pethtel, O. (2011). Age differences in trade-off decisions: Older adults prefer choice deferral. *Psychology and Aging, 26*(2), 269–273. doi:10.1037/a0021582.

Ende, J., Kazis, L., Ash, A., & Moskowitz, M. A. (1989). Measuring patients' desire for autonomy, decision-making, and information seeking preferences among medical patients. *Journal of General Internal Medicine, 4*(1), 23–30. doi:10.1007/bf02596485.

Finucane, M. L., Slovic, P., Hibbard, J. H., Peters, E., Mertz, C. K., & MacGregor, D. G. (2002). Aging and decision-making competence: An analysis of comprehension and consistency skills in older versus younger adults considering health-plan options. *Journal of Behavioral Decision Making, 15*(2), 141–164. doi:10.1002/bdm.407.

Frank, L., Smyer, M., Grisso, T., & Appelbaum, P. (1999). Measurement of advance directive and medical treatment decision-making capacity of older adults. *Journal of Mental Health and Aging, 5*(3), 257–274.

Frederick, S., Loewenstein, G., & O'Donoghue, T. (2002). Time discounting and time preference: A critical review. *Journal of Economic Literature, 40*(2), 351–401. doi:10.1257/002205102320161311.

Fried, T. R., & O'Leary, J. R. (2008). Using the experiences of bereaved caregivers to inform patient- and caregiver-centered advance care planning. *Journal of General Internal Medicine, 23*(10), 1602–1607. doi:10.1007/s11606-008-0748-0.

Gilinsky, A. S., & Judd, B. B. (1994). Working memory and bias in reasoning across the life span. *Psychology and Aging, 9*(3), 356–371. doi:10.1037/0882-7974.9.3.356.

Gould, O. N. (1999). Cognition and affect in medication adherence. In D. C. Park, R. W. Morrell, & K. Shifren

(Eds.), *Processing of medical information in aging patients: Cognitive and human factors perspectives* (pp. 167–183). Mahwah, NJ: Lawrence Erlbaum Associates Publishers.

Happé, F. G. E., Winner, E., & Brownell, H. (1998). The getting of wisdom: Theory of mind in old age. *Developmental Psychology, 34*(2), 358–362. doi:10.1037/0012-1649.34.2.358.

Healey, M. K., & Hasher, L. (2009). Limitations to the deficit attenuation hypothesis: Aging and decision making. *Journal of Consumer Psychology, 19*(1), 17–22. doi:10.1016/j.jcps.2008.12.003.

Hess, T. M. (2005). Memory and aging in context. *Psychological Bulletin, 131*(3), 383–406. doi:10.1037/0033-2909.131.3.383.

Hess, T. M., Rosenberg, D. C., & Waters, S. J. (2001). Motivation and representation processes in adulthood: The effects of social accountability and information relevance. *Psychology and Aging, 16*(4), 629–642. doi:10.1037//0882-7974.16.4.629.

Hudak, P. L., Clark, J. P., Hawker, G. A., Coyte, P. C., Mahomed, N. N., Kreder, H. J., & Wright, J. G. (2002). "You're perfect for the procedure! Why don't you want it?" Elderly arthritis patients' unwillingness to consider total joint arthroplasty surgery: A qualitative study. *Medical Decision Making, 22*(3), 272–278. doi:10.1177/02789x02022003009.

Hummert, M. L., Garstka, T. A., Shaner, J. L., & Strahm, S. (1994). Stereotypes of the elderly held by young, middle-aged, and elderly adults. *Journal of Gerontology, 49*(5), 240–249.

Isaacowitz, D. M., & Choi, Y. (2011). The malleability of age-related positive gaze preferences: Training to change gaze and mood. *Emotion, 11*(1), 90–100. doi:10.1037/a0021551.

Isen, A. M., & Labroo, A. A. (2003). Some ways in which positive affect facilitates decision making and judgment. In S. L. Schneider & J. Shanteau (Eds.), *Emerging perspectives on judgment and decision research* (pp. 365–393). New York, NY: Cambridge University Press.

Johnson, M. M. (1990). Age differences in decision making: A process methodology for examining strategic information processing. *Journal of Gerontology, 45*(2), P75–P78.

Kahneman, D. (2003). A perspective on judgment and choice—mapping bounded rationality. *American Psychologist, 58*(9), 697–720. doi:10.1037/0003-066x.58.9.697.

Kennedy, Q., Mather, M., & Carstensen, L. L. (2004). The role of motivation in the age-related positivity effect in autobiographical memory. *Psychological Science, 15*(3), 208–214.

Kim, S., Hasher, L., & Zacks, R. T. (2007). Aging and benefit of distractibility. *Psychonomic Bulletin and Review, 14*(2), 301–305. doi:10.3758/bf03194068.

Labouvie-Vief, G., Grühn, D., & Studer, J. (2010). Dynamic integration of emotion and cognition:

Equilibrium regulation in development and aging. In M. E. Lamb, A. M. Freund, & R. M. Lerner (Eds.), *The handbook of life-span development* (Vol. 2, pp. 79–115)., Social and emotional development Hoboken, NJ: Wiley.

Laganà, L., & Shanks, S. (2002). Mutual biases underlying the problematic relationship between older adults and mental health providers: Any solution in sight? *The International Journal of Aging & Human Development, 55*(3), 271–295. doi:10.2190/1lte-f1q1-v7hg-6bc9.

Löckenhoff, C. E. (2011). Age, time, and decision making: from processing speed to global time horizons. *Annals of the New York Academy of Sciences, 1235*, 44–56. doi:10.1111/j.1749-6632.2011.06209.x.

Löckenhoff, C. E., & Carstensen, L. L. (2007). Aging, emotion, and health-related decision strategies: Motivational manipulations can reduce age differences. *Psychology and Aging, 22*(1), 134–146. doi:10.1037/0882-7974.22.1.134.

Löckenhoff, C. E., & Carstensen, L. L. (2008). Decision strategies in health care choices for self and others: Older but not younger adults make adjustments for the age of the decision target. *Journals of Gerontology Series B-Psychological Sciences and Social Sciences, 63*(2), P106–P109.

Löckenhoff, C. E., De Fruyt, F., Terracciano, A., McCrae, R. R., De Bolle, M., Costa, P. T., et al. (2009). Perceptions of aging across 26 cultures and their culture-level associates. *Psychology and Aging, 24*(4), 941–954. doi:10.1037/a0016901.

Löckenhoff, C. E., O'Donoghue, T., & Dunning, D. (2011). Age differences in temporal discounting: The role of dispositional affect and anticipated emotions. *Psychology and Aging, 26*(2), 274–284. doi:10.1037/a0023280.

Löckenhoff, C. E., Maresca, S. N., & Reed, A. E. (2012). Who saves the best for last? Age differences in decisions about affective sequences. *Psychology and Aging, 27*, 840–848.

Luce, M. F. (2005). Decision making as coping. *Health Psychology, 24*(4), S23–S28. doi:10.1037/0278-6133.24.4.s23.

Mata, R., & Nunes, L. (2010). When less is enough: Cognitive aging, information search, and decision quality in consumer choice. *Psychology and Aging, 25*(2), 289–298. doi:10.1037/a0017927.

Mather, M., & Carstensen, L. L. (2005). Aging and motivated cognition: The positivity effect in attention and memory. *Trends in Cognitive Sciences, 9*(10), 496–502. doi:10.1016/j.tics.2005.08.005.

Mather, M., & Knight, M. (2005). Goal-directed memory: The role of cognitive control in older adults' emotional memory. *Psychology and Aging, 20*(4), 554–570. doi:10.1037/0882-7974.20.4.554.

Meyer, B. J. F., & Pollard, C. A. (2004). *Why do older adults make faster decisions about treatments for breast cancer.* Paper presented at the Cognitive Aging Conference.

Mikels, J. A., Löckenhoff, C. E., Maglio, S. J., Carstensen, L. L., Goldstein, M. K., & Garber, A. (2010). Following your heart or your head: Focusing on emotions versus information differentially influences the decisions of younger and older adults. *Journal of Experimental Psychology-Applied, 16*(1), 87–95. doi:10.1037/a0018500.

Moorman, S. M. (2011). Older adults' preferences for independent or delegated end-of-life medical decision making. *Journal of Aging and Health, 23*(1), 135–157. doi:10.1177/0898264310385114.

Nielsen, L., Knutson, B., & Carstensen, L. L. (2008). Affect dynamics, affective forecasting, and aging. *Emotion, 8*(3), 318–330. doi:10.1037/1528-3542.8.3.318.

Okun, M. A., & Rice, G. E. (2001). The effects of personal relevance of topic and information type on older adults' accurate recall of written medical passages about osteoarthritis. *Journal of Aging and Health, 13*(3), 410–429. doi:10.1177/089826430101300305.

Peters, E., Hess, T. M., Västfjäll, D., & Auman, C. (2007). Adult age differences in dual information processes: Implications for the role of affective and deliberative processes in older adults' decision making. *Perspectives on Psychological Science, 2*(1), 1–23. doi:10.1111/j.1745-6916.2007.00025.x.

Petrisek, A. C., Laliberte, L. L., Allen, S. M., & Mor, V. (1997). The treatment decision-making process: Age differences in a sample of women recently diagnosed with non recurrent, early-stage breast cancer. *Gerontologist, 37*(5), 598–608.

Pinquart, M., & Duberstein, P. R. (2004). Information needs and decision-making processes in older cancer patients. *Critical Reviews in Oncology Hematology, 51*(1), 69–80. doi:10.1016/j.critrevonc.2004.04.002.

Posma, E. R., van Weert, J. C. M., Jansen, J., & Bensing, J. M. (2009). Older cancer patients' information and support needs surrounding treatment: An evaluation through the eyes of patients, relatives and professionals. *BMC Nursing, 8*(1), 1. doi:10.1186/1472-6955-8-1.

Reed, A. E., Mikels, J. A., & Simon, K. I. (2008). Older adults prefer less choice than young adults. *Psychology and Aging, 23*(3), 671–675. doi:10.1037/a0012772.

Reyna, V. F., & Brainerd, C. J. (2011). Dual processes in decision making and developmental neuroscience: A fuzzy-trace model. *Developmental Review, 31*(2–3), 180–206. doi:10.1016/j.dr.2011.07.004.

Richter, D., & Kunzmann, U. (2011). Age differences in three facets of empathy: Performance-based evidence. *Psychology and Aging, 26*(1), 60–70. doi:10.1037/a0021138.

Ruffman, T., Henry, J. D., Livingstone, V., & Phillips, L. H. (2008). A meta-analytic review of emotion recognition and aging: Implications for neuropsychological models of aging. *Neuroscience and Biobehavioral Reviews, 32*(4), 863–881. doi:10.1016/j.neubiorev.2008.01.001.

Salthouse, T. A., & Davis, H. P. (2006). Organization of cognitive abilities and neuropsychological variables across the lifespan. *Developmental Review, 26*(1), 31–54. doi:10.1016/j.dr.2005.09.001.

Samanez-Larkin, G. R., Gibbs, S. E. B., Khanna, K., Nielsen, L., Carstensen, L. L., & Knutson, B. (2007). Anticipation of monetary gain but not loss in healthy older adults. *Nature Neuroscience, 10*, 787–791. doi:10.1038/nn1894.

Scheibe, S., & Carstensen, L. L. (2010). Emotional aging: Recent findings and future trends. *Journals of Gerontology Series B-Psychological Sciences and Social Sciences, 65*(2), 135–144. doi:10.1093/geronb/gbp132.

Schewe, C. D., & Meredith, G. (2004). Segmenting global markets by generational cohorts: Determining motivations by age. *Journal of Consumer Behaviour, 4*(1), 51–63. doi:10.1002/cb.157.

Shalowitz, D. I., Garrett-Mayer, E., & Wendler, D. (2006). The accuracy of surrogate decision makers—a systematic review. *Archives of Internal Medicine, 166*(5), 493–497.

Skurnik, I., Yoon, C., Park, D. C., & Schwarz, N. (2005). How warnings about false claims become recommendations. *Journal of Consumer Research, 31*(4), 713–724. doi:10.1086/426605.

Spencer, W. D., & Raz, N. (1995). Differential effects of aging on memory for content and context: A meta-analysis. *Psychology and Aging, 10*(4), 527–539. doi:10.1037/0882-7974.10.4.527.

Squiers, L., Rutten, L. J. F., Treiman, K., Bright, M. A., & Hesse, B. (2005). Cancer patients' information needs across the cancer care continuum: Evidence from the cancer information service. *Journal of Health Communication, 10*, 15–34. doi:10.1080/10810730500263620.

Stephens, E. C., & Johnson, M. M. S. (2000). Dr. Mom and other influences on younger and older adults' OTC medication purchases. *Journal of Applied Gerontology, 19*(4), 441–459.

Street, R. L., Voigt, B., Geyer, C., Manning, T., & Swanson, G. P. (1995). Increasing patient involvement in choosing treatment for early breast cancer. *Cancer, 76*(11), 2275–2285. doi:10.1002/1097-0142(19951201)76:11<2275:aid-cncr2820761115>3.0.co;2-s.

Urry, H. L., & Gross, J. J. (2010). Emotion regulation in older age. *Current Directions in Psychological Science, 19*(6), 352–357. doi:10.1177/0963721410388395.

Wennberg, J. E., O'Connor, A. M., Collins, E. D., & Weinstein, J. N. (2007). Extending the P4P agenda, part 1: How medicare can improve patient decision making and reduce unnecessary care. *Health Affairs, 26*(6), 1564–1574. doi:10.1377/hlthaff.26.6.1564.

Willis, S. L., Dolan, M. M., & Bertrand, R. M. (1999). Problem solving on health-related tasks of daily living. In D. C. Park, R. W. Morrell, & K. Shifren (Eds.), *Processing of medical information in aging patients: Cognitive and human factors perspectives* (pp. 199–219). Mahwah, NJ: Lawrence Erlbaum Associates Publishers.

Wilson, T. D., Lisle, D. J., Schooler, J. W., Hodges, S. D., Klaaren, K. J., & Lafleur, S. J. (1993). Introspecting about reasons can reduce post-choice satisfaction. *Personality and Social Psychology Bulletin, 19*(3), 331–339. doi:10.1177/0146167293193010.

Zwahr, M. D., Park, D. C., & Shifren, K. (1999). Judgments about estrogen replacement therapy: The role of age, cognitive abilities, and beliefs. *Psychology and Aging, 14*(2), 179–191. doi:10.1037/0882-7974.14.2.179.

Decision-Making in Adolescents and Young Adults

Bonnie Halpern-Felsher, Majel Baker and Sarah Stitzel

Fifteen-year-old Jasmine's pediatrician reports back that the biopsy of the abnormal lump located in her right underarm is most likely lymphoma. What is Jasmine thinking now? Does she understand her treatment options? Does she know the risks and benefits associated with each treatment option? What will her quality of life be if she chooses the most aggressive treatment? Would Jasmine seek out additional professional opinions, or advice from her parents and friends?

Tommy, a 14-year-old high school freshman, is being encouraged by his friends to smoke marijuana. He is really curious to try it, and is excited to experience a "high," but he has heard many harmful effects of this drug. What will he decide to do?

Alice, a 16-year old, is considering having sex with her boyfriend of one year. She knows about the risks such as sexually transmitted infections (STIs), pregnancy, and HIV/AIDS, but really wants to experience sex with her boyfriend. She is not sure what protection to use, and is unsure how to talk to her boyfriend or others about this decision.

These are all health-related decisions that adolescents face, some focusing more on decisions regarding risk behaviors and others addressing medical-related decisions. Adolescence, which begins with the onset of puberty (average age of 12) and continues to young adulthood (up until age 21–24), represents a unique period in life characterized by greater freedom to make autonomous and meaningful decisions compared to childhood. However, adolescence is also a time when some areas of decision-making remain limited until age 18 or older, such as when making decisions concerning consenting to or denying medical treatment, choosing whether or not to have an abortion, participating in research, and purchasing and using alcohol and tobacco. These decisions occur juxtaposed to significant physical, cognitive, emotional, and psychosocial changes, which are coupled with societal influences offering mixed messages that both encourage and restrict decision-making autonomy, especially decisions involving health-risk behaviors. The various contexts influencing adolescent and young adult decision-making include cultural messages that encourage autonomy and risk-taking, parental monitoring that seeks to prevent risky health decisions, and peers who can be both a positive and negative influence on health-related decisions. This chapter will explain the foundational processes and theories used to conceptualize and

B. Halpern-Felsher (✉) · S. Stitzel
Department of Pediatrics, Stanford University, Palo Alto, CA, USA
e-mail: bonnie.halpernfelsher@stanford.edu

M. Baker
Department of Psychology, University of Minnesota Twin Cities, Minneapolis, MN, USA
e-mail: bake0633@umn.edu

S. Stitzel
e-mail: stitz87@gmail.com

study adolescent and young adult health-related decision-making while also reviewing the most recent findings in the field.

Definitions and Models of Decision-making

The study of decision-making is multi-disciplinary, with perspectives ranging from personality psychology to evolutionary psychology to developmental psychology to neuroscience to public policy and legal rights. While there is no one commonly agreed upon definition of competent decision-making, most theories and empirical research focus on the *process* of decision-making rather than the resulting decisions. That is, adolescents can still make competent decisions to choose to participate in unprotected sex after weighing all the pros and cons and considering the consequences of their action or non-action. Some definitions of decision-making competence use adults as the standard by which to judge adolescents' decisions. Others use a more formalized model by which to assess decision-making. For example, in the health care arena, competency to make a decision focuses on the ability to understand the treatment or procedure, deliberating over the risks and benefits, and reaching a decision after deliberation, a process by which children as young as nine years old appear to be capable (Beidler and Dickey 2001; Martenson and Fagerskiold 2008). In the legal arena, decision-making competence is typically defined as decisions that are made knowingly, with a full understanding of the procedures, related outcomes, and alternative courses of action. Further, the individual is capable of, and ultimately does, make the decision without undue influence or control from others.

According to normative decision-making models, competent or mature decisions involve some variation of the following: considering the potential positive and negative consequences of engaging *or not* engaging in any particular behavior, perceptions of the likelihood of being vulnerable to those positive and negative consequences, desires to engage in the behavior despite possible negative consequences, intentions to engage in the given behavior, and combining all information to make a final decision. Normative decision-making, which is grounded in Rational Choice Theory, presupposes that individuals methodically weigh the risks and benefits of each decision in order to make a decision that maximizes the utility of their choice. While such rational processing may apply to some situations (e.g., deciding which driving route is the most efficient to get to a friend's house), people in general, and adolescents in particular, rarely apply such a deliberative, rational process to decision-making, especially when the decision involves emotional or impulsive components such as deciding whether or not to have sex or making other health-related decisions. Instead, adolescents often apply a less deliberate, more social, emotional, and reactive process to decision-making. This type of decision-making is more commonly applied when the outcomes are more uncertain, such as the case with many decisions concerning health care and engagement in health-related risky behaviors. The realization that both the deliberate and the emotional or reactive decisions may be co-occurring has spurred investigation of different decision-making processes and multiple paths to decision-making (Halpern-Felsher 2009). Such alternative decision-making processes are often referred to as "dual models" or "multiple models" of decision-making (e.g., Gerrard et al. 2008; Reyna 2008).

The research on dual (or multiple) models of decision-making have produced two similar but unique models that particularly describe adolescents: Fuzzy Trace Theory (Reyna 2008) and the Prototype Willingness Model (Gerrard et al. 2008). The central tenet of Fuzzy Trace Theory is that people use verbatim mental representations and heuristic-based representations to make decisions, and they use these mental resources interchangeably. The verbatim mental representation is exactly that—the literal meaning of the information presented (e.g., numbers, definitions) —but the heuristic shortcuts, or "gists," are mental representations that capture the meaning of the information. Consider how this process could affect health-related decisions: an adolescent learns from her doctor that her current risky sexual activities put her at a 12 % risk of contracting chlamydia, which she might interpret as "low risk of chlamydia" considering the risk is less than 50 %. However, the average risk for her age group could be 0.6 %, and so her risk for chlamydia is comparatively very high. Relying on her gist understanding of her infection risk as "low" could be detrimental to her adherence to other relevant health promotion behaviors her doctor recommends, such as using condoms consistently or having sex with fewer partners.

The prototype willingness model similarly maintains that reasoned, analytical pathways and image-based, heuristic pathways are both employed during decision-making. Adolescents have image-based prototypes of risk behaviors and of those who engage in risk behaviors (e.g., what a "typical" smoker looks like). Empirical evidence for this model supports the notion that the more favorable the prototype or image, the more willing the adolescent is to engage in the risk behavior, and it is this behavioral willingness that most directly predicts engagement in risky behavior when the opportunity is presented. Thus, for example, if an adolescent associates smoking positively, such as images associated with seeing a movie star smoke, then an adolescent would be more willing to smoke. The prototype willingness model also argues for a distinction between willingness and intentions. Thus, while an adolescent may not actively seek out or intend to engage in health-compromising behaviors, such as smoking, when the situation arises, such as peers smoking at an unsupervised house party, an adolescent's willingness to try smoking will predict if they take part in that behavior or not (see Gerrard et al. 2008, for a review).

Components of Decision-making Specific to Adolescents and Young Adults

For the purpose of having a more complete account of decision-making, one must also address psychosocial and cognitive factors that impact decision-making (Fischhoff 2008), as well as individual variation like gender and cultural background that impact judgment and decisions. One should also consider the substantial insight recent work in developmental neuroscience has brought to understanding adolescent decision-making. However, this chapter will forgo discussion of neuroscience of decision-making as the limited space allotted could not due the topic justice (see Steinberg 2008, 2010 for detailed reviews). In addition to psychosocial and cognitive influences, research suggests that the decision-making processes adolescents use, and therefore how inputs are differentially weighed in the decision-making equation, are specific to the domain and topic of decision-making (Adler et al. 2003; Reyna and Farley 2006). Specifically, how a decision is made varies if the decision occurs in a non-emergency situation, where there is time to carefully consider all risks and benefits (e.g., abortion-related or other health-related decisions), or in a heat-of-the-moment situation, where peer influences and heuristic reasoning may dominate the decision (e.g., sexual behavior or alcohol use).

Cognitive and psychosocial factors Extending beyond normative and dual-process models, consensus in the literature reveals several cognitive and psychosocial factors that have a prominent influence on decision-making in adolescents.

Cognitive Development. During adolescence, thinking becomes more abstract and less concrete, allowing adolescents the ability to consider multiple aspects of their actions and decisions at one time, assess potential positive and negative consequences of each decision, and plan for the future. Studies have shown that by age 16, adolescents' general cognitive abilities, such as the ability to understand risks, process information, and reason are essentially identical to those of adults. For example, in a study of 935 individuals ranging from age 10 to 30, Steinberg et al. (2009) found no significant differences in cognitive skills between older adolescents (as young as age 15) and adults.

Psychosocial Maturity. Cognitive changes are coupled with *psychosocial maturity or development*, including increased social and peer comparison, reduced impulsivity, greater peer affiliation, changes in susceptibility to peer pressure, greater ability to understand and plan for the future, and increased ability to consider and acknowledge other people's perspectives on the behavioral options. These adolescent changes typically translate into adolescents' desire to participate in, and eventually dictate, their decisions.

Although there are individual differences and within-age group variation, most adolescents reach a level of psychosocial maturity comparable to adults by age 16. Perspective taking is the ability to recognize how the thoughts and actions of one person can influence those of another, and to imagine how others might see them. Social perspective taking also involves the ability to recognize that other people may have different points of view or a different knowledge set from one's own. The ability to take others' perspective continues to develop in early adolescence, stabilizing and becoming similar to adults' abilities by age 16.

Susceptibility to peer pressure that is undesirable or goes against the adolescent's goals generally decreases by age 16, with many adolescents able to ameliorate the influence of peer pressure by age 12. Impulsivity refers to making decisions in a quick and reflexive fashion, without much thought or information. Impulsivity steadily declines from age 10 on (Steinberg et al. 2008). Future perspective taking includes the ability to project into the future, to consider possible positive and negative outcomes associated with choices, and to plan for the future. By age 16, adolescents have the ability to consider the future (Steinberg et al. 2009). However, the ability to consider possible positive and negative outcomes develops much earlier, with adolescents able to recognize behavior-related risk, including positive and negative outcomes associated with sexual behavior, by age 10–12.

The overall thrust of the aforementioned literature is that adolescents' abilities to process information rationally and to reason through a decision emerge as young as age 10 and are essentially identical to the abilities of adults by age 16. Their psychosocial maturity, such as their ability to consider long-term consequences and rewards, to resist impulsivity, and to resist peer pressure, are also similar to adults by age 16, but these abilities continue to develop into early adulthood.

Risk and benefit judgments In addition to understanding the complexity of the decision-making process, it is important to understand the way in which adolescents and young adults perceive or judge health and social risks and benefits in making their decisions. The perception that adolescents judge themselves as invulnerable to harm, oft circulated in the scientific and lay community, has been widely discounted by evidence that adolescents, like adults, actually *overestimate* their risk for negative outcomes (e.g., their risk of getting lung cancer if they smoke) compared to statistical data. However, adolescents, like adults, also demonstrate an optimistic bias in their estimation of risk: they judge their personal risk to be less than others' risks, controlling for behavioral experience, habits and histories (Gibbons et al. 2012; Halpern-Felsher 2009; Reyna and Farley 2006). Life experience plays a prominent role in risk perceptions. For instance, while adolescents are generally optimistic, adolescents who witness a great deal of neighborhood violence and who have experienced direct threats to their safety, indicate higher mortality judgments and also perceive a higher sense of mortality; such judgments are understandable given that violence and crime are much more salient to these youth compared to other youth (Fischhoff et al. 2010). Contrary to belief, research demonstrates that adolescents generally perceive greater risk than adults, and that perceptions of low risk actually predict the onset of risk behaviors. For example, Song et al. (2009) showed that adolescents who held the lowest perceptions of tobacco-related risks were significantly more likely to initiate smoking 6 months or more later than adolescents who held higher perceptions of risk.

Most literature focuses on how adolescents and young adults judge risks, but benefit perceptions are equally important and highly influential in the adolescent decision-making process. Benefit perceptions have been demonstrated to predict increased engagement in a variety of health-compromising behaviors including underage drinking (Goldberg et al. 2002), smoking (Song et al. 2009), and early sexual activity (Michels et al. 2005). Adolescents' perceptions of benefits are unique predictors of health decisions above and beyond their perceptions of risk, and changes (or no changes) in benefit perceptions over time are shown to be independent of changes in risk perceptions (Morrell et al. 2010). Additionally, the ordering of information about risks and benefits can significantly influence decision-making. For example, participants were twice as likely to refuse consent to treatment when hearing the risks after the benefits compared to those who heard the benefits after the risks (Bergus et al. 2002). The demonstrated influence of ordering risks and benefits further highlights the importance of collaboration and communication between all parties involved in making medical decisions so as to avoid these decision-making misperceptions and pitfalls.

Role of experience Experience and knowledge play an important role in adolescent decision-making, especially when considering perceptions of risk and benefits. Adolescents have less experience with and knowledge about making decisions compared to adults, and therefore have fewer opportunities to receive positive or negative feedback about their choices (Jacobs 2004; Halpern-Felsher 2009). This might lead adolescents to believe that they are less likely to experience the possible negative outcomes as a result of their decisions and subsequent actions. Experience could also result in increased engagement in risky behaviors if previous risk-taking was not met with negative consequences—this is referred to as a "downward shift in risk perception" and is supported by longitudinal research on alcohol and drug use, drinking and driving, and sexual activity (Albert and Steinberg 2011; Halpern-Felsher et al. 2001).

Although adolescents are not as well equipped to make decisions given that they have less knowledge and experience compared to adults, as adolescents mature and acquire more experience in certain areas, their opinions should be given more weight and have a greater decision impact (see Piker 2011, for a review). Consider an adolescent patient who has struggled with a disease over many years. Her experience would likely result in greater maturity and experience in her views about her treatment compared to someone who was recently diagnosed with the same or a similar disease, even if that person was older in age. The adults involved in making decisions about her treatment may not have her specific experience of suffering from and fighting the disease themselves, so the adolescent's input should be given more evidential weight when they make judgments regarding her best interests. This idea of "evidential decisional impact" should be viewed in conjunction with the type of decision that is being made and the proportionality of the risks and benefits. That is, with more complex decisions that have higher potential for harm, greater decisional control should be given to adolescents who have a higher level of maturity and experience (Piker 2011).

Gender and cultural factors There are very few studies examining gender differences in decision-making, but those that do have largely found decision-making processes to be similar between males and females. In regards to shared medical decision-making, the small research yields mixed results as to whether one gender is more communicative with doctors during the decision-making process (Moore and Kirk 2010). There does, however, seem to be a difference between boys and girls in perceptions of and concerns about health-related benefits and risks. Regardless of actual behavioral experience or intentions, boys tend to perceive that they are more likely to experience positive outcomes from engaging in risky behaviors, such as experiencing pleasure from unprotected sex, while girls more often perceive negative outcomes, such as getting pregnant, getting into an accident while drunk driving, or getting lung cancer from smoking (Halpern-Felsher 2009). Additional gendered decision-making considerations might arise with further domain-specific decision-making research.

For example, gender is a factor in the topic of fertility preservation during cancer treatment because studies of pediatric oncologists show that girls are more willing to discuss fertility than boys and also show more concern about this subject in comparison to boys (Quinn et al. 2011).

Research has also established certain racial, ethnic, and cultural disparities that can have an effect on the development of and capacity for decision-making among adolescents. It is important to note how these variations can influence adolescents' personal values, their autonomy, and goals for the future, and how these capacities correspond with their decision-making process. While generally decision-making is similar across racial/ethnic groups, there are some differences. For example, in some Native American and Asian cultures, decision-making is a group process, and the outcomes of each decision are expected to have an effect on the entire family group. Therefore, when making decisions, oftentimes individuals will heavily consider others' input and the potential impact on family members in addition to their own individual preferences (Halpern-Felsher 2009).

Overall and Age Differences in Adolescent and Young Adult Decision-making

Few studies have examined the extent to which individuals, and in particular adolescents and young adults, actually make use of the factors involved in the entire decision-making process as outlined by the health, legal, and normative models. The few articles that do exist yield mixed results regarding adolescents' and young adults' capacities to make decisions. Michels et al. (2005) conducted a qualitative study of the extent to which adolescents spontaneously thought about each of the components of the normative decision-making model when making decisions about sexual activity. They found that, despite speculation that adolescents are incapable of making competent and thoughtful decisions, adolescents went through a deliberate decisional process, including considering relational and contextual factors, future goals, risks and benefits, and other relevant factors before making a decision about whether or not to have sex.

The literature investigating age differences in decision-making competence similarly yields mixed results, with some studies suggesting that there are little to no age differences and other studies indicating that adolescents have less decision-making competence compared to young adults and adults. These studies also suggest that in addition to competence gradually increasing from adolescence into young adulthood, many of the other characteristics thought to define competent decision-making such as personal independence, the ability to resist peer pressure, and the ability to control impulses also increase with age and time (Halpern-Felsher 2009). General consensus in the research demonstrates that, contrary to typical conceptions of decision-making developing along a linear progression from nascent logical thinking to more rational adult thinking, children and adolescents actually increase their reliance on heuristics, or mental shortcuts, as they progress developmentally towards adulthood (Reyna 2012). It is ironic that adolescents are lampooned for making "irrational" decisions when adult decision-making could be considered "irrational" because of the prominent use of heuristics.

In general, adolescents' cognitive reasoning ability is equivalent to adult reasoning by age 15 or 16, while their psychosocial maturity (e.g., ability to resist peer pressure, focus on short-term rewards over long-term rewards; Gibbons et al. 2012; Steinberg et al. 2009), still continues into young adulthood. However, social components (i.e., the presence of peers, social comparison) and how adolescents perceive risks and rewards uniquely contribute to the decision-making equation for adolescents (Albert and Steinberg 2011; Gibbons et al. 2012). In sum, while the *process* of decision-making for youth is similar to the process in adults, youth appear to assign different weights to the components of decision-making, making them look like "poorer" decision makers compared to adults. For example, youth may consider maintaining a relationship with a boyfriend by having unprotected sex as more important than avoiding an STI using a condom.

Shared Decision-making

Given that adolescents and young adults should not and do not make decisions in a vacuum, it is imperative to consider the network of resources available to adolescents to aid (and sometimes hinder) their decision-making.

Shared Decision-making in the Medical Context

Shared decision-making, in which the physician and family share information and together take steps to build consensus about the preferred treatment plan and implementation of that plan, is viewed as an ideal process for medical decision-making (Charles et al. 1997; Lipstein et al. 2012; Spring 2008). An undeniably important factor when considering youth participation in medical decisions is decision-making competency. In general, competency in this context focuses on reaching a level of understanding to make a decision, and some research suggests children as young as nine years old may be capable of participating in health care decisions (Martenson and Fagerskiold 2008). Preliminary qualitative research suggests that youth do want to be involved in the medical decision-making process, and that being involved makes them feel valued and less anxious (Morrell et al. 2010). For example, based on studies of adolescents with cancer, adolescents' desires for information and active participation in decisions concerning preserving fertility during cancer treatment clearly parallel those of adults with cancer, and evidence on adolescent decision-making in oncology suggests that conversations about fertility preservation are appropriate for teenagers (see Quinn et al. 2011, for a review). Adolescents under the age of 18 are still considered children under their guardian's care, and unfortunately, reviews of the literature demonstrate the children are "rarely involved in the decision-making process and appear to occupy a marginalized position in health care" (Coyne 2008, pp. 1682). Moreover, it is often the case that parents and health care providers override minors' decisions or do not involve them in the decision-making process because they act "in the best interest" of the minor (Coyne 2008; Martenson and Fagerskiold 2008). Parents and health care professionals do not enable competent decision-making when they fail to fully provide adolescent patients with the information they need to make a decision or when they judge adolescents' competency for themselves based only on age. Because adolescents have fewer experiences on which to base their decisions, if treatment options have not been clearly addressed with adolescent patients, they will often adopt the morals and values of their parents and the health care system that is providing treatment (Quinn et al. 2011). Therefore, adolescents' decisions may be limited, only extending as far as their parents' comprehension, and teenagers' understanding of their options usually mirrors their parents' (Quinn et al. 2011).

Seeking Advice

Adolescence is a bridge between inchoate childhood capabilities and mature adult proficiencies: the adult-like capability of seeking out advice from knowledgeable sources emerges in adolescence, and advice seeking is a cornerstone of competent decision-making. To illustrate, research on adolescents' decision-making regarding abortions demonstrates that in this domain, adolescents seek consultation from their romantic partners, their parents, and health care professionals (Finken 2005; Henshaw and Kost 1992). In large national samples, 61–65 % of teens said that one or both of their parents knew about the abortion (Blum et al. 1987; Henshaw and Kost 1992). For adolescents who do not consult their parents, often for fear of negative consequences, a majority still seek advice from another adult (Finken 2005). The caveat here is that research also highlights the essential role confidentially plays in ensuring adolescents seek out appropriate advice. Studies show that adolescents are more likely to obtain care, disclose sensitive information, and return for future care if clinicians address confidentiality (see Berlan and Bravender 2009, for a review). Furthermore, when clinicians fail to address sensitive psychosocial and medical concerns, adolescents often actually avoid the health care system (Berlan and Bravender 2009). Uncertainties about the legality of adolescents' consenting for and receiving confidential care are common among adolescents, their parents, and clinicians; parents are often conflicted in their views about the role of privacy in their child's health care, which can create tension in the medical relationship (Berlan and Bravender 2009). Physicians are usually less aware of legal minor consent guidelines or may be preoccupied with the parents' reaction to confidential discussions, which is unfortunate considering that adolescents are more willing to disclose sensitive health information if they receive assurances of their confidentiality and privacy (Berlan and Bravender 2009).

Technology and Decision-making Aids

The modern age offers a growing range of opportunities to aid adolescent decision-making through social media and technology. Given that participation in social networking sites has more than quadrupled from 2005 to 2009, and given that age was the strongest predictor of social networking and blogging in a nationally representative study (Chou et al. 2009), technology has tremendous potential as a health decision-making resource among adolescents and young adults. These networks offer a wealth of resources for managing health, such as supplying medical information to facilitate quality decision-making as well as providing social

support from niche communities on social networking sites.

Some of the barriers to health services and opportunities to make more autonomous decisions that young people face include such practical barriers as cost, transportation, and a shortage of medical providers. Telemedicine has the potential to overcome access factors and to deliver health services by connecting patients and health care providers with various forms of technology such as telephone, texting, email, or video conferencing. This approach can be particularly advantageous as it increases access to services and providers and decreases travel and wait time (Garrett et al. 2011). For example, studies have shown telemedicine to have successful applications in the field of mental health (Garrett et al. 2011). Electronic aids such as video, telephone, texting, and use of the Internet not only help increase knowledge and self-efficacy in adolescents and young adults, but can also increase adherence to treatment recommendations (see Zebrack and Isaacson 2012, for a review). Furthermore, pilot studies reveal that these forms of media can result in higher levels of satisfaction and participation, as well as improve coping abilities, lower amounts of distress, and increased quality of life—all with the potential to provide support in a cost-efficient manner (Zebrack and Isaacson 2012). However, confidentiality is still a lynchpin for adolescent health services: a survey of adolescents' views on the potential use of telemedicine consultations for sexual health revealed that youth were concerned about confidentiality and security of webcam consultations (Garrett et al. 2011). These concerns were not specific to sexual health and may be mitigated if health care providers explicitly address privacy policies regarding young people, as well as establishing a trusting relationship with their adolescent patients.

It is important to note the limitations of modern technology, as the myriad of information on the Internet can easily confound adolescents and young adults with conflicting and possibly inaccurate information (Chou et al. 2009; Zebrack and Isaacson 2012). With regard to cancer treatment information, because adolescents and young adults are typically unable to distinguish accurate and useful information, most of them need assistance from adults to analyze and interpret the plethora of available material (Zebrack and Isaacson 2012) in order to make competent decisions. Nevertheless, social media and electronic communication tools can and should be harnessed in positive ways to help patients play a more active role in health-related decision-making.

Implications for Health Care Professionals, Parents, and Researchers

Including children and adolescents in the medical decision-making process has the potential to offer concrete medical advantages; for example, it is often the case that treatment success depends on the compliance of the patient to adhere to treatment (Spring 2008). There are important reasons for enabling and advocating for adolescents being actively involved in health and health care decisions including: enabling them to practice and develop their autonomy, enhancing their feelings of self-determination, decreasing behaviors of learned helplessness, (i.e., behaving helplessly because previous attempts at autonomy or action have been met with failure; Beidler and Dickey 2001), and participating in health promotion (e.g., understanding the need for condoms to reduce risk pregnancy and STIs). Health care professionals are very much in a position to enable adolescents to participate in medical decision-making by taking steps to overcome communication barriers. Such efforts could include using child-friendly medical terminology, avoiding jargon, and providing children with all the information they need to make decisions while adjusting for their health literacy levels (Morrell et al. 2010). It is the responsibility of health care professionals to act as patient

advocates (Beidler and Dickey 2001). Likewise, parents should play a prominent role in encouraging competent medical decision-making. Parental barriers to including adolescents in the decision-making process include dominating the conversation with the health care providers, interrupting and blocking interaction between the health care provider and the youth, or answering questions directed to the youth (for a review see Morrell et al. 2010). While encouraging youth participation and acknowledging their decision-making competency, professionals, and parents reasoning with youth should still understand adolescents' limitations in their decision-making capacities. For example, health care professionals and parents should not assume that youth understand all the information they are receiving as research shows adolescents interpret words about probability in a more varied fashion than do adults (Biehl and Halpern-Felsher 2001), which could lead to misinterpretation of health information. Nevertheless, given that adolescence is a middle ground between childhood and adulthood, health care professionals and parents should find a middle ground for adolescent decision-making that encourages autonomy while accommodating for adolescents' limitations (Piker 2011). Adolescents are far more competent to make health decisions than is acknowledged or realized by parents or health care providers. In fact, the Mature Minor Doctrine has been implemented by some states in an attempt to give minors more health-related decision power based on their age and maturity level (Schlam and Wood 2000; Quinn et al. 2011). This allows health care providers and courts to give minors the power to consent to treatment and even make end-of-life decisions or refuse treatment if they are competent and mature enough to do so (Piker 2011). To truly inform such discussions, more research on adolescent decision-making in the medical context is a necessity. There is little research, to these authors' knowledge, detailing the outcomes of

Table 1 Summary of chapter points regarding adolescent and young adult decision-making

• There is not a unified definition of "competent decision-making" in adolescents, but a general definition relevant to health care is: an adolescent's ability to understand the treatment or procedure, deliberate over the risks and benefits, and reach a decision after deliberation and consultation yet without undue influence or control from others
• Adolescents' abilities to understand risks, to process information rationally, and to reason through a decision are essentially identical to the abilities of adults by age 16. Their psychosocial maturity, such as their ability to consider long-term consequences and rewards, to resist impulsivity, and to resist peer pressure, are also similar to adults by age 16, but these abilities continue to develop into early adulthood
• Adolescents with more experience making decisions about their medical care should be afforded more weight in the decision process—consider the adolescent who has struggled with a disease over many years and the resulting maturity and life experience that could inform his/her decisions
• Shared decision-making is an ideal process for medical decision-making, in which physician and family share information and together take steps to build consensus about the preferred treatment plan and implementation
• Seeking advice is important to competent decision-making, and adolescents often seek advice from guardians and trusted adults. However, addressing confidentiality is essential: adolescents are more likely to obtain care, disclose sensitive information, and return for future care if clinicians address and provide confidential care
• Telemedicine provides many advantages for adolescents, including increased access to medical information, surmounting barriers like cost and transportation, and increased involvement and self-efficacy with their own health care. Addressing confidentiality is still paramount for adolescents with regards to telemedicine
• Health care professionals and parents should find a middle ground for adolescent decision-making that encourages autonomy while adjusting for adolescents' limitations

allowing adolescents to participate fully in medical decisions, including whether or not their participation leads to improved health and psychosocial outcomes. Such information on decision outcomes could prove extremely advantageous to health care professionals, parents, and policy-makers alike, as we continue to learn and understand the evolution and principles of adolescents' decision-making competences. Table 1 provides a summary of the points made in this chapter.

References

Albert, D., & Steinberg, L. (2011). Judgment and decision making in adolescence. *Journal of Research on Adolescence, 21*(1), 211–224.

Adler, N. E., Ozer, E. J., & Tschann, J. (2003). Abortion among adolescents. *American Psychologist, 58*(3), 211–217. doi:10.1037/0003-066X.58.3.211.

Berlan, E. D., & Bravender, T. (2009). Confidentiality, consent, and caring for the adolescent patient. *Current Opinion in Pediatrics, 21*, 450–456. doi:10.1097/MOP.0b013e32832ce009.

Biehl, M., & Halpern-Felsher, B. L. (2001). Adolescents' and adults' understanding of probability expressions. *Journal of Adolescent Health, 28*(1), 30–35.

Beidler, S. M., & Dickey, S. B. (2001). Children's competence to participate in healthcare decisions. *JONA's Healthcare, Law, Ethics, and Regulation, 3*(3), 80–87.

Bergus, G. R., Levin, I. P., & Elstein, A. S. (2002). Presenting risks and benefits to patients: The effect of information order on decision making. *Journal of General and Internal Medicine, 17*, 612–617.

Blum, R. M., Resnick, M. D., & Stark, T. A. (1987). The impact of a parental notification law on adolescent abortion decision-making. *American Journal of Public Health, 77*(5), 619–620.

Charles, C., Gafni, A., & Whelan, T. (1997). Shared decision-making in the medical encounter: What does it mean? (or it takes at least two to tango). *Social Science and Medicine, 44*(5), 681–692.

Chou, W. S., Hunt, Y. M., Beckjord, E. B., Moser, R. P., & Hesse, B. W. (2009). Social media use in the United States: Implications for health communication. *Journal of Medical Internet Research, 11*(4), e48. doi:10.2196/jmir.1249.

Coyne, I. (2008). Children's participation in consultations and decision-making at health service level: A review of the literature. *International Journal of Nursing Studies, 45*, 1682–1689.

Finken, L. (2005). The role of consultants in adolescents' decision making: A focus on abortion decisions. In Janis Jacobs & Paul Klaczynski (Eds.), *The development of judgment and decision making in children and adolescents* (pp. 255–278). Mahwah, NJ: Lawrence Erlbaum Associates Publishers.

Fischhoff, B. (2008). Assessing adolescent decision-making competence. *Developmental Review, 28*, 12–28.

Fischhoff, B., Bruine de Bruin, W., Parker, A. M., Millstein, S. G., & Halpern-Felsher, B. L. (2010). Adolescents' perceived risk of dying. *Journal of Adolescent Health, 46*, 265–269. doi:10.1016/j.jadohealth.2009.06.026.

Garrett, C. C., Hocking, J., Chen, M. Y., Fairly, C. K., & Kirkman, M. (2011). Young people's views on the potential use of telemedicine consultations for sexual health: Results of a national survey. *BMC Infectious Diseases, 11*(285), 1–11. doi:10.1186/1471-2334/11/285/prepub.

Gerrard, M., Gibbons, F. X., Houlihan, A. E., Stock, M. L., & Pomery, E. A. (2008). A dual-process approach to health risk decision making: The prototype willingness model. *Developmental Review, 28,* 29–61.

Gibbons, F. X., Kingsbury, J. H., & Gerrard, M. (2012). Social-psychology theories and adolescent health risk behavior. *Social and Personality Psychology Compass, 6* (2), 170–183. doi:10.1111/j.1751-9004.2011.00412.x.

Goldberg, J. H., Halpern-Felsher, B. L., & Millstein, S. G. (2002). Beyond invulnerability: The importance of benefits in adolescents' decisions to drink alcohol. *Health Psychology, 21,* 477–484.

Halpern-Felsher, B. (2009). Adolescent decision making: An overview. *The Prevention Researcher, 16*(2), 3–7.

Halpern-Felsher, B. L., Millstein, S. G., Ellen, J. M., Adler, N. E., Tschann, J. M., & Biehl, M. (2001). The role of behavioral experience in judging risks. *Health Psychology, 20*(2), 120–126. doi:10.1037//0278-6133.20.2.120.

Henshaw, S. K., & Kost, K. (1992). Parental involvement in minors' abortion decisions. *Family Planning Perspectives, 24*(5), 196–207, 213.

Jacobs, J. (2004). Perceptions of risk and social judgments: Biases and motivational factors. In R. J. Bonnie & M. E. O'Connell (Eds.), *Reducing underage drinking: A collective responsibility* (pp. 417–436). Washington, DC: The National Academies Press.

Lipstein, E. A., Brinkman, W. B., & Britto, M. T. (2012). What is known about parents' treatment decisions? A narrative review of pediatric decision making. *Medical Decision Making, 32,* 246–258. doi:10.1177/0272989X11421528.

Martenson, E. K., & Fagerskiold, A. M. (2008). A review of children's decision-making competence in health care. *Journal of Clinical Nursing, 17,* 3131–3141.

Michels, T. M., Kropp, R. Y., Eyre, S. L., & Halpern-Felsher, B. L. (2005). Initiating sexual experiences: How do young adolescents make decisions regarding early sexual activity? *Journal of Research on Adolescents, 15*(4), 583–607.

Moore, L., & Kirk, S. (2010). A literature review of children's and young people's participation in decisions relating to health care. *Journal of Clinical Nursing, 19*(15–16), 2215–2225. doi:10.1111/j.1365-2702.2009.03161.

Morrell, H. E. R., Song, A. V., & Halpern-Felsher, B. L. (2010). Predicting adolescent perceptions of the risk and benefits of cigarette smoking: A longitudinal investigation. *Health Psychology, 29*(6), 610–617.

Piker, A. (2011). Balancing liberation and protection: A moderate approach to adolescent health care decision-making. *Bioethics, 25*(4), 202–208. doi:10.1111/j.1467-8519.2009.01754.x.

Quinn, G. P., Murphy, D., Knapp, C., Stearsman, D. K., Bradley-Klug, K. L., Sawczyn, K., et al. (2011). Who decides? Decision making and fertility preservation in teens with cancer: A review of the literature. *Journal of Adolescent Health, 49,* 337–346.

Reyna, V. F. (2008). A theory of medical decision making and health: Fuzzy trace theory. *Medical Decision Making, 28,* 850–865. doi:10.1177/0272989X08327066.

Reyna, V. F. (2012). A new intuitionism: Meaning, memory, and development in fuzzy-trace theory. *Judgment and Decision Making, 7*(3), 332–359.

Reyna, V. F., & Farley, F. (2006). Risk and rationality in adolescent decision making: Implications for theory, practice, and public policy. *Psychological Science in the Public Interest, 7*(1), 1–44. doi:10.1111/j.1529-1006.2006.00026.x.

Schlam, L., & Wood, J. (2000). Informed consent to the medical treatment of minors: Law and practice. *Health Matrix, 10,* 141–174.

Spring, B. (2008). Health decision making: Lynchpin of evidence-based practice. *Medical Decision Making, 28,* 866–874.

Song, A. V., Morrell, H. E. R., Cornell, J. L., Ramos, M. E., Biehl, M., Kropp, R. Y., & Halpern-Felsher, B. L. (2009). Perceptions of smoking-related risks and benefits as predictors of adolescent smoking initiation. *American Journal of Public Health, 99,* 487–492.

Steinberg, L., Albert, D., Cauffman, E., Banich, M., Graham, S., & Woolard, J. (2008). Age differences in sensation seeking and impulsivity as indexed by behavior and self-report: Evidence for a dual systems model. *Developmental Psychology, 44*(6), 1764–1778. doi:10.1037/a0012955.

Steinberg, L., Cauffman, E., Woolard, J., Graham, S., & Banich, M. (2009). Are adolescents less mature than adults?: Minors' access to abortion, the juvenile death penalty, and the alleged APA "flip-flop." *American Psychologist, 64*(7), 583–594.

Steinberg, L., Graham, S., O'Brien, L., Woolard, J., Cauffman, E., & Banich, M. (2009). Age differences in future orientation and delay discounting. *Child Development, 80*(1), 28–44. doi:10.1111/j.1467-8624.2008.01244.x.

Steinberg, L. (2008). A social neuroscience perspective on adolescent risk-taking. *Developmental Review, 28,* 78–106.

Steinburg, L. (2010). A behavioral scientist looks at the science of adolescent brain development. *Brain and Cognition, 72,* 160–164.

Zebrack, B., & Isaacson, S. (2012). Psychosocial care of adolescent and young adult patients with cancer survivors. *Journal of Clinical Oncology, 30*(11), 1221–1226. doi:10.1200/JCO.2011.39.5467.

Decision Making in the Family

Laura A. Siminoff and Maria D. Thomson

Key Points

- Healthcare decision making research has traditionally focused on dyadic, patient–clinician processes of decision making, despite a growing recognition that patients often express a preference for and actively seek out family participation in healthcare decision making.
- While there are a limited number of theoretical frameworks available, most were not developed for healthcare decision contexts, include family members superficially or have not been extensively used or refined.
- Involvement of family members in healthcare decision making has been evaluated using both direct observation and self report measures. To date, self report instruments focus primarily on caregiver burden and needs.
- New models and measures of triadic (patient–family–clinician) communica-

tion are needed to provide a more accurate reflection of the healthcare decision making context. Assessment of triadic communication and decision making needs to move beyond assessments of caregiver burden to measure how individual and shared goals are negotiated, the definition of roles in the decision making process, and clinician acceptance of family member participation in healthcare decision making in a range of clinical contexts.

Introduction

Decision sciences are focused on understanding the fundamental cognitive and affective processes of how decisions are made and understanding the factors that shape decisions as individuals make choices in real-world situations. Although cognitive processes reside within individuals, almost all health decisions result from a procedure whereby individuals process information from multiple sources. Moreover, evidence indicates that affective factors also play an important role. Yet this complex process has been largely studied from the vantage of it being a highly individual process in which isolated patients interact with a health care practitioner to make health care decisions. This view of decision

M.D. Thomson
Department of Social and Behavioral Health, School of Medicine, Virginia Commonwealth University, PO Box 980149, Richmond, VA 23298-0149, USA
e-mail: maria.thomson@vcuhealth.org

L.A. Siminoff (✉)
College of Public Health, Temple University, 1101 W. Montgomery Avenue, 3rd Floor, Philadelphia, PA 19122 USA
e-mail: lasiminoff@temple.edu

© Springer Science+Business Media New York 2016
M.A. Diefenbach et al. (eds.), *Handbook of Health Decision Science*,
DOI 10.1007/978-1-4939-3486-7_13

making is an impoverished one. A patient and at least one companion, usually a family member, frequently attend clinical encounters. It is estimated that 15–30 % of general primary care visits are accompanied (Brown et al. 1998; Schilling et al. 2002; Botelho et al. 1996; Clayman et al. 2005) and that 50 % of patients report family involvement in their health care decisions (Sayers et al. 2006). The frequency and intensity of familial involvement is higher for individuals with serious illness; most cancer patient clinical encounters include a family member/companion (Eggly et al. 2012; Gleason et al. 2009) and overwhelmingly express a desire for family involvement in their healthcare decisions (Schafer et al. 2006).

The traditionally highly individualistic view of decision making derives from several sources. First, basic studies of cognitive processes naturally focus on tests with individuals. Second, western legal and ethical principals are based on the rights of individuals (Beuchamps and Childress 2008), divorced from the families in which most individuals are embedded. Notions of autonomy, specifically the doctrine of informed consent, is based entirely on a single patient interacting with the health system (generally a physician). This has led to discounting the role of families in the decision process. However, arguments have been made that family involvement is integral to promoting patients' overall well-being and agency (Kuczewski 1996; Sayers et al. 2006; Ho 2008). The relative neglect of this area may also be a result of the methodological and analytic difficulties entailed in studying decision making processes that are, at a minimum, triadic. Still, the lack of research in this area is notable given the documented importance of family support to overall quality of life (Street et al. 2009).

To date, the literature in this field has been mostly centered on the family role as surrogate decision makers. Families' decision-making behaviors have not been well studied except as they apply to decisions for minor children and decisions to terminate treatment for incompetent adults. Most studies have treated decision making as a purely dyadic interaction between an individual patient and physician. However, it is becoming increasingly apparent that families, as a unit, play an important role in the process of making decisions about care for and with adult patients (Rose 1999). This chapter focuses on how families influence and make decisions with decisionally intact individuals.

Theoretical Perspectives

A variety of behavioral theories have been applied to the study of decision making in health care. Of these, few are applicable specifically to family decision making. The following represent models that have been used in the literature or are relevant to the exploration of family decision making in heath care.

The Convergence Model of Communication

The convergence model, developed by Rogers and Kincaid (1981), describes a communication process between two or more participants within a social network. Through the creation and sharing of information (information exchange) participants attempt to reach mutual understanding that will then enable collective action (Rogers and Kincaid 1981). While Rogers and Kincaid provide a thorough description of the communication process, the Convergence model does not specifically address what happens if mutual understanding is not reached.

Family Centered Decision Making Model

From their work with South East Asian oncology patients, Back and Huak (2005) developed the Family-Centered Decision Making Model to understand family requests of nondisclosure of diagnosis and/or prognosis. The decision making process is conceptualized as shared between the physician and the family on behalf of, but with the consent and approval of, the patient (Back and Huak 2005). In this model the family is viewed as a unit in that decisions will not only impact the patient but also the entire family. Therefore, including endpoints in the decision making process such as familial harmony and maintenance of family relationships is highly valued. In a 12 month period in one oncology practice in South East Asia, Back and Huak (2005) reported 17 % of patient–family groups requested nondisclosure of diagnosis and 36.8 % requested nondisclosure of prognosis to the patient. Schafer et al. (2006) have cautioned that patient autonomy is at risk in this model and argue for the development of a shared decision making model that more clearly delineates patient autonomy and family participation in the decision making process.

Shared Decision Making

The model of shared decision making is described as a partnership featuring the two-way exchange of both information and preferences between patient and clinician comprised of four socially derived characteristics: (1) joint patient and physician involvement in decision making; (2) information sharing between these two actors; (3) expression of treatment preferences by both parties; (4) a treatment plan that is agreed on by both patient and physician (Charles et al. 1999; Towle and Godolphin 1999; Brown et al. 2004). In this model, involvement, information sharing, expressed preferences and agreement are negotiated during dyadic interactions. The model reflects increased emphasis on patient autonomy and coincides with a healthcare system that increasingly shifts responsibility for individual healthcare management to patients (Indeck and Bunney 1997) and caregiving to families (Siminoff et al. 2008; Lobchuk et al. 2012). Although the model is largely focused on individual decision makers, a feature of the shared decision making model is the involvement of the family during all stages of the process. In a revision of the SDM (Charles et al. 1999), Charles et al. explicitly acknowledge that the process of decision making, if not the actual decision taken,

allows for family participation. To date, such applications are lacking in the literature.

Family Systems Theory

A related theoretical framework is Family Systems Theory (FST). To our knowledge, this framework has not been applied specifically to health-related decision making, however it has been used to explore family functioning and health outcomes. FST provides a framework for understanding patterns of cognition, feelings, and behavior at various levels within the family system. Family systems have well-developed patterns of functioning including patterns of transactions and role definition. When changes occur in one part of the family system, change will also occur in other areas. Research findings suggest that the quality of communication and emotional support available in a family system predicts adjustment to cancer and caregiver burden (Gotcher 1993, 1995; Ballard-Reisch and Letner 2003; Mazanec and Bartel 2002; Walsh-Burke 1992; Fried et al. 2005). The FST may be a useful compliment to other existing models of decision making that do not specifically consider family members.

Measurement of Family Decision Making in Health Care

Decision making is ideally shared and the communication process is the primary vehicle for decision making, whether it is written, aural or oral communication. Communication is embedded within the doctor–patient–family relationship, and acknowledges decision making as a social process (Siminoff and Step 2005). Any number of combinations of the patient, clinician, and family may form information-based alliances in which the patient seeks medical help, provides active input (either as a primary agent, in conjunction with the family or may cede agency solely to the family) and then places him/herself into the care of the physician/health system. Applied research in decision making is the study of how the communication process, as the facilitating factor, drives decision making.

To accomplish this, researchers have relied on both direct observation of healthcare interactions and health care interactants' self-reports. The ability to capture live interactions and code them reliably has grown substantially with the assistance of digital and computer technologies. Various observational schemas have been developed over the years, but few depict process-based explanations that can assess individual, joint, and situational contributions to communication transactions, including verbal and nonverbal communication (Siminoff and Step 2011). Observational analysis schema include the Roter Interaction Analysis System (RIAS) designed to describe physician–patient interaction in terms of content and context of routine dialogue during medical care and the Medical Interaction Process System (MIPS) which measures communicated affect via ratings of each utterance for feeling (Ford et al. 2000). The Siminoff Communication Content & Affect Program (SCCAP), a newer computerized coding system, provides reliable measurement of communication variables including tailored content areas, relational and affective characterization of utterances, and observer ratings of speaker immediacy, affiliation, confirmation/disconfirmation, and persuasive behaviors. The SCCAP can also explicitly code multiple interactants in addition to the patients and a single clinician, including family members and multiple members of the healthcare team (Siminoff and Step 2011). Several systems have been developed to measure very specific aspects of the clinician–patient relationship or communication behaviors. For example, Street and colleagues have developed a coding scheme specifically focused on measuring patient centeredness (Street and Millay 2001).

Not all studies rely on observational methods. Instruments that characterize interactions across various dimensions exist, including ones that specifically measure families' roles in decision making. The Shared Care Instrument measures this construct across three dimensions-communication, decision making and reciprocity (Sebern

2008). The Family Decision Making Self-Efficacy scale is a reliable tool to understand the level of confidence that family members have for participating in health care decisions for terminally ill patients using two scenarios, one for patients with capacity and one for decisionally incapacitated patients (Nolan et al. 2009). The Cancer Communication Assessment Tool for Patients and Families (CCAT-PF) assesses level and type of congruence in patient–family caregiver communication. The 18 item scale assesses several domains including patient and family perspectives about physicians' decisions and communication and family support of patient decisions (Siminoff et al. 2008). A 2007 systematic review (Simon et al. 2007) found 18 instruments, including the Control Preference Scale (Degner and Sloan 1992), the Autonomy Preference Index and the Decisional Regret Scale (O'Connor 2009) relevant to decision studies, but not specific to family role in health care decision making. In fact, instrument development has been focused more on assessing family caregiver burden (Given et al. 1992, 2001; Oberst et al. 1989) and needs (Kristjanson et al. 1995, 1997).

Empirical Evidence for Family Decision Making in Health Care

There is considerable evidence that family participation in decision making is largely salutary, that families play a significant role in patient decision making and that their participation is welcomed by patients. Further, although concerns have been expressed that family members can overwhelm the patient's voice and are unwelcome by patients' physicians, most empirical studies do not bear out these concerns (Brown et al. 1998; Schilling et al. 2002; Clayman et al. 2005). A study of prostate cancer patients demonstrated that almost all patients (91 %) discussed decisions with a family member. Family caregivers reported that their role was to provide emotional support (98 %) and to assist with treatment decision making (Zeliadt et al. 2011). Similar findings have been reported irrespective of patient race or ethnicity (Rim et al. 2011) and patient gender (Gilbar and Gilbar 2009). The importance of family roles in decisions about screening behaviors has also been reported (Jones et al. 2010; Brittain et al. 2012). Racial/ethnic differences have been detected for certain decisions. In a study of African American versus White lung cancer caregivers, African Americans had higher expectations for treatment outcomes ($p \leq 0.05$) but poorer understanding of hospice and a stronger preference for hospice care outside the home ($p \leq 0.05$). African Americans have also been reported to be more likely to believe that the patient communicates with the family about cancer treatment to meet the family's expectations rather than seek emotional support ($p \leq 0.01$) and are less likely to be fully satisfied with the decision making process ($p \leq 0.05$) (Zhang et al. 2011).

Although the health system is focused on the information needs of the patient, family caregivers and patients report similar needs for information, communication and relationship building with the physician. A study of pain control in cancer patients found that alliances between patients and caregivers resulted in them 'teaming up' to get the information and pain relief medication needed from the physician (Kimberlin et al. 2004). Another study of the use of Complementary and Alternative Medicine (CAM) in patients found that caregivers frequently act as negotiators (Ohlen et al. 2006). However, alliances are not always formed between patients and caregivers, sometimes conflict exists. Patients may be reluctant to discuss illness and symptoms with caregivers. In a small study of lung cancer patients and their caregivers, 65 % of families reported various family disagreements that mainly concerned routine treatment decisions, discontinuation of therapeutic treatment, and use of hospice care. Furthermore, avoidance of family communication was associated with several underlying thought processes: avoidance of psychological distress; desire for mutual protection; and belief in positive thinking. Family communication was further hindered by the increasing difficulty of issues inherent to late-stage cancer (Zhang and Siminoff 2003). Because patient–family communication is critical to treatment and care decision making these communication 'glitches' can cause excessive stress for both patients and caregivers resulting in diminished quality of life (Fried et al. 2003; Zhang et al. 2011). Interestingly, younger caregivers have been found to experience greater stress and caregiver burden (Gaugler et al. 2005). Studies correlate increased frequency and depth of information sharing among family members with better overall adjustment and fewer conflicts in coping with the disease (Walsh-Burke 1992). In both primary care settings and in instances of a life threatening illness such as cancer, family members (or other care giving companions) presence has been shown to have a largely positive impact on communication and subsequent decision making. Families provide expanded medical histories and assist in question asking (Prohaska and Glasser 1996; Sanford et al. 2011; Kahana and Kahana 2003) and patients report that their presence during clinical encounters increases their understanding as do physicians, although to a lesser extent (Zeliadt et al. 2011; Gilbar and Gilbar 2009). However, when patients and caregivers are discordant, conflict can arise along with increased levels of psychosocial distress (Lobchuk et al. 2012; Siminoff et al. 2010).

Improving Family Decision Making

Few interventions have been designed and tested to specifically improve the family–patient decision making process. Most interventions with families are designed to alleviate caregiver burden and improve psychological outcome (Northouse et al. 2005). Although decision aids have been found to improve outcomes such as decisional satisfaction, knowledge and increase patient participation (Spiegle et al. 2012; O'Connor et al. 2011), decision aids and decision supports are typically designed to be used by a patient only or a patient with a clinician (Siminoff et al. 2006; Krones et al. 2008; Anderson et al. 2001; Man-Son-Hing et al. 1999; Allaire et al. 2011), reflecting the predominate paradigm of patient as a solitary decision making entity. Three notable exceptions were found in the literature, a decision aid designed to assist caregivers discuss terminal disease status with the patient (Yun et al. 2011), and the Comprehensive Health Enhancement Support System (CHESS), an interactive health communication system designed for patients, their family caregivers and clinicians (DuBenske et al. 2010) and a 90-min individualized educational session that taught basic problem-solving principles using a cognitive behavioral framework to patients with advanced cancer and their families, who were visiting a tertiary-care outpatient setting (Bucher et al. 2001).

Future Research Directions

The study of family decision making in health care requires the development of models and frameworks that specifically include family members or triadic communication in the decision making processes. The exclusion of family members from current models precludes important actors in the decision making process, focusing very narrowly on dyadic interactions that often do not accurately reflect the context in which decisions are made. Models that acknowledge the role that family members can have in the decision process will enable better understanding of how patient, family and healthcare provider negotiate the decision process including role definition for each member and definition of decisional goals. These are important but not well understood components of the decision making process that can influence health outcomes such as coping, quality of life, and decisional satisfaction. There is some evidence that patients and family members do not always agree on the roles they play in a decision. Schafer et al. (2006) found that among 50 patient–family pairs, most agreed (89 %) that shared physician–patient–family decision making was optimal yet family members (42 %) believed that their right to participate in decision making changed at the end of life compared to only 30 % of patients. Family decision making models will help to better understand the factors

that contribute to this type of communication disconnect and enable a more nuanced exploration of factors that facilitate and impede patient autonomy in the decision process as well as the incorporation of family or caregiver concerns.

It will also be important to systematically explore how physicians react to the presence of family members in different types of medical consultations. More work is needed in this area to understand physician behavior in these encounters, for example in what ways does the physician include or exclude family members in the decision making process? Are family members actively or passively included in elements of information provision, the discussion of treatment options and elicitation of goals, preference, concerns and other elements of relationship building? Skills training for healthcare providers may help physicians and other healthcare workers improve their ability to communicate and develop more meaningful care relationships with patients and their family members. More research is required to understand how physicians communicate when family members accompany patients and whether currently available physician communication skills training are also beneficial for communication in triadic encounters.

Additional research is needed in multiple health and disease contexts to understand how communication and decision making occur in diverse clinical and cultural contexts. Family decision making is likely very different depending on the type of clinical consultations, the health decision choices and the overall health and disease stage experienced by the patient. What is clear is that in an era when even complex treatment and care has shifted from the clinic to the home, understanding the role of families is a critical component of providing quality health care to patients.

References

Allaire, A. S., Labrecque, M., et al. (2011). Barriers and facilitators to the dissemination of DECISION+, a continuing medical education program for optimizing decisions about antibiotics for acute respiratory infections in primary care: A study protocol. *Implement Science, 6*, 3.

Anderson, H., Espinosa, E., et al. (2001). Evaluation of the chemotherapy patient monitor: An interactive tool for facilitating communication between patients and oncologists during the cancer consultation. *European Journal of Cancer Care (Engl), 10*(2), 115–123.

Back, M. F., & Huak, C. Y. (2005). Family centred decision making and non-disclosure of diagnosis in a South East Asian oncology practice. *Psychooncology, 14*(12), 1052–1059.

Ballard-Reisch, D. S., & Letner, J. A. (2003). Centering families in cancer communication research: Acknowledging the impact of support, culture and process on client/provider communication in cancer management. *Patient Education and Counseling, 50*(1), 61–66.

Beuchamps, T., & Childress, J. F. (2008). *Principles of biomedical ethics*. Oxford: Oxford University Press.

Botelho, R. J., Lue, B. H., et al. (1996). Family involvement in routine health care: A survey of patients' behaviors and preferences. *The Journal of Family Practice, 42*(6), 572–576.

Brittain, K., Loveland-Cherry, C., et al. (2012). Sociocultural differences and colorectal cancer screening among African American men and women. *Oncology Nursing Forum, 39*(1), 100–107.

Brown, J. B., Brett, P., et al. (1998). Roles and influence of people who accompany patients on visits to the doctor. *Canadian Family Physician, 44*, 1644–1650.

Brown, R. F., Butow, P. N., et al. (2004). Seeking informed consent to cancer clinical trials: Describing current practice. *Social Science and Medicine, 58*(12), 2445–2457.

Bucher, J. A., Loscalzo, M., et al. (2001). Problem-solving cancer care education for patients and caregivers. *Cancer practice, 9*(2), 66–70.

Charles, C., Gafni, A., et al. (1999). Decision-making in the physician-patient encounter: Revisiting the shared treatment decision-making model. *Social Science and Medicine, 49*(5), 651–661.

Clayman, M. L., Roter, D., et al. (2005). Autonomy-related behaviors of patient companions and their effect on decision-making activity in geriatric primary care visits. *Social Science and Medicine, 60*(7), 1583–1591.

Degner, L. S., & Sloan, J. A. (1992). Decision making during serious illness: What role do patients really want to play? *Journal of Clinical Epidemiology, 45*(9), 941–950.

DuBenske, L. L., Gustafson, D. H., et al. (2010). Web-based cancer communication and decision making systems: Connecting patients, caregivers, and clinicians for improved health outcomes. *Medical Decision Making, 30*(6), 732–744.

Eggly, S., Penner, L. A., et al. (2012). Patient, companion, and oncologist agreement regarding information discussed during triadic oncology clinical interactions. *Psychooncology, 22*, 637–645.

Ford, S., Hall, A., et al. (2000). The medical interaction process system (MIPS): An instrument for analysing interviews of oncologists and patients with cancer. *Social Science and Medicine, 50*(4), 553–566.

Fried, T. R., Bradley, E. H., et al. (2005). Unmet desire for caregiver-patient communication and increased caregiver burden. *Journal of the American Geriatrics Society, 53*(1), 59–65.

Fried, T. R., Bradley, E. H., et al. (2003). Valuing the outcomes of treatment: Do patients and their caregivers agree? *Archives of Internal Medicine, 163*(17), 2073–2078.

Gaugler, J. E., Hanna, N., et al. (2005). Cancer caregiving and subjective stress: A multi-site, multi-dimensional analysis. *Psycho-Oncology, 14*(9), 771–785.

Gilbar, R., & Gilbar, O. (2009). The medical decision-making process and the family: The case of breast cancer patients and their husbands. *Bioethics, 23*(3), 183–192.

Given, B. A., Given, C. W., et al. (2001). Family support in advanced cancer. *CA: A Cancer Journal for Clinicians, 51*(4), 213–231.

Given, C. W., Given, B., et al. (1992). The caregiver reaction assessment (CRA) for caregivers to persons with chronic physical and mental impairments. *Research in Nursing & Health, 15*(4), 271–283.

Gleason, M. E., Harper, F. W., et al. (2009). The influence of patient expectations regarding cure on treatment decisions. *Patient Education and Counseling, 75*(2), 263–269.

Gotcher, J. (1993). The effects of family communication on psychosocial adjustment of cancer patients. *Journal of Applied Communication Research, 21*(2), 176–188.

Gotcher, J. (1995). Well-adjusted and maladjusted cancer patients: An examination of communication variables. *Health Communication, 7*(1), 21–33.

Ho, A. (2008). Relational autonomy or undue pressure? Family's role in medical decision-making. *Scandinavian Journal of Caring Sciences, 22*(1), 128–135.

Indeck, B., & Bunney, M. (1997). Community resources. In V. T. DeVita, S. Hellman Jr., & S. A. Rosenberg (Eds.), *Cancer: Principles and practice of oncology* (5th ed., pp. 2891–2904). Philadelphia: Lippincott Williams & Wilkins.

Jones, R. A., Steeves, R., & Williams, I. (2010). Family and friend interactions among African-American men deciding whether or not to have a prostate cancer screening. *Urologic Nursing, 30*(3), 189–193.

Kahana, E., & Kahana, B. (2003). Patient proactively enhancing doctor-patient-family communication in cancer prevention and care among the aged. *Patient Education and Counseling, 50*(1), 67–73.

Kimberlin, C., Brushwood, D., et al. (2004). Cancer patient and caregiver experiences: Communication and pain management issues. *Journal of Pain and Symptom Management, 28*(6), 566–578.

Kristjanson, L. J., Atwood, J., et al. (1995). Validity and reliability of the family inventory of needs (FIN): Measuring the care needs of families of advanced cancer patients. *Journal of Nursing Measurement, 3*(2), 109–126.

Kristjanson, L. J., Leis, A., et al. (1997). Family members' care expectations, care perceptions, and satisfaction with advanced cancer care: Results of a multi-site pilot study. *Journal of Palliative Care, 13* (4), 5–13.

Krones, T., Keller, H., et al. (2008). Absolute cardiovascular disease risk and shared decision making in primary care: A randomized controlled trial. *Annals of Family Medicine, 6*(3), 218–227.

Kuczewski, M. G. (1996). Reconceiving the family: The process of consent in medical decision making. *Hastings Center Report, 26*(2), 30–37.

Lobchuk, M. M., McPherson, C. J., et al. (2012). A comparison of patient and family caregiver prospective control over lung cancer. *Journal of Advanced Nursing, 68*(5), 1122–1133.

Man-Son-Hing, M., Laupacis, A., et al. (1999). A patient decision aid regarding antithrombotic therapy for stroke prevention in atrial fibrillation: A randomized controlled trial. *JAMA, 282*(8), 737–743.

Mazanec, P., & Bartel, J. (2002). Family caregiver perspectives of pain management. *Cancer Practice, 10*(Suppl 1), S66–S69.

Nolan, M. T., Hughes, M. T., et al. (2009). Development and validation of the family decision-making self-efficacy scale. *Palliative Support Care, 7*(3), 315–321.

Northouse, L., Kershaw, T., et al. (2005). Effects of a family intervention on the quality of life of women with recurrent breast cancer and their family caregivers. *Psychooncology, 14*(6), 478–491.

O'Connor, A. M., Bennett, C. L., et al. (2009). Decision aids for people facing health treatment or screening decisions. *Cochrane Database of Systematic Reviews, 3*(3), CD001431.

O'Connor, P. J., Sperl-Hillen, J. M., et al. (2011). Impact of electronic health record clinical decision support on diabetes care: A randomized trial. *The Annals of Family Medicine, 9*(1), 12–21.

Oberst, M. T., Thomas, S. E., et al. (1989). Caregiving demands and appraisal of stress among family caregivers. *Cancer Nursing, 12*(4), 209–215.

Ohlen, J., Balneaves, L. G., et al. (2006). The influence of significant others in complementary and alternative medicine decisions by cancer patients. *Social Science and Medicine, 63*(6), 1625–1636.

Prohaska, T. R., & Glasser, M. (1996). Patients' views of family involvement in medical care decisions and encounters. *Research on Aging, 18*, 52–69.

Rim, S. H., Hall, I. J., et al. (2011). Considering racial and ethnic preferences in communication and interactions among the patient, family member, and physician following diagnosis of localized prostate cancer: Study of a US population. *International Journal of General Medicine, 4*, 481–486.

Rogers, E., & Kincaid, D. L. (1981). *Communication networks: Towards a new paradigm for research.* New York: The Free Press.

Rose, J. H. (1999). Book review: Communication and the cancer patient: Information and truth. *Journal of Ethics, Law and Aging, 5*(1), 71–73.

Sanford, J., Townsend-Rocchicciolli, J., et al. (2011). A process of decision making by caregivers of family members with heart failure. *Research Theory Nursing Practice, 25*(1), 55–70.

Sayers, S. L., White, T., et al. (2006). Family involvement in the care of healthy medical outpatients. *Family Practice, 23*(3), 317–324.

Schafer, C., Putnik, K., et al. (2006). Medical decision-making of the patient in the context of the family: Results of a survey. *Supportive Care in Cancer, 14*(9), 952–959.

Schilling, L. M., Scatena, L., et al. (2002). The third person in the room: Frequency, role, and influence of companions during primary care medical encounters. *Journal of Family Practice, 51*(8), 685–690.

Sebern, M. D. (2008). Refinement of the shared care instrument-revised: A measure of a family care interaction. *Journal of Nursing Measurement, 16*(1), 43–60.

Siminoff, L. A., Gordon, N. H., et al. (2006). A decision aid to assist in adjuvant therapy choices for breast cancer. *Psycho-Oncology, 15*(11), 1001–1013.

Siminoff, L. A., & Step, M. M. (2005). A communication model of shared decision making: Accounting for cancer treatment decisions. *Health Psychology: Official Journal of the Division of Health Psychology, American Psychological Association, 24*(4 Suppl), S99–S105.

Siminoff, L. A., & Step, M. M. (2011). A comprehensive observational coding scheme for analyzing instrumental, affective, and relational communication in health care contexts. *Journal of health communication, 16* (2), 178–197.

Siminoff, L. A., Wilson-Genderson, M., et al. (2010). Depressive symptoms in lung cancer patients and their family caregivers and the influence of family environment. *Psycho-Oncology, 19*(12), 1285–1293.

Siminoff, L. A., Zyzanski, S. J., et al. (2008). The cancer communication assessment tool for patients and families (CCAT-PF): A new measure. *Psycho-Oncology, 17*(12), 1216–1224.

Simon, D., Loh, A., et al. (2007). Measuring (shared) decision-making—A review of psychometric instruments. *Zeitschrift Arztliche Fortbildung Qualitatssich, 101*(4), 259–267.

Spiegle, G., Al-Sukhni, E., et al. (2012). Patient decision aids for cancer treatment: Are there any alternatives? *Cancer, 119*, 189–200.

Street, R. L, Jr., Makoul, G., et al. (2009). How does communication heal? Pathways linking clinician-patient communication to health outcomes. *Patient Education and Counseling, 74*(3), 295–301.

Street, R. L, Jr., & Millay, B. (2001). Analyzing patient participation in medical encounters. *Health Communication, 13*(1), 61–73.

Towle, A., & Godolphin, W. (1999). Framework for teaching and learning informed shared decision making. *BMJ (Clinical Research ed.), 319*, 766–771.

Walsh-Burke, K. (1992). Family communication and coping with cancer: Impact of the we can weekend. *Journal of Psychosocial Oncology, 10*(1), 63–81.

Yun, Y. H., Lee, M. K., et al. (2011). Use of a decision aid to help caregivers discuss terminal disease status with a family member with cancer: A randomized controlled trial. *Journal of Clinical Oncology, 29*(36), 4811–4819.

Zeliadt, S. B., Penson, D. F., et al. (2011). Provider and partner interactions in the treatment decision-making process for newly diagnosed localized prostate cancer. *BJU International, 108*(6), 851–856. (discussion 856–857).

Zhang, A. Y., & Siminoff, L. A. (2003). Silence and cancer: Why do families and patients fail to communicate? *Health Communication, 15*(4), 415–429.

Zhang, A. Y., Zyzanski, S. J., et al. (2011). Ethnic differences in the caregiver's attitudes and preferences about the treatment and care of advanced lung cancer patients. *Psycho-Oncology, 21*, 1250–1253.

Shared Decision-Making and the Patient-Provider Relationship

Kathryn J. Rowland and Mary C. Politi

Introduction

Approximately 82 % of Americans over age 40 have made a medical decision within the past 2 years across decisions ranging from initiating medications to type and timing of cancer screening to whether or not to have surgery (Zikmund-Fisher et al. 2010a). More than half (56 %) have made two or more health decisions in the past 2 years (Zikmund-Fisher et al. 2010a). Some health decisions are relatively simple to make based on strong data about a beneficial intervention with minimal associated risks, minimal lifestyle disruptions, and minimal costs. However, most medical decisions are burdened with unclear, conflicting, or unknown data (Esserman et al. 2009). Intervention options often require significant trade-offs between their associated benefits and risks. In these situations, shared decision making can assist clinicians and patients as they together weigh the scientific evidence with patient's preferences and goals to reach an agreement about health decisions with no clear

best option from an evidence standpoint. In this chapter, we will introduce the concept of shared decision making between patients and clinicians, and we will discuss current and future applications of shared decision making in clinical practice.

Supporting Good Quality Health Decisions

It is tempting to equate "good" medical outcomes with "good" healthcare decisions. In the era of CT scanners, robotic surgery, and genome mapping, patients often expect the certainty of medical success when treating diseases. However, over half of all medical interventions have unknown or uncertain benefits (Esserman et al. 2009). Even healthcare decisions made based on strong evidence can lead to unanticipated or anticipated negative effects. Invasive interventions may prolong a patient's duration of life but result in a significantly lower quality of life. Therefore, decisions could be perceived both positively and negatively by patients and clinicians depending on the context and aspect of the decision being evaluated (Politi and Street 2011). In this paper, we define quality medical decisions as those that are made based on the best available clinical evidence, incorporate patients values and preferences, involve patients in the decision making process, and are feasible to implement (Elwyn et al. 2000; Sepucha et al. 2007).

K.J. Rowland
Department of Surgery, Washington University School of Medicine, 660 South Euclid Avenue, Campus Box 8109, St. Louis, MO 63110, USA
e-mail: rowlandk@wudosis.wustl.edu

M.C. Politi (✉)
Division of Public Health Sciences, Department of Surgery, Washington University School of Medicine, 660 South Euclid Avenue, Campus Box 8100, St. Louis, MO 63112, USA
e-mail: mpoliti@wustl.edu

© Springer Science+Business Media New York 2016
M.A. Diefenbach et al. (eds.), *Handbook of Health Decision Science*,
DOI 10.1007/978-1-4939-3486-7_14

Unfortunately, good quality decisions in healthcare are not always the norm. Only 36 % of patients feel well informed when facing important medical decisions (Sepucha et al. 2010). Most patients want to be informed to some extent about their diseases, although preferences for the amount of involvement may vary by patient characteristics (Benbassat et al. 1998). Although a balanced discussion of the clinical evidence and incorporation of patient values and preferences are essential to quality medical decisions, clinicians are much more likely to actively discuss the advantages of a treatment rather than its potential harms (Zikmund-Fisher et al. 2010b), and they are more likely to express an opinion about a decision than solicit patients' preferences (Zikmund-Fisher et al. 2010b).

Lack of information and failure to solicit patient preferences can lead to significant discrepancies between a physician's assessments and recommendations and the actual implementation of appropriate care (Benbassat et al. 1998; Rimer et al. 2004). Most medical interventions require patient input and acceptance in order to be effective. For example, while clinicians can prescribe a medication or recommend surgery, the impetus is on the patient to fill and take the prescription or schedule and show up for surgery. These behaviors are unlikely to occur if a patient does not support or agree with his/her physician's recommendation.

Shared decision making can improve patients decision quality by improving their knowledge about the decision, clarifying their values for the possible outcomes of the decision, and improving the match between their values and choice. (Sepucha et al. 2004). Improving decision quality may improve the quality of overall care by better matching the right patients with the right care for them. The 2012 National Quality Strategy announced patient and family engagement (including shared decision making) as a priority in healthcare reform with the potential to eradicate disparities, reduce harm, increase underuse, and decrease overuse of interventions in the American healthcare system (Fenwick et al. 2001).

Shared Decision Making

Shared decision making is a collaborative approach during which clinicians and patients work together to reach an agreement regarding a healthcare decision (Charles et al. 1997; Edwards and Elwyn 2006; O'Connor et al. 2009). The process involves reviewing the best medical evidence, soliciting patient preferences and values, and addressing potential outcomes so that the patient can understand the implications of their choice before a joint decision is reached (Charles et al. 1997).

The process of shared decision making is especially important for patients facing preference-sensitive conditions where treatment options are accompanied with substantial trade-offs between benefits and risks to the patient. Compared to usual care, patients who participate in shared decision making demonstrate improved understanding of their choices and are more likely to receive treatment that is aligned with their personal preferences and values (Stacey et al. 2011a). Patients who receive more information regarding their treatment options may choose to receive a lower intensity of services than those who are less informed about options and their associated uncertainty (Stacey et al. 2011a). A study of patients with preference-sensitive conditions—including heart conditions, benign uterine conditions, benign prostatic hyperplasia, joint pain, and back pain—found that patients who received enhanced support through contact with health coaches (via telephone, mail, e-mail, or the internet) opted for fewer preference-sensitive surgeries, had fewer hospital admissions, and had lower overall medical costs (Veroff et al. 2013). In medical ethics, shared decision making has been advocated as the balancing force between the principles of patient autonomy and beneficence (Elwyn et al. 1999; Stiggelbout et al. 2012).

Quality shared decision making for complex decisions requires clinician and patient skills and engagement. Clinicians first must have the necessary clinical knowledge, reasoning, and judgment to correctly interpret medical evidence and its associated uncertainty (Dy and Purnell 2012). The content, quantity, and level of detail of information, verbal versus written form, and timing of presentation are all important considerations (Epstein et al. 2004). Framing of this information can also impact patients' understanding and decisions (Moxey et al. 2003). For example, presenting information in a formats using frequencies (e.g., X out of 100), pictorial representations of risk, and using both positive and negative frames are associated with improved patient knowledge (Edwards et al. 2001).

In addition, interpersonal skills including respect, empathy, and fidelity towards the patient are essential to establishing a relationship from which to engage in shared decision making (Dy and Purnell 2012). Shared decision making respects patient autonomy and seeks to foster a sense of partnership between clinician and patient. For this partnership to succeed, clinicians must elicit, understand, and validate the patient's perspective, involve the patient in care and decision making to the extent the patient desires to be, provide clear and understandable explanations, and foster trust and commitment (Epstein and Peters 2009). Lack of trust can inhibit shared decision making and patients' willingness to engage in the shared decision making process (Pearson and Raeke 2000; Poses et al. 1995).

Patients also require shared decision making skills, including an ability to understand clinical information, appreciate its significance, and apply the information to make value-consistent decisions (Dunn et al. 2006). In addition, patients need communication skills and self-efficacy to ask questions, state preferences, express concerns, and offer opinions (Street and Millay 2001). As a process, shared decision making requires communicating about the patient's

health condition, sharing both a patient's and his/her clinician's perspective on the decision, and reaching an agreement about the best treatment option for the individual patient (Politi and Street 2011). However, during the process, patients can disagree with some of what their clinician suggests about treatment or preferences for possible outcomes of treatment. Patients may fear being labeled as a "difficult patient," or feel as if they will receive inferior care if they express disagreement (Adams et al. 2012). Thus the process can present challenges even for patients with skills understanding clinical information and communicating their preferences.

Although patients typically want some level of involvement in medical decisions, the degree that a patient desires to be in control of the decisions may change across different medical scenarios (Deber et al. 1996). In one study, patients preferred clinicians to be more involved in decisions that ultimately impacted mortality, but preferred to remain in greater control of decisions impacting morbidity or quality of life (Deber et al. 1996). The act of involving the patient in the decision making process may be more important than whether the patient or clinician ultimately makes the final decision (Edwards and Elwyn 2006). For patients with reluctance or hesitance to engage in the process, encouragement and patient-centered communication can increase patient empowerment, self-efficacy, and involvement and improve decision making (Dy and Purnell 2012).

Decision aids may also facilitate the shared decision making process. Decision aids serve as balanced sources of information regarding the treatment options for a particular health condition (Stacey et al. 2011b). They aim to present information in plain language, describe alternatives to treat or manage a condition, and provide information about the risks and benefits to various treatment options. Decision aids can take the form of paper-based brochures or pamphlets, videos, or websites The use of decision aids in making treatment choices has been shown to increase patient knowledge of options, risks, and benefits, create more realistic expectations, lower decisional conflict, reduce uncertainty, enhance active patient participation, decrease the number of undecided patients, and improve agreement between values and choices (Stacey et al. 2011b).

Shared Decision Making in Practice

Future Opportunities for the Application of Shared Decision Making: High-Risk Surgical Procedures, Postoperative Care, and Surgical "Buy-in"

Shared decision making can be used to facilitate the implementation of care that aligns with patient preferences and values (Fenwick et al. 2001; Sepucha et al. 2004). While applicable to many medical care decisions, shared decision making is especially important for preference-sensitive decisions. In the past, shared decision making has been applied to medical decisions regarding screening, medical drug therapy initiation, and elective surgery. Decision aids designed to promote shared decision making have been developed for a variety of clinical decisions, including but not limited to prostate cancer screening and treatment, prenatal screening, obstetrical decisions, male newborn circumcision, vaccination, colon cancer screening, genetic testing, diabetes treatment, hormone replacement therapy, treatment for abnormal uterine bleeding, back surgery, breast cancer treatment, heart disease management, and osteoporosis treatment (Stacey et al. 2011b). However, discussions about high-risk surgical procedures, postoperative care, and surgical "buy-in" is one area in which shared decision making could greatly improve clinical care, but has yet to be applied.

Elective high-risk surgical procedures include many vascular procedures, cardiac surgery, thoracic surgery, transplant surgery, extensive abdominal operations, and neurosurgery. Such procedures are considered elective if the patient's life is not in immediate jeopardy (requiring emergent surgery) and if the operation is planned in advance. These high-risk elective procedures

have a high mortality rate (generally considered to be above 3 %) and may result in the need for prolonged postoperative intensive care unit stay and temporary or permanent respiratory failure requiring tracheostomy, renal failure requiring hemodialysis, use of artificial nutrition, and/or non-healing surgical wounds. Given the inherent risks of the surgery and postoperative care, and given the fact that these operations are planned in advance, discussion of the risks, benefits, and postoperative care is necessary for patients to make informed decisions about surgery.

Unfortunately, detailed discussion of risks, benefits, and postoperative care is often either left out of preoperative discussions or is very briefly discussed with patients. A study of surgeon-patient discussions regarding treatment for abdominal aortic aneurysms revealed that only a minority of discussions (29 %) addressed the disorder, the proposed procedure, the consequences and risks of surgery, the option of watchful observation, and individual prognosis (Knops et al. 2010). Moreover, 18 % of patients after aneurysm surgery indicated that they would not have undergone surgery had they understood the recovery process involved (Williamson et al. 2001). Even when patients are provided with adequate information, they may fail to comprehend important details necessary to make an informed decision (Mulsow et al. 2012). For example, among patients consenting to carotid endarterectomy, most had unrealistic expectations as to the risks and benefits of surgery and postoperative care (Lloyd et al. 2001); And a study of postoperative laparoscopic cholecystectomy patients found that while 84 % believed they were well informed and satisfied with the information provided to them, only 51 % demonstrated satisfactory knowledge of the procedure, and only 30 % could list a potential complication of the procedure (Kriwanek et al. 1998). A similar lack of understanding of the basic information required for surgical consent has been shown in patients undergoing coronary artery bypass grafting, carotid surgery, lower-limb bypass, hip arthroplasty, and varicose vein surgery (Dillon et al. 2005; Larobina et al.

2007; Mishra et al. 2006; Stanley et al. 1998; Turner and Williams 2002).

In addition, surgeons often assumed or infer patient preferences without explicitly discussing how patient preferences might affect surgery decisions and subsequent postoperative care. Surgical "buy-in" has been described by surgeons as the informal contract between surgeons and patients that commits a patient to the surgeon's anticipated postoperative care when the patient consent for an operative procedure (Schwarze et al. 2010). Surgeons often view this commitment to postoperative care as a packaged deal, a roughly 30 day commitment by the patient to receive intensive life-sustaining therapy, including mechanical ventilation, hemodynamic support, hemodialysis, artificial nutrition, and additional invasive procedures after a surgical intervention (Schwarze et al. 2010). While such anticipated postoperative care may involve preference-sensitive life-sustaining therapies, it is unclear if patients are aware of having consented to such care upon arrival in the operating room for a preference-sensitive, elective procedure (Schwarze et al. 2010).

Surgeons invest time, operating facilities, and resources (including scarce resources such as blood products) in their patients, and while poor outcomes are expected to occasionally occur, these outcomes are often viewed as personal failures of the surgeon (Schwarze et al. 2010). These factors all contribute to the sentiment of the surgeon to do everything possible to prolong the patient's life. However, many patients have strong opinions regarding the use of life-sustaining interventions. Surgeons performing such operations recognize the importance of preoperative discussion with patients prior to proceeding to the operating room (McKneally et al. 2009), but it is not clear that patients fully understand and consent to the plan for postoperative care that is assumed by the surgeon. The lack of patient input preoperatively results in patients proceeding with surgery and subsequently finding themselves in situations postoperatively where life-supporting therapy is implemented, potentially against their wishes.

In one study, none of the surgeons in the study reported formal documentation of this explicit contract (Schwarze et al. 2010). Some view the presence of a signed informed consent document as evidence that such a contract exists (Schwarze et al. 2010). Ideally, surgical consent should include a discussion of whether the patient authorizes the surgeon to treat complications after the procedure, including prolonged mechanical ventilation or intensive care unit stay (Bernat and Peterson 2006). Unfortunately, in many cases, patients remain uninformed and unaware of surgical "buy-in". Many suggest that informed consent should be a process and not simply a document. However, often, clinicians simply request signatures from patients without any engagement in shared decision making prior to signing informed consent documents (Weinstein et al. 2007).

To better communicate about surgical "buy-in" and engage in shared decision making about these high-risk elective procedures, clinicians could design improved informed consent documents for surgery that include postoperative care as a distinct entity on the forms. However, in current practice, patients feel misinformed about the surgeries themselves, much less the unaddressed issue of "buy-in" and postoperative care. In addition, focusing only on improving consent documents to include stipulations on postoperative care is likely to have little effect on current practice. One study demonstrated that 70 % of surgical patients do not read the informed consent form (Lavelle-Jones et al. 1993). Most adults admit that the forms are too long, intimidating, with small, crowded text and unexplained medical and legal terms (Han et al., in press), and the readability of these documents exceeds the average reading level in the United States (Einhorn and Hogarth 1986). Developing consent documents that pay attention to principles of health literacy (Lorenzen et al. 2008) and including personalized risk assessments (Krumholz 2010) can improve patient-centered decision making. Yet research suggests that going beyond improving informed consent documents and focusing on the informed consent process and discussion is needed to improve understanding and decision making (Flory and Emanuel 2004).

Patients express a strong desire to be informed about the risks of surgical procedures (Larobina et al. 2007). Surgeons greatly underestimate patients need for information relating to surgery and the perioperative period (Keulers et al. 2008). Some believe that providing patients with detailed information regarding the risks of procedures may increase anxiety, however this is not supported by the research (Garrud et al. 2001). Shared decision making can help improve the surgical "buy-in" and informed consent discussion by involving patients in conversations about surgery and all postoperative care, incorporating patients' values into the discussion, and agreeing on a plan based on possible outcomes of surgery and postoperative complications. Consenting to surgery with agreed upon limitations to postoperative care, or not consenting to the high-risk elective procedures are both reasonable options depending on patients' goals and values. Surgeons should include their patients in shared decision making to ensure that proceeding with surgery and postoperative care aligns with the patient's preferences. The major limitation of preoperative discussion of the patient's preferences about postoperative care is the lack of familiarity and experience that patients have with life-sustaining interventions. Patients sometimes report higher quality of life postoperatively than they would have predicted preoperatively when forced to deal with previously unimaginable situations (such as a colostomy or paraplegia) (Ubel et al. 2005). It is possible that patients opposed to life sustaining interventions preoperatively may support such measures postoperatively.

The role of decision aids and patient narratives during surgical "buy-in" might assist in this process, although the role of decision aids for informed consent remains unclear. In studies on surgical consent, paper based tools have been shown to have little effect on patient's understanding of surgical consent and are often too difficult to read (Mulsow et al. 2012). Multimedia interventions as an adjunct to informed consent have been shown to increase recall and knowledge (Danino et al. 2005; Evrard et al.

2005; Mulsow et al. 2012). However, these interventions have failed to have an effect on patient understanding of potential complications (Danino et al. 2005), with surgical patients who had adverse outcomes showing poor recollection of key messages in respect to complications (Evrard et al. 2005).

Challenges in Shared Decision Making

The above section described one potential application of shared decision making to an important clinical context. However, across many areas, shared decision making in clinical practice remains a challenge.

Work Flow and Time Limitations

Time constraints are the most frequently cited barrier to implementation of shared decision making in clinical practice (Legare et al. 2008). Despite the perceived time constraints, no robust evidence exists that more time is required to engage in shared decision making than to offer usual care (Legare et al. 2010, 2012; Stacey et al. 2011a). As Legare and Witteman argue, time constraints are the most frequently cited barrier to *any* change in clinical practice and implementation of shared decision making is no different in this sense than implementation of any other practice improvement (Legare and Witteman 2013).

Health Literacy Skills

Health literacy represents "the degree to which individuals have the capacity to obtain, process, and understand basic health information and services needed to make appropriate health decisions" (Einhorn and Hogarth 1986). In the shared decision making process, limited health literacy skills may affect a patient's ability to understand and process the medical information required to make an informed decision. Patients with limited health literacy skills have more difficulty understanding physician instructions (Schillinger et al. 2004; Williams et al. 2002), and ask fewer questions (Katz et al. 2007). Clinicians commonly overestimate patients' literacy levels (Bass et al. 2002; Powell and Kripalani 2005), and patients may hide their limited understanding out of embarrassment (Parikh et al. 1996). Patients with limited health literacy skills are overrepresented among those with chronic diseases (Dewalt et al. 2004; Howard et al. 2005). Health literacy skills are not related to the amount of information that patients desire, however, patients with lower literacy skills may have lower knowledge recall and might be less likely to want an active role in medical decision making (Lillie et al. 2007). Clarifying decision role preference, using everyday language/avoiding of medical jargon, limiting the amount of information discussed at each visit, and using teach-back techniques to confirm patient understanding can help this population (Kripalani and Weiss 2006).

Numeracy Skills

Shared decision making involves an understanding of treatment options and the associated benefits and harms, and the process often requires clinicians to communicate statistical information to patients. Low numeracy skills are pervasive across the US population (Nelson et al. 2008) and can present challenges when communicating and interpreting risk/benefit information. One study demonstrated that only 20 % of participants were able to convert the frequency 1 in 1000 to a percentage (Lipkus et al. 2001). Low numeracy skills cannot be predicted based on education or other sociodemographic characteristics (Nelson et al. 2008). When numeric data is available, risks and benefits of treatment options should be presented as frequencies (e.g., X out of 100 or X out of 1000) with a consistent denominator (Fagerlin et al. 2011). In some cases, qualitative "gist" understanding may result in superior quantitative processing (Nelson

et al. 2008; Reyna 2005). One drawback to the gist approach is that individuals may interpret qualitative values such as "not likely", "somewhat likely", and "very likely" or "high risk" or "low risk" differently from that of the clinician. As patients weigh the risks and benefits, it is important to reinforce the time interval over which risk occurs (Fagerlin et al. 2011). Risks may or may not be assumed immediately and may or may not dissipate over time, while the expected benefits of treatment may or may not be realized immediately or over the course of years, if at all. Research has demonstrated that patients with limited numeracy skills are less likely to prefer active roles in shared decision making, although education efforts to improve numeric understanding and using non-quantitative communication may foster the involvement of patients with limited numeracy skills during shared decision making (Galesic and Garcia-Retamero 2011).

Surrogate Decision Making

Surrogate decision making introduces additional challenges into the shared decision making process. Surrogates may not know patient preferences for a particular situation or may encounter difficulty in applying the patient's preferences rather than their own (Shah et al. 2009). Conflicts of interest, family conflict, emotions, and role expectations may affect decision making (Schenker et al. 2012). Research has shown that treatment options that seem reasonable for oneself may seem less appropriate when giving advice or acting on behalf of another (Zikmund-Fisher et al. 2006). Surrogate decisions can suffer from omission bias, where an error of omission is seen as preferable to an error of commission (Asch et al. 1994). For example, a parent may choose not to vaccinate a child (an omission) due to unsubstantiated or exaggerated fears that vaccination (a commission) will result in serious side effects. Research on surrogate decision making is recent and growing, and will help clinicians better learn how to incorporate surrogates into shared decision making with patients.

Teaching Shared Decision Making

Shared decision making has the potential to improve patient health while helping control healthcare costs (Frosch et al. 2011). Despite its promise, shared decision making has not been universally integrated into clinical practice (Pellerin et al. 2011). The Accreditation Council for Graduate Medical Education has recognized the need to train physicians in communication and interpersonal skills, and endorses such skills as a general competency requirement for medical education during residency. Despite this requirement, studies have demonstrated that physician residents overestimated the clarity to which they were able to communicate with patients and, on average, used two medical jargon terms per minute in interactions with standardized patients (Howard et al. 2013). While it is clear that clinicians need more training in clear communication and the shared decision making approach, the best interventions to teach such skills or to measure professional competency of such skills remains unclear (Epstein and Hundert 2002; Legare et al. 2010; Legare and Witteman 2013). Use of educational meetings, giving healthcare professionals feedback, giving healthcare professionals learning materials, and using patient decision aids have been tried to increase the adaptation of shared decision making by established healthcare professionals (Legare et al. 2010); standardized patients, workshops, and role modeling have been suggested for training resident physicians and medical students in the use of shared decision making (Kripalani and Weiss 2006; Lagan et al. 2013).

Conclusions

Shared decision making involves providing information to patients as to the benefits and risks associated with different treatment options and incorporating patient values into the treatment decision (Charles et al. 1997). Shared decision making respects patient autonomy and seeks to foster a sense of partnership between clinician and patient. For this partnership to succeed,

clinicians must elicit, understand, and validate the patient's perspective, involve the patient in care and decision making to the extent the patient desires to be, provide clear and understandable explanations, and foster a relationship of trust and commitment (Epstein and Peters 2009). The clinician-patient relationship can have a significant impact on medical decision making. In some settings, when discussions occur in clinical practice without a shared decision making approach, physician recommendations have been shown to lead patients to make decisions against what they would otherwise prefer (Gurmankin et al. 2002). In addition, there is a delicate balance between involving patients in medical decision making without leaving them feeling unsupported through the complex process of making sense of uncertain clinical evidence. Patients should feel empowered, and not abandoned, during the shared decision making process. Overall, the goal of shared decision making is to encourage a patient-clinician discussion that goes beyond factual information giving, resulting in the physician and patient understanding the patient's health condition, discussing each other's perspective about the decision and its associated uncertainty, incorporating patients' values into the decision, and agreeing on a decision and follow-up plan. In this chapter, we present current and future applications of shared decision making, and discuss some challenges incorporating shared decision making in clinical practice. Additional research, shared decision making training opportunities, and institutional policy approaches can illuminate possible solutions to these challenges.

Key Points

Shared decision making is a collaborative approach where physicians and patients work together to reach an agreement regarding a preference-sensitive healthcare decision where valid treatment options are accompanied by both risks and benefits.

The shared decision making process involves presenting the medical evidence clearly, soliciting patient preferences and values, and addressing potential outcomes so that the patient can appreciate the implications of their decision before an agreement is reached.

Shared decision making facilitates the implementation of care that aligns with patient preferences and values, and may increase patient compliance and adherence with medical treatment. Several innovative applications of shared decision making are discussed in this chapter.

One innovative application in the field of surgery is to practice shared decision making regarding high-risk surgical procedures and postoperative care. This chapter discusses how shared decision making could enhance informed consent and patient-centered care for high-risk surgical procedures that carry significant risk of need for intensive, life-sustaining, postoperative care.

References

Adams, J. R., Elwyn, G., Legare, F., & Frosch, D. L. (2012). Communicating with physicians about medical decisions: A reluctance to disagree. *Archives of Internal Medicine, 172,* 1184–1186.

Asch, D. A., Baron, J., Hershey, J. C., Kunreuther, H., Meszaros, J., et al. (1994). Omission bias and pertussis vaccination. *Medical Decision Making, 14,* 118–123.

Bass, P. F, 3rd, Wilson, J. F., Griffith, C. H., & Barnett, D. R. (2002). Residents' ability to identify patients with poor literacy skills. *Academic Medicine: Journal of the Association of American Medical Colleges, 77,* 1039–1041.

Benbassat, J., Pilpel, D., & Tidhar, M. (1998). Patients' preferences for participation in clinical decision making: A review of published surveys. *Behavioral Medicine, 24,* 81–88.

Bernat, J. L., & Peterson, L. M. (2006). Patient-centered informed consent in surgical practice. *Archives of Surgery, 141,* 86–92.

Charles, C., Gafni, A., & Whelan, T. (1997). Shared decision-making in the medical encounter: What does it mean? (Or it takes at least two to tango). *Social Science and Medicine, 44,* 681–692.

Danino, A. M., Chahraoui, K., Frachebois, L., Jebrane, A., Moutel, G., et al. (2005). Effects of an informational CD-ROM on anxiety and knowledge before aesthetic surgery: A randomised trial. *British Journal of Plastic Surgery, 58,* 379–383.

Deber, R. B., Kraetschmer, N., & Irvine, J. (1996). What role do patients wish to play in treatment decision making? *Archives of Internal Medicine, 156,* 1414–1420.

Dewalt, D. A., Berkman, N. D., Sheridan, S., Lohr, K. N., & Pignone, M. P. (2004). Literacy and health outcomes: A systematic review of the literature. *Journal of General Internal Medicine, 19,* 1228–1239.

Dillon, M. F., Carr, C. J., Feeley, T. M., & Tierney, S. (2005). Impact of the informed consent process on patients' understanding of varicose veins and their treatment. *Irish Journal of Medical Science, 174,* 23–27.

Dunn, L. B., Nowrangi, M. A., Palmer, B. W., Jeste, D. V., & Saks, E. R. (2006). Assessing decisional capacity for clinical research or treatment: A review of instruments. *The American Journal of Psychiatry, 163,* 1323–1334.

Dy, S. M., & Purnell, T. S. (2012). Key concepts relevant to quality of complex and shared decision-making in health care: A literature review. *Social Science and Medicine, 74,* 582–587.

Edwards, A., & Elwyn, G. (2006). Inside the black box of shared decision making: Distinguishing between the process of involvement and who makes the decision. *Health Expectations, 9,* 307–320.

Edwards, A., Elwyn, G., Covey, J., Matthews, E., & Pill, R. (2001). Presenting risk information—A review of the effects of "framing" and other manipulations on patient outcomes. *Journal of Health Communication, 6,* 61–82.

Einhorn, H. J., & Hogarth, R. M. (1986). Decision making under uncertainty. *Journal of Business, 59,* S225–S250.

Elwyn, G., Edwards, A., & Kinnersley, P. (1999). Shared decision-making in primary care: The neglected second half of the consultation. *British Journal of General Practice, 49,* 477–482.

Elwyn, G., Edwards, A., Kinnersley, P., & Grol, R. (2000). Shared decision making and the concept of equipoise: The competences of involving patients in healthcare choices. *British Journal of General Practice, 50,* 892–899.

Epstein, R. M., Alper, B. S., & Quill, T. E. (2004). Communicating evidence for participatory decision making. *JAMA: The Journal of the American Medical Association, 291,* 2359–2366.

Epstein, R. M., & Hundert, E. M. (2002). Defining and assessing professional competence. *JAMA: The Journal of the American Medical Association, 287,* 226–235.

Epstein, R. M., & Peters, E. (2009). Beyond information: Exploring patients' preferences. *JAMA: The Journal of the American Medical Association, 302,* 195–197.

Esserman, L., Shieh, Y., & Thompson, I. (2009). Rethinking screening for breast cancer and prostate cancer. *JAMA, 302,* 1685–1692.

Evrard, S., Mathoulin-Pelissier, S., Larrue, C., Lapouge, P., Bussieres, E., & Tunon De Lara, C. (2005). Evaluation of a preoperative multimedia information program in surgical oncology. *European Journal of Surgical Oncology: The journal of the European Society of Surgical Oncology and the British Association of Surgical Oncology, 31*, 106–110.

Fagerlin, A., Zikmund-Fisher, B. J., & Ubel, P. A. (2011). Helping patients decide: Ten steps to better risk communication. *Journal of the National Cancer Institute, 103*, 1436–1443.

Fenwick, E., Claxton, K., & Sculpher, M. (2001). Representing uncertainty: The role of cost-effectiveness acceptability curves. *Health Economics, 10*, 779–787.

Flory, J., & Emanuel, E. (2004). Interventions to improve research participants' understanding in informed consent for research: A systematic review. *JAMA: The Journal of the American Medical Association, 292*, 1593–1601.

Frosch, D. L., Moulton, B. W., Wexler, R. M., Holmes-Rovner, M., Volk, R. J., & Levin, C. A. (2011). Shared decision making in the United States: Policy and implementation activity on multiple fronts. *Zeitschrift fur Evidenz, Fortbildung und Qualitat im Gesundheitswesen, 105*, 305–312.

Galesic, M., & Garcia-Retamero, R. (2011). Do low-numeracy people avoid shared decision making? *Health psychology: Official Journal of the Division of Health Psychology, American Psychological Association, 30*, 336–341.

Garrud, P., Wood, M., & Stainsby, L. (2001). Impact of risk information in a patient education leaflet. *Patient Education and Counseling, 43*, 301–304.

Gurmankin, A. D., Baron, J., Hershey, J. C., & Ubel, P. A. (2002). The role of physicians' recommendations in medical treatment decisions. *Medical Decision Making, 22*, 262–271.

Han PK, Korbrin SC, Klein WMP, Davis WW, Stefanak M, Taplin SH. Perceived ambiguity about screening mammography recommendations: Association with future mammography uptake and perceptions. *Cancer Epidemiology Biomarkers and Prevention* (in press).

Howard, D. H., Gazmararian, J., & Parker, R. M. (2005). The impact of low health literacy on the medical costs of medicare managed care enrollees. *The American journal of medicine, 118*, 371–377.

Howard T, Jacobson KL, Kripalani S. (2013). Doctor talk: Physicians' use of clear verbal communication. *Journal of health communication*

Katz, M. G., Jacobson, T. A., Veledar, E., & Kripalani, S. (2007). Patient literacy and question-asking behavior during the medical encounter: A mixed-methods analysis. *Journal of General Internal Medicine, 22*, 782–786.

Keulers, B. J., Scheltinga, M. R., Houterman, S., Van Der Wilt, G. J., & Spauwen, P. H. (2008). Surgeons underestimate their patients' desire for preoperative information. *World Journal of Surgery, 32*, 964–970.

Knops, A. M., Ubbink, D. T., Legemate, D. A., de Haes, J. C., & Goossens, A. (2010). Information communicated with patients in decision making about their abdominal aortic aneurysm. *European Journal of Vascular and Endovascular Surgery: The Official Journal of the European Society for Vascular Surgery, 39*, 708–713.

Kripalani, S., & Weiss, B. D. (2006). Teaching about health literacy and clear communication. *Journal of General Internal Medicine, 21*, 888–890.

Kriwanek, S., Armbruster, C., Beckerhinn, P., Blauensteier, W., & Gschwantler, M. (1998). Patients' assessment and recall of surgical information after laparoscopic cholecystectomy. *Digestive surgery, 15*, 669–673.

Krumholz, H. M. (2010). Informed consent to promote patient-centered care. *JAMA: The Journal of the American Medical Association, 303*, 1190–1191.

Lagan, C., Wehbe-Janek, H., Waldo, K., Fox, A., Jo, C., & Rahm, M. (2013). Evaluation of an interprofessional clinician-patient communication workshop utilizing standardized patient methodology. *Journal of Surgical Education, 70*, 95–103.

Larobina, M. E., Merry, C. J., Negri, J. C., & Pick, A. W. (2007). Is informed consent in cardiac surgery and percutaneous coronary intervention achievable? *ANZ Journal of Surgery, 77*, 530–534.

Lavelle-Jones, C., Byrne, D. J., Rice, P., & Cuschieri, A. (1993). Factors affecting quality of informed consent. *BMJ, 306*, 885–890.

Legare, F., Ratte, S., Gravel, K., & Graham, I. D. (2008). Barriers and facilitators to implementing shared decision-making in clinical practice: Update of a systematic review of health professionals' perceptions. *Patient Education and Counseling, 73*, 526–535.

Legare F, Ratte S, Stacey D, Kryworuchko J, Gravel K, et al. (2010). Interventions for improving the adoption of shared decision making by healthcare professionals. *Cochrane Database Syst Rev*, CD006732

Legare, F., Turcotte, S., Stacey, D., Ratte, S., Kryworuchko, J., & Graham, I. D. (2012). Patients' perceptions of sharing in decisions: A systematic review of interventions to enhance shared decision making in routine clinical practice. *Patient, 5*, 1–19.

Legare, F., & Witteman, H. O. (2013). Shared decision making: Examining key elements and barriers to adoption into routine clinical practice. *Health Affairs (Millwood), 32*, 276–284.

Lillie, S. E., Brewer, N. T., O'Neill, S. C., Morrill, E. F., Dees, E. C., et al. (2007). Retention and use of breast cancer recurrence risk information from genomic tests: The role of health literacy. *Cancer Epidemiology, Biomarkers and Prevention: A Publication of the American Association for Cancer Research, Cosponsored by the American Society of Preventive Oncology, 16*, 249–255.

Lipkus, I. M., Samsa, G., & Rimer, B. K. (2001). General performance on a numeracy scale among highly educated samples. *Medical Decision Making, 21*, 37–44.

Lloyd, A., Hayes, P., Bell, P. R., & Naylor, A. R. (2001). The role of risk and benefit perception in informed consent for surgery. *Medical Decision Making, 21,* 141–149.

Lorenzen, B., Melby, C. E., & Earles, B. (2008). Using principles of health literacy to enhance the informed consent process. *AORN Journal, 88,* 23–29.

McKneally, M. F., Martin, D. K., Ignagni, E., & D'Cruz, J. (2009). Responding to trust: Surgeons' perspective on informed consent. *World Journal of Surgery, 33,* 1341–1347.

Mishra, P. K., Ozalp, F., Gardner, R. S., Arangannal, A., & Murday, A. (2006). Informed consent in cardiac surgery: Is it truly informed? *Journal of Cardiovascular Medicine (Hagerstown), 7,* 675–681.

Moxey, A., O'Connell, D., McGettigan, P., & Henry, D. (2003). Describing treatment effects to patients. *Journal of General Internal Medicine, 18,* 948–959.

Mulsow, J. J., Feeley, T. M., & Tierney, S. (2012). Beyond consent—Improving understanding in surgical patients. *American Journal of Surgery, 203,* 112–120.

Nelson, W., Reyna, V. F., Fagerlin, A., Lipkus, I., & Peters, E. (2008). Clinical implications of numeracy: Theory and practice. *Annals of Behavioral Medicine: A Publication of the Society of Behavioral Medicine, 35,* 261–274.

O'Connor AM, Bennett CL, Stacey D, Barry M, Col NF, et al. (2009). Decision aids for people facing health treatment or screening decisions. *Cochrane Database Syst Rev,* CD001431

Parikh, N. S., Parker, R. M., Nurss, J. R., Baker, D. W., & Williams, M. V. (1996). Shame and health literacy: The unspoken connection. *Patient Education and Counseling, 27,* 33–39.

Pearson, S. D., & Raeke, L. H. (2000). Patients' trust in physicians: Many theories, few measures, and little data. *Journal of General Internal Medicine, 15,* 509–513.

Pellerin, M. A., Elwyn, G., Rousseau, M., Stacey, D., Robitaille, H., & Legare, F. (2011). Toward shared decision making: Using the OPTION scale to analyze resident-patient consultations in family medicine. *Academic Medicine: Journal of the Association of American Medical Colleges, 86,* 1010–1018.

Politi, M. C., & Street, R. L, Jr. (2011). The importance of communication in collaborative decision making: Facilitating shared mind and the management of uncertainty. *Journal of Evaluation in Clinical Practice, 17,* 579–584.

Poses, R. M., Cebul, R. D., & Wigton, R. S. (1995). You can lead a horse to water-improving physicians' knowledge of probabilities may not affect their decisions. *Medical Decision Making, 15,* 65–75.

Powell, C. K., & Kripalani, S. (2005). Brief report: Resident recognition of low literacy as a risk factor in hospital readmission. *Journal of General Internal Medicine, 20,* 1042–1044.

Reyna, V. F. (2005). Fuzzy-trace theory, judgment, and decision-making: A dual-processes approach. In C. Izawa & N. Ohta (Eds.), *Human learning and memory: Advances in theory and applications* (pp. 239–256). Mahwah, NJ: Erlbaum.

Rimer, B. K., Briss, P. A., Zeller, P. K., Chan, E. C., & Woolf, S. H. (2004). Informed decision making: What is its role in cancer screening? *Cancer, 101,* 1214–1228.

Schenker, Y., Crowley-Matoka, M., Dohan, D., Tiver, G. A., Arnold, R. M., & White, D. B. (2012). I don't want to be the one saying 'we should just let him die': Intrapersonal tensions experienced by surrogate decision makers in the ICU. *Journal of General Internal Medicine, 27,* 1657–1665.

Schillinger, D., Bindman, A., Wang, F., Stewart, A., & Piette, J. (2004). Functional health literacy and the quality of physician-patient communication among diabetes patients. *Patient Education and Counseling, 52,* 315–323.

Schwarze, M. L., Bradley, C. T., & Brasel, K. J. (2010). Surgical "buy-in": The contractual relationship between surgeons and patients that influences decisions regarding life-supporting therapy. *Critical Care Medicine, 38,* 843–848.

Sepucha, K., Ozanne, E., Silvia, K., Partridge, A., & Mulley, A. G, Jr. (2007). An approach to measuring the quality of breast cancer decisions. *Patient Education and Counseling, 65,* 261–269.

Sepucha, K. R., Fagerlin, A., Couper, M. P., Levin, C. A., Singer, E., & Zikmund-Fisher, B. J. (2010). How does feeling informed relate to being informed? The DECISIONS survey. *Medical Decision Making, 30,* 77S–84S.

Sepucha KR, Fowler FJ, Jr., Mulley AG, Jr. (2004). Policy support for patient-centered care: The need for measurable improvements in decision quality. *Health Affair (Millwood),* Suppl Variation, VAR54-62

Shah, S. G., Farrow, A., & Robinson, I. (2009). The representation of healthcare end users' perspectives by surrogates in healthcare decisions: A literature review. *Scandinavian Journal of Caring Sciences, 23,* 809–819.

Stacey D, Bennett CL, Barry MJ, Col NF, Eden KB, et al. (2011a). Decision aids for people facing health treatment or screening decisions. *Cochrane Database Syst Rev,* CD001431

Stacey D, Bennett CL, Barry MJ, Col NF, Eden KB, et al. (2011b). Decision aids for people facing health treatment or screening decisions. *Cochrane Database of Systematic Reviews, 10,* Article No.: CD001431

Stanley, B. M., Walters, D. J., & Maddern, G. J. (1998). Informed consent: How much information is enough? *The Australian and New Zealand Journal of Surgery, 68,* 788–791.

Stiggelbout, A. M., Van der Weijden, T., De Wit, M. P., Frosch, D., Legare, F., et al. (2012). Shared decision making: Really putting patients at the centre of healthcare. *BMJ, 344,* e256.

Street, R. L, Jr., & Millay, B. (2001). Analyzing patient participation in medical encounters. *Health Commun, 13,* 61–73.

Turner, P., & Williams, C. (2002). Informed consent: Patients listen and read, but what information do they retain? *The New Zealand medical journal, 115*, U218.

Ubel, P. A., Loewenstein, G., Schwarz, N., & Smith, D. (2005). Misimagining the unimaginable: The disability paradox and health care decision making. *Health Psychology: Official Journal of the Division of Health Psychology, American Psychological Association, 24*, S57–S62.

Veroff, D., Marr, A., & Wennberg, D. E. (2013). Enhanced support for shared decision making reduced costs of care for patients with preference-sensitive conditions. *Health Affair (Millwood), 32*, 285–293.

Weinstein, J. N., Clay, K., & Morgan, T. S. (2007). Informed patient choice: Patient-centered valuing of surgical risks and benefits. *Health Affair (Millwood), 26*, 726–730.

Williams, M. V., Davis, T., Parker, R. M., & Weiss, B. D. (2002). The role of health literacy in patient-physician communication. *Family Medicine, 34*, 383–389.

Williamson, W. K., Nicoloff, A. D., Taylor, L. M, Jr., Moneta, G. L., Landry, G. J., & Porter, J. M. (2001). Functional outcome after open repair of abdominal aortic aneurysm. *Journal of Vascular Surgery, 33*, 913–920.

Zikmund-Fisher, B. J., Couper, M. P., Singer, E., Levin, C. A., Fowler, F. J, Jr., et al. (2010a). The DECISIONS study: A nationwide survey of United States adults regarding 9 common medical decisions. *Medical Decision Making, 30*, 20S–34S.

Zikmund-Fisher, B. J., Couper, M. P., Singer, E., Ubel, P. A., Ziniel, S., et al. (2010b). Deficits and variations in patients' experience with making 9 common medical decisions: The DECISIONS survey. *Medical Decision Making, 30*, 85S–95S.

Zikmund-Fisher, B. J., Sarr, B., Fagerlin, A., & Ubel, P. A. (2006). A matter of perspective: Choosing for others differs from choosing for yourself in making treatment decisions. *Journal of General Internal Medicine, 21*, 618–622.

Legal Aspects of Healthcare Decision-Making

15

Rebecca Saracino, Elissa Kolva and Barry Rosenfeld

In June of 1987, Dr. William Behringer tested positive for the Human Immunodeficiency Virus (HIV) and was diagnosed with Acquired Immunodeficiency Syndrome (AIDS) (*Behringer v. The Medical Center at Princeton* 1991). Behringer was a practicing surgeon at the Medical Center at Princeton, which is also where he was diagnosed. Within hours of receiving his diagnosis, Behringer received an outpouring of phone calls and communication from staff at the Medical Center, friends in the community, and within a matter of days, from patients. These calls, while expressing concern for his wellbeing, indicated that his friends, colleagues, and patients were aware of his diagnosis. The Medical Center subsequently suspended his surgical privileges and canceled all of his scheduled operations. The Board of Directors at the Medical Center insisted on the use of a revised informed consent form that included

R. Saracino
Department of Psychology, Fordham University, Dealy 226 441 East Fordham Road, Bronx, NY 10458, USA
e-mail: rjames11@fordham.edu

E. Kolva
Department Medicine, University of Colorado, Denver, Anschutz Medical Campus, 1665 Aurora Court, Aurora, CO 80045, USA
e-mail: elissa.kolva@ucdenver.edu

B. Rosenfeld (✉)
Department of Psychology, Fordham University, 441 East Fordham Road, Bronx, NY 10458, USA
e-mail: rosenfeld@fordham.edu

Behringer's diagnosis. It read: "I have also been informed by Dr. Behringer that he has a positive blood test indicative of infection with HIV which is the cause of AIDS. I have also been informed of the potential risk of transmission of the virus" (*Behringer v. The Medical Center at Princeton* 1991, p. 5). Dr. Behringer's surgical privileges were eventually reinstated, however due to patient reactions to the consent form, he never performed another surgery. Behringer died two years after receiving his initial diagnosis.

Before his death, Behringer initiated a lawsuit against the Medical Center, arguing that they breached confidentiality when they shared his AIDS diagnosis with the hospital staff and patients, and that the law of informed consent did not require him to disclose his condition. The Superior Court of New Jersey upheld the Medical Center's decision to mandate disclosure of Behringer's diagnosis in the consent form despite the fact that there was only a 1 in 1300 chance that any individual patient would contract HIV during a surgical procedure (*Behringer v. The Medical Center at Princeton* 1991). The Court's ruling highlights the implications, for both patients and healthcare providers, of the ever-expanding boundaries of informed consent. In *Behringer,* the doctor's right to privacy was deemed secondary to the rights of his patients, and this disclosure had an obvious and tangible impact on the decision-making of Behringer's prospective patients.

© Springer Science+Business Media New York 2016
M.A. Diefenbach et al. (eds.), *Handbook of Health Decision Science*,
DOI 10.1007/978-1-4939-3486-7_15

The legal issues surrounding healthcare decision-making have important implications for both patients and clinicians. This chapter introduces the legal doctrine of informed consent and its relationship to an individuals' ability to make treatment decisions for him or herself. Seminal legal cases are used to highlight the evolution of informed consent, including the information that should be disclosed in the informed consent process. This includes information about positive and negative treatment outcomes, disclosure about the level of uncertainty inherent in many procedures, as well as the disclosure of provider- and institution-specific personal, professional, and economic factors. Next, the legal standards and procedures used to assess and determine competence are discussed along with patient rights to refuse treatment, and the legal implications of a finding of incompetence. Finally, advice for providers surrounding the assessment of decision-making capacity is provided.

Origins of Informed Consent

The goal of informed consent is to promote patient autonomy and rational decision-making. Healthcare providers have an obligation to ensure that patients are capable of providing informed consent. This entails ensuring that each patient is aware of his or her condition, understands his or her treatment options, and can exercise free will. Additionally, providers have an ethical responsibility to protect their patients from harm (Appelbaum et al. 1987; Faden et al. 1986). Providers attempt to resolve the tension that can arise between patient autonomy and their obligation to protect patients from harm by providing accurate information about the patient's health, obtaining voluntary, informed consent and when necessary, assessing the patient's decision-making capacity.

The doctrine of informed consent is based on three core elements or prongs. First, consent must be voluntarily provided. Second, the patient must be provided with sufficient knowledge to make a decision as discussed above. Third, the

patient must have sufficient decisional capacity to make a competent decision (Melton et al. 2007). The doctrine of informed consent imposes tort liability on a clinician who treats a patient that has not validly given his or her consent. Accordingly, it is critical for healthcare providers to ensure that adequate information has been disclosed and that the patient has sufficient decision-making capacity to give valid consent.

Rooted in the English common law, informed consent stems from the tort of trespass for assault and battery. In the first recorded case to apply this principle to health care, *Slater v. Baker & Stapleton* (1767), two physicians were accused of breaking a patient's healing fracture without his consent. The *Slater* judge cited the physicians' failure to obtain the patient's consent in stating "indeed it is reasonable that a patient should be told what is about to be done to him that he may take courage and put himself in such a situation as to enable him to undergo the operation" (p. 37). Although this language was referenced in early US court cases, (*Mohr v. Williams* 1905; *Pratt v. Davis* 1906), the legal foundation of informed consent would not be crystallized for another 150 years (Appelbaum et al. 1987).

The origin of the doctrine of informed consent in US law is typically attributed to the seminal opinion delivered by New York State Court of Appeals Judge (later U.S. Supreme Court Justice) Benjamin Cardozo in *Schloendorff v. Society of N.Y. Hospital* (1914). Mary Schloendorff was informed by her physicians that an exploratory examination was needed to determine the nature of a lump in her stomach. During the examination, the physicians identified the lump as a fibroid tumor and removed it, despite the fact that the plaintiff had only consented to the examination, not intervention. Ms. Schloendorff subsequently developed gangrene in her arm that caused her intense pain and suffering and necessitated the amputation of several fingers. In her civil lawsuit against the hospital, the court ruled that the physicians' actions went beyond mere negligence and constituted an act of trespass. Judge Cardozo's ruling stated, "every human being of adult years and sound mind has a right to determine what shall be done with his own body; and a surgeon who performs an operation without his patient's consent, commits an assault, for which he is liable in damages" (p. 93).

The doctrine of informed consent was extended to research participation following recognition of the atrocities and human rights abuses carried out by Nazi Germany during World War II, specifically that concentration camp prisoners were forced to endure inhumane, often fatal experiments without their consent (Appelbaum et al. 1987). In *United States v. Karl Brandt* (1947), 23 German physicians were tried for crimes against humanity (Slovenko 2005). Following these trials, which resulted in guilty verdicts for 15 of the 23 doctors (including seven death sentences), two American physicians (who had served as witnesses for the prosecution) authored the Nuremberg Code, detailing guidelines for ethical human experimentation (Slovenko 2005). These guidelines emphasized the importance of informed consent as a requirement for ethical research conduct and emphasized the rights of the participants over the interests of science (Appelbaum et al. 1987). The Nuremberg Code states that research participants should be informed of the "nature, duration and purpose of the experiment; the method and means by which it is to be conducted; all inconveniences and hazards reasonably to be expected; and the effects upon his person which may possibly come from his participation in the experiment" (Reiser et al. 1977, pp. 272–273). These criteria, in conjunction with the requirement that research participation be voluntary, influenced the development of the doctrine of informed consent with regard to patient care.

In the decade following the Nuremburg trials, a series of legal cases outlined the contours of how and what information healthcare providers are expected to communicate to their patients (i.e., the knowledge requirement for informed consent). In *Salgo v. Leland Stanford Jr. University Board of* Trustees (1957), the California Court of Appeals stipulated that consent must be "informed", which they defined as

providing the patient with "any facts which are necessary to form the basis of an intelligent consent by the patient to the proposed treatment" (p. 578). This standard was elaborated in *Canterbury v. Spence* (1972), in which the United States Court of Appeals for the District of Columbia concluded that a physician should inform his or her patient of any potential risks that a reasonable person would likely find significant when making a medical decision. The court stated, "true consent to what happens to one's self is the informed exercise of a choice, and that entails an opportunity to evaluate knowledgably the options available and the risks attendant upon each. The average patient has little or no understanding of the medical arts, and ordinarily only his physician to whom he can look for enlightenment with which to reach an intelligent decision" (p. 780). This "reasonable person" standard for the disclosure of information has become a central element of modern tort law, including serving as the standard against which to judge whether a clinician's disclosure of the risks of a medical procedure are sufficient (Mazur 2003). However, no clinician can definitively avoid liability without disclosing every known risk and alternative (Merz 1991). The California Supreme Court noted this dilemma in stating "One cannot know with certainty whether a consent is valid until a lawsuit has been filed and resolved" (*Moore v. Regents* 1990, p. 936).

More recently, case law has expanded the contours of disclosure in the process of informed consent, by expanding the range of information that might be considered relevant to the patient (as evident in the Behringer case previously described). Twerski and Cohen (1999) labeled this wave of case law the "second revolution" in informed consent. For example, cases have indicated the need to disclose the treatment provider's experience (or lack thereof), his or her success using a proposed intervention, and the economic interests of the institution in which treatment might occur (Petrila 2003). Each of these components has potential implications for the informed consent process and will be explored in detail in the following section.

Knowledge

Communication of risks, benefits, and uncertainty. The knowledge prong of the legal doctrine of informed consent requires that patients be informed about the possible benefits and risks of each treatment option (including the option of foregoing treatment altogether) before a valid decision can be reached (Whitney et al. 2003). Despite these established guidelines, the discussion of possible negative treatment outcomes occurs with much less frequency than that of positive outcomes. Zikmund-Fisher et al. (2010) surveyed more than 3000 individuals who had made decisions about initiating prescription medications, cancer screening, and elective surgeries. Participants indicated that providers discussed positive treatment outcomes in 90 % of cases, while negative outcomes were only discussed 49–55 % of the time. This discrepancy in the discussion of risks and benefits in the informed consent process underscores the inconsistencies, or lack of standardization, in the way that providers often approach disclosure.

Despite numerous recommendations as to what information regarding risks and benefits should be conveyed to patients, very little is actually known about the best ways to communicate uncertainty to patients during informed consent (Politi et al. 2007). In fact, a full disclosure of *all* of the benefits and risks of a medical treatment, as well as the uncertainties associated with each element, may actually overwhelm the patient and hinder effective decision-making. Patients are also prone to misinterpret the uncertainties that often accompany information disclosures, such as believing that they are likely to benefit from experimental treatments even when the likelihood of direct personal health benefits is extremely low (Appelbaum et al. 1987). Ethical concerns have been posed around the "therapeutic misconceptions" that lead some patients to consent to Phase I clinical trials (i.e., those intended primarily to assess the potential toxicity of a novel intervention; Joffe et al. 2001), as many patients believe that they are likely to benefit from experimental treatments (Appelbaum et al. 1987). Patients are not the only party susceptible to these misconceptions. In a study that surveyed both physicians and participants involved in clinical trials, less than half of physicians recognized that the main reason for clinical trials was to benefit *future* patients (Joffe et al. 2001). Moreover, up to one-third of physicians were unsure whether the treatments assessed in these clinical trials were unproven and whether the treatment involved any incremental risk or potential discomfort for their patients. Again, these findings demonstrate some of the challenges inherent in the requirement that physicians provide adequate knowledge to their patient in obtaining informed consent.

Personal characteristics. Recently, the issue of whether the disclosure of provider personal or professional characteristics should be included in informed consent has been contested in the courts. Thus far, courts have generally overturned laws that force practitioners to disclose personal information such as physical or mental deterioration or contagious disease status (Furrow 1998). However, several courts have expanded the obligations of physicians by requiring the disclosure of personal health information to patients. In the case described at the beginning of this chapter, information regarding an AIDS diagnosis was determined to be relevant to informed consent (*Behringer v. The Medical Center at Princeton* 1991). Similarly, an appellate court in Louisiana found that a surgeon was required to disclose his history of alcoholism to his patients (*Hidding v. Williams* 1991). The court concluded that a reasonable patient might have refused treatment due to knowledge of the physician's illness. Taken together, these cases highlight the expanding boundaries of the legal doctrine of informed consent.

Provider experience and success. Physicians may also be required to disclose information to patients related to their experience and success with specific procedures as part of the informed consent process. The specific standards vary by state, with some requiring no such disclosures (e.g., Pennsylvania) and others (e.g., California, Massachusetts) having legislation that mandates access to reports on physician performance (Gable 1998). In *Johnson v. Kokemoor* (1996), the Wisconsin Supreme Court ruled that a physician is required to respond accurately to a patient who inquires about his or her experience performing surgery. This ruling resulted from a case in which a physician recommended neurosurgery to the plaintiff in order to clip an aneurysm. He exaggerated his experience with the procedure and told the patient that there was only a 2 % risk of death from the surgery. However, the death rate was actually closer to 30 % when performed by inexperienced surgeons. The physician also failed to disclose the availability of more experienced surgeons at a nearby facility. Due to surgical complications, the plaintiff became quadriplegic with vision and speech impairments. The court found that the physician's failure to disclose his lack of experience, the availability of more experienced physicians, and inaccurate disclosure of mortality rates violated the doctrine of informed consent (*Johnson v. Kokemoor* 1996). In contrast, the Supreme Court of Pennsylvania ruled that a patient's request for physician-related information was not relevant to the informed consent process (*Duttry v. Patterson* 2001). Petrila (2003) contends that all patients have a right to inquire about physician characteristics and to legal recourse, but underscores the difficulty of deciding how much information should be provided. While the trend appears to be moving towards making more information available to patients, deciding where to draw the line between relevant and excessive disclosure, and just what is and is not germane to making an informed decision remains subject to debate.

Economic interests. Due to the expanding influence of managed care companies, their financial agreements with healthcare providers, and the potential for these relationships to influence treatment recommendations, case law now requires that the economic interests of healthcare providers be included in the informed consent process (Petrila 2003). In *Moore v. Regents* (1990), the California Supreme court held that

physicians were required to disclose their economic self-interest in cells cultivated from a patient during treatment for leukemia. The defendants used these cells in research that had the potential to be very profitable. The court found that failure to disclose economic self-interest in obtaining the cells violated informed consent, including a failure to disclose facts material to informed consent and related to the medical procedure. Similarly, due to the increasing demands of managed care, some providers now have contractual obligations to insurance companies that may discourage them from delivering the best possible care to their patients (Petrila 2003). In *Neade v. Portes* (1999), a patient with heart disease died after he was denied further hospitalization and an angiogram despite not having been examined by the physician who refused his treatment. The wife of the deceased patient sued the physician because he failed to disclose that the patient's health maintenance organization (HMO) provided financial incentives to limit specialist referrals and procedures. The appellate court upheld the lower court's ruling, citing the ethical code of the American Medical Association, which states that physicians cannot withhold services from patients based on financial incentives, and asserted that the provider should have disclosed this incentive during the informed consent (*Neade v. Portes* 1999). However, the Illinois Supreme Court later deemed this finding impractical, stating that it would place too much burden on the provider, who cannot be expected to be familiar with each patient's HMO and its policies (*Neade v. Portes* 2000). Still, other courts have upheld rulings regarding the disclosure of economic incentives and cost-containment strategies imposed by insurance companies.

In sum, the knowledge prong of the legal doctrine of informed consent has expanded over recent decades to include information about the personal characteristics, experience, and economic interests of healthcare providers. There are now wide variations across jurisdictions in terms of precisely what information might be considered integral to any given treatment decision. This creates new challenges for healthcare providers, who must be aware of the expectations regarding disclosure of information, both related to the treatment as well as to their own experience and interests, and for patients, who must be active participants in their own healthcare decision-making.

Decision-Making Capacity

The evolution of the patient-physician relationship over the last half century has placed patients in the role of autonomous consumers, providing consent to treatments and working collaboratively with their physicians (Gaston and Mitchell 2005). Patients are expected to weigh the relative benefits and risks of proposed treatments and integrate this information with their personal values (Whitney et al. 2003). Thus, in order for consent to be truly "informed", the patient must have sufficient decision-making capacity to participate in the process.

The array of legal cases that have shaped the doctrine of informed consent has provided considerable guidance as to how decision-making capacity should be conceptualized and assessed, as well as when a formal assessment is required. In general, an assessment of decision-making capacity is required whenever a patient's ability to make an important decision about medical treatment is questioned. The critical question for the clinician is determining whether the patient has sufficient decisional capacity to make a "competent" decision (Petrila 2003). In the medical decision-making literature, capacity is a clinical term that generally refers to the patient's cognitive abilities, or in the medical treatment setting, the ability to make a given treatment decision (Rosenfeld 2004). In contrast, competence is a legal term that refers to a patients' legal authority to make decisions for him or herself. Competency is typically determined by a judge but in many cases physicians will merely seek guidance from a family member without a formal adjudication of incompetency (Rosenfeld 2004). When a patient lacks sufficient capacity to make a competent decision, alternative provisions must

be implemented in order to ensure that the decision has been made by a competent individual.

Legal Determination of Competence

Most patients do not require a formal clinical evaluation of decision-making capacity when making healthcare decisions. Legally, adults are presumed to be competent unless proven otherwise. This reflects the priority placed on the right to self-determination by the judicial system. Thus, the capacity of an adult with no obvious cognitive, psychiatric, or physical limitations, who is accepting the treatment recommendation of a physician, is rarely questioned. Conversely, the incompetence of a nonresponsive patient is undeniable. As a result, disputes about decisional capacity are relatively uncommon, as there is usually agreement between the physician, patient, and family members involved in the patient's care. Moreover, concerns about a patient's decision-making capacity in the medical setting are generally handled through collaboration between the patient's family and treating clinician when the patient is unable to participate fully (Appelbaum 2007; Lo 1990). The utilization of a substitute decision maker in the absence of a judicial ruling of incompetence is known as de facto incompetence (Melton et al. 2007), whereas de jure incompetence refers to a formal judicial finding of incompetence. Disagreements may arise, such as when a patient refuses to accept a potentially beneficial treatment favored by family members, or when disagreements exist among family members as to whether their relative's expressed wishes should be respected. In these instances, the court is forced to adjudicate the patient's decision-making competence. Hence, although assessments of decisional capacity may be initiated by the treating clinician (often in response to a refusal of recommended treatment), only a judge or other legal decision maker can formally adjudicate a person incompetent. The court's decision will typically include both a determination of competence or incompetence and, in the case of incompetence, the appointment of a surrogate decision maker or guardian.

Legal Standards of Competence

There are no universally accepted standards for competency. Thus, the standards employed by courts differ between, and sometimes even within jurisdictions (Appelbaum et al. 1987). These standards have generally been grouped by legal scholars into five broad categories: ability to express a choice, ability to understand and recall information disclosed, ability to provide rational reasons for one's choice, ability to appreciate the significance of the decision, and ability to rationally manipulate information into a decision that is consistent with one's values and preferences (Appelbaum and Grisso 1988; Appelbaum et al. 1987; Roth et al. 1977). These are typically thought of as representing a hierarchy of "tests" of competence, with more rigorous tests applied to more important decision.

Expressing a choice. The simplest test of competency is the ability to articulate a choice. Applying this standard, incompetence would occur only in cases in which the individual was incapable of articulating a choice (either verbally or behaviorally) or adhering to a decision long enough for the choice to be implemented. Hence, a finding of incompetence is typically due to impaired consciousness (e.g., coma, excessive sedation), severe thought disorder, or extreme short-term memory impairment (Appelbaum and Grisso 1988). Roth et al. (1977) described an early case in which this legal standard was used to prohibit the sterilization of mentally retarded individuals unless they expressed a genuine desire to undergo the procedure (Wyatt v. Aderholt 1974). Despite the important decision that underlay the early application of this standard, at present this low threshold is generally only considered appropriate for decisions in which the risks and benefits are modest. Nevertheless, some commentators have argued that it should be used more often, as it offers the most protection for patient autonomy (Saks 1991).

Understanding information. Perhaps the most widely used standard for assessing decision-making competence is the ability to understand information relevant to the decision. According to

this standard, the patient must understand the information that has been disclosed before he or she can be permitted to accept or reject a proposed treatment. This test of competence is typically assessed by asking the individual to simply repeat or paraphrase previously disclosed information and thus relies heavily on memory, attention, and general intelligence (Appelbaum and Grisso 1988). Indeed, many healthcare providers utilize this standard, whether knowingly or intuitively, by asking their patients to repeat information that has just been disclosed as a means of testing their understanding of the information. The most common source of impairments in "understanding" are intellectual disabilities or disorders that disrupt memory, although extremely psychotic or severely depressed patients may also have difficulty satisfying this standard (Appelbaum and Grisso 1988).

Ability to provide rational reasons. The ability to provide rational reasons for one's decision is also easily evaluated by clinicians and has often been deemed acceptable in court decisions, but is frequently maligned by legal theorists and mental health clinicians (Appelbaum and Grisso 1988; Roth et al. 1977). Like understanding, this standard is relatively easily ascertained and has an obvious intuitive appeal, as asking "why" is a natural extension of asking patients what decision they intend to choose. However, the requirement that one's patient provide a "rational" explanation for his or her decision may undercut the emphasis on autonomy that forms the basis for informed consent. Patients who are confused or have distorted thinking (e.g., psychosis or severe depression) may be unable to meet the demands of this standard, however even mentally intact individuals who have idiosyncratic values or belief systems may also "fail" this legal standard if improperly applied (i.e., if the clinician's own values form the basis for determining what is "rational"). Moreover, because evaluators may fail to distinguish between the decision-making process and outcome, theorists have increasingly dismissed the ability to provide rational reasons as a valid test of competence.

Appreciating the situation. A somewhat more abstract test of competence rests on the patient's ability to assign personal meaning to the information that has been presented. "Appreciation" refers to the ability of an individual to understand the implications of his or her treatment decisions, which includes acknowledging the illness and the possible effects each alternative has for one's life (often including the effects that a decision might have on others). For example, in *United States v. George* (1965), a US District Court in Connecticut applied an early example of this standard, finding that the patient (Mr. George) was competent to refuse life-saving treatments because his refusal rested on his religious beliefs. His refusal of a life-saving blood transfusion on religious grounds was described as an idiosyncratic decision that would not be widely accepted by others, yet he demonstrated an appreciation of the nature of his circumstances and the implications of his choice. Patients who lack abstract reasoning abilities due to a cognitive or psychiatric disorder, or have a delusional perception of their health state, may fail to meet this standard of competence even when they appear to understand the risks and benefits of the treatment.

Rational manipulation of information. Arguably the most rigorous standard for assessing decisional competence, "reasoning" requires an ability to rationally manipulate the information that has been presented. Under this standard, patients are required to demonstrate not only an understanding and appreciation of the information disclosed, but are able to balance the pros and cons of treatment alternatives in the context of their own personal goals and values. This standard differs from the ability to provide rational reasons in that patients need not offer a rationale that would be accepted by others, but rather need only offer a rationale that is consistent with their own values, even if others might not accept their logic. For example, medically ill patients with advanced disease are routinely allowed to refuse life-sustaining interventions provided they can demonstrate that the refusal of treatment is in keeping with their values and personal beliefs (e.g., regarding the relative merits of extending life given worsening physical limitations and symptoms). Because of the emphasis on rationality, patients with thought disorder, confusion,

delirium, dementia, or even significant mood or anxiety symptoms may fail to meet this rigorous standard.

Application of legal standards of competence. Although the courts have given little guidance for determining which test of competence is appropriate for a particular treatment decision, many experts agree that more stringent requirements for competence should be applied to more important decisions (Grisso and Appelbaum 1998; Rosenfeld 2004). Yet increasing the cognitive demands upon a patient for a determination of competence may have the unintended effect of diminishing self-determination and autonomy. Roth et al. (1977) recommended that a more stringent level of competency might be appropriate, not only for decisions that involve considerable risk, but depending on whether the patient accepts or rejects the treatment. They suggested that a lower standard should be applied to a decision to accept treatment and a more stringent standard should be applied to reject recommended treatment, presumably because of the differing implications of these decisions. Although debates continue as to how a "sliding scale" of competence should be operationalized, the idea of matching the legal test or standard with the seriousness of the consequences that hinge on a patient's decision was endorsed by the Presidential Commission for the Study of Ethical Problems in Medicine and Biomedical and Behavioral Research (1982) and has often been applied by the courts.

Despite the intuitive appeal of a sliding scale of competence, the hierarchical nature of these tests of competence may be clearer in theory than in practice. Grisso and Appelbaum (1995) compared the different legal standards for competence in their study of an instrument designed to assess four of these standards (expression of a choice, understanding, appreciation, and rational manipulation of information). They found that the different tests of competence do not necessarily form a coherent hierarchy, as patients who appeared impaired according to a "lower" test (e.g., understanding) were not necessarily impaired on a more stringent test (e.g., rational manipulation of information). On the other hand, the use of compound tests (i.e., requiring that patients meet more than one test of competence) inevitably increases the number of patients classified as impaired. Clearly, further research is needed to better understand the cognitive processes that underlie these tests of competence.

Competence and the Right to Refuse Treatment

Prior to the 1970s, psychiatric hospitals were penalized for failing to involuntarily medicate their patients (see Isaac and Brakel 1992). It was assumed that once a patient was involuntarily committed to the hospital, psychoactive medication could be administered freely without consulting the patient or his or her family. This practice changed following the US Supreme Court's decision in *Rennie v. Klein* (1978), when the Court ruled that an involuntarily committed psychiatric patient still retained the right to refuse medication provided he or she did not pose a risk of harm to themselves or others. Before employing the coercive power of the state to force a patient to take medication, the government must clear the procedural hurdle of proving that the patient lacks competence to make his or her own decisions.

The guardian of a legally incompetent patient also has the ability to refuse treatments, provided this refusal is consistent with the presumed wishes of the incompetent patient (Wortzel 2006). In *Superintendent of Belchertown State School v. Saikewicz* (1977) the guardian of a legally incompetent man with profound mental retardation was able to refuse life-prolonging treatment for his ward's incurable acute myeloblastic leukemia. In their decision, the court recognized that the guardian has the right to make decisions in accordance with what the patient would want if he or she were competent (a process termed substituted judgment). Guardians may make almost any medical decisions for an incompetent patient except for the refusal or deprivation of life-saving treatment (*Charles S. Soper, as Director of Newark Developmental Center* et al. *v. Dorothy Storar* 1981).

Although some jurisdictions require the surrogate decision maker to attempt to replicate the decision that the patient, if competent, would make, other jurisdictions apply a "best interest" standard, asking the surrogate to make decisions that are in the patient's best interest. Of course, substitute judgment is simpler when an advance directive (AD) is in place to specify treatment preferences. However, even when an AD exists, questions inevitably remain as to what and how a surrogate should decide on behalf of the incompetent patient. ADs rarely provide specific instructions pertinent to a particular decision in a specific set of circumstances, instead providing broad guidance regarding preferences.

Guardianship. The designation of a particular individual as a guardian may be specified in an AD or "living will," or left to the discretion of the court. If no decision maker is specified, in many cases the burden of surrogate decision-making is left to family members, with the hierarchy of surrogacy dictated by state law. In most states, the order of surrogacy for an adult is as follows: spouse, adult children, parents, siblings, and then other relatives (Appelbaum 2007). However, many courts have ignored the preferences of the incompetent patient's relatives and appointed an independent guardian. For example, in cases involving the decision to terminate life-sustaining interventions, the courts have occasionally rejected the decision of a family member, even when evidence exists to indicate that the decision reflects the patients' preferences (e.g., *Cruzan v. Harmon* 1988; *In re O'Connor* 1988). Moreover, when caregivers have divergent opinions about what treatments should be sought, legal intervention is typically necessary. Because guardianship entails a loss of autonomy, the courts have typically required a high standard of proof—clear and convincing evidence—before such decisions can be made (Tor and Sales 1994).

The court also has the power to limit the ability of the guardian to make treatment decisions on behalf of the patient. In the case of Richard Roe (*In the Matter of Guardianship of Richard Roe III* 1981), a father was appointed guardian of his son (Roe), who suffered from schizophrenia and had been declared legally incompetent. However, despite being appointed guardian, the father was not allowed to make decisions regarding his son's medication (i.e., to authorize medication over his son's objections), only his financial decisions. The court stated that "a guardian of a mentally ill person does not have inherent authority to consent to the forcible administration of antipsychotic medication to his noninstitutionalized ward in the absence of an emergency" (p. 417).

Clinician Assessment of Decision-Making Capacity

In most instances, questions of competence are not decided by the legal system. Indeed, if physicians sought a judicial review every time there was a question of incompetence, both the legal and medical systems would be overwhelmed. In medical settings, a patient's capacity to make a given treatment decision is often assessed by the treating clinician, such as in cases in which the patient consents to or refuses a recommended treatment (Grisso and Appelbaum 1995). The goal of these assessments is to balance the tension between a desire to protect the patient from harm and respect for the patient's autonomy (Emanuel and Scandrett 2010; Moye and Marson 2009).

The critical question for the clinician is whether the patient has sufficient decisional capacity to make a competent decision, as defined by the legal standards previously described (Petrila 2003). There is often considerable variability in the assessment of decision-making capacity, due in part to the paucity of well-accepted assessment methods. Ideally, clinicians assess decision-making capacity in their own patients, allowing for a more thorough understanding of the patient's goals and values, and enabling them to frame the current decision in the context of past decisions. This context may enable the clinician to determine when a decision seems to diverge from goals and values that the patient has expressed in the past. However, in some instances patients must make

important treatment decisions in an emergent situation, often with a doctor they have only recently been introduced to, effectively removing the patient's life-context from the assessment process. Moreover, when a long-standing physician–patient relationship exists, treating clinicians may be vulnerable to the temptation of projecting their own feelings or expectations onto their patients, or misinterpreting psychological changes that influence decision-making (Rosenfeld 2004). For example, treating physicians may interpret their patient's onset of depressive symptoms as a natural reaction to declining health rather than identifying depression as a potentially treatable disorder that has clouded the patient's judgment.

Perhaps more importantly, relatively few clinicians are familiar with the process, or legal standards, for assessing decision-making capacity. Indeed, many institutions utilize specialized professionals for the assessment of decision-making capacity—at least for instances when capacity is unclear or a patient's refusal of recommended treatment raises concern. Such institutional services are typically the domain of a Consultation-Liaison (C-L) service, and are ideally staffed by psychiatrists or psychologists who have learned, among other specialized evaluation skills, techniques for assessing decision-making capacity. Although C-L services may not have any context for understanding a patient's decision, the sophistication and expertise brought to bear on the assessment process typically outweighs the potential for diminished contextual information. This reliance on mental health professionals who have learned specialized evaluation skills and techniques for assessing decision-making capacity can increase the reliability and validity of capacity assessments.

Summary

Over the past few decades, researchers, clinicians, and legal scholars have become increasingly focused on issues related to decision-making in medical settings. The legal doctrine of informed consent guides both clinical and legal decisions regarding whether consent is valid, whether the information provided to patients is sufficient, and whether the patient has sufficient decisional capacity to reach a legally valid decision. As recent legal cases have demonstrated, the doctrine of informed consent is continuously evolving, as are the techniques for assessing decisional capacity. Thus, clinicians must be aware of what information must be provided to their patients during informed consent as well as how to assess the decisional capacity of these patients. In addition to the actual communication of relevant information, the patient-physician interaction is an important component of medical decision-making. A number of research studies have demonstrated that as quality of communication with providers increases, both patient satisfaction and treatment adherence increase (Zikmund-Fisher et al. 2010). Similarly, when patients discuss their healthcare preferences with their providers, they tend to be more confident and pleased with their decisions, regardless of the eventual outcome (Zikmund-Fisher et al. 2010). Incorporating family or significant others into the decision process, or what has become known as "shared decision-making," has also emerged as an important area of study and may lead to greater patient satisfaction with the treatment decision-making process. In addition, some novel interventions such as video vignettes showing end of life care options for advanced dementia patients have demonstrated efficacy in improving health literacy and eliminating uncertainty in decision-making (Volandes et al. 2009). Despite these advances, continued research is needed to determine the optimal strategies, and methods for helping patients make informed decisions about their medical care.

This chapter provides broad guidelines regarding the legal parameters of decisional competence and considerable variations exist across jurisdictions. Clinicians must familiarize themselves with these variations in order to adequately research, assess, and make decisions about the complex issues involved in obtaining legally valid informed consent.

Practice Recommendations

- Be aware that legal standards of informed consent vary by jurisdiction and are constantly evolving
  - Keep up to date with your State and Federal statutes
  - Communicate with your institution to determine if specific information should be provided to patients
- Encourage patients to be proactive in planning their medical treatment
  - Have discussions early on with patients about developing clear ADs
  - Involve family members in the shared-decision-making process
- Patients can benefit tremendously from discussions with healthcare providers
  - A discussion of patient values can help identify information about risks and benefits that will be most helpful
- Clinicians should be aware that cognitive impairment can be subtle and undetectable without direct measurement
  - Never assume that a patient does not have capacity simply because he or she has a diagnosis that MAY impact competence (i.e., Alzheimer's disease, Parkinson's disease, Schizophrenia)
- Decision-making capacity is dynamic and specific to individual decisions. Thus it should be frequently assessed with respect to changes in cognitive status (i.e., delirium).

References

Appelbaum, P. S. (2007). Clinical practice: Assessment of patients' competence to consent to treatment. *New England Journal of Medicine, 357*, 1834–1840.

Appelbaum, P. S., & Grisso, T. (1988). Assessing patients' capacities to consent to treatment. *The New England Journal of Medicine, 319*, 1635–1638.

Appelbaum, P. S., Lidz, C. W., & Meisel, A. (1987). *Informed consent: Legal theory and clinical practice.* New York: Oxford University Press.

Behringer v. *The Medical Center at Princeton,* Superior Court of New Jersey, 592 A.2d 1251 (1991).

Canterbury v. Spence, 464 F.2d 772 (D.C. Cir. 1972).

Charles S. Soper, as *Director of Newark Developmental Center* et al. *v. Dorothy Storar,* N.Y., 420 N.E.2d 64, (1981).

Cruzan v. Harmon, 760 S.W. 2d 408 (Mo. 1988).

Duttry v. Patterson, 771. A.2d 1255 (Pa. 2001).

Emanuel, L., & Scandrett, K. G. (2010). Decisions at the end of life: Have we come of age? *BMC Medicine, 8,* 57.

Faden, R. R., Beauchamp, T. L., & King, N. M. P. (1986). *A history and theory of informed consent.* New York: Oxford University Press.

Furrow, B. (1998). Doctors' dirty little secrets: The dark side of medical privacy. *Washburn Law Journal, 37,* 283–316.

Gaston, C. M., & Mitchell, G. (2005). Information giving and decision-making in patients with advanced cancer: A systematic review. *Social Science and Medicine, 61,* 2252–2264.

Gable, W. (1998). Review of selected 1997 California legislation: public access to physicians' history and background. *McGeorge Law Review, 29,* 427–438.

Grisso, T., & Appelbaum, P. S. (1995). Comparison of standards for assessing patients' capacities to make treatment decisions. *American Journal of Psychiatry, 152,* 1033–1037.

Grisso, T., & Appelbaum, P. S. (1998). *Assessing competence to consent to treatment: A guide for physicians and other health professionals.* New York: Oxford University Press.

Hidding v. Williams, 578 So. 2d 1192 (Court of Appeal of Louisiana, 5th Circuit, 1991).

In re O'Connor, 531 NE2d 607 (N.Y. 1988).

In the Matter of Guardianship of Richard Roe III, 421 N. E.2d 40 (Mass. 1981).

Isaac, R. J., & Brakel, S. J. (1992). Subverting good intentions: A brief history of mental health law reform. *Cornell Journal of Law and Public Policy, 2,* 89–119.

Joffe, S., Cook, F., Cleary, P. D., Clark, J. W., & Weeks, J. C. (2001). Quality of informed consent in cancer clinical trials: A cross sectional survey. *The Lancet, 358,* 1772–1777.

Johnson v. Kokemoor, 545 n.w. 2d 495 (Wis. 1996).

Lo, B. (1990). Assessing decision-making capacity. *Law, Medicine and Health Care, 18,* 193–201.

Mazur, D. J. (2003). Influence of the law on risk and informed consent. *British Medical Journal, 327,* 731–734.

Melton, G. B., Petrila, J., Poythress, N. G., & Slobogin, C. (2007). *Psychological evaluations for the courts.* New York: The Guilford Press.

Merz, J. F. (1991). An empirical analysis of the medical informed consent doctrine: Search for a "standard" of disclosure, *Risk: Issues in Health and Safety, 2,* 1–27.

Mohr v. Williams, 104 N.W. 12 (Minn. 1905).

Moore v. Regents of the University of California, 793 P. 2d 479 (Cal. 1990).

Moye, J., & Marson, D. C. (2009). Assessment of decision-making capacity in older adults: An emerging area of practice and research. *The Journal of Lifelong Learning in Psychiatry, 7,* 88–97.

Neade v. Portes, 710 N.E. 2d 418 (Ill. App. 3d 1999).

Neade v. Portes, 739 N.E. 2d 496 (Ill. 2000).

Petrila, J. (2003). The emerging debate over the shape of informed consent: Can the doctrine bear the weight? *Behavioral Sciences and the Law, 21,* 121–133.

Politi, M. C., Han, P. K., & Col, N. F. (2007). Communicating uncertainty of harms and benefits of medical interventions, *Medical Decision Making,* 681–695.

Pratt v. Davis, 118 161, 79 N.E. 562 (Ill. App. 1906).

President's Commission for the Study of Ethical Problems in Medicine and Biomedical and Behavioral Research. (1982). United States Code Annotated. U S. 1982; Title 42 Sect. 300v.

Reiser, S. J., Dyck, A. J., & Curran, W. J. (1977). *Ethics in medicine: Historical perspectives and contemporary concerns.* Cambridge, MA: MIT Press.

Rennie v. Klein, 462 F Supp 1131(D NJ, 1978), 476 F Supp 1294 (D NJ, 1979), affirmed in part, 653 F 2d 836 (3rd Cir, 1981), vacated and remanded, 102 S Ct 3506 (1982), 700 F 2d 266 (3rd Cir, 1983).

Rosenfeld, B. (2004). *Assisted suicide and the right to die: The interface of social science, public policy, and medical ethics.* Washington, DC: American Psychological Association.

Roth, L. H., Meisel, A., & Lidz, C. W. (1977). Tests of competency to consent to treatment. *American Journal of Psychiatry, 134,* 279–284.

Saks, E. R. (1991). Competency to refuse treatment. *North Carolina Law Review, 69,* 945–999.

Salgo v. Leland Stanford Jr. University Board of Trustees, 154 2d 560 (Cal. App. 1957).

Schloendorff v. Society of New York Hospital, 211 125, 105 NE 92 (NY 1914).

Slater v. Baker & Stapleton, 95 860 (Eng. 1767).

Slovenko, R. (2005). The evolution of standards for experimental treatment or research. *The Journal of Psychiatry and Law, 33,* 129–174.

Superintendent of Belchertown State School et al. *v. Joseph Saikewicz,* 370 N.E.2d 417, (Mass. 1977).

Tor, P. B., & Sales, B. D. (1994). A social science perspective on the law of guardianship: Directions for improving the process and practice. *Law and Psychology Review, 18,* 1–41.

Twerski, A. D., & Cohen, N. B. (1999). The second revolution in informed consent: Comparing physicians to each other. *Northwestern University Law Review, 94,* 1–54.

United States v. George, 239 F.Supp. 752 (D. Conn.1965).

United States v. Karl Brandt et al., in U.S. Adjutant General's Department, Trials of War Criminals before the Nuremberg Military Tribunals under Control Council Law No. 10 (October 1946–April 1949) (Vol. 2). *The Medical Case.* Washington, D.C.: U.S. Government Printing Office, 1947.

Volandes, A. E., Barry, M. J., Chang, Y., & Paasche-Orlow, M. K. (2009). Improving decision making at the end of life with video images. *Medical Decision Making, 30*, 29–34.

Whitney, S. N., McGuire, A. L., & McCullough, L. B. (2003). A typology of shared decision making, informed consent, and simple consent. *Annals of Internal Medicine, 140*, 5–9.

Wortzel, H. (2006). The right to refuse treatment. *Psychiatric Times, 23*, 30–32.

Wyatt v. Aderholt, 503 F.2d 1305, 1308 (5th Cir. 1974).

Zikmund-Fisher, B. J., Couper, M. P., Singer, E., Ubel, P. A., Ziniel, S., Fowler, F. J., & Fagerlin, A. (2010). Deficits and variations in patients' experience with making 9 common medical decisions: The DECISIONS survey. *Medical Decision Making, 30*, 20–34.

Part IV
Applied Decision Making

Decision Tools for HealthCare Professionals

16

Ambili Ramachandran, Shivani Reddy
and Devin M. Mann

Key Points

- Shared decision making is often used in situations of clinical equipoise—where there is no clear recommended course of management based on existing scientific evidence and the "right" decision depends on a patient's values.
- In shared decision making, a patient and a provider deliberate healthcare options together by considering the risks and benefits for a decision based on a patient's particular values and a provider's medical expertise.
- Decision aids are tools to facilitate shared decision making. Most decision aids present essential health information, highlight that a decision must be made that depends on the values and preferences of the patient, list the options available, describe the potential benefits, and harms of the various options, and help patients clarify their personal values.
- Effectively communicating the chance of benefit or harm in decision aids can be challenging, and decision aids rely on graphical and pictorial approaches. Decision aids can appear in a variety of formats, can contain a range of information and exercises, and can be used in many different clinical situations.
- Values clarification distinguishes decision aids from patient educational materials, and is accomplished through implicit techniques, deliberation exercises, or patient narratives.
- High-quality decision aids demonstrate an increase in patient knowledge, more accurate risk perception by patients, appropriate patient involvement in decision making, and lower measures of decisional conflict for patients. International standards have been developed for evaluating the quality of decision aids.
- Barriers to the implementation of decision aids exist for patients, providers, and healthcare systems, such as attitudes and readiness toward shared decision making, health literacy, and workflow limitations.
- Future research on decision aids should examine their impact on outcomes such as cost or visit time, their usability in diverse populations, and their effectiveness at achieving patient-centered care when implemented into routine practice.

A. Ramachandran
Department of Medicine, Boston University School of Medicine, 801 Massachusetts Avenue, Boston, MA 02118, USA
e-mail: ambili@bu.edu

S. Reddy
RTI International, 1440 Main Street, #302, Waltham, MA 02451, USA
e-mail: sreddy@bu.edu

D.M. Mann (✉)
Department of Medicine, Boston University School of Medicine, 801 Massachusetts Avenue, Suite 470, Boston, MA 02118, USA
e-mail: dmann@bu.edu

© Springer Science+Business Media New York 2016
M.A. Diefenbach et al. (eds.), *Handbook of Health Decision Science*,
DOI 10.1007/978-1-4939-3486-7_16

Shared Decision Making

SP is a 41-year-old Caucasian female with hypertension and diabetes. She is generally compliant with her medications and somewhat reluctantly keeps up with cervical cancer screening. At her scheduled primary care visit, she asks if she should get a mammogram. Her older sister has been getting mammograms since she turned 40, though a close friend said her doctor recommended waiting until she turned 50. SP has no first-degree relatives with breast cancer and a normal clinical breast exam at the present visit. She expresses concerns about her breasts being "squished" by the mammogram machine, but is also nervous about the possibility of having cancer. How do you counsel her?

The doctor–patient relationship is in the midst of a paradigm shift. Historically, the expertise of clinicians has conferred upon them the responsibility of medical decision making, with the authority to direct clinical management of patients who play a relatively passive role. This type of decision making is referred to as paternalism, in which the physician unilaterally makes decisions about patient care. Patients are obligated to comply with the doctor's plan, contributing little input beyond informed consent. While a paternalistic model of decision making may be necessary in certain clinical situations, such as emergency care, there has been a growing movement to include patient preferences and values into his or her ultimate treatment choices (Bowling and Ebrahim 2001). In a model of shared decision making, the office visit is reconceptualized as the meeting of two experts, where the doctor provides knowledge of medical conditions and care, and the patient provides information about his or her attitudes toward illness and treatment (Coulter 2010).

Several factors have influenced the shifting balance of power between clinicians and patients, including patients' rights advocacy and the changing nature of medical care (Charles et al. 1997). Informed consent for procedures represents a minimum of shared decision making, by informing patients of the risks, benefits, and alternatives of treatment choice. The patients' rights movement has progressed beyond simple informed consent, advocating for increased patient involvement in medical decisions based on ethical principles of autonomy and self-determination (Elwyn et al. 2012). Simply put, patients have a right to be equal partners in decisions that concern their health, even if the physician's medical expertise and experience exceeds that of the patient.

At the same time that healthcare consumers are calling for more participation in their care, the nature of that medical care has evolved. There has been a shift from acute care to chronic disease management. The vast numbers of patients with cardiovascular disease, diabetes, hypertension, obesity, and dementia—numbers that are only rising with an aging population—expand the goal of medical care from curing disease to managing diseases that will likely persist throughout the patient's lifetime. The successful management of chronic disease cannot be achieved by physician directive alone; it relies on patient self-management, patients acquiring the skills and knowledge to effectively take care of their chronic illness outside the setting of the doctor's office. A collaborative model of decision-making fosters patient participation in his or her illness, which is necessary for monitoring and adherence to a plan of care (Charles et al. 1997). A collaborative model of decision making may better foster patient participation in his or her illness. Some studies show that patient–physician collaboration may improve patient adherence to medications, behaviors, and appointment attendance (Arbuthnott and Sharpe 2009; Ludman et al. 2003), while others do not (Branda et al. 2013; Mullan et al. 2009; Weymiller et al. 2007). Further research is needed to determine the impact on health outcomes (Heisler et al. 2009).

Furthermore, many medical decisions today are characterized by equipoise, an unknown balance of benefit and harm to the patient for a given diagnostic or treatment decision (Elwyn et al. 2009). In our example above of patient SP, the decision to screen for breast cancer with mammography between the age of 40 and 50 is fraught with uncertainty for both the provider and the patient. There is conflicting evidence regarding the reduction of breast cancer mortality with screening for women in this age group. The decision-maker must balance the risk of missing a lethal breast cancer diagnosis with the risk of a false positive test leading to unnecessary procedures and psychological harm, and the additional possibility of treating a potentially benign breast cancer like ductal carcinoma in situ (Mathieu et al. 2010). Clinical guidelines offer minimal guidance in the setting of conflicting medical evidence, manifest by recommendations that vary for different professional societies. For example, the American College of Radiology recommends yearly mammograms beginning at age 40, while the United States Preventive Services Task Force (USPSTF) recommends biennial screening between the ages of 50 and 74. The explosive expansion of diagnostic and treatment modalities further complicates decision making. When is genetic testing for BRCA1/2 appropriate? What is the role of MRI in breast cancer screening? When should prophylactic treatments like tamoxifen be considered? What type of surgery should be considered if a breast cancer is found? In an age of accelerating medical innovation, the questions that patients and providers confront will only multiply.

In the face of growing uncertainty in medicine, shared decision making offers clinicians and patients a means to negotiate a mutually derived treatment plan. Patients and physicians come to a decision by incorporating not only available clinical evidence, but an understanding of the patient's values as well. A patient may view the harms and benefits of medical care in different ways based on his or her value system. Patient SP's preference for limiting discomfort from tests (suggested by her reluctance to participate in relatively noninvasive screening tests) may outweigh the anxiety of potentially having breast cancer that is undetected, or she may prefer screening despite the possibility of ultimately unnecessary procedures. In the absence of a clear-cut clinical guideline, eliciting patient values can lead to a decision that is satisfying for both the patient and the provider.

Beyond an ethical imperative to involve patients in their care, evidence shows that patients may benefit from shared decision making in many ways. In a Cochrane review of 86 randomized control studies, patients who engaged in shared decision making had higher knowledge scores, were able to more accurately perceive risk and benefits, and made decisions that more closely aligned with their values. When general health outcomes, such as quality of life, physical function, or mental health function, have been assessed, decision aids were associated with similar outcome scores as usual care. In select studies, condition-specific outcomes have been found to be improved with use of decisions aids, but the effect is not consistent (Stacey et al. 2011).

At its core, shared decision making incorporates sharing medical information with patients, clarifying patient values, and supporting patients in deliberation when presented with medical decisions that have multiple reasonable treatment options. The minimal criteria for shared decision making are that the decision making process involves at least two participants (the patient and provider), both parties engage in the decision making process, the provider lays out treatment options with risks, benefits, and alternatives, and both parties endorse a treatment decision (Charles et al. 1997). Shared decision making moves beyond patient education about a specific disease process, an activity that many clinicians already incorporate into daily practice. With shared decision making, the provider emphasizes to the patient that a diagnostic or treatment choice exists for which the medical community does not have a clear recommendation, and that the risks and benefits of each option will be weighed differently based on the patient's values. Providers help patients to deliberate, guiding patients on how to structure the decision making process. By helping patients become aware of their preferences, and understand their options in the context of these preferences, physicians become teachers of not only medical knowledge, but of decision making skills (Elwyn et al. 2012).

Several groups have shown support for shared decision making, from patients and professionals to policy makers. A growing community of researchers from across the world is invested in the advancement of a collaborative model of decision making. Groups such as the Ottawa Health Research Institute in Canada, Informed Health Choice in the UK, the Center for Shared Decision Making, and Foundation for Informed Medical Decision Making in the United States are involved in research and initiatives to implement shared decision making into clinical practice. International conferences also offer the opportunity to share ideas and research, including the Society for Medical Decision Making and International Shared Decision Making (Coulter 2010). Many researchers are involved in the International Patient Decision Aids Standards (IPDAS) collaboration, which works to establish an international standard of quality for the development of decision aids.

Decision aids, or decision support interventions, are tools used to facilitate shared decision making. Most decision aids are targeted for "preference-sensitive" decisions; decisions with equipoise where the evidence-based course of action is unclear. Preference-sensitive decisions are characterized by discrete decision points where a specific option must be selected rather than a continuous self-management "decision" such as whether to exercise or eat healthy or adhere to an agreed upon regimen. In preference-sensitive situations the harms and benefits of treatment need to be evaluated through the lens of a patient's value system (Elwyn et al. 2009). Patient SP is the type of patient who may well benefit from the use of a decision aid to help her and her provider come to a decision about whether screening for breast cancer would be appropriate at her age. In contrast, for clinical situations where strong recommendations exist, clinicians may need to focus on strategies to promote behavioral change and self-management (Van der Weijden et al. 2012). For example, there is a high degree of certainty that a 60-year-old female patient with several first-degree relatives with breast cancer should undergo mammography. If the patient is ambivalent, a motivational interviewing approach, rather than shared decision making, may be more appropriate to elicit underlying causes for the patient's resistance to screening or in other situations where medical evidence is stronger. In contrast, this chapter will focus on preference-sensitive decisions, for which decision aids are ideally suited.

Decision Aids as Implementation Tools of Shared Decision Making

What Are Decision Aids?

Decision aids are a type of decision support tool designed to facilitate shared decision making. Their purpose is "to help people make specific and deliberative choices among options by providing information about the options and outcomes that are relevant to a person's health status" (Elwyn et al. 2010).

In the case of SP, she is faced with a medical decision for which there is no "right" answer, but one where her personal values—to avoid the discomfort of a screening test, to avoid a treatable disease—help determine the best course of action. In this situation, a decision aid could be employed to engage both her and her provider in the decision making process. A decision aid presents the risks of not screening, and the number of procedures that may occur as a result of false positive results. The decision aid also provides a mechanism to generate patient–centered pros and cons of testing and helps the patient and provider weigh patient values enabling both parties to reach a suitable, satisfying decision.

Unlike health educational materials, which only deliver general information about a disease such as its causes, diagnosis, and treatment, decision aids explicitly communicate that a healthcare choice must be made and emphasize the importance of individual values in choosing among potential options (Stacey et al. 2011). They can be used for treatment decisions, such as whether to use aspirin or warfarin to prevent stroke in a low-risk patient with atrial fibrillation, or for screening decisions, such as whether a woman should get a screening mammogram at a particular age. In these scenarios, clinical equipoise exists and the desirable or "right" decision is dependent on individual, personal values (Elwyn et al. 2009). Values are difficult to assess, and decision aids provide a tool to do so in a structured fashion.

Decision aids are also distinct from clinical practice guidelines that support providers with population-based recommendations on the appropriate course of action based on the most current evidence. When there is low uncertainty about the evidence and little equipoise in the decision to be made, guidelines can deliver strong recommendations, and the focus of patient–provider interactions is on how best to support the patient in adhering to the recommended behavior or treatment. For example, there is strong evidence to support screening mammography in women between the ages of 50 and 70 and patients should be encouraged to seek this screening test (U.S. Preventive Services Task Force 2009).

However, when the evidence is less certain and only weak recommendations may be provided, then the right course of action may be more preference-sensitive and the discussion shifts to what matters most to the patient. A decision aid helps to individualize the choice and prepares the patient to engage in the decision making process with her provider (van der Weijden et al. 2012). In the case of SP, recent guidelines from the USPSTF would suggest that she should not get a screening mammogram at age 40, but there is substantial debate among clinicians about this recommendation and many providers rely on patient preferences to guide the decision for when to initiate mammography outside the clear-cut window.

Decision aids come in many varieties and are intended for use at different time points in the patient–provider interaction. For example, decision aids may be used before an office visit in preparation for an anticipated decision, such whether to have an amniocentesis to screen for chromosomal abnormalities in a fetus. They may be used spontaneously during a clinical encounter as the decision arises, such as when a new medication is recommended during a clinic visit. They can be used after the clinical visit when a decision point has been reached and the patient needs to consider his options prior to proceeding. Decision aids can appear in various media, including printed pamphlets, cards, booklets, audio, or videotapes, and, increasingly, online interactive web sites (or combinations of these formats). Such online tools allow patients to use the decision aid independently from their clinical encounter, to use it repeatedly, or to share it with family members who are also involved in making the decision (Elwyn et al. 2010). A decision aid can take many forms based on the needs of the shared decision making scenario. Nevertheless, there are common elements to decision aids that provide a structure for understanding and creating these important shared decision making tools.

Elements of a Decision Aid

The common elements of a decision aid are discussed below and a summary is presented in Table 16.1 (Elwyn 2006a; Stacey et al. 2011).

Basic Health Information

Similar to general health educational materials, the decision aid should include factual information about the health condition, such as how it is acquired or diagnosed, the incidence or prevalence rates of the condition in the population, common symptoms, and the importance of treating or preventing the condition or its sequelae. The information should be in sufficient detail to allow for informed decision making, and based on the most recent scientific evidence. Ideally this information is presented in a simple, literacy- and numeracy-appropriate manner so that it is easily understood by most patients.

Recognize that a Decision Must Be Made

Where decision aids diverge from health educational materials, however, is their focus on the preference-sensitive decision. Decision aids should indicate the state of clinical equipoise (that there is more than one medically reasonable option) and explain that the "right" decision

Table 16.1 Elements of a decision aid

Element	Description	Example: early stage breast cancer	
Basic information about the health condition	Objective information such as how a disease is acquired or diagnosed, incidence or prevalence rates of the condition, common symptoms, and why the condition should be treated or prevented	Breast cancer occurs when abnormal cells grow out of control in the breast. It is highly curable if found early	
Recognizing that a decision needs to be made	Defines the state of clinical equipoise for this condition. May acknowledge scientific uncertainty about outcomes	There are two common treatment options for early stage breast cancer: (1) lumpectomy and radiation (2) mastectomy. One treatment option is not superior to the other.	
List and describe the options available	Clearly delineates potential options, such as different medications, surgical procedures, or the option of no new action (status quo)	Lumpectomy and radiation	Mastectomy
Benefits and Harms	Benefits and harms of the potential options. May present statistical probabilities for the outcomes. May acknowledge scientific uncertainty about outcomes	• Conserves natural breast appearance and sensation • Same survival as mastectomy • Slightly higher risk of cancer recurrence in that breast, which would necessitate a mastectomy • Radiation risks including fatigue and skin discoloration	• Avoids daily radiation • Lower chance of cancer recurrence • Same survival as lumpectomy and radiation • Disappointment with breast appearance, even with reconstruction • Altered sensitivity of breast tissue • Without reconstruction, there is uneven weight on the chest, potentially causing neck or back pain • Risks associated with additional reconstructive surgery
Values clarification	Implicit: suggested by the benefits and harms outlined. Explicit: deliberative exercises such as balance sheets, interactive weighing of decision attributes, or numeric rating of decision factors according to personal values	• I don't mind trying breast-conserving surgery first and having a mastectomy if it's needed to remove all of the cancer • I really want to keep most of my breast • I am worried about problems after mastectomy, such as neck and back pain • Time and travel for radiation treatment isn't a concern	• I am worried that breast-conserving surgery will not remove all of the cancer • Keeping my breast is not as important as getting rid of all the cancer • I am worried about having radiation treatment or side effects such as fatigue and skin changes • I'm worried about the inconvenience of radiation treatment, such as extra time and daily travel

(continued)

Table 16.1 (continued)

Element	Description	Example: early stage breast cancer
Patient narratives (optional)	Stories describing others' experiences with the given decision to help patients imagine future outcomes, to clarify values, or to reiterate factual information	
Guidance in next steps of decision making	If ready to make a decision, indicate preference If not ready to make a decision, indicate what the patient needs to do next, such as to talk to family members or gather more information about the options	• I am ready to make a decision • I want to discuss the options with others, like my spouse, my doctor, or with breast cancer survivors • I want to learn more about my options

depends on an individual's values. Therefore, the clinician cannot make this decision without guidance from the patient, who is the expert on his or her values, and the patient cannot necessarily make the decision alone without more objective information from the clinician about the options.

List the Options Available

Decision aids delineate the options available to the patient. One of these options may be the status quo, or no new action whatsoever. Scientific uncertainty may be acknowledged at this point. For example, the state of science may not be able to distinguish yet if one option is superior to another, or it may not be certain how a given individual will respond to the one treatment compared to the other. Each option should be presented with equal footing in an unbiased fashion to allow for the patient's values and preferences to drive the shared decision making process.

Benefits and Harms

The advantages and disadvantages of the available options are clearly stated and compared. While presenting risk and benefit information, decision aids strive to make the patient well informed without biasing his or her decision in one direction or another.

Communicating risk information

Communicating risk information in a manner that is accessible and comprehensible can be challenging. Numeric risk can be misinterpreted if presented as a relative risk (50 % reduction in risk) instead of an absolute risk (risk decreases from 10 to 5 %) (Epstein et al. 2004). More complex ideas like number needed to treat are even harder to convey accurately. Graphical displays can rapidly communicate these numbers and ideas, and decision aids employ some of the most common, effective graphic formats.

One of the most popular forms is the icon array: a set of individual icons, such as faces or dots, to represent probabilities at the individual level. Figure 16.1 is taken from a decision aid for initiation of statin therapy to lower cholesterol and reduce the risk of cardiovascular events (Mann et al. 2010; Weymiller et al. 2007). Faces are shown to depict 100 hypothetical patients with a low (15 % or less) but measurable risk for a heart attack. In the "no statin" panel, ten frowning red faces represent those patients predicted to have a heart attack out of 100 patients who do not take statins. In the "yes statin" panel, there are eight frowning red faces representing patients expected to have a heart attack despite taking a statin and two smiling yellow faces representing patients who avoided a heart attack by taking a statin. The 90 smiling green faces in

Fig. 16.1 Example of icon array. The figures display the risk of a heart attack, with or without statin therapy, in an individual with an average (<15 %) risk of heart disease. Icon arrays rapidly convey the change in absolute risk (in this case, 2 out of a 100 people avoid a heart attack because of statin therapy)

What is my risk of having a heart attack in the next 10 years?

The risk for 100 people like you who **DO NOT** take statins.

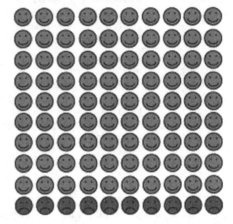

NO STATIN

90 people **DO NOT** have a heart attack (green)

10 people **DO** have a heart attack (red)

The risk for 100 people like you who **DO** take statins.

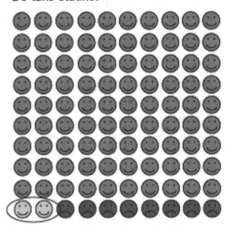

YES STATIN

90 people still **DO NOT** have a heart attack (green)

2 people **AVOIDED** a heart attack (yellow)

8 people still **DO** have a heart attack (red)

98 people experienced **NO BENEFIT** from taking statins

had a heart attack

avoided a heart attack

didn't have a heart attack

both panels show those patients not expected to have a heart attack regardless of statin therapy.

Icon arrays give an opportunity to depict both the numerator (the number of people affected) and the denominator (the population at risk). When numerator information alone is shown (e.g., 10 vs. 8 patients), risks tend to be overestimated. Compared to percentage information, icon arrays have been shown to help patients generate more accurate risk estimations (Ancker et al. 2006). Risk perception is equally accurate whether icons show more humanistic faces or abstract dots or asterisks, though users may prefer the display with human features.

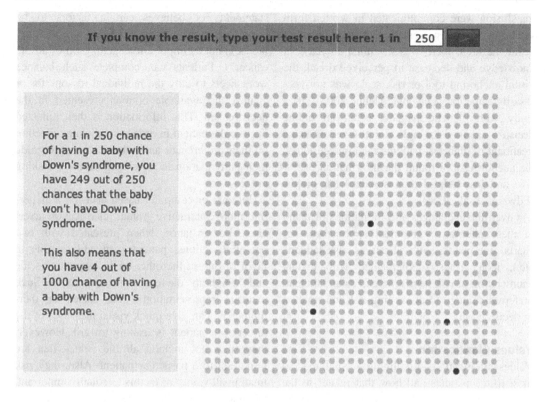

Fig. 16.2 Example of icon array with random distribution of affected individuals

Icon arrays can display affected individuals in random order instead of in summed arrangement (Fig. 16.2). Such a strategy helps convey the nature of chance in predicting outcomes, and is sometimes used in genetic counseling. However, it comes at the cost of compromising users' comprehension of risk since it relies on counting the individual icons and removes the advantage of quickly visually comparing one array to another in terms of area or number (Ancker et al. 2006).

Another popular graphical format for representing risk information is the bar chart. Bar charts and icon arrays are both examples of part-to-whole displays that are visually appealing, easy to process, and convey both absolute and relative risk (Ancker et al. 2006). Bar charts are usually preferred by patients, but are vulnerable to axis distortion in which the scale or range of the axes can mislead interpretation of the data (Edwards et al. 2006). In fact, formats preferred by patients, such as simpler designs, are

not always associated with increased accuracy of risk perception. Other formats for conveying risk information, such as survival curves, are often highly dependent on education level and are understood better after teaching (Ancker et al. 2006). Such graphics may still be useful in decision aids, but they limit independent use of the tool and demand more guidance in interpretation from the provider.

A third technique is to compare the probabilities in the given situation to other familiar situations, such as the chance of having a motor vehicle crash. These comparisons can be made in text, so-called "anchoring" descriptions, or graphically using risk scales or risk ladders, where familiar and unfamiliar risks are presented together so that the relative magnitude of risk can be compared. In theory, this allows patients to use a well-known reference as a way of helping them frame and comprehend the new risk information. In practice, however, there may not be a substantial advantage. When risks of blood transfusion were communicated in written form versus a visual presentation alongside other health hazards, there was a similar increase in knowledge and decrease in perceived dread; the visual anchoring tool or risk scale was not necessarily superior (Lee and Mehta 2003). In a study with diabetic patients using an online decision aid tool for tight control versus usual treatment of diabetes, patients randomized to use the anchoring tool found the information excessive and less helpful than standard bar graphs (Edwards et al. 2006).

Given the challenges and limitations of many of these alternative graphical approaches (bar charts, line charts, survival curves, risk ladders, etc.), icon arrays supplemented with textual enumeration of risk have emerged as an efficient, preferred strategy to conveying risk information in decision aids.

Values Clarification

Values clarification—highlighting what matters most to the patients and how that relates to the available options—is a key distinguishing feature of decision aids. Values clarification can be implicit or explicit. Implicit values clarification may highlight benefits or harms that many patients may find significant without formally leading the patient through a values clarification process. For example, the Diabetes Choice decision aid is comprised of six cards displaying several important features of possible new medications for the patient: side effects, risk of hypoglycemia, effect on weight, self-monitoring demands, daily routine, and impact on hemoglobin A1c (a long-term measure of glycemic control) (Mullan et al. 2009). During their use of the decision aid with their clinician, diabetic patients decide which cards they wish to discuss in detail, implicitly acknowledging—to themselves and to their provider—which drug characteristics are most meaningful to them (e.g., side effects) and what they value (e.g., freedom from the possibility of gastrointestinal problems).

Explicit values clarification usually entails patient deliberation exercises. For example, a patient may be asked to indicate numerically or graphically to what extent she agrees with certain statements or believes certain factors to be important to her decision (e.g., "Keeping my breast is not as important as getting rid of all the cancer"). Patients can complete such balance worksheets to tally the individual reasons for or against the available options presented in the decision aid. This information is then reflected back to the patient in order to stimulate reflection on their preferences and values in order to guide their participation in the shared decision making process.

Internet or computer-based decision aids permit more interactive values clarification exercises. For instance, when presented with two potential options, patients can add reasons in favor of one or the other on an interactive scale and "weigh up" the reasons for their choice. Such pictorial representations, like scales or thermometers, can give quick visual measures of the direction a patient is leaning toward. However, they may not include all the values that are important to a particular patient. Also, they risk treating all values or factors as equally important, whereas there may be a single value or belief that trumps all others (e.g., refusal to accept a blood transfusion regardless of the circumstances). Other deliberation exercises are designed to accommodate these situations by allowing patients to assign the greatest weight to their most important value or to indicate that they are able to make a decision after enumerating only one or two salient values. When completed, these values clarification exercises and worksheets can be shared with the provider to facilitate further discussion and decision making.

The role of patient narratives

There remains ongoing debate among developers, researchers, and consumers about the appropriate role of patient narratives in decision aids. Narratives are first-person stories that may appear in various forms in decision aids (text, audio, or video). These stories can serve various purposes. They may describe what it is like to live with a certain condition ("Having atrial fibrillation means I have an irregular heart beat and can sometimes feel palpitations") or reiterate facts about the condition and the options

("My doctor told me I could have a stroke because of a-fib, but that there are medications I can take to reduce that risk"). Patients can describe the values that were important to them in making their decisions ("My mother had a stroke and was bedridden until she died, and I would never want that to happen to me, so I chose to take the blood thinner, even if that meant accepting a small risk of serious bleeding") and comment on their satisfaction or certainty of their decision ("When I must go to the clinic every week to have my labs checked, I sometimes wonder if this was the right decision"). More than just restating information or ideas found in other sections of the decision aid, these testimonials share the experiences of people who faced the same decision, people who may have already encountered the hypothetical outcomes presented in the decision aid.

These stories are important because they can be more powerful and persuasive than mere statistics, and patients have expressed an interest in narratives when making health decisions (Khangura et al. 2008; Volandes et al. 2009). When choosing among potential options, patients are asked to imagine what it would be like to undergo unfamiliar procedures or states—what would it feel like to have a mastectomy, or take cholesterol-lowering medication every day, or to live with the anxiety of an uncertain diagnosis? Such future affective forecasting can be difficult, and narratives can help patients better envision their potential future states and clarify their values (Elwyn et al. 2010). Narratives can also effectively promote behavior change. In a randomized trial among adults who had not undergone colon cancer screening, subjects who were exposed to written testimonials from patients living with advanced colorectal cancer expressed less ambivalence about screening and were more likely to report completion of a colorectal cancer screening test 6-months post-intervention compared to patients who did not view the testimonials (Lipkus 2007).

Still, these testimonials can also unduly influence patients' decisions. Cognitive psychology research has long documented the persuasive potential of narratives or testimonials. More

recently, Ubel et al. (2001) showed that participants were more likely to choose the option for which more positive stories were presented, compared to when equal numbers of stories were presented for the two options, despite unchanged statistical probabilities. Moreover, testimonials may under-represent different points of view, and divert attention away from the facts. According to one international quality standard for decision aids, patient narratives are not essential to decision aids. However, if they are included, then a range of positive and negative experiences should be featured and it should be clear whether patients gave informed consent for their stories and received any financial incentive to share their stories (O'Connor and Elwyn 2005).

In a review of publically available decision aids, Khangura and colleagues found that 84 % of decision aids featured narratives (Khangura et al. 2008). In their analysis, stories both for and against the most intensive option were featured in all of the decision aids, though not always in an equal or balanced fashion. Only half of the sampled decision aids described patients' satisfaction with their decisions, either the decision itself ("I'm very satisfied that I decided to have the surgery…") or with the decision-making process ("I wished that it had been explained to me at the time so I could have made the choice to have it done or not"). If satisfaction was discussed, either positive experiences were presented exclusively, or positive experiences exceeded negative experiences. Statements regarding patient consent or financial compensation for sharing stories were nearly completely absent. By these measures, currently available decision aids may not be utilizing patient narratives in an even-handed manner.

What balance or range of experiences would be appropriate for patient stories? It may not be enough to show an equal number of stories for the various possible options and outcomes. Perhaps instead the proportion of stories should reflect the statistical probabilities of the possible outcomes. Or perhaps it should reflect the frequency with which patients choose the various options. The tendency to show positive satisfaction with decisions may reflect self-selection bias among the patients who agree to share their stories or may reflect bias on the part of decision aid developers. The use of patient narratives offers great potential to enhance the power of decision aids, but much research remains to be done to determine how best to employ this potential.

Evaluating the Quality of Decision Aids

In the end, the goal of a decision aid is to support the patient and his or her provider in reaching a high-quality decision. In these situations, where there is inherently no "correct" course of action, what constitutes a "good" decision? Both the final choice and the process of choosing should be considered. One may consider a decision "good" when there is congruence between a patient's values and the option he chooses, that is, the chosen option maximizes what is important to the patient and minimizes that which he wishes to avoid. To arrive at this decision, the patient should attain adequate knowledge of the given options and their key features, and should be involved in the decision making to the extent that he or she desires (Elwyn 2006a).

Knowledge and Risk Perception

Thus, when evaluating the quality of decision aids, one would like to see that patients have greater knowledge of their health condition, their options, and the risks and benefits of those options after using the decision aid compared to before using the decision aid or compared to patients not exposed to the decision aid. In other words, patients should be more informed decision-makers as a result of the tool. In systematic reviews, this increase in disease-specific knowledge is indeed observed, compared to patients receiving usual care (O'Connor et al. 2009; Stacey et al. 2011). For example, a Cochrane review of decision aids found that, on a standardized knowledge scale of 100 hundred points, patient who used decision aids scored 13 points higher than patients who experienced usual care. Patients using decision aids also had more accurate risk perceptions, especially when probabilities were depicted

quantitatively rather than qualitatively. However, although these statistically significant differences have been measured among decision aids collectively, it is difficult to know if these changes are clinically meaningful to the decision making process or applicable to all decision aids. Does answering one more question correctly on a ten item survey, a 10 % increase in knowledge, practically translate to better comprehension of a patient's underlying illness or treatment choice? Further research is needed to better understand the relationship between patient knowledge and decision making.

Patient Involvement

Again, decision aids are intended as tools to facilitate the implementation of shared decision making, that collaborative process between a patient and his or her provider to reach a decision that reflects the patient's values. How can one know if shared decision making has occurred? In order to measure the extent to which clinicians involve patients in decision making, researchers developed the OPTION scale (observing patient involvement in decision making). The OPTION scale is a validated, reliable instrument that measures 12 observable clinician behaviors that one would expect to occur during a shared decision making process (Elwyn et al. 2005). Each action is rated from zero (if it is not observed) to four (if it is observed and executed to high standard). Some of these behaviors (e.g., stating that there is more than one option for the problem, explaining the benefits and harms of the options) are precisely what decision aids aim to do. Other behaviors (e.g., verifying that the patient has understood the information, giving an opportunity to ask questions, indicating that a decision-making or decision-deferring stage has been reached) constitute general communication and decision-negotiation skills.

In trials of decision aids where clinical encounters are recorded by audio or video, use of decision aids is associated with higher OPTION scores compared to usual care encounters. That is, decision aids do indeed promote and enable the behaviors that constitute shared decision making. Furthermore, patients exposed to decision aids were approximately 37 % more likely to adopt an active role in decision making compared to patients exposed to usual care, but just as likely to assume a collaborative or shared role. Based on these studies, patients appear less likely to defer entirely to their providers and more likely to participate in decision making when decision aids are used (Stacey et al. 2011). Although patient participation has been measured in a minority of studies, the evidence favors a small but positive effect of decision aids on patient involvement, thereby promoting shared decision-making.

Decisional Conflict

In addition to being knowledgeable, informed of risks, and adequately involved in their decisions, patients engaged in making high-quality decisions should experience low decisional conflict. Decisional conflict is not merely recognition that advantages and disadvantages exist for any given option, or that there are "conflicting" options available. It is an undesirable state of discomfort and internal conflict experienced when facing a difficult decision (LeBlanc et al. 2009). Decisional conflict is a measure of the confidence and security in one's decision, and, in research studies of decision aids, is measured by the Decisional Conflict scale (DCS), a validated tool that "discriminates between those who make or delay decisions, is sensitive to change, and discriminates between different decision support interventions" (O'Connor et al. 2009). The DCS is composed of five subscales: personal uncertainty, feeling uninformed, unclear about personal values, inadequate support in decision making, and perception that one has made an ineffective decision. High scores reflect higher decisional conflict, that is, greater insecurity and lower confidence in one's decision; specifically, scores greater than 38 on the total 100-point scale are associated with delays in decision making. Low scores (i.e., less than 25 out of 100 points) are associated with less conflict and greater likelihood of executing a decision (O'Connor 1995). Overall, decision aids are associated with lower DCS scores, with

significant differences compared to usual care noted for the subscales of "feeling uninformed" and "unclear about personal values." These results suggest that decision aids help patients feel more comfortable with their decision by clarifying their values and increasing their knowledge (O'Connor et al. 2009; Stacey et al. 2011). In a Cochrane review of decision aids, compared to usual care, users of decision aids had DCS scores that were only 6 % lower (Stacey et al. 2011). Thus, while decision aids may reduce some measures of discomfort that patients have about their decisions and create a greater sense of understanding, the general impact may not be dramatic.

Other Outcomes

Trials of decision aids have assessed differences between usual care and decision aid groups in level of satisfaction with the decision-making process or with the chosen decision itself, but taken together, these studies have not found significant differences in decisional satisfaction. Nor have conclusive differences been detected in terms of level of anxiety or regret, as might be expected if patients are more informed and involved in their health decisions.

Likewise, one might expect decision aids to have a potential impact on healthcare costs or length of time for healthcare visits. As of yet, no clear trend has emerged. The few studies that have looked at patients' adherence to their chosen option at some time point after exposure to the decision have found either no difference in adherence compared to the usual care group or marginally increased adherence (Man-Son-Hing et al. 1999; Mullan et al. 2009; Stacey et al. 2011). Finally, long-term patient outcomes such as adverse event rates or survival have been infrequently assessed, since most trials of decision aids are short-term studies only, and no pattern has emerged in systematic reviews.

International Quality Standards

Given the burgeoning array of decision aids in recent years from academic, commercial, and nonprofit organizations, there has been a need to measure and compare the quality of these tools.

Table 16.2 Select criteria from the International Patient Decision Aid Standards (IPDAS)

I. Content: the patient decision aid...	– Provides information about options in sufficient detail for decision making – Includes methods for clarifying and expressing patients' values: describes the procedures and outcomes to help patients imagine what it is like to experience their physical, emotional, and social effects; asks patients to consider which positive and negative features matter most – Includes structured guidance in deliberation and communication: provides steps to make a decision, includes tools (e.g., worksheets, question lists) to discuss options with others
II. Development process: the patient decision aid...	– Presents information in a balanced manner: shows negative and positive features with equal detail – Has a systematic development process: has peer review by experts not involved in development; is field tested with users – Uses up to date scientific evidence: provides references to evidence used, describes quality of scientific evidence, uses evidence from studies of patients similar to target audience – Uses plain language: written at grade 8 equivalent level or less; provides ways to help patients understand information other than reading (e.g., audio, video)
III. Effectiveness: the patient decision aid helps patients to...	– Recognize a decision needs to be made – Know options and their features – Understand that values affect the decision – Be clear about option features that matter most – Discuss values with their practitioner – Become involved in preferred ways

The IPDAS Collaboration was established in 2003 from a group of researchers, clinicians, decision aid developers, and policy makers whose objective was to create quality criteria for decision aids. They proposed a checklist of 64 criteria in three domains (content, development process, and effectiveness) against which to measure decision aids (see Table 16.2 for examples of criteria).

Depending on the format and length of the decision aid, these standards may or may not be fulfilled. Many decision aids have not been formally tested in clinical trials, therefore effectiveness data are unavailable, and, until recently, less attention has been paid to the development process or theoretical underpinnings of creating decision aids. Still, while not prescriptive, these criteria do set a benchmark for a comprehensive, high-quality decision aid, and facilitate comparisons between competing instruments.

In the next section, several example decision aids are presented, and their key attributes are discussed to illustrate some different ways of executing the common elements of decision aids.

Decision Aid Examples

As discussed above, decision aids come in different forms, though they share common elements to facilitate shared decision making between patients and providers. In this section, we give a few examples of decision aids for preference-sensitive decisions, highlight common elements of decision aids, and comment on the quality of, and evidence for, supporting the decision aid. These examples were selected because they illustrate the diversity of clinical situations in which decision aids can be used, such as cancer screening, prenatal testing, and medication management. They also demonstrate the range of decision aid formats and the variety of information and exercises that can be included.

The Australian Screening Mammography Decision Aid

Our case patient SP and her physician are faced with the decision to screen for breast cancer between the ages of 40- and 50-years old. This decision is complicated by conflicting clinical guidelines, risk of unnecessary procedures and over-diagnosis, and risk of missing a lethal breast cancer. In short, the decision to screen for breast cancer between 40 and 50 years of age is a preference-sensitive decision for which a decision aid may be helpful.

A mammography screening decision aid developed by the Screening and Test Evaluation Program at the University of Sidney has been studied for use in women 40–50-years old and older than 70-years old [Screening and Test Evaluation Program (STEP) 2003]. This decision aid is both paper–based and web-based and provides little *health information* on the pathophysiology or treatment of breast cancer, nor the specific diagnostic modalities after abnormal mammogram. However, the decision aid does highlight risk factors that may increase a woman's personal risk of breast cancer and links to an online breast cancer risk calculator. Website links are also provided to the National Cancer Institute in the U.S. and the National Breast and Ovarian Cancer Centre in Australia.

The decision aid does clearly *present a choice* that needs to be made and stresses the uncertainty of the decision. ("Remember there is no right or wrong answer about whether to start having screening mammograms.") The *benefits and harms* of screening are not listed specifically but addressed through risk communication and values clarification tools. A major focus of the Australian screening mammogram decision aid is *conveying risks* of screening and not screening. Risks of breast cancer diagnosis and breast cancer death with and without screening are portrayed with icon arrays in summed arrangement and absolute risk reductions (Fig. 16.3). Additionally, risk of further testing in the absence of disease and risk of anxiety and worry are also communicated.

A *values clarification* worksheet reviews risk factors that may increase a patient's personal risk for breast cancer, such as family history, early age of menarche, and age of first child bearing,

and then asks the patient how the specific risks presented in the decision aid make her feel about screening. The patient can respond along a graded scale from "Start screening now" to "Consider screening later." The patient may also include her own reasons. After considering her risks weighed against her values, the patient is asked if she is leaning in favor of or against screening (Fig. 16.4). In other words, the patient is asked to commit to a decision.

The Australian Screening mammogram decision aid was evaluated in a randomized control trial of 321 women between the ages of 38 and 45. Patients in the decision aid group had higher knowledge scores after using the decision aid and more women had made a decision about screening (82 % vs. 61 %). Of the women who had made a decision, more decided against screening, 48 % versus 35 % in the control group (Mathieu et al. 2010). The online decision aid was an adaptation of a paper- based decision aid for women over the age of 70 deciding to continue screening. An earlier randomized control trial of the mammography decision aid in an older population of women illustrated increases in knowledge of the benefits and harms of screening, clearer values, and more women making an informed choice, though at 1 month there was no difference in the number of women participating in screening between the intervention and control groups (Mathieu and Barratt 2007).

In summary, the content of the Australian Screening mammogram decision aid primarily focuses on risk assessment and values clarification. The decision aid does not delve into detailed patient education about breast cancer, and in this way draws a clear distinction between decision aids and patient education brochures. While the latter often contain facts about the disease, diagnostic procedures, and treatment, decision aids focus on medical uncertainty and what this means to the patient. While there is some evidence of improvement in the decision-making process by increasing patient knowledge and reducing indecision, the relationship between knowledge and decisional conflict is

AUSTRALIAN SCREENING MAMMOGRAPHY DECISION AID TRIAL

A decision aid for women aged 40
thinking about starting
mammography screening

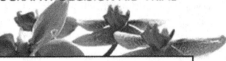

What else happens to 1000 women aged 40 who *have* screening mammograms every two years for 10 years?

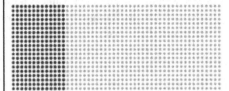

● 21 women are diagnosed with breast cancer over the next 10 years
- 12 women will have their cancer detected by screening
- 9 women develop symptoms and are diagnosed with breast cancer between screening mammograms

● 239 women have extra tests after an abnormal mammogram. The extra tests will show these women don't have breast cancer. Aside from the inconvenience of attending for these tests, some women will worry long after they have had them[4]

● 740 women are correctly reassured they do not have breast cancer

What else happens to 1000 women aged 40 who *do not have* screening mammograms during the next 10 years?

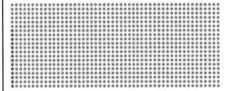

● 14 women develop symptoms and are diagnosed with breast cancer

● 986 women continue with their daily activities without being affected by breast cancer or attending for screening for the next 10 years

---

In summary, screening 1000 women aged 40 every 2 years for next 10 years results in

- 0.5 less deaths from breast cancer » Find out why
- 7 extra women diagnosed with breast cancer » Find out why
- 239 women having tests after an abnormal mammogram without having breast cancer found. They may worry from these 'false alarms' » Find out why
- 740 women are correctly reassured they do not have breast cancer
- 9 women have breast cancer diagnosed between screens, even though they regularly attend screening » Find out why

» Next

Fig. 16.3 Australian screening mammography decision and trail

For 1000 women aged 40 who commence screening:

0.5 death from breast cancer is avoided because of screening.
This makes me feel I want to...

Start screening now ○ ○ ○ ○ ○ ○ ○ ○ ○ ○   Consider screening later

7 more women are diagnosed with breast cancer over the next 10 years because of screening.
This makes me feel I want to...

Start screening now ○ ○ ○ ○ ○ ○ ○ ○ ○ ○   Consider screening later

239 women will have extra tests because of screening.
This makes me feel I want to...

Start screening now ○ ○ ○ ○ ○ ○ ○ ○ ○ ○   Consider screening later

740 women are reassured they do not have breast cancer because of screening.
This makes me feel I want to...

Start screening now ○ ○ ○ ○ ○ ○ ○ ○ ○ ○   Consider screening later

Others: | Please describe them here |

This makes me feel I want to...

Start screening now ○ ○ ○ ○ ○ ○ ○ ○ ○ ○   Consider screening later

After weighing up the points, from the last two steps, tick the box that best describes which way you are leaning:

○ I will start having a mammogram every 2 years
○ I will have a mammogram now and reconsider in 2 years
○ I am undecided
○ I will not have a mammogram now but I may reconsider in two years
○ I will not have a mammogram now but I may reconsider later when 50

You can write in this space any questions you still have. You could contact us, ask your doctor or ask your local BreastScreen Australia service.

| Please describe them here |

Fig. 16.4 Risks of breast cancer diagnosis and breast cancer death with and without screening

uncertain, as is the impact on healthcare outcomes. Future research is needed to determine if use of this decision aid would change measures such as screening rates, rates of unnecessary procedures, or breast cancer diagnoses or mortality.

Amniodex

Amniodex (www.amniodex.com) is a decision aid developed by the researchers at Cardiff University for women contemplating amniocentesis to determine risk of a fetal chromosome abnormality. An amniocentesis may be offered after a screening blood test, a mid-pregnancy ultrasound suggestive of a fetal anomaly, or a previous history of chromosomal abnormality (ACOG Committee on Practice Bulletins 2007). The risks associated with amniocentesis, such as miscarriage and infection, may be interpreted differently by patients with different value systems. For some women, the small chance of miscarriage (Driscoll and Gross 2009) may be worth the benefit of learning if a fetus has a developmental disability, while another women might find this risk unacceptable. A decision aid is well suited to this preference-sensitive decision.

Amniodex is a web-based decision aid that may be used independently by a patient prior to or after a clinic visit. The decision aid presents **basic health information** about the procedure, including indications for amniocentesis, how the test is done, the types of tests performed [polymerase chain reaction (PCR) or Karyotype], and what symptoms women can expect post procedure. Information is presented in text and figures, as well as one short video of a patient describing her experience of the procedure. ("Amniocentesis can be uncomfortable but not painful.") Furthermore, the decision aid provides resources to help a patient decide to continue or terminate a pregnancy, and lists organizations that can support patients in preparing for a child with congenital anomalies.

The decision aid clearly **recognizes that there is a choice** to be made, and that no right or wrong decision exists. Under the heading "It's Your Choice," the decision aid relates how preference-sensitive decisions can be fraught with anxiety and emotion. Screening pathway flow diagrams also visually depict when a decision is required, emphasizing the decision points and **highlighting the patient's options** of accepting or declining a screening test or amniocentesis (Fig. 16.5).

Amniodex explicitly lays out the **harms and benefits** of an amniocentesis, listing intended benefits such as learning if the fetus has an inherited condition and making choices about a pregnancy. The risks are also clearly presented, including miscarriage, infection, premature delivery, and false negative or inconclusive results.

Fig. 16.5 Screening pathway flow diagram

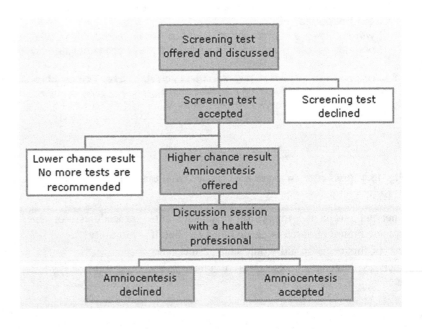

Amniodex *communicates the risk* of Downs Syndrome based on personalized information, allowing the user to enter her test results into the tool and better understand what her risk of having a baby with Down's Syndrome might be. The decision aid uses both absolute risk ratios and an icon array in random arrangement (Fig. 16.2). As discussed earlier, random arrangements may better convey chance, though may diminish understanding of absolute risk.

Amniodex approaches *values clarification* in several ways—"Weighing it up," "Your most important reason," a values clarification worksheet, and patient narratives. Regarding "Weighing it up," reasons for and against amniocentesis are listed and as the patient identifies reasons for and against an amniocentesis, a graphic display of a scale weighs pros and cons for the patient (Fig. 16.6). Alternatively, on the "Your most important reason" screen, the patient is encouraged to rank the factors that are most important in their decision. The values clarification worksheet lists reasons to have and not have an amniocentesis and how the patient feels about the risks associated with screening and not screening.

Additionally, several *patient narratives* are presented in streaming videos. The decision aid gives examples of women who did and did not choose an amniocentesis, women who had a miscarriage and did not, as well as women who had different feelings about these outcomes. Both positive and negative experiences are presented to address the inherent bias of one patient's story. With all values clarification tools, the patient is asked if she has made a decision at the end of the exercise and, if not yet, toward which direction she is leaning.

Amniodex contains robust information about the reasons to screen for Down Syndrome and

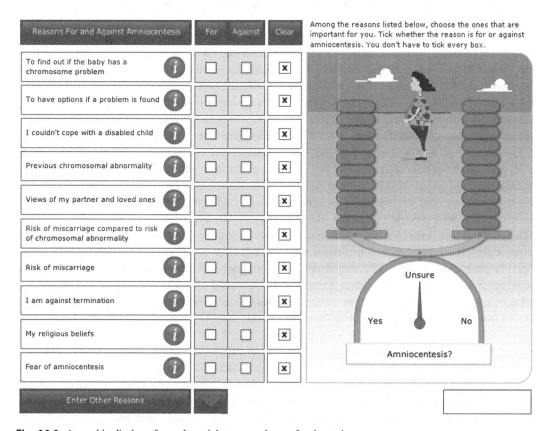

Fig. 16.6 A graphic display of a scale weighs pros and cons for the patient

content about the choices available to women and families. Risk perception is presented in the most evidence-based format, as percentages and icon arrays (Ancker et al. 2006) though, as mentioned above, random arrangement has strengths and weaknesses. A review of current recommendations and research also highlights the challenge of maintaining decision aids when sensitivity of screening tests, risk assessments, and guideline recommendations change over time. For example, in 2007, the American College of Obstetricians and Gynecologists issued updated guidelines for the screening of fetal chromosomal abnormalities, which include to offer screening to all women regardless of maternal age, to begin offering screening in the first trimester, and to consider using the results of integrated first and second trimester screening versus stepwise serum screening by semester to guide invasive diagnostic testing for chromosomal abnormalities (ACOG Committee on Practice Bulletins 2007). The estimated risk of Down syndrome cited in Amniodex, the decision flow chart, and risk of miscarriage would need significant revision to remain clinically relevant over time. Clinician adherence to ACOG guidelines has increased over time (Cleary-Goldman et al. 2006; Driscoll et al. 2009), and decision support tools will need to be updated in a timely manner to support continued use.

The decision aid was developed with the input of several stakeholders, researchers, doctors, and patients (Durand et al. 2012; Durand 2012), which is an important consideration in quality evaluation by international standards (Elwyn 2006a). Amniodex provides several tools for values clarification, though which method best supports patients in unclear. The abundance of information and values clarification exercises could be counterproductive, the sheer number of options from which to choose detracting from the main focus of integrating enhanced knowledge and self-reflection to arrive at one decision. Still, in field-testing, some women wanted more information than was available in the decision aid (Durand 2012). Currently, there is little evidence of how this decision aid impacts the decision-making process or healthcare outcomes. Future research is needed to study the effect of the decision aid on patients' knowledge of options, congruence of values and decision made, and outcomes such as rates of invasive screening procedures and miscarriage.

Diabetes Medication Choice

The number of medications available to treat type 2 diabetes mellitus has increased considerably in recent years. Medical societies differ in their recommendations for which medications to use when starting or intensifying treatment, although all agree that regimens should be personalized to individual patients (Handelsman et al. 2011; Qaseem et al. 2012; Standards of medical care in diabetes 2012). This situation presents an ideal opportunity for shared decision making, not only because of the state of clinical equipoise, but because diabetes is a chronic medical condition that relies on patient self-management and essentially lifelong administration of medications.

The Diabetes Medication Choice (DMC) decision aid is a product of the Mayo Clinic's Knowledge and Evaluation Research Unit in Rochester, Minnesota (see Fig. 16.7). Researchers designed the tool to be used during the clinical visit rather than as a stand-alone decision aid, like Amniodex. DMC includes six laminated, color-coded "issue cards" describing features of five diabetes medications (metformin, insulin, glitazones, exenatide, and sulfonylureas). The six issues highlighted are weight change, low blood sugar or hypoglycemia, side effects, daily administration routine, daily sugar testing or monitoring, and change in blood sugar or hemoglobin A1c reduction. In practice, the clinician would offer all six issue cards and invite the patient to select which card they wished to talk about first. The patient and provider would then discuss the advantages and disadvantages of the medications according to that feature (Mullan et al. 2009).

The brevity of the DMC demands greater involvement by the clinician since the cards do not contain enough *information in sufficient*

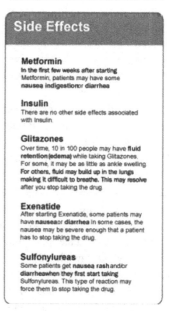

Fig. 16.7 Diabetes medication choice decision aid

detail for the patient to make a decision on his or her own. For example, basic information like which medications are oral and which are injections is only implied on one of the cards. There is no general educational information about diabetes mellitus or the importance of blood glucose control within the decision aid. It is up to the clinician to communicate why a *decision must be*

made and how the patient's values impact the decision; the DMC cards do not convey this message.

The cards succinctly present the five potential medication *options*, and the structure of the issue cards enables quick comparisons between the drugs, which are always listed in the same order and arranged directly on top of one another.

Harms and benefits are distributed across the six cards according to the issue that the cards emphasize. Information is displayed both in text and graphically when possible. For example, self-monitoring demands are displayed according to a weekly calendar and weight change is shown both by direction (weight gain or loss) and magnitude. Risk of hypoglycemia is shown in an icon array of 100 circles with different colors to indicate the probability of minor or severe events. By *communicating risk* in these multiple ways, DMC satisfies some of the IPDAS criteria for decision aid content (see next section for more detail about IPDAS criteria).

The DMC does not have explicit *values clarification* exercises; instead, the patient implies what she values based on what cards she elects to talk about (e.g., choosing the weight change card first implies that that factor is important to her). There is also no *guided deliberation* contained in the cards; again, the clinician must take a more active role in helping the patient think about the benefits and risks of the various options.

The cards have a clear, simple design that developers chose after iterative testing with clinicians and patients (Breslin et al. 2008). Indeed, the development process used to create this decision aid tool was particularly strong and in accordance with IPDAS criteria. The developers were aware of the limitations of the minimalist DMC decision aid structure, but their purpose was to create a tool that clinicians could feasibly use during the short, time-limited space of a clinic visit and that would prepare the stage for more detailed, personalized discussions that may take place over more than one visit.

Empiric testing of the DMC has shown results similar to conclusions drawn from reviews of several decision aids. In a pilot randomized trial of the DMC decision aid, patients with diabetes exposed to the tool had higher knowledge scores than usual care patients, but similar scores of decisional conflict (Mullan et al. 2009). Encounters were video-recorded and rated according to the OPTION scale; by this measure, patients using the DMC decision aid were more involved in the decision-making process compared to usual care patients. Investigators hypothesized that use of the decision aid would increase medication adherence since patients were more engaged in determining their treatment. Yet, based on pharmacy records and self-report, the patients exposed to the decision aid did not have superior adherence compared to control patients, although adherence was very high in both groups, suggesting a ceiling effect. There was also no difference between the groups in hemoglobin A1c values at 6-months post-intervention.

Still, the fact that the DMC has undergone effectiveness testing is one of its strengths. Based on ongoing evaluation, changes have been made to the DMC. For example, since the cost of medications is a common, important factor for many patients, a cost issue card has recently been added to the tool. The DMC has also been studied in nonacademic and rural settings in a cluster randomized controlled trial, with similar findings in knowledge transfer, decisional conflict, adherence, and clinical outcomes, illustrating that decision aids may be implemented in real world settings as well (Branda et al. 2013).

Limitations and Future Directions

As discussed above, decision aids are a tool for shared decision making that go beyond merely educating a patient about her condition, but also acknowledging that a decision must be made, one where her personal values and beliefs determine the optimal choice. Though there are certain common elements to these tools, the examples included above reflect the diversity, strengths, and weaknesses in decision aid designs. In this final section, we comment on a few areas of ongoing inquiry in decision aid science and discuss barriers to implementation of decision aids and shared decision making.

Standards of Quality for Decision Aids

As mentioned, in response to the need for quality standards to evaluate and compare decision aids, the IPDAS Collaboration created a collection of criteria by which to judge these interventions. IPDAS is an international, multidisciplinary network of researchers, policy makers, and patient advocates. The IPDAS quality criteria or checklist was developed in 2006 using the Delphi method based on expert opinion (Elwyn 2006b). By creating a uniform standard, the checklist has been a valuable contribution to the field of decision aid research, and the IPDAS criteria have been employed in recent reviews of decision aids (O'Connor et al. 2007; Stacey et al. 2011).

However, the checklist has its limitations (Bekker 2010). It implies that all criteria are equally important to the quality of a decision aid, rather than helping to identify what elements of the decision aid are truly essential and effective. Such a checklist suggests that a quality decision aid should satisfy all criteria, although one could imagine a decision aid that fulfills only some of the criteria (e.g., Diabetes Medication Choice) and yet is still a valuable tool for shared decision making. Conversely, a given decision aid may fulfill most of the technical criteria, but not be effective in practice. Critics note that there is still considerable debate about what constitutes a good decision and as yet limited evidence that decision aids developed using IPDAS criteria result in higher quality decisions than decision aids created without the criteria (Bekker 2010). At the least, IPDAS criteria will likely reduce variation in the quality of decision aids, and hopefully stimulate more rigorous development and testing of these decision tools.

Decision aids have been found to increase knowledge, decrease decisional conflict, increase the accuracy of risk perceptions, and increase informed value-based choices (Stacey et al. 2011). Still, there are several areas where uncertainty remains and further research is needed. For instance, what is the effect of decision aids on cost and cost-effectiveness of care (Oshima Lee and Emanuel 2013)? There may be cost savings if implementation of decision aids is associated with greater adherence to medication use, greater patient involvement in their own care, or decreased total consultation time, but a

consistent change has not been found for these measures. A randomized controlled trial that compared two levels of care management support found that subjects in the arm where shared decision making and decision aids were used had fewer hospital admissions and fewer preference-sensitive surgeries, including almost 21 % fewer preference-sensitive heart surgeries. The authors estimated that the enhanced support including shared decision making would result in a net savings of $18 per subject per month (Veroff et al. 2013). The effect of decision aids on patient health outcomes also remains largely unknown since most effectiveness trials are for short-term outcomes only.

Given the high expectations for decision aid performance in practice and the standards of quality proposed by IPDAS, it is not surprising that quality decision aids take a great deal of time and effort to produce. The resource-intensive nature of decision aid development may explain why many are created in the private sector, either by not-for-profit foundations or academic–commercial partnerships (Coulter 2010). Even when guided by templates like the Ottawa Decision Support Framework, it can be challenging for a clinical group to create their own decision aid, and they may instead adapt an existing one to their purpose.

However, decision aids have limited flexibility. They can become obsolete, as new evidence emerges, in a shorter time than it takes to develop them and therefore must be constantly updated. While online content may be more nimble, other formats, like pen-and-paper aids or video-based aids, may not be so easily changed. Decision aids are designed for fairly specific clinical scenarios and are not interchangeable. Often, the content is tailored to or derived from a particular population, and may not apply to patients of different ages, racial or ethnic backgrounds, or with certain medical co-morbidities. This shortcoming can potentially limit the applicability of decision aids to diverse patient populations.

Engaging hard-to-reach populations
For example, most existing decision aids have been designed for and tested among relatively

well-educated, non-minority populations; the challenge remains how to design decision aids with similar elements that are accessible to users with lower health literacy. Health literacy may be defined as "the degree to which individuals have the capacity to obtain, process, and understand [the] basic health information and services needed to make appropriate health decisions" (Parker and Ratzan 2010). Understanding the content of decision aids relies not only on literacy for the written word, but numeracy skills and comprehension of mathematical concepts. It is worth noting that IPDAS criteria include standards for phrasing in plain language and delivering content in ways that do not rely on reading ability (O'Connor and Elwyn 2005). As more and more decision aids are Internet-based, digital literacy will also be expected.

One approach to adapt decision aids for patients with lower literacy capitalizes on the power of patient narratives with entertainment education, or "edutainment." For example, researchers developed a decision aid for women with early stage breast cancer deciding on breast-conserving surgery or modified radical mastectomy that featured didactic soap opera episodes linked to interactive learning modules (Jibaja-Weiss et al. 2011). Available in English or Spanish, the computer-based decision aid was fully narrated with limited screen text. It was designed to resemble the familiar appearance of a television screen and required minimal, simple navigation, but still contained essential elements of a decision aid, such as values clarification.

Similar to trials of other decision aids, a randomized controlled trial of this "edutainment" breast cancer surgery decision aid among urban, uninsured women found a greater increase in knowledge, greater feelings of being informed about their options, and a clearer sense of their personal values among decision aid users compared to usual care (Jibaja-Weiss et al. 2011). Women rated the decision aid favorably on entertainment value and ease of use. Unlike other decision aids for this same surgical decision, however, women in the intervention group were more likely to choose the invasive mastectomy option rather than breast-conserving surgery than

women in the control group, raising questions about how effectively risks and benefits were communicated via the novel decision aid (Jibaja-Weiss et al. 2011; Waljee et al. 2007). The authors note that mastectomy rates have been increasing overall in the US, and acknowledge that greater understanding of the treatment options does not necessarily lead most women to choose the less radical approach.

Patients with lower literacy may stand to benefit the most from decision aids. Low health literacy is associated with poorer health outcomes as well as minority race and ethnicity, older age, and lower socioeconomic status (Paasche-Orlow and Wolf 2010). By increasing patient knowledge, conveying risks and benefits, clarifying values, and enabling patients to be involved in the decision-making process to the extent that they desire, decision aids have the potential to increase shared decision making within a population historically disadvantaged in the patient–provider dyad.

Barriers to Implementation of shared decision making

Time
An overarching obstacle to implementation of shared decision making—with or without decision aids as a tool—is the lack of time available to providers, staff, and patients to put shared decision making into practice. Time constraints was the most frequently cited impediment in a systematic review of providers' perceived barriers and facilitators to implementing shared decision making (Légaré et al. 2006b). Providers may need more time to use decision aids in the clinic, to address questions appropriately raised by decision aids, or to engage in the thoughtful conversations anticipated in collaborative decision making. Not only providers, but nurses and other staff may have more work related to administering or distributing decision aids (e.g. helping a patient use a clinic computer or watch a preconsultation video). Even patients may be burdened by the additional time required by some decision aids. A web log analysis of an

online decision aid found that patients who spent more time using the aid were better informed than those who hastily completed it (Coulter 2010). Though some studies of decision aids have measured change in consultation time from usual care to use of decision aid, the range is wide and variable, from a potential time saved of 8 min to an extra 23 min of care (Stacey et al. 2011). Although it is not clear if shared decision making is associated with a net time savings or time cost, the perceived time demand alone creates a formidable hurdle. While time is a barrier that affects all aspects of delivering shared decision making, other barriers are unique to providers, patients, and the healthcare system itself.

Provider Factors

Implementing shared decision making requires physicians to have knowledge of the concept and the attitude that patient involvement is integral to patient care. A lack of awareness of and familiarity with shared decision making can obviously limit the use of decision aids in clinical practice; a provider who is unfamiliar with decision aids will be less likely to know how to use them or evaluate them for use in everyday practice.

As discussed in the introduction, shared decision making represents a significant shift from a traditional paternalistic model of care, and such change can encounter strong cultural resistance from the medical community. In a review by Gravel et al., provider attitudes toward shared decision making were a commonly cited barrier to implementation of shared decision making in clinical practice, specifically that shared decision making was not applicable for certain patients and clinical situations, or physicians did not agree with asking patients about their preferred role in decision making (Légaré et al. 2006a). Combining a lack of physician buy-in with uncertainty of whether decision aids change health outcomes results in professional skepticism that can limit the utilization of decision support tools.

Finally, even if providers agree with the moral imperative to include patients in decision making, the prospect of additional demands on stretched resources or disrupted workflow can limit the deployment of decision aids (Coulter 2010). Many physicians want to personally evaluate decision aids prior to distribution; finding the time to do this can be difficult and delay adoption of decision aids into practice (Feibelmann et al. 2011; Silvia et al. 2008a). Furthermore, there is little evidence from randomized controlled trials on the best ways to promote physician adoption of shared decision making (Légaré et al. 2010). While education, feedback, and the use of decision aids may be important tools, the authors of this review caution those motivated to include shared decision making into practice to be aware of the lack of evidence and weigh the pros and cons of integrating decision support interventions (Légaré et al. 2010).

Patient Factors

Shared decision making is predicated on the assumption that patients are able and willing to engage in the process with their clinicians, but patients may differ in the level of involvement they wish to have and thus may pose additional barriers to the implementation of shared decision tools in practice. Surveys of patients suggest that most would defer the role of medical problem solving—making diagnoses, determining treatment options—to the expertise of their physicians. Nevertheless, they had a strong interest overall in being informed and would prefer to share or take a more dominant role when it came to making treatment decisions (Deber and Kraetschmer 1996). In a population-based survey of US adults, nearly all respondents wanted their physicians to offer them choices and ask for their opinions regarding their medical care (Levinson et al. 2005). However, about half of those surveyed preferred to leave ultimate medical decisions to their doctor and to rely on doctors' knowledge rather than seek out information on their own. Higher educational attainment, better self-reported health, and female sex were associated with a preference for more active patient involvement in medical decision making, whereas Hispanic and African-American respondents were more likely to prefer greater physician involvement.

Indeed, preferences and readiness for shared decision making may vary according to other patient-level factors such as cultural background, health literacy (as discussed above), and age. In qualitative interviews with older adults regarding medication-related decision making, a range of attitudes toward shared decision making emerged (Belcher et al. 2006). Some seniors expressed the opinion that patients *do not want* to be part of decision making, for example, due to anxiety about their illness or passive acceptance of a physician's judgment. Others stated that patients *were not able* to be part of decision making due to lack of knowledge or efficacy, or because the physician should "know best." Still others voiced a belief that a patient *should* participate in decision making since the patient knows her body and health best. In the aforementioned population-based survey, preference for patient involvement increased until age 45, at which point the effect declined, favoring greater physician involvement with older patient age. This trend may change with the Baby Boomer generation, a cohort that has taken a more active role in their own health and healthcare than their predecessors.

Patients' likelihood of adopting decision aids and shared decision making may additionally depend on the particular clinical scenario. A diagnosis of breast cancer or prostate cancer may be frightening and overwhelming to a patient, who would prefer to yield the decision-making role entirely to their provider (Silvia et al. 2008b). Furthermore, asking a patient to engage in shared decision making may be misinterpreted as abdicating responsibility for that decision or potentially abandoning the patient to make the decision independently, rather than an invitation to collaborate with the clinician. Thus, overcoming patient barriers of adoption of shared decision making may depend on a strong patient-provider relationship. Trust in a provider may lead a patient to be receptive to shared decision making and more comfortable expressing their beliefs and preferences. On the other hand, trust may also cause a patient to cede the decision to his faithful provider (Belcher et al. 2006). In one survey, patients were more likely to prefer shared decision making, compared to the extremes of paternalism or consumerism, if they received ongoing care from a well-regarded physician, suggesting that continuity of care and regular primary care would facilitate shared decision making (Murray et al. 2007).

shared decision making places patients in an unfamiliar role with new expectations. Patients are confronted with the uncertainty inherent in preference-sensitive situations as well as the general uncertainty regarding outcomes that is often present, but arguably under-acknowledged, in much of medical care. Such uncertainty may be uncomfortable and dissatisfying. In shared decision making, patients are expected to take a more active role by contributing their unique values, beliefs, and preferences to the process. In doing so, patients are expected to engage in a fair degree of self-reflection—"What *is* most important to me?" This requires a level of self-knowledge and insight not needed in the passive, paternalistic model of decision making. Decision aids are designed to promote such values clarification, though further patient-facing interventions may be needed to promote patient receptiveness to shared decision making.

System factors

The system in which providers practice can present barriers to the implementation of shared decision making and the use of decision aids. While the support of clinical leadership and well-intentioned physicians is important, it is not enough to ensure the dissemination and sustained use of decision support tools. The support of ancillary staff—including nurses, social workers, and patient educators—must be considered, since they will also carry the additional administrative burden of maintaining and distributing decision aids, in addition to providing direct patient support (Coulter 2010). In the Breast Cancer Initiative to promote the use of decision aids in the community setting, over 80 % of healthcare workers who distributed decision aids and responded to study questionnaires about implementation were non-physicians (Feibelmann et al. 2011).

The development of infrastructure to support decision making has increased over the last several years, including the growth of decision aid libraries and development of international standards for decision aids (O'Connor et al. 2007). Future work involves establishing economic incentives for providers to adopt shared decision making, establishing national certification standards for providers and healthcare organizations, and leveraging health information technology to cue decisions aids in preference-sensitive clinical situations. Furthermore, we need a better understanding of where decision aids fit within the clinical workflow of a healthcare organization—is it at the point of care in the clinic, through a healthcare plan call center, or via an electronic patient portal? Should a decision aid be introduced in primary care or in subspecialty care, where many decisions about elective procedures or specialized medications are made? Should they be required across a healthcare organization or targeted to specific medical and surgical conditions where most of the research now focuses (O'Connor et al. 2007)? Decision aids have been tested primarily in idealized research settings thus far, but are now being integrated into practice. Future study of decision aids will need to use the lens of implementation science to examine how well decision aids perform in routine care.

Conclusion

There is great public, political, and commercial interest in producing, disseminating, and adopting decision aids, the tools of shared decision making. However, as future research and projects proceed, we should keep in mind that decision aids are only a means to an end and are appropriate for preference-sensitive situations only. Efforts to implement decision aids should be grounded in the principles of delivering patient-centered care, providing support to promote healthcare decisions that are consistent with patient values, when that support is desired. Understanding the role of decision aids in shared decision making is an ongoing pursuit and a significant part of the research agenda for patient-centered care.

References

ACOG Committee on Practice Bulletins. (2007). ACOG practice bulletin no. 77: Screening for fetal chromosomal abnormalities. *Obstetrics and Gynecology, 109* (1), 217–227.

Ancker, J. S., Senathirajah, Y., Kukafka, R., & Starren, J. B. (2006). Design features of graphs in health risk communication: A systematic review. *Journal of the American Medical Informatics Association, 13*(6), 608–618. doi:10.1197/jamia.M2115.

Arbuthnott, A., & Sharpe, D. (2009). The effect of physician–patient collaboration on patient adherence in non-psychiatric medicine. *Patient Education and Counseling, 77*(1), 60–67. doi:10.1016/j.pec.2009.03.022.

Bekker, H. L. (2010). The loss of reason in patient decision aid research: Do checklists damage the quality of informed choice interventions? *Patient Education and Counseling, 78*(3), 357–364. doi:10.1016/j.pec.2010.01.002.

Belcher, V. N., Fried, T. R., Agostini, J. V., & Tinetti, M. E. (2006). Views of older adults on patient participation in medication-related decision making. *Journal of General Internal Medicine, 21*(4), 298–303.

Bowling, A., & Ebrahim, S. (2001). Measuring patients' preferences for treatment and perceptions of risk. *Quality in Health Care, 10*(suppl 1), i2–i8.

Branda, M. E., LeBlanc, A., Shah, N. D., Tiedje, K., Ruud, K., Van Houten, H., & Montori, V. M. (2013). Shared decision making for patients with type 2 diabetes: A randomized trial in primary care. *BMC Health Services Research, 13*(1), 301. doi:10.1186/1472-6963-13-301.

Breslin, M., Mullan, R. J., & Montori, V. M. (2008). The design of a decision aid about diabetes medications for use during the consultation with patients with type 2 diabetes. *Patient Education and Counseling, 73*(3), 465–472.

Charles, C., Gafni, A., & Whelan, T. (1997). Shared decision-making in the medical encounter: What does it mean? (Or it takes at least two to tango). *Social Science and Medicine, 44*(5), 681–692. doi:10.1016/S0277-9536(96)00221-3.

Cleary-Goldman, J., Morgan, M. A., Malone, F. D., Robinson, J. N., D'Alton, M. E., & Schulkin, J. (2006). Screening for Down syndrome. *Obstetrics and Gynecology, 107*(1), 11–17. doi:10.1097/01.AOG.0000190215.67096.90.

Coulter, A. (2010, July). Implementing shared decision making in the UK—Health Foundation. *Health Foundation.* Retrieved November 12, 2012, from http://www.health.org.uk/publications/implementing-shared-decision-making-in-the-uk

Deber, R. B., & Kraetschmer, N. (1996). What role do patients wish to play in treatment decision making? *Archives of Internal Medicine, 156*(13), 1414–1420. doi:10.1001/archinte.1996.00440120070006.

Driscoll, D. A., & Gross, S. (2009). Prenatal screening for aneuploidy. *New England Journal of Medicine, 360* (24), 2556–2562. doi:10.1056/NEJMcp0900134.

Driscoll, D. A., Morgan, M. A., & Schulkin, J. (2009). Screening for Down syndrome: changing practice of obstetricians. *American Journal of Obstetrics and Gynecology, 200*(4), 459.e1–459.e9. doi:10.1016/j.ajog.2008.12.027

Durand, M.-A. (2012). Stakeholder field-testing of amnioDex, a person-centered decision support intervention for amniocentesis. *The International Journal of Person Centered Medicine, 2*(3), 568–576.

Durand, M.-A., Wegwarth, O., Boivin, J., & Elwyn, G. (2012). Design and usability of heuristic-based deliberation tools for women facing amniocentesis. *Health Expectations, 15*(1), 32–48. doi:10.1111/j.1369-7625.2010.00651.x.

Edwards, A., Thomas, R., Williams, R., Ellner, A. L., Brown, P., & Elwyn, G. (2006). Presenting risk information to people with diabetes: evaluating effects and preferences for different formats by a web-based randomised controlled trial. *Patient Education and Counseling, 63*(3), 336–349. doi:10.1016/j.pec.2005.12.016.

Elwyn, G. (2006a). Developing a quality criteria framework for patient decision aids: Online international Delphi consensus process. *BMJ, 333*(7565), 417. doi:10.1136/bmj.38926.629329.AE.

Elwyn, G. (2006b). Developing a quality criteria framework for patient decision aids: Online international Delphi consensus process. *BMJ, 333*(7565), 417. doi:10.1136/bmj.38926.629329.AE.

Elwyn, Glyn, Frosch, D., & Rollnick, S. (2009). Dual equipoise shared decision making: Definitions for decision and behaviour support interventions. *Implementation Science, 4*(1), 75. doi:10.1186/1748-5908-4-75.

Elwyn, G., Frosch, D., Thomson, R., Joseph-Williams, N., Lloyd, A., Kinnersley, P., et al. (2012). Shared decision making: A model for clinical practice. *Journal of General Internal Medicine, 27*(10), 1361–1367. doi:10.1007/s11606-012-2077-6

Elwyn, Glyn, Frosch, D., Volandes, A. E., Edwards, A., & Montori, V. M. (2010). Investing in deliberation: A definition and classification of decision support interventions for people facing difficult health decisions. *Medical Decision Making: An International Journal of the Society for Medical Decision Making, 30*(6), 701–711. doi:10.1177/0272989X10386231.

Elwyn, G., Hutchings, H., Edwards, A., Rapport, F., Wensing, M., Cheung, W.-Y., & Grol, R. (2005). The OPTION scale: Measuring the extent that clinicians involve patients in decision-making tasks. *Health Expectations: An International Journal of Public Participation in Health Care and Health Policy, 8*(1), 34–42. doi:10.1111/j.1369-7625.2004.00311.x.

Epstein, R. M., Alper, B. S., & Quill, T. E. (2004). Communicating evidence for participatory decision making. *JAMA: The Journal of the American Medical Association, 291*(19), 2359–2366. doi:10.1001/jama.291.19.2359.

Feibelmann, S., Yang, T. S., Uzogara, E. E., & Sepucha, K. (2011). What does it take to have sustained use of decision aids? A programme evaluation for the Breast Cancer Initiative. *Health Expectations, 14*, 85–95. doi:10.1111/j.1369-7625.2010.00640.x.

Gravel, K., Légaré, F., Graham, I. D., et al. (2006a). Barriers and facilitators to implementing shared decision-making in clinical practice: a systematic review of health professionals' perceptions. *Implement Science, 1*(1), 16.

Gravel, K., Légaré, F., & Graham, I. D. (2006b). Barriers and facilitators to implementing shared decision-making in clinical practice: a systematic review of health professionals' perceptions. *Implementation Science, 1*(1), 16. doi:10.1186/1748-5908-1-16.

Handelsman, Y., Mechanick, J., Blonde, L., Grunberger, G., Bloomgarden, Z., Bray, G., et al. (2011). American Association of clinical endocrinologists medical guidelines for clinical practice for developing a diabetes mellitus comprehensive care plan. *Endocrine Practice, 17*, 1–53.

Heisler, M., Tierney, E., Ackermann, R. T., Tseng, C., Narayan, K. M. V., Crosson, J., et al. (2009). Physicians' participatory decision-making and quality of diabetes care processes and outcomes: results from the triad study. *Chronic Illness, 5*(3), 165–176. doi:10.1177/1742395309339258

Jibaja-Weiss, M. L., Volk, R. J., Granchi, T. S., Neff, N. E., Robinson, E. K., Spann, S. J., et al. (2011). Entertainment education for breast cancer surgery decisions: A randomized trial among patients with low health literacy. *Patient Education and Counseling, 84* (1), 41–48. doi:10.1016/j.pec.2010.06.009

Khangura, S., Bennett, C., Stacey, D., & O'Connor, A. M. (2008). Personal stories in publicly available patient decision aids. *Patient Education and Counseling, 73* (3), 456–464. doi:10.1016/j.pec.2008.07.035.

LeBlanc, A., Kenny, D. A., O'Connor, A. M., & Légaré, F. (2009). Decisional conflict in patients and their physicians: A dyadic approach to shared decision making. *Medical Decision Making, 29*(1), 61–68. doi:10.1177/0272989X08327067.

Lee, D. H., & Mehta, M. D. (2003). Evaluation of a visual risk communication tool: Effects on knowledge and perception of blood transfusion risk. *Transfusion, 43* (6), 779–787.

Légaré, F., Ratte, S., Stacey, D., Kryworuchko, J., Gravel, K., Graham, I. D., & Turcotte, S. (2010). Interventions for improving the adoption of shared decision making by healthcare professionals. *Cochrane Database of Systematic Reviews, 5.* doi:10.1002/14651858.CD006732.pub2

Levinson, W., Kao, A., Kuby, A., & Thisted, R. A. (2005). Not all patients want to participate in decision making. *Journal of General Internal Medicine, 20*(6), 531–535. doi:10.1111/j.1525-1497.2005.04101.x.

Lipkus, I. M. (2007). Numeric, verbal, and visual formats of conveying health risks: Suggested best practices and future recommendations. *Medical Decision Making, 27*(5), 696–713. doi:10.1177/0272989X07307271.

Ludman, E., Katon, W., Bush, T., Rutter, C., Lin, E., Simon, G., et al. (2003). Behavioural factors associated with symptom outcomes in a primary care-based depression prevention intervention trial. *Psychological Medicine, 33*(6), 1061–1070. doi:10.1017/S003329170300816X

Mann, D. M., Ponieman, D., Montori, V. M., Arciniega, J., & McGinn, T. (2010). The statin choice decision aid in primary care: A randomized trial. *Patient Education and Counseling, 80*(1), 138–140. doi:10.1016/j.pec.2009.10.008.

Man-Son-Hing, M., Laupacis, A., O'Connor, A. M., Biggs, J., Drake, E., Yetisir, E., & Hart, R. G. (1999). A patient decision aid regarding antithrombotic therapy for stroke prevention in atrial fibrillation: A randomized controlled trial. *JAMA: The Journal of the American Medical Association, 282*(8), 737–743.

Mathieu, E., & Barratt, A. (2007). Informed choice in mammography screening: A randomized trial of a decision aid for 70-year-old women. *Archives of Internal Medicine, 167*(19), 2039–2046. doi:10.1001/archinte.167.19.2039.

Mathieu, E., Barratt, A. L., McGeechan, K., Davey, H. M., Howard, K., & Houssami, N. (2010). Helping women make choices about mammography screening: An online randomized trial of a decision aid for 40-year-old women. *Patient Education and Counseling, 81*(1), 63–72. doi:10.1016/j.pec.2010.01.001.

Mullan, R. J., Montori, V. M., Shah, N. D., Christianson, T. J. H., Bryant, S. C., Guyatt, G. H., et al. (2009). The diabetes mellitus medication choice decision aid: a randomized trial. *Archives of Internal Medicine, 169* (17), 1560.

Murray, E., Pollack, L., White, M., & Lo, B. (2007). Clinical decision-making: Patients' preferences and experiences. *Patient Education and Counseling, 65* (2), 189–196. doi:10.1016/j.pec.2006.07.007.

O'Connor, A. M. (1995). Validation of a decisional conflict scale. *Medical Decision Making: An International Journal of the Society for Medical Decision Making, 15*(1), 25–30.

O'Connor, A. M, & Elwyn, G. (2005). International Patient Decision Aid Standards (IPDAS) Collaboration.

O'Connor, A. M., Stacey, D., Barry, M. J., Col, N. F., Eden, K. B., Entwistle, V., et al. (2007). Do patient decision aids meet effectiveness criteria of the international patient decision aid standards collaboration? A systematic review and meta-analysis. *Medical Decision Making, 27*(5), 554–574.

O'Connor, A. M., Wennberg, J. E., Legare, F., Llewellyn-Thomas, H. A., Moulton, B. W., Sepucha, K. R., et al. (2007). Toward the "Tipping Point": decision aids and informed patient choice. *Health Affairs, 26*(3), 716–725. doi:10.1377/hlthaff.26.3.716

O'Connor, A. M, Bennett, C. L., Stacey, D., Barry, M., Col, N. F., Eden, K. B., et al. (2009). Decision aids for people facing health treatment or screening decisions. *Cochrane Database of Systematic Reviews (Online),* (3), CD001431. doi:10.1002/14651858.CD001431.pub2

Oshima Lee, E., & Emanuel, E. J. (2013). Shared decision making to improve care and reduce costs. *The New England Journal of Medicine, 368*(1), 6–8. doi:10.1056/NEJMp1209500.

Paasche-Orlow, M. K., & Wolf, M. S. (2010). Promoting health literacy research to reduce health disparities. *Journal of Health Communication, 15*(Suppl 2), 34–41. doi:10.1080/10810730.2010.499994.

Parker, R., & Ratzan, S. C. (2010). Health literacy: A second decade of distinction for Americans. *Journal of Health Communication, 15*(sup2), 20–33. doi:10.1080/10810730.2010.501094.

Qaseem, A., Humphrey, L. L., Sweet, D. E., Starkey, M., & Shekelle, P. (2012). Oral pharmacologic treatment of type 2 diabetes mellitus: A clinical practice guideline from the American College of Physicians. *Annals of Internal Medicine, 156*(3), 218–231. doi:10.1059/0003-4819-156-3-201202070-00011.

Screening and Test Evaluation Program (STEP). (2003). Australian screening mammography decision aid— The University of Sydney. Retrieved January 3, 2013, from http://www.mammogram.med.usyd.edu.au/

U.S. Preventive Services Task Force. (2009). Screening for breast cancer: U.S. Preventive Services Task Force recommendation statement. *Annals of Internal Medicine, 151*(10), 716–726, W–236. doi:10.1059/0003-4819-151-10-200911170-00008

Silvia, K. A., Ozanne, E. M., & Sepucha, K. R. (2008a). Implementing breast cancer decision aids in community sites: Barriers and resources. *Health Expectations, 11*(1), 46–53. doi:10.1111/j.1369-7625.2007.00477.x.

Silvia, K. A., Ozanne, E. M., & Sepucha, K. R. (2008b). Implementing breast cancer decision aids in community sites: Barriers and resources. *Health Expectations: An International Journal of Public Participation in Health Care and Health Policy, 11*(1), 46–53. doi:10.1111/j.1369-7625.2007.00477.x.

Stacey, D., Bennett, C. L., Barry, M. J., Col, N. F., Eden, K. B., Holmes-Rovner, M., et al. (2011). Decision aids for people facing health treatment or screening decisions. In The Cochrane Collaboration & D. Stacey (Eds.), *Cochrane database of systematic reviews.* Chichester, UK: Wiley. Retrieved from http://doi.wiley.com/10.1002/14651858.CD001431.pub3

Standards of medical care in diabetes. (2012). *Diabetes Care, 35 Suppl 1,* S11–63. doi:10.2337/dc12-s011

Ubel, P. A., Jepson, C., & Baron, J. (2001). The inclusion of patient testimonials in decision aids: Effects on treatment choices. *Medical Decision Making: An International Journal of the Society for Medical Decision Making, 21*(1), 60–68.

Van der Weijden, T., Boivin, A., Burgers, J., Schüne-mann, H. J., & Elwyn, G. (2012). Clinical practice guidelines and patient decision aids. An inevitable relationship. *Journal of Clinical Epidemiology, 65*(6), 584–589. doi:10.1016/j.jclinepi.2011.10.007.

Veroff, D., Marr, A., & Wennberg, D. E. (2013). Enhanced support for shared decision making reduced costs of care for patients with preference-sensitive conditions. *Health Affairs, 32*(2), 285–293. doi:10. 1377/hlthaff.2011.0941.

Volandes, A. E., Paasche-Orlow, M. K., Barry, M. J., Gillick, M. R., Minaker, K. L., Chang, Y., et al. (2009). Video decision support tool for advance care planning in dementia: randomised controlled trial.

BMJ: British Medical Journal, 338. Retrieved from http://www.ncbi.nlm.nih.gov/pmc/articles/ PMC2688013/

Waljee, J. F., Rogers, M. A. M., & Alderman, A. K. (2007). Decision aids and breast cancer: Do they influence choice for surgery and knowledge of treatment options? *Journal of Clinical Oncology, 25* (9), 1067–1073. doi:10.1200/JCO.2006.08.5472.

Weymiller, A. J., Montori, V. M., Jones, L. A., Gafni, A., Guyatt, G. H., Bryant, S. C., et al. (2007). Helping patients with type 2 diabetes mellitus make treatment decisions: statin choice randomized trial. *Archives of Internal Medicine, 167*(10), 1076–1082. doi:10.1001/ archinte.167.10.1076

Using the Veterans Health Administration as a Laboratory for Integrated Decision Tools for Patients and Clinicians

17

Sara J. Knight

- The Veterans Health Administration (VHA) offers an extraordinary laboratory for research on integrated decision support through its Electronic Health Record and close alignment of research with VHA clinical and operational priorities.
- Significant research advancements have been accomplished in integrated decision support systems and patient-facing decision aids.
- Further evidence is needed on integration of patient-facing decision aids with the Electronic Health Record, incorporation of patient preference information in individual health decisions, and implementation of patient-facing decision aids and patient preferences in clinical settings.

In his second inaugural address close to the end of the Civil War, Abraham Lincoln asserted the nation's responsibility to Veterans "To care for him who shall have borne the battle and for his widow, and his orphan, ..." The contemporary Department of Veterans Affairs (VA) affirms this commitment and, among the three administrative branches of the VA, the Veterans Health Administration (VHA) fulfills this mission through "exceptional healthcare to improve Veterans health and wellbeing." The VHA vision shown below emphasizes patient-centered, evidence-based, collaborative healthcare in a system that seeks continuous quality improvement.

VHA will continue to be the benchmark of excellence and value in health care and benefits by providing exemplary services that are both patient centered and evidence based. This care will be delivered by engaged, collaborative teams in an integrated environment that supports learning, discovery and continuous improvement. It will emphasize prevention and population health and contribute to the nation's well-being through education, research and service in National emergencies.
http://www.va.gov/health/aboutVHA.asp

S.J. Knight (✉)
Health Services Research and Development Program, Birmingham VA Medical Center, Birmingham, AL, USA
e-mail: sara.knight@va.gov

S.J. Knight
Department of Medicine, Division of Preventive Medicine, University of Alabama at Birmingham, MT 638 1720 2nd Ave S, Birmingham 35294, AL, USA

Integrated decision support is a key approach to accomplishing this mission. VHA decision support systems provide a platform to engage clinicians and patients in making health decisions that incorporate the best evidence on diagnostic and treatment options, the patient's clinical information and risk factors, and patient values, goals, and preferences for care. The early adoption of health

© Springer Science+Business Media New York 2016
M.A. Diefenbach et al. (eds.), *Handbook of Health Decision Science*, DOI 10.1007/978-1-4939-3486-7_17

239

information technology in the VHA, such as the electronic health record (EHR), has facilitated the use of decision support systems in clinical settings (Hurdle et al. 2003; Hynes et al. 2010). The Veterans Health Information Systems and Technology Architecture (VistA) EHR was designed with the explicit goal of improving care coordination and continuous quality improvement, providing even greater integration of information on the patient experience in care and supporting a team-based approach to healthcare services (Fig. 17.1). A significant advancement in the VistA system is currently underway and the next generation EHR—VistA Evolution—will provide even more extensive and deeper integration of patient goals for care through clinician notes based

on interviews with patients and through patient notes entered directly into My HealtheVet Personal Health Record (Charters and Nazi 2007; Nazi et al. 2010). The system will also allow direct communication between VHA clinicians and their Veteran patients through mobile devices and applications and with clinicians providing care to Veterans outside the VHA (Chumbler et al. 2010).

This chapter describes VHA as an early adopter of the knowledge and technology, such as the EHR and patient-facing personal health records, and the clinical service structures, such as integrated primary care, that have created an extraordinary laboratory for applied research and development in health decision making, particularly in the area of decision support for both

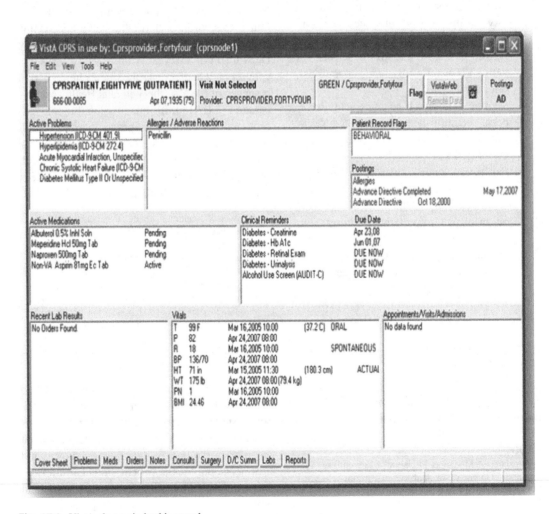

Fig. 17.1 VistA electronic health record

clinicians and patients. The chapter will consider major contributions of the VHA investigators including the development of decision support tools, decision aids for patients, and approaches to incorporate patient values, goals, and preferences in health decisions. The central focus will be on research conducted by VHA investigators and funded by the VHA Office of Research and Development Health Services Research and Development Service (HSR&D). The chapter presents a description of the VHA environment —its structure and population served—to build the foundation for the work and to articulate the value and generalizability of VHA studies. The primary intent is to illustrate the applied research that is conducted in the VHA rather than to provide a systematic review of evidence supporting an approach to health decision making. Rather, the chapter offers a perspective on the innovations to decision support that have emerged through VHA funded research.

The VHA Environment for Decision Support

The VA healthcare system has its roots in soldier's homes established to provide care for wounded Veterans of the Civil War with the national VA healthcare system being established in 1930. The contemporary VHA is an integrated healthcare system, the largest in the nation, organized as one of three administrative units in the VA along with Veterans Benefits Administration (VBA) and the National Cemetery Administration. The VHA is responsible for providing extensive acute and chronic health and social services to Veterans, unparalleled educational opportunities for physicians and other health professionals, and a research service to build scientific evidence to improve the health care and health outcomes of Veterans. The close alignment of clinical services, health professional education, and research in the VHA is a structural characteristic that is highly favorable to research that is connected with operational and clinical priorities, including the development and

testing of integrated decision support (Cox et al. 2011; Kizer and Dudley 2009).

The VHA cares for 8 million Veterans of the 22 million Veterans in the US. Veterans cared for in the VHA tend to be older and sicker than those who receive care outside the VHA and compared to nonVeterans and, for this reason, the VHA provides a setting to understand key questions about how complex information on the risks and potential benefits of a diagnostic or treatment approach are best communicated to those of lower educational status and lower health literacy. Health care for Veterans in the contemporary VHA system is provided in 152 medical centers, more than 800 community-based outpatient facilities, 135 community living centers, and 103 residential rehabilitation centers. In these facilities, the VHA offers extensive primary care, specialty care, and social services. When services are not available in the VHA, care is coordinated through facilities and health professionals located outside the VA, often academic medical centers that are affiliated with the VHA. This extensive national system provides an unparalleled opportunity to examine wide dissemination of decision support tools and systems on a national scale.

The VHA Office of Research and Development (ORD), especially through the HSR&D, has funded much of the foundational work in health decision making conducted by VHA researchers. The Quality Enhancement Research Initiative (QUERI) program within HSR&D has been responsible for the implementation of health decision making interventions, including decision aids and decision support in clinical settings throughout VHA (McQueen et al. 2004; Solberg 2009; Stetler et al. 2008). Researchers in the HSR&D service are encouraged to collaborate with VHA clinical and operational stakeholders with the goal of accelerating the implementation of research findings (Anderson et al. 2013; Damush et al. 2010). In January 2014, a search of HSR&D-funded projects using the search terms of decision support, shared decision making, informed decision making, decision aids, and patient preferences indicated that between 1995

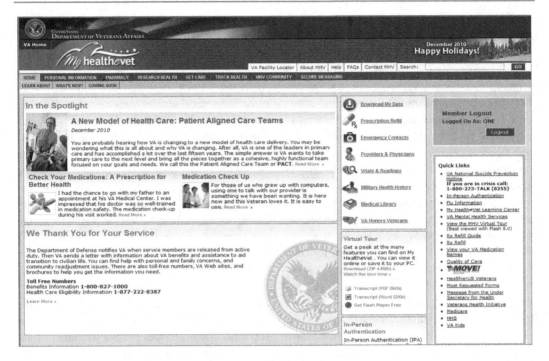

Fig. 17.2 MyHealth*e*Vet patient web portal

and 2014, HSR&D had funded over 170 projects relevant to health decision making.

In the 1990s, the VHA began a major realignment of its resources to serve Veterans reorganizing into regional care units to improve quality, safety, and efficiency, adopting evidence-based guidelines and clinical performance measures for clinicians and managers, and shifting its emphasis to primary care (Jha et al. 2003; Kizer and Dudley 2009). At this time, the VHA made a major investment in an electronic health record system (EHR)—the Computerized Patient Record System (CPRS), one of the earliest healthcare systems to do so (Hurdle et al. 2003; Wenzel 2002). The VHA EHR has facilitated scientific and management research and quality improvement, with many studies focusing on clinical decision support technology (Hynes et al. 2000; McQueen et al. 2004; Stetler et al. 2008). The use of the EMR for decision support and other clinician and patient-centered decision tools has rapidly expanded with the transformation of primary care in the VHA, (Yano et al. 2007) and with the introduction of the Patient

Aligned Care Team (PACT), that emphasizes team-based care and care management (Damush et al. 2010; Piette et al. 2011). The PACT has made greater use of e-health such as a Patient Web portal, health risk appraisal, secure messaging with health professionals, and e-consults involving patients and clinicians (Chumbler et al. 2010; Haggstrom et al. 2011; McInnes et al. 2011) (see Figs. 17.2 and 17.3).

Clinical Decision Support Systems

The VHA EHR and the organization of the VHA around primary care has offered a unique opportunity to build, test, and implement integrated decision support tools that work with the EHR. Decision support systems support decision processes often through analytic approaches to access, retrieve, and combine data over a range of databases and other diverse sources of information. In the VHA, decision support systems are often used to implement evidence-based clinical practice by automating the incorporation of

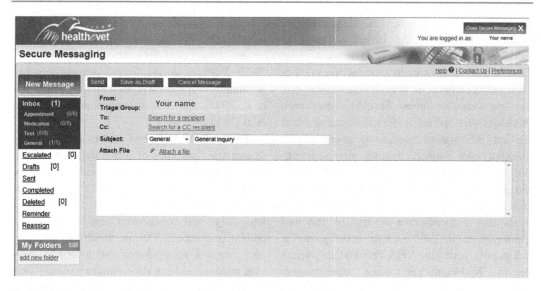

Fig. 17.3 Secure messaging: patient and health professional communication

evidence-based practice recommendations with patient-specific information from the VHA EHR.

One of the challenges of adding a DSS to an existing EHR such as VistA is in the integration of relational database architecture that can organize and analyze diverse data with a legacy system that was developed using earlier technology. VistA was developed over the course of thirty years using hierarchical architecture and now consisting of over 100 applications with diverse purposes, such as the EHR Graphical User Interface (GUI)/Computerized Patient Record System (CPRS), the Personal Health Record, VistA Imaging, and Order Entry/Result Reporting.

Among the first to address the computing barriers to providing decision support using VistA, The Assessment and Treatment of Hypertension Evidence-Based Automation (ATHENA) project developed at the Palo Alto VA Medical Center and led by Mary K. Goldstein, MD, has become one of the most widely recognized decision support systems incorporated in the VA EHR (Advani et al. 2003, 2004; Goldstein et al. 2004). A key innovation of ATHENA is in its use of the EON architecture developed at Stanford that serves a mediational function in working with the complex hierarchical structures of VistA (Advani et al. 1999;

Musen et al. 1996). ATHENA automates activities associated with evidence-based guidelines allowing the guidelines to be used and applied in the context of patient-specific clinical data in the medical record ultimately generating a treatment recommendation and monitoring the quality of treatment received. From the perspective of the patient and clinician, ATHENA provides comprehensive patient-centered information, when and where it is needed, and ensures the quality of the resulting treatment recommendation.

The ATHENA model and processes for development are described in the literature and extensions of the model have been applied in hypertension interventions designed for both patients and their clinicians (Bosworth et al. 2009, 2011), and in other health conditions including opioid management for noncancer pain (Michel et al. 2008; Midboe et al. 2011; Trafton et al. 2010). Similar decision support tools have been used to intervene in stroke prevention (Anderson et al. 2013; Damush et al. 2010).

Early research and development identified barriers to the implementation of integrated VHA decision support. To build capacity to test and refine these systems for implementation, HSR&D recruited and funded investigators and research centers that would support research in informatics, systems redesign, and human factors engineering. For example, the human factors laboratory located at the HSR&D Center in Indianapolis found that decision support using CPRS did not allow simultaneous access to other information in the EHR when another dialog box was open on the screen. Similarly, dropdown checklists that opened in CPRS obscured other relevant information needed to complete the checklist tasks. Further, clinicians were unable to close the dropdown menu until the checklist task had been completed. Refinements to integrated decision support in CPRS have eliminated these issues that reduced ease of use of the tool (Anderson et al. 2013). Other investigators at Indianapolis tested the VHA Personalized Health Record MyHealtheVet using observational methods and focusing on key activities including login and registration, prescription refill, health tracking(e.g., colonoscopy, physical activity), and health information seeking. Quantitative efficiency measures and qualitative observations using video recordings were analyzed. Usability barriers were identified, including difficulties with registration, privacy concerns, and lack of ability to share results of health tracking or information with members of the healthcare team (Haggstrom et al. 2011).

Patient-Facing Decision Aids

VHA investigators have contributed to the development and testing of decision aids for patients with much of this work focusing on improving the access for Veterans many of whom have lower health literacy and lower educational status than others cared for outside the VHA. Investigators have developed educational content, preference assessment methods, and algorithms that integrate information about clinical characteristics, patient preferences, and expected outcomes. Decision aids that provide information on prostate cancer, colorectal cancer, and lung cancer screening and treatment have been tested in randomized controlled trials. Studies have focused on prostate cancer screening, (Costanza et al. 2011; Partin et al. 2004; Schapira and VanRuiswyk 2000), treatment for

localized prostate cancer, (Kim et al. 2001; Knight et al. 2002; Schapira et al. 1997), medication management for arthritis, (Fraenkel et al. 2007; Rochon et al. 2012), post-menopausal hormone therapy for women Veterans, (Schapira et al. 2007), and advance care planning (Sudore et al. 2014).

These HSR&D funded studies have demonstrated the feasibility of using decision aids in clinical settings and among patients who have limitations in health literacy, and the efficacy of decision aids especially in increasing patient knowledge and engagement, and in modifying patient preferences. Despite feasibility and efficacy, implementing shared and informed decision making has been slow even in a setting such as the VHA where information processes are highly integrated and where funding mechanisms exist to support implementation. To date, there is little wide dissemination of decision aids in the VHA, and integration of decision aids in the EHR and the MyHealtheVet personal health record has not been achieved to date.

It is not clear why decision aids have not been integrated in the EHR and MyHealtheVet. Studies by Fagerlin and colleagues have suggested that providing information-based decision aids in VA clinical settings does not increase patient and clinician discussion of patient values, preferences, and goals for care. In a multisite randomized controlled trial to compare a low literacy decision aid for localized prostate cancer treatment decisions to a standard decision aid used by a national organization, decision aids were provided to Veterans scheduled for a prostate cancer biopsy. Patient and physician discussions were recorded during the first post-biopsy visit for those who were to receive a prostate cancer diagnosis. An early analysis of the transcripts of 40 visits at one of the site identified five major communication activities that occurred during discussions that lasted an average 21 min (range 8–37 min)—diagnosis delivery, risk classification, options talk, decisions talk, and next steps. Patient speech was infrequent from diagnosis delivery to options talk. Physicians elicited patient questions and concerns following their communication about treatment options (options talk), but physician elicitation of patient preferences and patient expression of preferences was rare even during the decisions talk activity (Henry et al. 2013).

It is perhaps not surprising that patient preferences are not clearly expressed by patients or well understood by the health professionals who care for them. Examination of clinician and patient ratings of patient preferences has shown poor agreement even when clinicians judge their own patients (Bennett et al. 1997; Elstein et al. 2004, 2005). The structure of care and its financing both within and outside the VHA provide little support for visits to discuss treatment decision making, and clinicians have little time to interact with patients even in the context of an emotionally challenging diagnosis such as cancer (Atkins and Kupersmith 2010).

Conceptualizing and Measuring Patient Values, Goals, and Preferences

While VHA research has contributed to integrated decision support and has enhanced clinical decision making, a gap remains in understanding patient values, goals, and preferences for health care. A clear approach to incorporate patient preferences in clinical decision making is critically needed in performance measurement. Concerns have been raised about the potential for unintended consequences with the use of inflexible quality standards that do not take into account individual patient characteristics including their interests and preferred activities. An extensive literature now documents the potential for harm with the use of a one-size-fits all approach to performance standards in prevention, diagnosis, and treatment (Kerr and Hayward 2013; Kerr et al. 2001; Walter et al. 2001, 2004, 2013). In addition, an understanding of patient preferences is important in health decisions where multiple options exist and where trade-offs need to be considered among treatment characteristics and potential outcomes in making a choice (Fraenkel 2013).

HSR&D investigators have focused on methods for obtaining information about patient preferences that do not rely solely on patient and clinician interaction through office visits. Formal assessment of patient preferences is illustrated by the work of Knight, Bennett, and colleagues to develop decision aids for Veterans diagnosed with localized prostate cancer (Kim et al. 2001; Knight et al. 2002). In a VHA pre-implementation study, this group tested a decision aid that included a Markov model that integrated clinical risk information and patient preferences for localized prostate cancer treatment formally assessed using utilities elicitation. The primary challenges that limited the feasibility of this approach occurred in assessing patient preferences. The standard time trade-off utilities elicitation measure used in this study resulted in a large proportion of refusals to make a hypothetical trade of years of life for quality of life and preference reversals, where the combination of two side effects were preferred to one (Knight et al. 2002). Consistent with these issues, concerns with reliability and validity of utilities elicitation measures have been observed by others (Souchek et al. 2000).

Liana Fraenkel, MD, MPH, and colleagues at the West Haven VA Medical Center have provided extensive information on Veterans preferences for healthcare choice-based methods across a wide range of conditions including rheumatoid arthritis, osteoarthritis, lupis, hepatitis C, and osteoporosis (Fraenkel et al. 2001, 2002, 2004a, 2005, 2010). Choice-based methods, including adaptive conjoint analysis, discrete choice experiments (DCE), and choice-based conjoint (CBC), havebeen used to quantify preferences for characteristics of consumer products and services, health care, and policy. When applied in health care, the approach assumes that decision alternatives, such as treatment options, can be decomposed into their associated characteristics, including potential outcomes and expected side effects. Choice-based conjoint analysis examines the trade-offs that are made among sets of possible characteristics. Based on the analysis of these trade-offs, information on the relative utility or importance of each characteristics compared to the others included in the model can be generated.

These measures have been used by Fraenkel and others to identify patient priorities for treatment (Fraenkel et al. 2004b), and to describe the types of information physicians find valuable in making treatment decision recommendations (Fraenkel et al. 2006). The work of Fraenkel and others supports the feasibility of administering the choice tasks in clinical settings with patients. In addition, there is evidence on the feasibility and usability of choice-based approachesto support patient decision making in computer-based decision tools (Fraenkel 2013; Fraenkel and McGraw 2007). However, little evidence is available as yet to support use of these methods in individual decision making.

Saul Weiner, MD, MPH, and others at the HSR&D Center of Innovation in Chicago have proposed a complementary perspective on incorporating patient experience, values, and interests in treatment planning. This approach termed "contextualizing care" is at the heart of patient-centered care. It involves "adapting the best evidence to the care of the individual patient." (Weiner et al. 2007, 2010, 2013b). Weiner's work emphasizes the importance of considering contextual factors, such as lifestyle preferences, family interests, and work demands in understanding health communication and in making treatment recommendations. Rather than directly assessing patient preferences, communication between patient and physician or other health professionals is evaluated for indications of contextual characteristics important to decision making (Weiner et al. 2013a, 2014). This conceptualization of individualized care has the advantage of capturing a wide range of potentially relevant data to use in treatment decision making. Because of the potential complexity and time involved in the assessment of context, additional research is needed on the feasibility and validity of using contextual factors in decision support tools and in patient-facing decision aids.

Closing Comments

The VHA mission, its structure of close alignment of research with health professional education and clinical and operational offices, and its investment in transformational processes of care including an electronic medical record system has created a platform that allows enormous creativity in applying decision support systems to patient health decisions at the point of care. In this chapter, the VHA environment for integrated decision support was described and three major domains of research were examined including integrated decision support systems, patient-facing decision aids, and assessment of patient values, goals, and preferences. The VHA HSR&D Service has developed capacity in informatics, systems redesign, and human factors engineering that has facilitated the advancement of decision support and patient-facing decision aids. Future opportunities for research include development work to design and test methods to incorporate patient values, goals, and preferences in decision support tools and decision aids and work to move both decision aids and patient preference assessment into implementation in clinical settings.

References

Advani, A., Goldstein, M., Shahar, Y., & Musen, M. A. (2003). Developing quality indicators and auditing protocols from formal guideline models: Knowledge representation and transformations [Research support, U.S. Gov't, Non-P.H.S. research support, U.S. Gov't, P.H.S.]. *AMIA... Annual Symposium proceedings/AMIA Symposium. AMIA Symposium* (pp. 11–15).

Advani, A., Jones, N., Shahar, Y., Goldstein, M. K., & Musen, M. A. (2004). An intelligent case-adjustment algorithm for the automated design of population-based quality auditing protocols [Research support, N.I.H., Extramural research support, U.S. Gov't, Non-P.H.S. research support, U.S. Gov't, P.H.S.]. *Studies in Health Technology and Informatics, 107*(Pt 2), 1003–1007.

Advani, A., Tu, S., O'Connor, M., Coleman, R., Goldstein, M. K., & Musen, M. (1999). Integrating a modern knowledge-based system architecture with a legacy VA database: The ATHENA and EON projects at stanford [Research support, U.S. Gov't, Non-P.H.S. research support, U.S. Gov't, P.H.S.]. *Proceedings/ AMIA ... Annual Symposium. AMIA Symposium* (pp. 653–657).

Anderson, J. A., Godwin, K. M., Saleem, J. J., Russell, S., Robinson, J. J., & Kimmel, B. (2013). Accessibility, usability and usefulness of a web-based clinical decision support tool to enhance provider-patient communication around self-management to prevent (STOP) stroke. *Health Informatics Journal*. doi:10. 1177/1460458213493195

Atkins, D., & Kupersmith, J. (2010). Implementation research: A critical component of realizing the benefits of comparative effectiveness research. *American Journal of Medicine, 123*(12 Suppl 1), e38–e45. doi:10. 1016/j.amjmed.2010.10.007

Bennett, C. L., Chapman, G., Elstein, A. S., Knight, S. J., Nadler, R. B., Sharifi, R., et al. (1997). A comparison of perspectives on prostate cancer: Analysis of utility assessments of patients and physicians [Comparative Study]. *European Urology, 32*(Suppl 3), 86–88.

Bosworth, H. B., Olsen, M. K., Dudley, T., Orr, M., Goldstein, M. K., Datta, S. K. ... Oddone, E. Z. (2009). Patient education and provider decision support to control blood pressure in primary care: A cluster randomized trial [Randomized Controlled Trial]. *American Heart Journal, 157*(3), 450–456. doi:10.1016/j.ahj.2008.11.003

Bosworth, H. B., Powers, B. J., Olsen, M. K., McCant, F., Grubber, J., Smith, V. ... Oddone, E. Z. (2011). Home blood pressure management and improved blood pressure control. Results from a randomized controlled trial. *Archives of Internal Medicine, 171*(13), 1173–1180. doi:10.1001/archinternmed.2011.276

Charters, K. G., & Nazi, K. (2007). Personal health record evaluation: My HealtheVet and RE-AIM. *AMIA Annual Symposium proceedings* (p. 899).

Chumbler, N. R., Haggstrom, D. A., & Saleem, J. (2010). Implementation of health information technology in veterans health administration to support transformational change: Telehealth and personal health records. *Medical Care*. doi:10.1097/MLR.0b013e3181d558f9

Costanza, M. E., Luckmann, R. S., Rosal, M., White, M. J., LaPelle, N., Partin, M. ... Foley, C. (2011). Helping men make an informed decision about prostate cancer screening: A pilot study of telephone counseling [Research Support, N.I.H., Extramural]. *Patient Education and Counseling, 82*(2), 193–200. doi:10.1016/j.pec.2010.05.011

Cox, M., Kupersmith, J., Jesse, R. L., & Petzel, R. A. (2011). Commentary: Building human capital: Discovery, learning, and professional satisfaction. *Academic Medicine, 86*(8), 923–924. doi:10.1097/ACM. 0b013e3182223b8e.

Damush, T. M., Jackson, G. L., Powers, B. J., Bosworth, H. B., Cheng, E., Anderson, J. ... Plue, L. (2010). Implementing evidence-based patient self-management programs in the Veterans Health Administration: Perspectives on delivery system design considerations. *Journal of General Internal Medicine, 25*(Suppl 1), 68–71. doi:10.1007/s11606-009-1123-5

Elstein, A. S., Chapman, G. B., Chmiel, J. S., Knight, S. J., Chan, C., Nadler, R. B. ... Bennett, C. L. (2004). Agreement between prostate cancer patients and their clinicians about utilities and attribute importance [Research support, U.S. Gov't, Non-P.H.S.]. *Health Expectations: An International Journal of Public Participation in Health Care and Health Policy, 7*(2), 115–125. doi:10.1111/j.1369-7625.2004.00267.x

Elstein, A. S., Chapman, G. B., & Knight, S. J. (2005). Patients' values and clinical substituted judgments: The case of localized prostate cancer. *Health psychology: Official journal of the Division of Health Psychology, American Psychological Association, 24* (4 Suppl), S85–S92. doi:10.1037/0278-6133.24.4.S85.

Fraenkel, L. (2013). Incorporating patients' preferences into medical decision making [Research support, N.I. H., Extramural]. *Medical Care Research and Review: MCRR, 70*(1 Suppl), 80S–93S. doi:10.1177/1077558712461283

Fraenkel, L., Bodardus, S., & Wittnik, D. R. (2001). Understanding patient preferences for the treatment of lupus nephritis with adaptive conjoint analysis [Multicenter study research support, Non-U.S. Gov't research support, U.S. Gov't, Non-P.H.S.]. *Medical Care, 39*(11), 1203–1216.

Fraenkel, L., Bogardus, S., & Concato, J. (2002). Patient preferences for treatment of lupus nephritis [Research support, Non-U.S. Gov't research support, U.S. Gov't, Non-P.H.S.]. *Arthritis and Rheumatism, 47*(4), 421–428. doi:10.1002/art.10534.

Fraenkel, L., Bogardus, S. T., Concato, J., Felson, D. T., & Wittink, D. R. (2004a). Patient preferences for treatment of rheumatoid arthritis [Comparative study research support, U.S. Gov't, Non-P.H.S.]. *Annals of the Rheumatic Diseases, 63*(11), 1372–1378. doi:10. 1136/ard.2003.019422

Fraenkel, L., Bogardus, S. T, Jr., Concato, J., & Wittink, D. R. (2004b). Treatment options in knee osteoarthritis: The patient's perspective [Comparative study research support, Non-U.S. Gov't research support, U.S. Gov't, Non-P.H.S.]. *Archives of Internal Medicine, 164*(12), 1299–1304. doi:10.1001/archinte.164. 12.1299

Fraenkel, L., Chodkowski, D., Lim, J., & Garcia-Tsao, G. (2010). Patients' preferences for treatment of hepatitis C [Research support, N.I.H., extramural research support, U.S. Gov't, Non-P.H.S.]. *Medical Decision Making: An International Journal of the Society for Medical Decision Making, 30*(1), 45–57. doi:10.1177/0272989X09341588

Fraenkel, L., Constantinescu, F., Oberto-Medina, M., & Wittink, D. R. (2005). Women's preferences for prevention of bone loss [Research support, U.S. Gov't, Non-P.H.S.]. *The Journal of Rheumatology, 32*(6), 1086–1092.

Fraenkel, L., & McGraw, S. (2007). Participation in medical decision making: The patients' perspective [Research support, N.I.H., extramural research support, Non-U.S. Gov't]. *Medical decision making: An international journal of the Society for Medical Decision Making, 27*(5), 533–538. doi:10.1177/0272989X07306784

Fraenkel, L., Rabidou, N., & Dhar, R. (2006). Are rheumatologists' treatment decisions influenced by patients' age? [Multicenter study research support, N.

I.H., Extramural]. *Rheumatology, 45*(12), 1555–1557. doi:10.1093/rheumatology/kel144

Fraenkel, L., Rabidou, N., Wittink, D., & Fried, T. (2007). Improving informed decision-making for patients with knee pain [Randomized controlled trial research support, N.I.H., extramural research support, Non-U.S. Gov't]. *The Journal of rheumatology, 34*(9), 1894–1898.

Goldstein, M. K., Coleman, R. W., Tu, S. W., Shankar, R. D., O'Connor, M. J., Musen, M. A. … Hoffman, B. B. (2004). Translating research into practice: Organizational issues in implementing automated decision support for hypertension in three medical centers [Research support, U.S. Gov't, Non-P.H.S. research support, U.S. Gov't, P.H.S.]. *Journal of the American Medical Informatics Association: JAMIA, 11*(5), 368–376. doi:10.1197/jamia.M1534

Haggstrom, D. A., Saleem, J. J., Russ, A. L., Jones, J., Russell, S. A., & Chumbler, N. R. (2011). Lessons learned from usability testing of the VA's personal health record [Research support, Non-U.S. Gov't research support, U.S. Gov't, Non-P.H.S.]. *Journal of the American Medical Informatics Association: JAMIA, 18*(Suppl 1), i13–i17. doi:10.1136/amiajnl-2010-000082

Henry, S. G., Czarnecki, D., Kahn, V. C., Chou, W. Y., Fagerlin, A., Ubel, P. A. … Holmes-Rovner, M. (2013). Patient-physician communication about early stage prostate cancer: Analysis of overall visit structure. *Health Expectations: An International Journal of Public Participation in Health Care and Health Policy,*. doi:10.1111/hex.12168

Hurdle, J. F., Weir, C. R., Roth, B., Hoffman, J., & Nebeker, J. R. (2003). Critical gaps in the world's largest electronic medical record: Ad Hoc nursing narratives and invisible adverse drug events [Research support, U.S. Gov't, Non-P.H.S.]. *AMIA Annual Symposium proceedings/AMIA Symposium. AMIA Symposium* (pp. 309–312).

Hynes, D. M., Cowper, D., Kerr, M., Kubal, J., & Murphy, P. A. (2000). Database and informatics support for QUERI: Current systems and future needs. Quality enhancement research initiative [Review]. *Medical care, 38*(6 Suppl 1), I114–I128.

Hynes, D. M., Weddle, T., Smith, N., Whittier, E., Atkins, D., & Francis, J. (2010). Use of health information technology to advance evidence-based care: Lessons from the VA QUERI program [Comparative study multicenter study research support, U.S. Gov't, Non-P.H.S.]. *Journal of General Internal Medicine, 25*(Suppl 1), 44–49. doi:10.1007/s11606-009-1144-0

Jha, A. K., Perlin, J. B., Kizer, K. W., & Dudley, R. A. (2003). Effect of the transformation of the veterans affairs health care system on the quality of care [Comparative Study]. *The New England Journal of Medicine, 348*(22), 2218–2227. doi:10.1056/NEJMsa021899

Kerr, E. A., & Hayward, R. A. (2013). Patient-centered performance management: Enhancing value for patients and health care systems [Research support,

N.I.H., extramural research support, U.S. Gov't, Non-P.H.S.]. *JAMA, the Journal of the American Medical Association, 310*(2), 137–138. doi:10.1001/jama.2013.6828

Kerr, E. A., Krein, S. L., Vijan, S., Hofer, T. P., & Hayward, R. A. (2001). Avoiding pitfalls in chronic disease quality measurement: A case for the next generation of technical quality measures [Research support, U.S. Gov't, Non-P.H.S.]. *The American Journal of Managed Care, 7*(11), 1033–1043.

Kim, S. P., Knight, S. J., Tomori, C., Colella, K. M., Schoor, R. A., Shih, L. … Bennett, C. L. (2001). Health literacy and shared decision making for prostate cancer patients with low socioeconomic status [Research support, Non-U.S. Gov't research support, U.S. Gov't, Non-P.H.S.]. *Cancer investigation, 19*(7), 684–691.

Kizer, K. W., & Dudley, R. A. (2009). Extreme makeover: Transformation of the veterans health care system [Review]. *Annual Review of Public Health, 30*, 313–339. doi:10.1146/annurev.publhealth.29.020907.090940

Knight, S. J., Nathan, D. P., Siston, A. K., Kattan, M. W., Elstein, A. S., Collela, K. M. … Golub, R. M. (2002). Pilot study of a utilities-based treatment decision intervention for prostate cancer patients [Comparative study research support, U.S. Gov't, Non-P.H.S.]. *Clinical Prostate Cancer, 1*(2), 105–114.

McInnes, D. K., Solomon, J. L., Bokhour, B. G., Asch, S. M., Ross, D., Nazi, K. M., et al. (2011). Use of electronic personal health record systems to encourage HIV screening: An exploratory study of patient and provider perspectives. *BMC Research Notes, 4*, 295. doi:10.1186/1756-0500-4-295

McQueen, L., Mittman, B. S., & Demakis, J. G. (2004). Overview of the veterans health administration (VHA) quality enhancement research initiative (QUERI). *Journal of the American Medical Informatics Association, 11*(5), 339–343. doi:10.1197/jamia.M1499

Michel, M., Trafton, J., Martins, S., Wang, D., Tu, S., Johnson, N., et al. (2008). Improving patient safety using ATHENA-decision support system technology: The opioid therapy for chronic pain experience. In K. Henriksen, J. B. Battles, M. A. Keyes & M. L. Grady (Eds.), *Advances in patient safety: New directions and alternative approaches* (Vol. 4: Technology and medication safety). Rockville, MD.

Midboe, A. M., Lewis, E. T., Cronkite, R. C., Chambers, D., Goldstein, M. K., Kerns, R. D., et al. (2011). Behavioral medicine perspectives on the design of health information technology to improve decision-making, guideline adherence, and care coordination in chronic pain management. *Translational Behavioral Medicine, 1*(1), 35–44. doi:10.1007/s13142-011-0022-6

Musen, M. A., Tu, S. W., Das, A. K., & Shahar, Y. (1996). EON: A component-based approach to automation of protocol-directed therapy [Research support, U.S. Gov't, Non-P.H.S. research support, U.

S. Gov't, P.H.S.]. *Journal of the American Medical Informatics Association: JAMIA, 3*(6), 367–388.

Nazi, K. M., Hogan, T. P., Wagner, T. H., McInnes, D. K., Smith, B. M., Haggstrom, D. ... Weaver, F. M. (2010). Embracing a health services research perspective on personal health records: Lessons learned from the VA My HealtheVet system. *Journal of General Internal Medicine, 25*(Suppl 1), 62-67. doi:10.1007/s11606-009-1114-6

Partin, M. R., Nelson, D., Radosevich, D., Nugent, S., Flood, A. B., Dillon, N. ... Wilt, T. J. (2004). Randomized trial examining the effect of two prostate cancer screening educational interventions on patient knowledge, preferences, and behaviors [Clinical Trial Randomized Controlled Trial Research Support, U.S. Gov't, Non-P.H.S.]. *Journal of General Internal Medicine, 19*(8), 835–842. doi:10.1111/j.1525-1497.2004.30047.x

Piette, J. D., Holtz, B., Beard, A. J., Blaum, C., Greenstone, C. L., Krein, S. L. ... Kerr, E. A. (2011). Improving chronic illness care for veterans within the framework of the patient-centered medical home: Experiences from the ann arbor patient-aligned care team laboratory [Review]. *Translational Behavioral Medicine, 1*(4), 615–623. doi:10.1007/s13142-011-0065-8

Rochon, D., Eberth, J. M., Fraenkel, L., Volk, R. J., & Whitney, S. N. (2012). Elderly patients' experiences using adaptive conjoint analysis software as a decision aid for osteoarthritis of the knee. *Health Expectations: An International Journal of Public Participation in Health Care and Health Policy,*. doi:10.1111/j.1369-7625.2012.00811.x

Schapira, M. M., Gilligan, M. A., McAuliffe, T., Garmon, G., Carnes, M., & Nattinger, A. B. (2007). Decision-making at menopause: A randomized controlled trial of a computer-based hormone therapy decision-aid [Randomized controlled trial research support, U.S. Gov't, Non-P.H.S.]. *Patient Education and Counseling, 67*(1–2), 100–107. doi:10.1016/j.pec.2007.02.007

Schapira, M. M., Meade, C., & Nattinger, A. B. (1997). Enhanced decision-making: The use of a videotape decision-aid for patients with prostate cancer [Research support, U.S. Gov't, Non-P.H.S.]. *Patient Education and Counseling, 30*(2), 119–127.

Schapira, M. M., & VanRuiswyk, J. (2000). The effect of an illustrated pamphlet decision-aid on the use of prostate cancer screening tests [Clinical trial randomized controlled trial research support, U.S. Gov't, Non-P.H.S.]. *The Journal of Family Practice, 49*(5), 418–424.

Solberg, L. (2009). Lessons for non-VA care delivery systems from the U.S. department of veterans affairs quality enhancement research initiative: QUERI series. *Implement Science, 4*, 9. doi:10.1186/1748-5908-4-9

Souchek, J., Stacks, J. R., Brody, B., Ashton, C. M., Giesler, R. B., Byrne, M. M. ... Wray, N. P. (2000).

A trial for comparing methods for eliciting treatment preferences from men with advanced prostate cancer: Results from the initial visit [Clinical trial randomized controlled trial research support, U.S. Gov't, Non-P.H.S.]. *Medical care, 38*(10), 1040–1050.

Stetler, C. B., Mittman, B. S., & Francis, J. (2008). Overview of the VA quality enhancement research initiative (QUERI) and QUERI theme articles: QUERI series. *Implement Science, 3*, 8. doi:10.1186/1748-5908-3-8

Sudore, R. L., Knight, S. J., McMahan, R. D., Feuz, M., Farrell, D., Miao, Y., et al. (2014). A novel website to prepare diverse older adults for decision making and advance care planning: A pilot study [Research support, Non-U.S. Gov't research support, U.S. Gov't, Non-P.H.S.]. *Journal of Pain and Symptom Management, 47*(4), 674–686. doi:10.1016/j.jpainsymman.2013.05.023

Trafton, J., Martins, S., Michel, M., Lewis, E., Wang, D., Combs, A. ... Goldstein, M. (2010). Evaluation of the acceptability and usability of a decision support system to encourage safe and effective use of opioid therapy for chronic, noncancer pain by primary care providers [Evaluation studies research support, Non-U.S. Gov't]. *Pain Medicine, 11*(4), 575–585. doi:10.1111/j.1526-4637.2010.00818.x

Walter, L. C., Davidowitz, N. P., Heineken, P. A., & Covinsky, K. E. (2004). Pitfalls of converting practice guidelines into quality measures: Lessons learned from a VA performance measure [Research support, Non-U.S. Gov't research support, U.S. Gov't, Non-P.H.S. research support, U.S. Gov't, P.H.S.]. *The Journal of the American Medical Association, 291*(20), 2466–2470. doi:10.1001/jama.291.20.2466

Walter, L. C., Eng, C., & Covinsky, K. E. (2001). Screening mammography for frail older women: What are the burdens? [Research support, Non-U.S. Gov't research support, U.S. Gov't, P.H.S.]. *Journal of General Internal Medicine, 16*(11), 779–784.

Walter, L. C., Fung, K. Z., Kirby, K. A., Shi, Y., Espaldon, R., O'Brien, S. .... Hoffman, R. M. (2013). Five-year downstream outcomes following prostate-specific antigen screening in older men [Research support, N.I.H., extramural research support, U.S. Gov't, Non-P.H.S.]. *JAMA Internal Medicine, 173*(10), 866–873. doi:10.1001/jamainternmed.2013.323

Weiner, S. J., Kelly, B., Ashley, N., Binns-Calvey, A., Sharma, G., Schwartz, A., et al. (2014). Content coding for contextualization of care: Evaluating physician performance at patient-centered decision making [Research support, U.S. Gov't, Non-P.H.S.]. *Medical Decision Making: An International Journal of the Society for Medical Decision Making, 34*(1), 97–106. doi:10.1177/0272989X13493146

Weiner, S. J., Schwartz, A., Cyrus, K., Binns-Calvey, A., Weaver, F. M., Sharma, G., et al. (2013a). Unannounced standardized patient assessment of the roter interaction analysis system: The challenge of measuring patient-centered communication [Research support, U.S. Gov't, Non-P.H.S.]. *Journal of General Internal Medicine, 28*(2), 254–260. doi:10.1007/s11606-012-2221-3

Weiner, S. J., Schwartz, A., Sharma, G., Binns-Calvey, A., Ashley, N., Kelly, B. ... Harris, I. (2013b). Patient-centered decision making and health care outcomes: An observational study [Research support, U.S. Gov't, Non-P.H.S.]. *Annals of Internal Medicine, 158*(8), 573–579. doi:10.7326/0003-4819-158-8-201304160-00001

Weiner, S. J., Schwartz, A., Weaver, F., Goldberg, J., Yudkowsky, R., Sharma, G. ...Abrams, R. I. (2010). Contextual errors and failures in individualizing patient care: A multicenter study [Case reports multicenter study randomized controlled trial research support, U.S. Gov't, Non-P.H.S.]. *Annals of Internal Medicine, 153*(2), 69–75. doi:10.7326/0003-4819-153-2-201007200-00002

Weiner, S. J., Schwartz, A., Yudkowsky, R., Schiff, G. D., Weaver, F. M., Goldberg, J., et al. (2007). Evaluating physician Performance at individualizing care: A pilot study tracking contextual errors in medical decision making [Randomized controlled trial research support, Non-U.S. Gov't research support, U. S. Gov't, Non-P.H.S.]. *Medical Decision Making: An International Journal of the Society for Medical Decision Making, 27*(6), 726–734. doi:10.1177/0272989X07306113

Wenzel, G. R. (2002). Creating an interactive interdisciplinary electronic assessment. *Computers, Informatics, Nursing: CIN, 20*(6), 251–260.

Yano, E. M., Simon, B. F., Lanto, A. B., & Rubenstein, L. V. (2007). The evolution of changes in primary care delivery underlying the Veterans Health Administration's quality transformation [Multicenter study research support, U.S. Gov't, Non-P.H.S.]. *American Journal of Public Health, 97*(12), 2151–2159. doi:10.2105/AJPH.2007.115709

Tailored Communications for Health-Related Decision-Making and Behavior Change

18

Seth M. Noar and Nancy Grant Harrington

Take Home Points for Reader

- Traditionally, health education programs were directed toward either general audiences or more targeted audiences.
- Tailoring is a newer practice in health communication, where messages are designed for an *individual*.
- Tailoring was made possible by computer technology, which allowed for complex algorithms that could select particular messages, from *messages libraries,* based upon an assessment of the individual.
- Tailoring has now been applied across a wide range of communication channels, including Internet and mobile channels.
- Tailoring results in messages that are more relevant to the individual, and as a result are more likely to be attended to and processed by the individual.

- Tailored health programs have been found to be efficacious across a wide range of health behaviors.
- Further work is needed to better understand the mechanisms underlying effective tailoring and to understand how to best disseminate tailored programs so that they can reach more people.

Traditionally, health education and health communication efforts have been directed toward either a general audience or a particular target audience. While this approach is efficient with regard to *reaching* audiences, it may often not be efficient with regard to public health *impact.* That is, if impact is defined as population reach x efficacy (Abrams et al. 1996), interventions must not only *reach* large audiences but also must be *efficacious* in changing those audiences' beliefs and behaviors. Several decades of research have taught us that general audience approaches to health communication are unlikely to be efficacious, while the efficacy of targeted health communication approaches varies (Noar et al. 2009; Snyder et al. 2004; Strecher 2009).

A newer practice in health communication, and one that has shown much promise over the past two decades, is tailored communication. Tailored communication has been defined as "any combination of strategies and information intended to reach one specific person, based on characteristics that are unique to that person,

S.M. Noar (✉)
School of Media and Journalism and Lineberger Comprehensive Cancer Center, University of North Carolina at Chapel Hill, 363 Carroll Hall (CB 3365), Chapel Hill, NC 27599-3365, USA
e-mail: noar@email.unc.edu
URL: http://noar.web.unc.edu/

N.G. Harrington
Department of Communication, University of Kentucky, Lexington, KY, USA
e-mail: nancy.harrington@uky.edu

© Springer Science+Business Media New York 2016
M.A. Diefenbach et al. (eds.), *Handbook of Health Decision Science*,
DOI 10.1007/978-1-4939-3486-7_18

Fig. 18.1 Level of customization of health content for general audience, group targeted, and individually tailored interventions. *Note* This figure was adapted from Kreuter et al. (1999) and Hawkins et al. (2008)

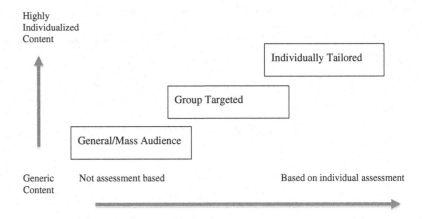

related to the outcome of interest, and derived from an individual assessment" (Kreuter et al. 1999, p. 277). Tailored communications are uniquely individualized to each person, whereas targeted messages are developed to be effective with an entire segment of the population. Targeting and tailoring can be thought of on a continuum of message design that ranges from the most generic mass audience communications, which are meant for everyone, to the more customized targeted communications, which are meant for a specific group of people, and finally to the most customized tailored communications, which are meant for individuals. To achieve their customization, tailored communications require an assessment of the individual (see Fig. 18.1).

Message tailoring operates on the premise that although targeting (at the group level) may enhance the perceived relevance of a health message for members of a group, there will still be a "mismatch" between a message designed for an entire group and some members of that group. Interestingly, while most advertising uses group-targeting practices, advertisers are increasingly using new technologies to provide tailored communications. For example, websites such as Amazon.com assess a person's browsing and buying tendencies and make tailored recommendations for what that person may be interested in buying. Netflix and Tivo use similar tailoring practices, making personalized suggestions for what movies one should rent or

television programs to record and watch. Even supermarket scanning technology assesses the kinds of items shoppers typically purchase and provides customized coupons at the checkout that reflect buying tendencies. While tailored health communication and this type of advertising tailoring uses *transparent* means, it is worth noting that advertisers are increasingly applying this type of tailoring in a more covert manner. That is, there have been several recent reports indicating that customized advertising is greatly increasing on the Internet, using location data and data that are accessed from one's personal computer (e.g., recent web pages viewed, search queries conducted, items bought, etc.) (Turow 2012). This kind of information is sometimes accessed *without* a person's knowledge, raising ethical and privacy-related concerns.

In the health promotion area, a perfect storm that ultimately led to the development of tailored communication interventions occurred: first, recognition of the poor outcomes of many health promotion programs using print materials (e.g., self-help manuals); second, development of stage-based theories such as the transtheoretical model (Prochaska et al. 1992), which suggested that because people are often at differing stages in the change process, they require different, more individualized messages; and third, technological developments in computer technology that made tailoring on a large scale basis possible. The first studies in the message tailoring area compared print materials tailored on determinants from health behavior theories (e.g., transtheoretical model, health belief model, social cognitive theory, theory of reasoned action) (Ajzen and Fishbein 1980; Bandura 1986; Prochaska et al. 1992; Rosenthal 1974) to materials that were more generic or targeted in nature and found that tailored materials led to more behavior change in areas such as smoking cessation and dietary practices (Skinner et al. 1999). The success of these early studies ultimately led to a burgeoning literature on tailored health communication. Tailoring has since been applied across many other communication channels, to more than 20 health behaviors, and to a number of populations (Noar et al. 2009). More recently tailoring applications in the area of Internet-based interventions (Lustria et al. 2009) and text messaging interventions (Fjeldsoe et al. 2012) have been rapidly growing.

How Tailoring Operates

How is a tailored intervention typically implemented? The process is depicted in Fig. 18.2 (also see Dijkstra and De Vries 1999; Kreuter et al. 2000). First, an individual is assessed using standardized measures on a variety of characteristics that are relevant to the behavior under study (e.g., demographic, behavioral, cultural, psychosocial characteristics). As the tailoring literature has been greatly driven by the transtheoretical (or stages of change) model and other psychosocial theories, such assessments often measure variables from one or more behavioral theories. Assessments can be made in a variety of ways—for example, via telephone, mail, local computer/kiosk, Internet, or in person. These data are then processed and, when the intervention relies on computer technology (which represents the vast majority of studies), decision rules (computer algorithms) select the particular messages that are most appropriate for the individual. These messages are derived from a *message library*, which consists of hundreds or even thousands of messages created for the program. In some cases, additional libraries may exist,

such as an image library that contains a variety of images to be matched to participant characteristics (e.g., gender, race, age). When delivery of tailored messages is done by a counselor or health educator, the same process of matching assessment to feedback is conducted, but typically without the use of computerized algorithms.

Delivery of tailored content varies depending on what channel is used. In the case of tailored print materials, a feedback report is compiled (again by the computer program), printed out, and presented to the participant in person or through the mail. Tailored computer programs that run on local computers, kiosks, or over the Internet operate in a similar fashion, except that the feedback messages are presented onscreen (immediately after assessment); in some cases, the feedback also may be printed. Computer-based programs have the opportunity to use interactivity and multimedia and thus may have additional content libraries (e.g., video library). Finally, counselors or health educators can deliver tailored messages over the telephone or in person. While most counseling interventions would *not* be considered tailored because of lack of a standardized assessment and subsequent matching of that assessment to tailored feedback, a small number of studies that used standardized measures for assessment and counselors/health educators to deliver feedback based on assessment can be considered tailored interventions (Brinberg and Axelson 1990; Brinberg et al. 2000). It is worth noting that the cost-effectiveness of tailoring may be reduced when human counselors are used for delivery of intervention feedback rather than print materials or the Internet. Finally, automated voice programs can also tailor content that is delivered in audio form over the telephone.

Tailoring Channels

The current discussion highlights the many assessment and delivery channels that tailored interventions have used to date. Table 18.1 provides a list of channels and channel attributes; an *X* indicates positive attributes of the channels, whereas a missing *X* indicates a negative

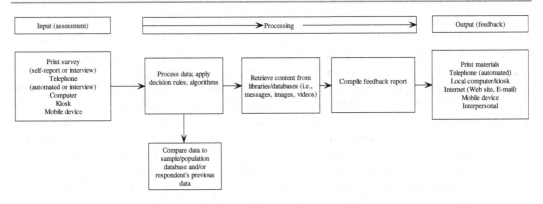

Fig. 18.2 Overview of the tailoring process

Table 18.1 Comparison of six delivery channels for tailored health communication programs

Attributes	Delivery channel					
	Print	Telephone (automated)	Local computer/kiosk	Internet (web site, e-mail)	Mobile device	Interpersonal
Low cost	X	X				
Broad reach	X	X		X		
Ease of updates		X		X	X	NA
Ease of access		X				
Ease of multiple assessments/exposures				X	X	
No internet connection necessary	X	X	X		X	X
No technical support necessary						X
No training/supervision necessary	X	X	X	X	X	
No computer skills necessary	X	X				X
High intervention fidelity	X	X	X	X	X	
Durability	X	X	X	X		NA
Portability of report	X				X	
Synchronous feedback						X
Interactivity			X	X	X	NA
Multimedia			X	X	X	NA
Visuals	X		X	X	X	NA

Note Each *X* indicates a positive attribute of the particular channel

attribute. While this list is not exhaustive, it provides a comparison of basic advantages and disadvantages of the major tailoring delivery channels at present. The list also provides generalizations; therefore, there may be exceptions. For example, print and telephone are generally viewed as lower cost options than computer and Internet; however, there are circumstances in which this may not be the case, such as when the number of participants in a program becomes very large and an Internet-based program may become more cost effective than a print-based program. Similarly, as time passes and programming and technical support become less costly, the Internet may overtake print as a more cost effective channel, regardless of the number of participants in a program.

A logical question that has been raised in this area is which delivery channel is "best." For the most part, the limited evidence to date does not suggest the clear superiority of one channel over another. The few trials that have conducted head-to-head tests comparing print, Internet, and telephone programs have found all of them to demonstrate short-term efficacy (Kroeze et al. 2008a; Marcus et al. 2007), and two meta-analyses support this conclusion (Krebs et al. 2010; Sohl and Moyer 2007). There is some evidence that print interventions may lead to longer maintenance of behavioral changes than telephone (Marcus et al. 2007) or web delivery (Kroeze et al. 2008a). However, a study comparing an online tailored web site with motivational interviewing (interpersonal tailoring) found both interventions to be equally effective (Prochaska et al. 2008).

The broader answer to this question may be that differing channels will suit differing circumstances (which seems quite apropos given the concept of tailoring). For instance, for program applications that demand interactivity and/or multimedia, local computer, mobile device, or Internet interventions may be best. However, these applications are not without their disadvantages, including requirements for ongoing technical assistance for the program, significant development costs, and a level of skill on the part of the user. Alternatively, channels such as mail (print materials) and telephone are lower cost options that are capable of reaching large numbers of individuals who are likely to have access to these media. On the downside, however, is the fact that these kinds of programs are not capable of approaching the kind of sophistication of media that is easily achieved with computer delivery.

Applications of Theory

To date, numerous behavioral theories have been used to inform tailored interventions. Constructs from such theories are often used in the tailoring process itself, a strategy referred to as *behavioral construct tailoring* (Kreuter et al. 2000). Theory can also be used in other ways, however, such as providing detailed message design guidance in intervention development (Harrington and Noar 2012).

Reviews of the tailoring literature indicate that the transtheoretical model and stages of change may be the most dominant theoretical perspective in this literature (Noar et al. 2007, 2011; Richards et al. 2007). This is not surprising, given the influential role that this model played early in the tailoring literature (Noar et al. 2007). In fact, many of the first tailored interventions applied stages of change (Campbell et al. 1994; Skinner et al. 1994) or the full transtheoretical model (Prochaska et al. 1993). Many other widely used theories have also been applied in this literature, however, including social cognitive theory, the health belief model, and the theory of planned behavior (Lustria et al. 2009; Noar et al. 2007, 2011; Richards et al. 2007; Sohl and Moyer 2007).

It is important to note that tailored interventions often apply multiple theories to inform a single tailored intervention (Noar et al. 2009; Richards et al. 2007). Also, it cannot be assumed that because a particular intervention is "based on" a theory that the intervention tailors messages on the basis of all of that theory's core constructs (Noar et al. 2007) (also see Painter et al. 2008). Instead, theory has been used in a very eclectic and utilitarian manner in this literature, with select constructs from a variety of theories often informing one intervention. While theoretical purists may object to this manner of using theory, others defend the use of theoretical constructs for interventions on the basis of their empirical usefulness (Bartholomew et al. 2006; Kreuter et al. 2000) or suggest that the use of multiple theories that make complementary contributions can strengthen interventions (Glanz and Bishop 2010).

Table 18.2 Summary of meta-analyses of tailored interventions

Authors	Summary of studies	Mean ES	Key findings
Noar et al. (2007)	57 studies of print-tailored behavior change interventions—primarily smoking cessation, diet, and mammography screening	$d = .15$	Effects greater when (a) demographic and particular psychosocial variables used in tailoring, (b) particular print formats used, (c) more than one intervention session
Sohl and Moyer (2007)	28 studies of print, telephone, and interpersonal mammography screening interventions	$d = .21$	Effects greater when (a) health belief model used, (b) physician recommendation a part of intervention, (c) recent mammography used as outcome variable. No significant difference by tailoring channels
Krebs et al. (2010)	88 studies of print, computer, and automated telephone tailored interventions, primarily smoking, physical activity, and diet	$d = .17$	Effects greater over time when dynamic tailoring (where participant re-assessed before each feedback report) applied rather than static tailoring (multiple reports tailored from baseline data). Intervening on multiple behaviors did not undermine intervention efficacy. No significant difference by tailoring channels
Lustria et al. (2013)	40 studies of web-tailored interventions, primarily physical activity, diet, and smoking	$d = .14$	Effects of interventions sustained at longer-term follow-up ($d = .16$). Intervening on multiple behaviors did not undermine intervention efficacy

Note ES = effect size

Evidence of Efficacy

Two decades of literature provides a strong empirical basis upon which to judge the efficacy of computer tailored interventions (CTIs). Early in the literature, a number of seminal studies demonstrated efficacy and thus provided reasons for optimism (Campbell et al. 1994; Prochaska et al. 1993; Skinner et al. 1994). Subsequently, narrative reviews of the literature concluded that CTIs generally were successful in affecting health behavior change in diverse areas (Skinner et al. 1999), including smoking cessation (Strecher 1999), nutrition (Brug et al. 1999), and cancer prevention (Rimer and Glassman 1999). There have also been more recent systematic reviews that have concluded that CTIs are generally efficacious (Kroeze et al. 2006; Neville et al. 2009; Richards et al. 2007). Perhaps most importantly, four meta-analytic projects have

examined the literature and provided a more fine-grained analysis of CTI efficacy. We describe these meta-analyses in greater detail next (also see Table 18.2).

Noar et al. (2007) conducted a meta-analysis of 57 studies that tested the ability of tailored print materials to affect health behavior change. The studies primarily consisted of smoking cessation (26 %), diet (23 %), and mammography screening (21 %) interventions. The overall effect size in this study was $r = .074$ for tailored interventions compared with no-treatment control and alternative interventions, which converts to $d = .15$. Perhaps more importantly, a subsequent analysis that excluded studies containing only no-treatment control comparison conditions revealed that tailored interventions still outperformed generic or targeted interventions ($r = .058$ or $d = .12$).

Across behaviors, smoking and diet had the largest effect sizes, followed by mammography screening and then exercise. Also, a variety of intervention characteristics moderated intervention efficacy. For example, studies that generated tailored reports in the form of pamphlets/leaflets and newsletters/magazines had significantly larger effect sizes than those generating letters or manuals. In addition, those interventions with more than one contact with participants had significantly larger effects than those with just one contact. Finally, studies tailoring on particular theoretical (i.e., attitudes, self-efficacy, stage of change) and other (i.e., demographic) factors had larger effect sizes than those not tailoring on these variables (Noar et al. 2007).

That same year, Sohl and Moyer (2007) published a meta-analysis of 28 tailored intervention studies focused on increasing mammography screening within print, telephone, and in-person interventions. Results indicated a statistically significant overall effect of the tailored interventions compared with no-treatment control and alternative interventions, with an odds ratio (OR) equal to 1.42 (which converts to $d = .21$). Telephone, in person, and print tailored interventions all had similar impact. In addition, studies that tailored on variables from the health belief model had significantly greater impact than those that did not, and interventions were significantly more effective when a physician recommendation was part of the intervention. Also, studies that measured *recent* mammography as opposed to *regular* mammography tended to have larger effect sizes.

More recently, Krebs et al. (2010) conducted a meta-analysis of 88 studies testing tailored interventions delivered using print (75 %), computer (22 %), and automated telephone (3 %) channels. Behaviors examined in this review were diet, smoking, physical activity, and mammography screening, and some studies intervened on more than one behavior at a time. Overall, there was a statistically significant effect of tailored interventions on health behavior change ($d = .17$), and this effect did not vary significantly across tailoring channels. Effects were similar across behaviors, with dietary fat reduction being most efficacious ($d = .22$). In addition, interventions that focused on multiple behaviors did *not* have smaller effects than those focusing on a single behavior.

Krebs et al.'s (2010) meta-analysis also examined tailoring effects over time. Results revealed that effects tended to peak between 4–12 months and then gradually decline over time. Interestingly, there was also evidence that dynamically tailored interventions (those reassessing individuals before providing new tailored feedback) had significantly larger effects at most timepoints (including 13–24 month follow-up) than statically tailored interventions (those providing new tailored feedback based on the same baseline assessment). Indeed, only dynamically tailored interventions demonstrated statistically significant effects at long-term follow-up.

Most recently, Lustria and colleagues conducted a meta-analysis of web-delivered, tailored health behavior change interventions (Lustria et al. 2013). The 40 studies primarily consisted of physical activity (42 %), diet (25 %), and smoking (18 %) interventions. The overall weighted mean effect size in this study was $d = .14$. Studies that contained a longer term follow-up timepoint (53 % of studies) also exhibited a significant effect at the follow-up timepoint, $d = .16$. This bodes well for maintenance of intervention effects using tailored interventions, as it suggests no decay of intervention effects over the course of the study. Another key finding is the fact that multiple behavior interventions had similar effects as single behavior interventions, suggesting that intervening on multiple behaviors may *not* undermine behavior change.

Overall, these meta-analyses suggest that tailored interventions have often been successful in stimulating behavior change, and they each contribute to our knowledge about what may make efficacious interventions. The evidence to date suggests that messages that are more customized to an individual are more successful in influencing health behavior change (Noar et al. 2007) and that carefully constructed interventions can maintain changes over the longer term (Krebs et al. 2010; Lustria et al. 2013). Effect sizes across all of these meta-analyses were similar (ranging from $d = .14–.21$), giving us some indication of what the "typical" effect of a tailored intervention may be. Other important findings from these meta-analyses indicate that tailoring channel does not in and of itself appear to make a difference, but how tailoring is carried out (e.g., choice of theoretical constructs, dynamic vs. static tailoring, design of print materials) does appear to have a measurable impact on the efficacy of a tailored intervention. Finally, tailoring may be a promising strategy for those who wish to intervene on multiple behaviors (Krebs et al. 2010; Lustria et al. 2013), although a meta-analysis focused only on multiple behavior interventions would better enable us to understand the effects of such interventions.

Future Directions

Cumulative Science of Tailoring

New research on tailored health communication is critical to advance the field. The field is currently shifting from research that addresses *whether* tailoring works to research that addresses *under what conditions* it works. Many of the meta-analyses discussed in this chapter have conducted analyses to explore this question. In addition, recent conceptual work has distinguished among the various types of personalization and feedback strategies that tailored interventions can deliver (Dijkstra 2008; Hawkins et al. 2008). This "new language" will help tailoring researchers better disentangle the various components of tailored messages in order to advance an understanding of how tailoring operates most effectively (see Table 18.3).

In addition, an important observation about tailored interventions is the following: To date, tailoring has almost entirely been conceived of as a way to customize intervention *content* to

Table 18.3 Contemporary terminology and definitions in tailoring research

Term	Definition	Hypothetical example
Content matching	Matching appropriate intervention content (based on key theoretical determinants) to the individual	–
Feedback	Providing messages to participants about their psychological or behavioral states	–
Descriptive	Repeating back objective data to the participant	"You told us that you never use condoms when you have sex"
Comparative normative	Comparing a participants' data to those of their peers	"Your answers indicate that compared to other people like you, you underestimate the benefits of using condoms"
Comparative progress	Comparing participants' data to their data at a previous timepoint	"Your answers indicate that compared to your last visit, you are using condoms less often"
Evaluative	Providing judgments or interpretations of participants' data	"By not using condoms when you have sex, you are putting yourself at risk for contracting sexually transmitted diseases"
Personalization	Incorporating recognizable aspects of participants to convey (implicitly or explicitly) that the messages are specifically designed for them	–
Identification	Using a participant's name or other unique identifier(s)	Person's name, age, or preferred brand of condom is integrated into messages
Raising expectation of customization	Making participants explicitly aware that the intervention was designed uniquely for them	"This program will ask you questions and provide feedback designed especially for you on the basis of your answers"
	Contextualization	Framing messages in a context that is meaningful to participants
Embedding gender- or	race/ethnicity-matched images in intervention messaging	

Note Definitions are based on Hawkins et al. (2008) and Dijkstra (2008); for in-depth discussion of these tailoring mechanisms, refer to these publications individuals. As a result, nearly all tailoring has focused on what scholars believe to be the behavioral determinants of tailoring, which come from the theories of behavior and behavior change described earlier in this chapter (also see Noar and Zimmerman 2005). Many other factors affect how health content will be received, however, and a number of these communication-oriented factors could also be tailored on. Table 18.4 lists four domains that can be considered in tailoring (Noar et al. 2009; Rimer and Kreuter 2006). To date, the literature has focused almost entirely on the first row (*content*) and often neglected the other three domains in tailoring. The potential here is enormous: Not only could CTIs ultimately deliver the right *content* to the individual but also they could deliver it in a way that best ensures that content is attended to, cognitively processed, and perceived as personally relevant.

That specific studies are beginning to examine the kinds of questions raised by Hawkins et al. (2008), Noar et al. (2009), Rimer and Kreuter (2006), and others (Dijkstra 2008; Strecher 2009) is promising. For example, newer studies are examining novel constructs on which to tailor—especially constructs in the areas of cultural tailoring (Kreuter et al. 2005; Resnicow et al. 2008; van der Veen et al. 2010), environmental tailoring (van Stralen et al. 2009, 2010), and message framing (Latimer et al. 2008; Ruiter et al. 2010). Research is also examining the effects of different types of tailoring personalization and feedback on intervention efficacy (de Vet et al. 2008; Dijkstra 2005; Kroeze et al. 2008b; Strecher et al. 2008), mediators and moderators of effective tailoring (Campbell et al. 2008; Ko et al. 2010, 2011; Strecher et al. 2006), different ways of delivering multiple behavior change interventions (Vandelanotte et al. 2008), and even brain responses to tailoring (Chua et al. 2009). Additional studies are needed to help build a cumulative science of best practices in tailoring. As this work is conducted, we strongly encourage researchers to follow recommended guidelines for reporting studies of tailored interventions (Harrington and Noar 2012).

Dissemination of Interventions

A second key area for future research on tailored interventions is the area of dissemination. While many tailored programs have shown efficacy in research trials, few have been disseminated into practice. Why is this the case? Key barriers include the following: (1) many platforms for dissemination (worksites, clinics, etc.) want an intervention that covers many behaviors, while most tailored interventions focus on a single behavior; (2) many of the computer platforms upon which tailored interventions were developed are now out of date; (3) ongoing technical assistance is needed for such interventions, but resources are not always available for such support; (4) intellectual property issues arise in the case of some tailored interventions; and (5) it is not clear whether a tailored intervention developed in one context or region of the country would work as effectively in another context or region of the country. Some of these barriers have resulted from the fact that many tailored interventions were *not* developed with dissemination in mind, and in that manner future studies will benefit from a more careful consideration of dissemination issues early in the development process (National Cancer Institute 2008; Vinson et al. 2011). Also, dissemination and implementation research specifically on the topic of tailored interventions will also be necessary (Rabin and Glasgow 2012).

Many of these barriers are surmountable, of course, and progress is being made toward potential solutions. Approaches include (1) increasing development of multiple behavior interventions that address many health behaviors in the context of a single program; (2) developing open source software that can be shared among developers of tailored interventions to provide a common platform for such interventions; (3) conducting studies to research the best manner in which to disseminate tailored interventions; (4) partnering with nonprofit and private sector agencies that have an interest in disseminating such interventions; and (5) increasing the dialogue among technical developers about the

Table 18.4 Domains in which tailoring can be achieved and associated theories and variables

Purpose	Theories	Variable types	Specific constructs/variables	Outcomes
Match content to individual's information needs and interests	Transtheoretical model and stages of change Health belief model Social cognitive theory Theory of reasoned action Theory of planned behavior	Psychosocial variables, past behavior	Attitudes, beliefs, self-efficacy, social norms, perceived susceptibility, perceived severity, behavioral intentions, stage of change, previous behavior	Argument strength (content was convincing)
Place information in a meaningful context	Audience segmentation Personalization Culturally oriented theories	Demographic, cultural variables	Gender, age, race Gender norms, cultural norms, ethnic identity, racial pride, religiosity, collectivism	Perceived relevance (intervention was designed for me and reflects my beliefs and values)
Use design, production, and channel elements to capture and keep individual's attention	Activation model Sensation-seeking targeting Limited capacity model	Message design variables ("look and feel")	Message sensation value	Attention (intervention kept my attention)
Present information in type and structure preferred by individual	Exemplification Theory/narratives Entertainment education Message framing Emotional appeals	Message structure variables (type of appeal)	Narrative versus statistical Gain versus loss framing Fear, guilt, warmth, and other appeals	Message processing (thought about information, recalled information later on)

best ways to create sustainable interventions and provide technical support over the long term. The ultimate impact of tailored interventions on lifestyle behaviors could be substantial, but this impact is only possible if such programs are exported from the confines of funded research to the field setting. Although we are not there yet, efforts are underway to move us closer to the goal of bringing more of these efficacious programs into the public domain.

While reaching many of the above goals will take time, there has been some substantive movement toward dissemination. Dr. Victor Strecher and his colleagues in the Center for Health Communications Research at the University of Michigan have developed open source software for the creation of CTIs (Center for Health Communications Research 2011). The software, called the Michigan Tailoring System, is free to use and is open source, making modifications to it possible by any technical developer. Also, Dr. Marci Campbell and her colleagues in the Communications for Health Applications and Interventions (CHAI) core at the University of North Carolina at Chapel Hill have developed *Tailortool*, an open source software toolkit that enables the creation and delivery of CTIs over the Web (Communication for Health Applications and Interventions 2011). *Tailortool* allows a user to develop CTIs that are delivered in a newsletter format on the computer (in PDF format), which can then be printed or saved electronically for later reading. Also in existence are open source interactive voice response programs that are available for use in developing and delivering CTIs (Vinson et al. 2011). Moreover, while public sector dissemination has so far been a challenge to achieve, companies such as Health Media (founded in 1998; http://www.healthmedia.com/) and Pro-Change Behavior Systems (founded in 1997; http://www.prochange.com/) have been successfully developing and disseminating CTIs in the private sector.

Conclusion

In this chapter, we have provided an overview of tailored health communication research, providing a brief history of its genesis, highlighting its theoretical foundations, and summarizing what we know about tailoring effects. We have described the basic process of how tailoring operates and the channels through which tailored interventions may be delivered. We also have identified important directions for future research, including the importance of building a cumulative science of tailoring and translating our knowledge to applied settings.

Tailored health communication interventions represent a cutting edge approach to integrating persuasive message design with theoretical and technological developments. Ongoing research in this area offers an exceptional opportunity to extend health decision science by increasing our understanding of how to design and deliver tailored messages to individuals in order to help them make good health decisions. We look forward to continued advancements in this vibrant area of research.

References

Abrams, D. B., Orleans, C. T., Niaura, R. S., Goldstein, M. G., Prochaska, J. O., & Velicer, W. F. (1996). Integrating individual and public health perspectives for treatment of tobacco dependence under managed health care: A combined step care and matching model. *Annals of Behavioral Medicine, 18*, 290–304.

Ajzen, I., & Fishbein, M. (1980). *Understanding attitudes and predicting social behavior* (Paperback ed.). Englewood Cliffs, N.J.: Prentice-Hall.

Bandura, A. (1986). *Social foundations of thought and action: A social cognitive theory.* Englewood Cliffs, N.J.: Prentice-Hall.

Bartholomew, L. K., Parcel, G. S., Kok, G., & Gottlieb, N. H. (2006). *Planning health promotion programs: An intervention mapping approach* (2nd ed.). San Francisco, CA US: Jossey-Bass.

Brinberg, D., & Axelson, M. L. (1990). Increasing the consumption of dietary fiber: A decision theory analysis. *Health Education Research, 5*, 409–420.

Brinberg, D., Axelson, M. L., & Price, S. (2000). Changing food knowledge, food choice, and dietary fiber consumption by using tailored messages. *Appetite, 35*, 35–43.

Brug, J., Campbell, M., & van Assema, P. (1999). The application and impact of computer-generated personalized nutrition education: A review of the literature. *Patient Education and Counseling, 36*, 145–156.

Campbell, M. K., DeVellis, B. M., Strecher, V. J., Ammerman, A. S., DeVellis, R. F., & Sandler, R. S. (1994). Improving dietary behavior: The effectiveness of tailored messages in primary care settings. *American Journal of Public Health, 84*, 783–787.

Campbell, M. K., McLerran, D., Turner-McGrievy, G., Feng, Z., Havas, S., Sorensen, G. ... Nebeling, L. (2008). Mediation of adult fruit and vegetable consumption in the national 5 a day for better health community studies. *Annals of Behavioral Medicine, 35*, 49–60.

Center for Health Communications Research. (2011). *The Michigan tailoring system.* Retrieved May 11, 2011, from http://chcr.umich.edu/mts/

Chua, H. F., Liberzon, I., Welsh, R. C., & Strecher, V. J. (2009). Neural correlates of message tailoring and self-relatedness in smoking cessation programming. *Biological Psychiatry, 65*, 165–168.

Communication for Health Applications and Interventions. (2011). *The chai core.* Retrieved May 11, 2011, from http://www.chaicore.com/

de Vet, E., de Nooijer, J., de Vries, N. K., & Brug, J. (2008). Testing the transtheoretical model for fruit intake: Comparing web-based tailored stage-matched and stage-mismatched feedback. *Health Education Research, 23*, 218–227.

Dijkstra, A. (2005). Working mechanisms of computer-tailored health education: Evidence from smoking cessation. *Health Education Research, 20*, 527–539.

Dijkstra, A. (2008). The psychology of tailoring-ingredients in computer-tailored persuasion. *Social and Personality Psychology Compass, 2*, 765–784.

Dijkstra, A., & De Vries, H. (1999). The development of computer-generated tailored interventions. *Patient Education and Counseling, 36*, 193–203.

Fjeldsoe, B. S., Miller, Y. D., & Marshall, A. L. (2012). Text messaging interventions for chronic disease management and health promotion. In S. M. Noar &

N. G. Harrington (Eds.), *eHealth applications: Promoting strategies for behavior change* (pp. 167–186). New York: Routledge.

Glanz, K., & Bishop, D. B. (2010). The role of behavioral science theory in development and implementation of public health interventions. *Annual Review of Public Health, 31*, 399–418.

Harrington, N. G., & Noar, S. M. (2012). Reporting standards for studies of tailored interventions. *Health Education Research, 27*, 331–342.

Hawkins, R. P., Kreuter, M., Resnicow, K., Fishbein, M., & Dijkstra, A. (2008). Understanding tailoring in communicating about health. *Health Education Research, 23*, 454–466.

Ko, L. K., Campbell, M. K., Lewis, M. A., Earp, J., & DeVellis, B. (2010). Mediators of fruit and vegetable consumption among colorectal cancer survivors. *Journal of Cancer Survivorship, 4*, 149–158.

Ko, L. K., Campbell, M. K., Lewis, M. A., Earp, J. A., & Devellis, B. (2011). Information processes mediate the effect of a health communication intervention on fruit and vegetable consumption. *Journal Of Health Communication, 16*, 282–299.

Krebs, P., Prochaska, J. O., & Rossi, J. S. (2010). A meta-analysis of computer-tailored interventions for health behavior change. *Preventive Medicine, 51*, 214–221.

Kreuter, M. W., Farrell, D., Olevitch, L., & Brennan, L. (2000). *Tailoring health messages: Customizing communication with computer technology.* Mahwah, N.J.: Lawrence Erlbaum.

Kreuter, M. W., Strecher, V. J., & Glassman, B. (1999). One size does not fit all: The case for tailoring print materials. *Annals of Behavioral Medicine, 21*, 276–283.

Kreuter, M. W., Sugg-Skinner, C., Holt, C. L., Clark, E. M., Haire-Joshu, D., Fu, Q. … Bucholtz, D. (2005). Cultural tailoring for mammography and fruit and vegetable intake among low-income African-American women in urban public health centers. *Preventive Medicine, 41*, 53–62.

Kroeze, W., Oenema, A., Campbell, M., & Brug, J. (2008a). The efficacy of web-based and print-delivered computer-tailored interventions to reduce fat intake: Results of a randomized, controlled trial. *Journal of Nutrition Education and Behavior, 40*, 226–236.

Kroeze, W., Oenema, A., Dagnelie, P. C., & Brug, J. (2008b). Examining the minimal required elements of a computer-tailored intervention aimed at dietary fat reduction: Results of a randomized controlled dismantling study. *Health Education Research, 23*, 880–891.

Kroeze, W., Werkman, A., & Brug, J. (2006). A systematic review of randomized trials on the effectiveness of computer-tailored education on physical activity and dietary behaviors. *Annals of Behavioral Medicine, 31*, 205–223.

Latimer, A. E., Williams-Piehota, P., Katulak, N. A., Cox, A., Mowad, L., Higgins, E. T., & Salovey, P. (2008).

Promoting fruit and vegetable intake through messages tailored to individual differences in regulatory focus. *Annals of Behavioral Medicine, 35*, 363–369.

Lustria, M. L., Cortese, J., Noar, S. M., & Glueckauf, R. L. (2009). Computer-tailored health interventions delivered over the web: Review and analysis of key components. *Patient Education and Counseling, 74*, 156–173.

Lustria, M. L., Noar, S. M., Cortese, J., Van Stee, S. K., Glueckauf, R. L., & Lee, J. (2013). A meta-analysis of web-delivered tailored health behavior change interventions. *Journal of Health Communication, 18*, 1039–1069.

Marcus, B. H., Lewis, B. A., Williams, D. M., Dunsiger, S., Jakicic, J. M., Whiteley, J. A. … Parisi, A. F. (2007). A comparison of Internet and print-based physical activity interventions. *Archives of Internal Medicine, 167*, 944–949.

Marcus, B. H., Napolitano, M. A., King, A. C., Lewis, B. A., Whiteley, J. A., Albrecht, A. … Papandonatos, G. D. (2007). Telephone versus print delivery of an individualized motivationally tailored physical activity intervention: Project STRIDE. *Health Psychology, 26*, 401–409.

National Cancer Institute. (2008). *Computerized tailored interventions workgroup meeting, executive summary. Accessed April 1, 2008:* http://cancercontrol.cancer.gov/d4d/info_computer_meeting.html. Washington, DC: US Department of Health & Human Services.

Neville, L. M., O'Hara, B., & Milat, A. J. (2009). Computer-tailored dietary behaviour change interventions: A systematic review. *Health Education Research, 24*, 699–720.

Noar, S. M., Benac, C. N., & Harris, M. S. (2007). Does tailoring matter? Meta-analytic review of tailored print health behavior change interventions. *Psychological Bulletin, 133*, 673–693.

Noar, S. M., Harrington, N. G., & Aldrich, R. S. (2009). The role of message tailoring in the development of persuasive health communication messages. *Communication Yearbook, 33*, 72–133.

Noar, S. M., Harrington, N. G., Van Stee, S. K., & Aldrich, R. S. (2011). Tailored health communication to change lifestyle behaviors. *American Journal of Lifestyle Medicine, 5*, 112–122.

Noar, S. M., & Zimmerman, R. S. (2005). Health behavior theory and cumulative knowledge regarding health behaviors: Are we moving in the right direction? *Health Education Research, 20*, 275–290.

Painter, J. E., Borba, C. P. C., Hynes, M., Mays, D., & Glanz, K. (2008). The use of theory in health behavior research from 2000 to 2005: A systematic review. *Annals of Behavioral Medicine, 35*, 358–362.

Prochaska, J. O., Butterworth, S., Redding, C. A., Burden, V., Perrin, N., Leo, M. … Prochaska, J. M. (2008). Initial efficacy of MI, TTM tailoring and HRI's with multiple behaviors for employee health promotion. *Preventive Medicine, 46*, 226–231.

Prochaska, J. O., DiClemente, C. C., & Norcross, J. C. (1992). In search of how people change: Applications to addictive behaviors. *American Psychologist, 47,* 1102–1114.

Prochaska, J. O., DiClemente, C. C., Velicer, W. F., & Rossi, J. S. (1993). Standardized, individualized, interactive, and personalized self-help programs for smoking cessation. *Health Psychology, 12,* 399–405.

Rabin, B. A., & Glasgow, R. E. (2012). Dissemination and implementation of eHealth interventions. In S. M. Noar & N. G. Harrington (Eds.), *eHealth applications: Promising strategies for behavior change* (pp. 221–245). New York: Routledge.

Resnicow, K., Davis, R. E., Zhang, G., Konkel, J., Strecher, V. J., Shaikh, A. R. ... Wiese, C. (2008). Tailoring a fruit and vegetable intervention on novel motivational constructs: results of a randomized study. *Annals of Behavioral Medicine, 35,* 159–169.

Richards, K. C., Enderlin, C. A., Beck, C., McSweeney, J. C., Jones, T. C., & Roberson, P. K. (2007). Tailored biobehavioral interventions: A literature review and synthesis. *Research & Theory for Nursing Practice, 21,* 271–285.

Rimer, B. K., & Glassman, B. (1999). Is there a use for tailored print communications in cancer risk communication? *Journal of the National Cancer Institute, 91,* 140.

Rimer, B. K., & Kreuter, M. W. (2006). Advancing tailored health communication: A persuasion and message effects perspective. *Journal of Communication, 56,* S184–S201.

Rosenthal, I. M. (1974). The health belief model and preventive health behavior. *Health Education Monographs, 2,* 354–387.

Ruiter, R. A. C., Werrij, M. Q., & de Vries, H. (2010). Investigating message-framing effects in the context of a tailored intervention promoting physical activity. *Health Education Research, 25,* 343–354.

Skinner, C. S., Campbell, M. K., Rimer, B. K., Curry, S., & Prochaska, J. O. (1999). How effective is tailored print communication? *Annals of Behavioral Medicine, 21,* 290–298.

Skinner, C. S., Strecher, V. J., & Hospers, H. (1994). Physicians' recommendations for mammography: Do tailored messages make a difference? *American Journal of Public Health, 84,* 43–49.

Snyder, L. B., Hamilton, M. A., Mitchell, E. W., Kiwanuka-Tondo, J., Fleming-Milici, F., & Proctor, D. (2004). A meta-analysis of the effect of mediated health communication campaigns on behavior change in the United States. *Journal of Health Communication, 9,* 71–96.

Sohl, S. J., & Moyer, A. (2007). Tailored interventions to promote mammography screening: A meta-analytic review. *Preventive Medicine, 45,* 252–261.

Strecher, V. J. (1999). Computer-tailored smoking cessation materials: A review and discussion. *Patient Education and Counseling, 36,* 107–117.

Strecher, V. J. (2009). Interactive health communications for cancer prevention and control. In S. M. Miller, D. J. Bowen, R. T. Croyle, & J. H. Rowland (Eds.), *Handbook of cancer control and behavioral science: A resource for researchers, practitioners, and policymakers* (pp. 547–558). Washington, DC US: American Psychological Association.

Strecher, V. J., McClure, J. B., Alexander, G. L., Chakraborty, B., Nair, V. N., Konkel, J. M. ... Pomerleau, O. F. (2008). Web-based smoking-cessation programs: Results of a randomized trial. *American Journal of Preventive Medicine, 34,* 373–381.

Strecher, V. J., Shiffman, S., & West, R. (2006). Moderators and mediators of a Web-based computer-tailored smoking cessation program among nicotine patch users. *Nicotine & Tobacco Research, 8,* S95–s101.

Turow, J. (2012). *The daily you: How the new advertising industry is defining your identity and your worth.* New Haven, CT: Yale University Press.

van der Veen, Y. J. J., de Zwart, O., Mackenbach, J., & Richardus, J. H. (2010). Cultural tailoring for the promotion of hepatitis B screening in Turkish Dutch: A protocol for a randomized controlled trial. *BMC Public Health, 10,* 674.

van Stralen, M. M., de Vries, H., Bolman, C., Mudde, A. N., & Lechner, L. (2010). Exploring the efficacy and moderators of two computer-tailored physical activity interventions for older adults: A randomized controlled trial. *Annals of Behavioral Medicine, 39,* 139–150.

van Stralen, M. M., de Vries, H., Mudde, A. N., Bolman, C., & Lechner, L. (2009). The working mechanisms of an environmentally tailored physical activity intervention for older adults: A randomized controlled trial. *International Journal of Behavioral Nutrition And Physical Activity, 6,* 83.

Vandelanotte, C., Reeves, M. M., Brug, J., & De Bourdeaudhuij, I. (2008). A randomized trial of sequential and simultaneous multiple behavior change interventions for physical activity and fat intake. *Preventive Medicine, 46,* 232–237.

Vinson, C., Bickmore, T., Farrell, D., Campbell, M., An, L., Saunders, E., & Shaikh, A. (2011). Adapting research-tested computerized tailored interventions for broader dissemination and implementation. *Translational Behavioral Medicine, 1,* 93–102.

Overcoming the Many Pitfalls of Communicating Risk

19

Erika A. Waters, Angela Fagerlin
and Brian J. Zikmund-Fisher

Introduction to Risk, Risk Perceptions, and Risk Communication

Risk is a complex concept that has multiple uses and meanings that are dependent upon the specific characteristics of the situation in question. For example, "Death is a risk of driving," "Driving is risky," and "The risk of accidental death is 10 %" are all legitimate statements, but they carry very different meanings. For our purposes, we define *risk* as a non-certain chance of experiencing a negative event. The focus of risk communication is the translation of such risk concepts into risk perceptions.

Perceptions of risk (also referred to as perceptions of susceptibility, likelihood, and, more recently, *feelings* of risk and vulnerability) are important because they can influence health-related decisions and behaviors (e.g., Brewer et al. 2007). However, they are inherently subjective concepts. Although it is possible to calculate an estimate of the probability of experiencing a particular outcome, the *meaning* of that probability to an individual varies based on a variety of intrapersonal, interpersonal, contextual, and societal factors (Slovic 2000). For example, a 1 % chance of a sore arm following immunization carries a different subjective meaning to a tennis player about to compete or to a concert pianist than it does to a soccer player, an opera singer, or even the pianist while on vacation. Thus, the feeling and meaning of a 1 % risk are influenced by the context in which it arises. In addition, the way in which information about risk is communicated (e.g., specific formats or strategies) can change perceived risk. The malleability of risk perceptions mean that any conveyance of risk information should be preceded by a thoughtful examination of the intended goals and purpose of the communication. This seems like an obvious first step, but it is one that is often neglected.

The goals of risk communication include: to inform, to change knowledge and beliefs, and/or to change behavior (Brewer 2011). The specific

E.A. Waters (✉)
Division of Public Health Sciences, Washington University in St. Louis, Saint Louis, MO, USA
e-mail: waterse@wudosis.wustl.edu

A. Fagerlin
Department of Population Health Sciences, University of Utah, Salt Lake City, UT, USA
e-mail: angie.fagerlin@hsc.utah.edu

B.J. Zikmund-Fisher
Department of Internal Medicine, University of Michigan, Ann Arbor, MI, USA
e-mail: bzikmund@umich.edu

B.J. Zikmund-Fisher
Center for Bioethics and Social Sciences in Medicine, Ann Arbor, MI, USA

B.J. Zikmund-Fisher
Department of Health Behavior and Health Education, University of Michigan, Ann Arbor, MI, USA

© Springer Science+Business Media New York 2016
M.A. Diefenbach et al. (eds.), *Handbook of Health Decision Science*,
DOI 10.1007/978-1-4939-3486-7_19

goal(s) of any given communication determines which strategies are most appropriate. Simply informing people of a risk may be useful in certain contexts, such as raising awareness of a hazard. However, raising awareness is usually intended to be only an intermediate step on the way to other goals. Changing beliefs and knowledge can be an appropriate goal when there is uncertainty about whether a particular decision should be recommended for everyone. For example, helping women with a BRCA1 mutation become more knowledgeable about the risks and benefits of prophylactic mastectomy, hormone therapy, and active surveillance may enable them to make an informed decision about managing their elevated breast cancer risk. Whether these informed decisions are the same as or different than the decisions they would have made otherwise will depend on the situation. Communications whose goals are to change behavior should be reserved for situations in which there is *no* uncertainty about whether a specific behavior should be recommended for all members of a given population, such as discouraging tobacco use. It should be recognized, however, that risk communication campaigns alone may not be the most efficient approaches to changing behavior.

The goals of the communication also influence the precision with which risk should be conveyed (Zikmund-Fisher, in press). For example, awareness of a risk requires only that people understand that there is a *possibility* of experiencing the hazard, not the exact probability (e.g., "You might develop cancer"). In contrast, helping people understand the tradeoffs among treatment options that have multiple risks and benefits requires more precise information (e.g., "The medication will reduce the risk of cancer by 10 % and will increase the risk of blood clot by 2 %"). Communicators who have taken the time to identify the goals of the communication effort and the degree of precision required to achieve those goals will be one step closer to conveying risk information in a way that is meaningful and useful to the public.

Theoretical Perspectives on Risk Perceptions and Decision Making

Many health behavior and decision theories have roots in economic models of "rational" and "normative" decision making (Conner and Norman 1995). These models assert that individuals make decisions based on which option is expected to yield the highest utility (i.e., subjective value x probability of occurrence). However, the ways in which individuals conceptualize, process, and use information about health risks are influenced by a variety of factors that are not included in these theories. Nonetheless, these additional factors provide necessary insight into the decision-making processes people use about risks, and understanding these factors can yield practical guidance for risk communicators.

Intuitive and Affective Information Processing

Psychology has a long tradition of distinguishing between two modes of cognition: a more deliberative and rational mode, and a more automatic and intuitive mode (see Smith and DeCoster 2000 for a review). Although many of these *dual process* theories posit that each mode operates independently, some researchers suggest that the more intuitive system operates concurrently with the deliberative system (see Reyna, Chap. 6, this volume and Ancker et al. 2006; Betsch and Glockner 2010; Kahneman and Frederick 2002).

Affect and emotions are important "companion[s] to thought" (Zajonc 1980, p. 154) that can influence risk judgments and decisions by changing how people evaluate the utility of a decision's consequences (Loewenstein et al. 2001). In addition to this "emotions as output" perspective, however, emotions can also act as input to risk decisions by providing necessary information and guidance, acting as "common currency" for comparing qualitatively different options, focusing the perceiver's attention on new information, and motivating behavior (Peters et al. 2006a). In fact, consistent with dual process theories discussed above, a "risk as feelings" process (e.g., Loewenstein et al. 2001) likely operates in parallel with cognitive evaluations of likelihood and potential consequences. Several recent studies have shown that these risk *feelings* were more predictive of health behavior and intentions than cognitive likelihood estimates (e.g., Janssen et al. 2011). Consequently, assessing the extent to which a communication makes people "feel" vulnerable and "at risk" is legitimate and often informative when designing or evaluating risk communication efforts. For a more comprehensive discussion of the role of affect in decision making, see Peters, Chap. 8 in this volume.

Context

Contextual factors inherent in the development and implementation of risk communication efforts can influence risk perceptions and health-related decisions. Because people have internal constructs of uncertainty that are not equivalent to mathematical probabilities, numeric statements of risk provided in isolation can be ambiguous from an intuitive perspective even though they are numerically precise (Windschitl et al. 2002). Such information has low "evaluability" (Hsee et al. 1999); it lacks inherent meaning, is difficult to interpret as good or bad, and is therefore less useful for decision making. Adding information that helps people place the risk in context increases evaluability and, consequently, facilitates the decision-making process. These contextual features can take many forms, including providing a standard of comparison (such as the risk of another group or another disease) or category labels (such as "high risk") (Zikmund-Fisher, in press). Critically, however, the intuitive assessment or comparative gist that a person takes away from risk data depends on which of the many potential comparison standards they are provided (e.g., the risk

of the average person, the risk faced by a different ethnic group, or the risk of a different disease) (Windschitl et al. 2002).

Expertise is another contextual feature that affects risk perceptions and health-related decisions. Much research demonstrates that laypeople and experts draw different conclusions about the same health hazard (for a review, see Finkel 2008). For example, laypeople and epidemiologists rated the statement, "According to the average cancer rate for the state as a whole, one would expect to find five cases of cancer on a block this size" (Levy et al. 2008, p. 1534) as "very reassuring," while laypeople rated it as "alarming."

There are several possible reasons for such discrepancies. First, experts and laypeople likely draw different evaluative meaning from the information provided because laypeople lack reference standards against which to evaluate it. In the absence of such context, *any* number of cases may seem alarming. In fact, most types of likelihood information are more meaningful to those with more expertise. In addition, laypeople and experts often hold different mental models or representations of a hazard (Fischhoff 1999; Leventhal et al. 2003). Mental models are complex, may or may not be correct, and can include a variety of topics including likelihood information, the time course of the risk, whether the risk can be mitigated or the illness can be treated, and potential causal factors. Whereas expert mental models change over time as new scientific discoveries are made, lay mental models are constructed based on many types of information sources, including the media, interpersonal interactions, and personal experiences (Gullion et al. 2008). Laypeople may also place greater importance on features of the hazard other than probability, such as the severity or catastrophic potential of the consequences, than experts do (Slovic 2000).

Communications that ignore the differences between lay and expert mental models are unlikely to influence laypeople's perceptions and behaviors regarding risk. The controversy surrounding the 2009 U.S. Preventive Services Task

Force recommendation to provide mammographic screening to women aged 40–49 only after considering the patient's individual values regarding harms and benefits (rather than making an outright recommendation to screen) is a likely example of this problem (Squiers et al. 2011). The experts on the panel based their recommendation on several scientific studies and placed great importance on the relatively small magnitude of the risk reduction conferred by screening for any individual woman. The resulting conversation in mass media focused less on the scientific evidence and more on the idea previously advanced by the public health community that delayed screening will cause more breast cancer deaths. The result was confusion among the women to whom the recommendation was targeted.

Summary

Meaningful comprehension of risk information is more than cognition; it also involves incorporating information provided by intuitive and affective processes, as well as contextual features that shape one's perspective. In the next section, we describe strategies to avoid common pitfalls that risk communicators can encounter, as well as specific strategies to overcome them.

Strategies to Avoid Common Risk Communication Pitfalls

Adhere to Basic Good Practices in Communication

Communicating risk is seldom straightforward, but there are three lessons we can take from the broader communication literature. Each lesson requires communicators to invest a little more time and resources into the project, but they are essential to conveying information in a way that is meaningful and useful to the audience. First, know whether the communication is intended to inform, persuade, or change behavior (Brewer 2011). Second, know as much about the target

audience as possible. This includes not only basic demographic information such as age, gender, race, and ethnicity, but also data about their knowledge, attitudes, and if possible, their mental models of the risk. This information will clarify content needs to be conveyed and how it might need to be framed. Third, test communications prior to deploying them in the field or clinic. At a minimum, conduct focus groups or semi-structured individual interviews to assess whether the message is being interpreted as intended (e.g., cognitive interviews; Willis 2004).

Recognize Numeracy Limitations

A concern that is more specific to *risk* communication than communication in general is numeracy, which is the ability to understand and use numerical information effectively when making health-related decisions. Numeracy serves several functions that are essential to making informed health decisions (Lipkus and Peters 2009). In addition to facilitating computation, interpretation, and acceptance of numerical data, it encourages people to seek out and deeply process more information, helps people draw evaluative meaning from likelihood information, and promotes behavior change. Consequently, people with limited numeracy may experience a variety of negative consequences compared to people with adequate numeracy, including inflated risk perceptions, differential sensitivity to risk communication formats, more difficulty understanding medical instructions, lower engagement in health behaviors and shared decision making activities, and poorer health (e.g., Nelson et al. 2008).

Unfortunately, many people have limited numeracy (Kutner et al. 2006). In fact, nearly 22 % of US adults sampled in a large national survey could not identify whether 1 in 10, 1 in 100, or 1 in 1000 represented the largest risk (National Cancer Institute 2009). Although people with limited formal education and who are members of underserved populations are more vulnerable to experiencing low numeracy, low numeracy is found across all segments of society. Thus, risk communications should be designed with the assumption that the audience will have limited numeracy (see below for details).

Avoid Defining Effective Risk Communication as Recall of Likelihood Information

Well-meaning risk communicators might attempt to assess the extent to which their communication has been understood and/or accepted by asking people to recall the risk information provided. However, in general, accurate recall is not necessarily equivalent to information comprehension, changed beliefs, or likelihood of making a good health decision (Brewer 2011; McGuire 1984; Windschitl 2002). Providing likelihood information often alters risk beliefs only to a limited extent (Lerman 1995). For example, although participants who were provided with personalized feedback about their risk of developing colorectal cancer could recall the risk information they were provided, approximately half did not believe what they were told (Weinstein et al. 2004). These discrepancies could be attributable to many factors, including the audience processing the information defensively (McQueen et al. 2012), the expert communicator not conveying the information in a way that is consistent with the lay audience's mental model of the risk (Fischhoff 1995, 1999), or the communication evoking the incorrect gist meaning from audience members due to limitations in numeracy or unnecessarily complex communications (Zikmund-Fisher, in press).

Provide Specific Risk Reduction Recommendations

Regardless of whether the goal of the communication is to inform, change beliefs, or change behavior, it is important to inform people of strategies that they can take to reduce their risk (e.g., stop smoking) (Weinstein et al. 1989). This is important for two reasons. The most obvious is

because people may not know *how* to reduce their risk, and informing them provides them with the tools needed to take action. The second reason is to help people effectively manage the worry and anxiety produced by the threatening information, rather than trying to control their feelings by less constructive means (e.g., by ignoring the risk; Leventhal et al. 2003).

Use Risk Communication Strategies that Increase Comprehension and Evaluative Meaning

(a) **Numerical formats**. Numerical risk information can be conveyed using a variety of formats. Percentages, natural frequencies (e.g., N in 1000), and the 1 in N format provide information about risk magnitude. Natural frequencies, which explicitly define the reference class, facilitate Bayesian reasoning and help older and less numerate adults calculate the positive predictive value of medical screening tests (Galesic et al. 2009; Gigerenzer 1996). They also appear to result in more consistent risk perceptions between people with higher and lower numeracy skills (Peters et al. 2006b). However, recent work suggests that the simplicity of percentages may be valuable when communicating many risks at once. In one study, the risks, and benefits of a hypothetical prescription medication were presented to participants via a carefully constructed table named a "Drug Facts Box" (Woloshin and Schwartz 2011). Participants who viewed the risks and benefits as percentages (rather than natural frequencies) were slightly more likely to comprehend the information overall. Compared to the natural frequency condition, the percentages condition also prompted participants to judge the benefits as less beneficial and the harms as less harmful. They were also more likely to indicate that the benefits outweighed the side effects of treatment. When choosing between presenting percentages and natural frequencies, the most appropriate format is likely dependent on the purpose of the communication, audience characteristics, and what the audience is expected to do with the information (Cuite et al. 2008).

Despite its current use in certain medical specialties, we and others specifically argue that the 1 in *N* format should be retired and its use classified as poor care (Cuite et al. 2008; Zikmund-Fisher 2011). Because the 1-in-*X* format varies the risk denominator, it is makes comparisons more difficult (Cuite et al. 2008), often leads to exaggerated perceptions of risk (Pighin et al. 2011), and is particularly difficult for less numerate people (Lipkus et al. 2001). In fact, many people interpret 1-in-*X* statistics in the *opposite* direction as is required (e.g., by viewing a 1 in 600 risk as double a 1 in 300 risk rather than half as large) (Cuite et al. 2008).

Information about the change in magnitude of a risk can be provided as relative risk, pairs of absolute risk statistics, Number Needed to Treat/Harm (NNT/NNH), or incremental risk. Evidence suggests that the NNT/NNH format (the inverse of the absolute risk change) should also be avoided for patient communications because it has the same potential for misinterpretation as 1-in-*X* formats and hence is more difficult than other formats to use when comparing treatment effectiveness or benefit (Sheridan et al. 2003). Incremental risk (also described as the absolute risk difference) is conceptually appealing, but visual displays (see below) may be necessary to help people understand what they are considering (Zikmund-Fisher et al. 2008a).

In general, we advise conveying information about changes in risk using absolute risk totals or differences. Never provide *only* relative risk reduction/increase information, because it can be misleading. A 50 % reduction in breast cancer risk may initially seem important, but it seems less impressive when we learn that the woman's absolute risk of breast cancer is 2 %. The power of relative risk reduction information to encourage treatment utilization is considerable. A large meta-analysis revealed that treatments whose benefits are described in terms of relative risk reduction are viewed more favorably than treatments described in terms of absolute benefit by both the general public and physicians (Covey 2007). Importantly, adding absolute risk information to relative risk reduction information eliminates this effect.

Lastly, we note the importance of identifying both risk events (i.e., the probability of the hazard occurring) and nonevents (i.e., the probability of the hazard *not* occurring). This can be thought of as providing both negative and positive frames (e.g., 30 % mortality = 70 % survival) or, to frame the issue as natural frequencies, as clarifying what happens to the whole population, not just one group. Extensive research demonstrates that describing risks in terms of the probability that a negative event will occur is perceived more negatively than the probability that the event will not occur. Such framing can affect perceptions of treatment risks and benefits among both laypeople and physicians. For example, samples of ambulatory patients, graduate students, and physicians viewed lung cancer treatments more favorably when efficacy information was provided in terms of the likelihood of living versus the likelihood of dying (McNeil et al. 1982). It is possible that people with low numeracy are more vulnerable to framing effects, but the data are mixed (Garcia-Retamero and Galesic 2010a; Peters et al. 2011). Regardless, clarification of such part-whole relationships is an essential part of risk communication (Lipkus and Hollands 1999).

(b) **Timeframe**. Any communication of risk must inform the audience about the timeframe over which the risk is relevant (Waters et al. 2009). For example, a 5 % chance of developing breast cancer during a five year time interval (which, if continued, will accumulate into a much larger risk over time) is very different than a 5 % chance spread out over a lifetime. Neglecting to provide a timeframe deprives decision makers of the knowledge needed to draw evaluative meaning from the information.

In general, communicators should use timeframes for risk communication that are somewhat restricted in duration to increase concreteness (Woloshin et al. 2002). Using similar time frames when communicating multiple risks and benefits will also help increase evaluability. In addition, focusing on short-term consequences helps people to act instead of postponing a decision about risk due to their inherent tendency to discount future rewards (e.g., longer life) in favor for more immediate rewards (e.g., pleasure from smoking cigarettes). This *temporal discounting* may be especially problematic among people with limited numeracy (Nelson et al. 2008). However, the needs of the audience are paramount. Whereas "lifetime risk" can be difficult for younger people to conceptualize, it may be more relevant for older people.

(c) **Interpretive labels**. Interpretive labels can be used in a variety of ways, including to describe the nature of the hazard (e.g., normal, abnormal), the magnitude of the probability (e.g., low, high), and the severity of the consequences (e.g., good, bad). In general, interpretive labels increase the evaluative meaning of many types of quantitative information. Without such labels, people may place widely different interpretations on the same risk number. In one study, some participants rated an 8 % risk as "extremely small," whereas others rate it as "extremely large" (Waters et al. 2007a). However, including interpretive labels can improve decision making. For example, labels such as "excellent" and "poor" can help people use numerical information to make better judgments about the quality of health care services, regardless of their numeracy levels (Peters et al. 2009). Indeed, labels may be especially important for people with low numeracy, who often have difficulty deriving gist meanings about risk data in their absence.

Our recommendation for adding interpretive labels to quantitative risk information is not without reservation. Like numbers, labels are vulnerable to wide variations in their perceived magnitude (Windschitl and Wells 1996). For example, asking people to provide a probability estimate that corresponds with a interpretive labels such as *likely*, *often*, *rarely*, and *unlikely* results in wide variation (Budescu and Wallsten 1985). In addition, interpretive labels may alter perceptions about the potential risks and benefits of a procedure and steer people toward action or inaction even when detailed numeric information is provided (Zikmund-Fisher et al. 2007a). Consequently, risk communicators should be thoughtful when using labels and, as always, test the communication prior to dissemination.

(d) **Comparative information**. Providing information that allows people to compare the risk of the hazard with another meaningful data point is an extremely powerful way to increase the ability to draw evaluative meaning from numbers. However, the meaning that people will take away from such comparisons depends heavily on what type of comparative data are provided (Windschitl et al. 2002). Several types of comparisons are often considered, and each has its own unique set of benefits and drawbacks. Consequently, comparative information should be provided only after careful consideration.

The most frequent comparator is the "average person's risk." For example, a woman who learns that her chances of developing breast cancer over the next 5 years are 6 % is likely to interpret that risk very differently if she is told that the average woman's risk is 12 % than if she is told that the average woman's risk is 3 % (Fagerlin et al. 2007). Even if the individual's personal risk is exactly the same in both contexts, women who were told that they were at above average risk perceived greater benefit from taking a pill to reduce their risk and were more willing to endorse taking such a pill than those believed that they were at below average risk. In effect, average risk presentations may be seen as evoking a social norm that implies that people should take action if they have more risk than most others face (Cialdini 2008). However, comparisons do not always act in predictable ways. Another study that communicated counts of risk factors rather than risk percentages found that providing information about the average person's number of risk factors increased participants' intentions to undergo colorectal cancer screening, but it did so *regardless* of whether the participants was told that the average person had more or fewer risk factors (Lipkus and Klein 2006). Nevertheless, communicators should be aware that telling someone that they are at below average risk for a hazard might discourage them from taking preventive action.

Communicators can also provide comparative information about the individual's risk of experiencing other types of hazards. One study found that comparing the risk of cancer conferred by exposure to ethylene oxide emissions to the risk of death from other hazards such as food poisoning and lightening strikes was viewed very favorably compared to several other types of comparison scenarios (Roth et al. 1990). Such comparison information might be particularly helpful for individuals with limited numeracy (Keller et al. 2009). However, research that examines this issue is limited, so the extent to which these findings generalize across populations and hazards is unclear.

Other types of comparative information include reference standards (e.g., normal ranges), though these do not help people know whether an out-of-range value is actually of concern. In situations where the purpose of a communication is to provide clear signals for action, thresholds for recommended action (e.g., begin radon remediation if household levels are greater than 4 pCi/l) clearly translate numerical data into evaluative meaning (Weinstein et al. 1989). Here again, though, thresholds essentially convert interval data into binary data, and the loss of fidelity between high and borderline values can sometimes be problematic.

(e) **Graphic displays**. There is a large literature demonstrating that adding a graphic display to probabilistic information can affect information comprehension, perceptions of risk, and health-related decisions and behaviors (for reviews, see Ancker et al. 2006; Garcia-Retamero et al. 2012; Lipkus 2007; Lipkus and Hollands 1999). There are many types of graphs, including bar charts, line graphs, icon arrays/pictographs (i.e., a matrix of shaded and unshaded objects such as stick figures or squares), bubble graphs, speedometers, and risk ladders. However, not all graphs are equally useful (Hawley et al. 2008), since different visuals create convey different "gist" messages about the same risk statistic. For example, line graphs emphasize risk trends (Lipkus and Hollands 1999), but icon arrays are particularly good at showing both specific risk magnitudes and part-whole relationships (Ancker et al. 2006; Hawley et al. 2008; Lipkus and Hollands 1999).

Because graphs can convey slightly different meanings, the choice of *which* graph to use must be based on thoughtful consideration of the goal of the communication and the needs of the audience. For example, although both stacked bar graphs and icon arrays can help people evaluate whether or not a treatment's benefits outweigh its risks, only icon arrays can reduce the undue importance people place on side effects (Waters et al. 2007b). Yet, tables that summarize all of a treatment's risks and benefits concisely (e.g., Woloshin and Schwartz 2011) may be more useful than pages of graphics showing the same data.

Regardless of the type of graph, care should be taken during the design process to avoid misleading the audience. For example, we discourage practices such as truncating the y-axis of a bar or line graph to emphasize the magnitude of a difference. Many people fail to account for the amount of time displayed in line graphs such as survival curves (Zikmund-Fisher et al. 2007b), and care must be taken to reinforce this dimension. Conversely, graphs that emphasize part-whole relationships highlight the number of people at risk *and* not at risk (e.g., icon arrays) can help people draw balanced evaluative meanings by providing both positive and negative frames for comparison (Hawley et al. 2008; Stone et al. 2003). Such visuals appear particularly important when communicating incremental risk in order to clarify the relationship between the size of the baseline risk and the risk difference (Zikmund-Fisher et al. 2008a, b).

Lastly, we note that the effectiveness of risk graphics depends on not just individual numeracy but also the complementary construct of graphical literacy (Gaissmaier et al. 2012; Galesic and Garcia-Retamero 2011). Although graphics like icon arrays can improve knowledge and recall among people with lower numeracy abilities (e.g., Garcia-Retamero and Galesic 2010b; Keller et al. 2009), recent work shows that less numerate people can learn effectively from risk graphics if they have good graphical literacy skills (Galesic and Garcia-Retamero 2011).

(f) **Cognitive effort**. A critical, but underappreciated, principle of effective risk communication involves limiting the amount of cognitive effort that is required for people to understand their messages. Providing less information in a more intuitive way helped people understand complex information about hospital cost and quality and to choose the hospital with the highest quality (Peters et al. 2007). Reducing cognitive effort was very important for less numerate people, who appeared to have particular difficulty finding decision critical information located within large tables and interpreting statistics framed so that lower numbers actually represented better outcomes.

This "less is more" principle is especially important when the information is complex. For example, when providing information about the risks and benefits of a treatment, limiting the number of numerical calculations that participants are required to perform increases their ability to determine whether or not the treatment is beneficial (Waters et al. 2006). Women facing breast cancer treatment decisions involving risk tradeoffs who viewed graphs describing only survival risk statistics had better risk recall than participants who viewed graphs that included data about survival, mortality due to cancer, and mortality due to all causes, Zikmund-Fisher et al. (2010). Similarly, risk assessment tools that provide estimates that are excessively complex (i.e., are more specific than integers) may lose credibility among audience members without increasing accurate recall (Witteman et al. 2011).

Limiting how much risk information is provided at one time may also be useful. For example, one study compared presenting survival information about adjuvant treatment options following breast cancer surgery sequentially (one at one time) versus all at once. Sequential presentations resulted in higher knowledge and enabled less numerate women's treatment choices to become sensitive to the magnitude of achievable treatment benefit (Zikmund-Fisher et al. 2011).

In general, enabling patients to engage in less cognitive effort when making decisions is beneficial. However, it would be premature to say that all risk communicators need to do is provide the most basic information. We again emphasize the importance of considering the goals of the communication, the task that the individual needs to complete, and the amount of precision required

to achieve that task. In some situations, such as motivating homeowners to test for radon, only a broad gist-level understanding may be required. In others, such as those that require patients to trade off multiple risks and benefits of different treatment options, patients may need to understand more detailed numerical information (Zikmund-Fisher, in press). It is clear that much more research is necessary to understand cognitive burden and to find the balance between too much and too little information.

Conclusions and Implications for Practice

Risk communication is a challenging task, in part because risk is abstract. People do not literally experience risk (although, as noted above, they may experience anticipatory emotions about risk). What people do experience are outcomes, the good or bad things that happen to us. As a result, we all seek certainty—we want to know what will or will not happen to us. Yet the uncertainty present in the world means that risk communication is fundamentally about clarifying the many shades of "maybe." For example, it requires someone to understand that a 6 % risk is much less likely than a 60 % risk in the mathematical probability sense of those terms, yet also accept the possibility that the 6 % risk event might happen while the 60 % might not.

Our discussion has highlighted the theoretical background of risk communication and presented practical guidance for clinicians, health educators, and anyone who wishes to help people make sense of their health risks. Box 1 summarizes our most critical messages: People only need risk data for specific purposes, and the design of optimal risk communications depends on identifying those purposes and systematically choosing numerical formats, visual displays, comparative data, and other elements that will lead message recipients to the same "gist" understanding of the risk that the communicator has.

Although the field of risk communication has seen enormous recent growth in its evidence base to support improved practices, many important questions do remain. For example, although much work has explored the use of static visual displays, only a few papers have explored the use of animated or interactive displays to communicate risk (e.g., Kaphingst et al. 2009). The interaction between numeracy and different risk communication methods is another important area of research. While it is clear that some risk communication approaches benefit less numerate people more than they do people with higher numeracy skills, it remains unclear whether presentations designed for a low numeracy audience might sometimes be nonoptimal for more numerate recipients.

One major question is how, or even whether, to address uncertainty about risk, often referred to as ambiguity or second-order uncertainty. Discussing ambiguity can be important since it is related to the strength of evidence supporting a risk estimate. In formal risk analyses, such uncertainty about risk estimates can be explored systematically through sensitivity analyses. However, the practical relevance of communicating ambiguity is less clear. A long-standing line of psychological research shows that in most situations people are ambiguity-averse. That is, people will prefer precisely known risks versus ambiguous risks even if they known risk are worse. Several researchers have explored novel visual displays and other approaches to discussing ambiguity, with mixed success (Han et al. 2012; Politi et al. 2007; Ancker et al.s 2011 #2176). Our perspective is that communication of risk ambiguity may be necessary in certain contexts, but many communication situations would be well served by simpler "gist" statements that certain risks are more "well known" versus others.

The ultimate measure of effective risk communication is whether it translates risk data first into risk meaning and then into risk actions. We care about improving risk understanding not as a goal in and of itself, but because of what that understanding can accomplish: improved and value-concordant healthcare decisions, willingness to undertake preventive actions to prevent or mitigate future harms, and an improved ability to make sense of the inherent uncertainty in the world. So perhaps a metaphor for risk communication techniques is of a roadmap. Like maps, risk communications can be very useful for guiding people, but only if you know where you want to send them and you select approaches that can take them in the right direction without getting them lost along the way.

Practice Recommendations

- Have clear and narrow goals for any risk communication.
    - Understand that changing beliefs may not change behavior.
- Use minimalist design: "less is more."
    - Understand that less numerate people need simpler and more focused communications in order to use risk information in decision making.
    - Understand that while quantitative risk data are helpful for some types of risk communication, they may inhibit meaningful understanding in other situations.
- Make sure that your communication evokes the intended emotional and/or evaluative "gist" meaning.
    - "Gist" often matters more than specific numerical recall or knowledge.
- Select the numerical formats, comparative data, and/or visual formats that align best with the intended "gist" and target goals.
    - Comparing one risk number versus another increases evaluability but also creates strong emotional meanings that may or may not be helpful.
    - Visuals (e.g., icon arrays, bar graphs) can clarify risk data and especially part-whole relationships, but different graphics emphasize different gist meanings (e.g., levels of risk vs. incremental risk vs. trends of risk over time).

- Avoid 1-in-X formats that change the risk denominator.
- Test the communication with the target audience prior to dissemination
  - Understand that the meaning you intend to convey may not be the meaning that your audience infers.

Acknowlegments Erika Waters was supported by Mentored Research Scholar Grant MRSG-11-214-01-CPPB and Brian Zikmund-Fisher was supported by Mentored Research Scholar Grant MRSG-06-130-01-CPPB from the American Cancer Society.

References

Ancker, J. S., Senathirajah, Y., Kukafka, R., & Starren, J. (2006). Design features of graphs in health risk communication: A systematic review. *Journal of the American Medical Informatics Association, 13*(6), 608–618.

Ancker, J. S., Weber, E. U., Kukafka, R. (2011). Effects of game-like interactive graphics on risk perceptions and decisions.*Medical Decision Making, 31*(1), 130–42. doi:10.1177/0272989X10364847

Betsch, T., & Glockner, A. (2010). Intuition in judgment and decision making: Extensive thinking without effort. *Psychological Inquiry, 21*(4), 279–294.

Brewer, N. T. (2011). Goals. In B. Fischhoff, N. T. Brewer, & J. S. Downs (Eds.), *Communicating risks and benefits: An evidence-based user's guide* (pp. 3–10). Silver Spring, MD: U.S. Department of Health And Human Services, Food and Drug Administration.

Brewer, N. T., Chapman, G. B., Gibbons, F. X., Gerrard, M., & McCaul, K. D. (2007). A meta-analysis of the relationship between risk perception and health behavior: The example of vaccination. *Health Psychology, 26*(2), 136–145.

Budescu, D. V., & Wallsten, T. S. (1985). Consistency in interpretation of probabilistic phrases. *Organizational Behavior and Human Decision Processes, 36*, 391–485.

Cialdini, R. (2008). *Influence: Science and practice* (5th ed.). Boston: Pearson.

Conner, M., & Norman, P. (Eds.). (1995). *Predicting health behaviour*. Buckingham/Philadelphia: Open University Press.

Covey, J. (2007). A meta-analysis of the effects of presenting treatment benefits in different formats. *Medical Decision Making, 27*, 638–654.

Cuite, C., Weinstein, N. D., Emmons, K., & Colditz, G. (2008). A test of numeric formats for risk communication. *Medical Decision Making, 28*(3), 377–384.

Fagerlin, A., Zikmund-Fisher, B. J., & Ubel, P. A. (2007). "If I'm better than average, then I'm ok?": Comparative information influences beliefs about risk and benefits. *Patient Education and Counseling, 69*(1–3), 140–144.

Finkel, A. M. (2008). Perceiving others' perceptions of risk: still a task for Sisyphus. *Annals of the New York Academy of Sciences, 1128*, 121–137.

Fischhoff, B. (1995). Risk perception and communication unplugged: Twenty years of progress. *Risk Analysis, 15*(2), 137–145.

Fischhoff, B. (1999). Why (cancer) communication can be hard. *Journal of the National Cancer Institute Monographs, 25*, 7–13.

Gaissmaier, W., Wegwarth, O., Skopec, D., Muller, A. S., Broschinski, S., & Politi, M. C. (2012). Numbers can be worth a thousand pictures: Individual differences in understanding graphical and numerical representations of health-related information. *Health Psychology, 31*(3), 286–296.

Galesic, M., & Garcia-Retamero, R. (2011). Graph literacy: A cross-cultural comparison. *Medical Decision Making, 31*(3), 444–457.

Galesic, M., Gigerenzer, G., & Straubinger, N. (2009). Natural frequencies help older adults and people with low numeracy to evaluate medical screening tests. *Medical Decision Making, 29*(3), 368–371.

Garcia-Retamero, R., & Galesic, M. (2010a). How to reduce the effect of framing on messages about health. *Journal of General Internal Medicine, 25*(12), 1323–1329.

Garcia-Retamero, R., & Galesic, M. (2010b). Who profits from visual aids: Overcoming challenges in people's understanding of risks. *Social Science and Medicine, 70*(7), 1019–1025.

Garcia-Retamero, R., Okan, Y., & Cokely, E. T. (2012). Using visual aids to improve communication of risks about health: A review. *Scientific World Journal, 2012*, 562637. doi:10.1100/2012/562637.

Gigerenzer, G. (1996). The psychology of good judgment: Frequency formats and simple algorithms. *Medical Decision Making, 16*(3), 273–280.

Gullion, J. S., Henry, L., & Gullion, G. (2008). Deciding to opt out of childhood vaccination mandates. *Public Health Nursing, 25*(5), 401–408.

Han, P. K., Klein, W. M., Killam, B., Lehman, T., Massett, H., & Freedman, A. N. (2012). Representing randomness in the communication of individualized cancer risk estimates: Effects on cancer risk perceptions, worry, and subjective uncertainty about risk. *Patient Education and Counseling, 86*(1), 106–113.

Hawley, S. T., Zikmund-Fisher, B. J., Ubel, P., Jancovic, A., Lucas, T., & Fagerlin, A. (2008). The impact of the format of graphical presentation on health-related knowledge and treatment choices. *Patient Education and Counseling, 73*, 448–455.

Hsee, C. K., Blount, S., Loewenstein, G. F., & Bazerman, M. H. (1999). Preference reversals between joint and separate evaluations of options: a review and theoretical analysis. *Psychological Bulletin, 125*(5), 576–590.

Janssen, E., van Osch, L., de Vries, H., & Lechner, L. (2011). Measuring risk perceptions of skin cancer: Reliability and validity of different operationalizations. *British Journal of Health Psychology, 16*(Pt 1), 92–112.

Kahneman, D., & Frederick, S. (2002). Representativeness revisited: Attribute substitution in intuitive judgment. In T. Gilovich, D. Griffin, & D. Kahneman (Eds.), *Heuristics and biases* (pp. 49–61). New York, NY: Cambridge University Press.

Kaphingst, K. A., Persky, S., McCall, C., Lachance, C., Beall, A. C., & Blascovich, J. (2009). Testing communication strategies to convey genomic concepts using virtual reality technology. *J Health Commun, 14*(4), 384–399.

Keller, C., Siegrist, M., & Visschers, V. (2009). Effect of risk ladder format on risk perception in high- and low-numerate individuals. *Risk Analysis, 29*(9), 1255–1264.

Kutner, M., Greenberg, E., Jin, Y., & Paulsen, C. (2006). *The health literacy of America's adults: Results from the 2003 national assessment of adult literacy.* Washington, DC: U.S. Department of Education, National Center for Health Statistics.

Lerman, C. (1995). Effects of individualized breast cancer risk counseling: A randomized trial. *Journal of the National Cancer Institute, 87*, 286–292.

Leventhal, H., Brissette, I., & Leventhal, E. A. (2003). The common-sense model of self-regulation of health and illness. In L. D. Cameron & H. Leventhal (Eds.), *The self-regulation of health and illness behaviour* (pp. 42–65). New York, NY: Routledge.

Levy, A. G., Weinstein, N., Kidney, E., Scheld, S., & Guarnaccia, P. (2008). Lay and expert interpretations of cancer cluster evidence. *Risk Analysis, 28*(6), 1531–1538.

Lipkus, I. M. (2007). Numeric, verbal, and visual formats of conveying health risks: Suggested best practices and future recommendations. *Medical Decision Making, 27*(5), 696–713.

Lipkus, I. M., & Hollands, J. G. (1999). The visual communication of risk. *Journal of the National Cancer Institute Monographs, 25*(1), 149–163.

Lipkus, I. M., & Klein, W. M. (2006). Effects of communicating social comparison information on risk perceptions for colorectal cancer. *Journal of Health Communication, 11*(4), 391–407.

Lipkus, I. M., & Peters, E. (2009). Understanding the role of numeracy in health: Proposed theoretical framework and practical insights. *Health Education Behavior, 36*(6), 1065–1081.

Lipkus, I. M., Samsa, G., & Rimer, B. K. (2001). General performance on a numeracy scale among highly educated samples. *Medical Decision Making, 21*(1), 37–44.

Loewenstein, G. F., Hsee, C. K., Weber, E. U., & Welch, N. (2001). Risk as feelings. *Psychological Bulletin, 127*(2), 267–286.

McGuire, W. J. (1984). Public communication as a strategy for inducing health-promoting behavior change. *Preventive Medicine, 13*(3), 299–313.

McNeil, B. J., Pauker, S. G., Sox, H., & Tversky, A. (1982). On the elicitation of preferences for alternative therapies. *New England Journal of Medicine, 306*(21), 1259–1262.

McQueen, A., Vernon, S. W., & Swank, P. R. (2012). Construct definition and scale development for defensive information processing: An application to colorectal cancer screening. *Health Psychology,*. doi:10.1037/a0027311.

National Cancer Institute. (2009). *Health information national trends survey (HINTS) items for years 2003–2007.* Retrieved June 7, 2010, from http://hints.cancer.gov/questions/all-questions1.jsp

Nelson, W., Reyna, V. F., Fagerlin, A., Lipkus, I., & Peters, E. (2008). Clinical implications of numeracy: Theory and practice. *Annals of Behavioral Medicine, 35*, 261–274.

Peters, E., Dieckmann, N., Dixon, A., Hibbard, J. H., & Mertz, C. K. (2007). Less is more in presenting quality information to consumers. *Medical Care Research Reviews, 64*(2), 169–190.

Peters, E., Dieckmann, N. F., Vastfjall, D., Mertz, C. K., Slovic, P., & Hibbard, J. H. (2009). Bringing meaning to numbers: the impact of evaluative categories on decisions. *Journal of Experimental Psychology Applied, 15*(3), 213–227.

Peters, E., Hart, P. S., & Fraenkel, L. (2011). Informing patients: The influence of numeracy, framing, and format of side effect information on risk perceptions. *Medical Decision Making, 31*(3), 432–436.

Peters, E., Vastfjall, D., Garling, T., & Slovic, P. (2006a). Affect and decision making: A "hot" topic. *Journal of Behavioral Decision Making, 19*(2), 79–85.

Peters, E., Vastfjall, D., Slovic, P., Mertz, C. K., Mazzocco, K., & Dickert, S. (2006b). Numeracy and decision making. *Psychological Science, 17*(5), 407–413.

Pighin, S., Savadori, L., Barilli, E., Cremonesi, L., Ferrari, M., & Bonnefon, J. F. (2011). The 1-in-X effect on the subjective assessment of medical probabilities. *Medical Decision Making, 31*(5), 721–729.

Politi, M. C., Han, P. K. J., & Col, N. F. (2007). Communicating the uncertainty of harms and benefits of medical interventions. *Medical Decision Making, 27*, 681–695.

Roth, E., Morgan, M. G., Fischhoff, B., Lave, L., & Bostrom, A. (1990). What do we know about making risk comparisons? *Risk Analysis, 10*(3), 375–387.

Sheridan, S. L., Pignone, M. P., & Lewis, C. L. (2003). A randomized comparison of patients' understanding of number needed to treat and other common risk reduction formats. *Journal of General Internal Medicine, 18*, 884–892.

Slovic, P. (2000). *The perception of risk.* London: Earthscan Publications Ltd.

Smith, E. R., & DeCoster, J. (2000). Dual-Process models in social and cognitive psychology: Conceptual integration and links to underlying memory systems. *Personality and Social Psychology Review, 4*(2), 108–131.

Squiers, L. B., Holden, D. J., Dolina, S. E., Kim, A. E., Bann, C. M., & Renaud, J. M. (2011). The public's response to the U.S. preventive services task force's 2009 recommendations on mammography screening. *American Journal of Preventive Medicine, 40*(5),497–504.

Stone, E. R., Sieck, W. R., Bull, B. E., Yates, J. F., Parks, S. C., & Rush, C. J. (2003). Foreground:background salience: Explaining the effects of graphical displays on risk avoidance. *Organizational Behavior and Human Decision Processes, 90*, 19–36.

Waters, E. A., Sullivan, H. W., Nelson, W., & Hesse, B. W. (2009). What is my cancer risk? Identifying how internet-based cancer risk calculators convey individualized risk estimates to the public. *Journal of Medical Internet Research, 11*(3), e33. doi:10.2196/jmir.1222

Waters, E. A., Weinstein, N. D., Colditz, G. A., & Emmons, K. (2006). Formats for improving risk communication in medical tradeoff decisions. *Journal of Health Communication, 11*(2), 167–182.

Waters, E. A., Weinstein, N. D., Colditz, G. A., & Emmons, K. (2007a). Aversion to side effects in preventive medical treatment decisions. *British Journal of Health Psychology, 12*, 383–401.

Waters, E. A., Weinstein, N. D., Colditz, G. A., & Emmons, K. (2007b). Reducing aversion to side effects in preventive medical treatment decisions. *Journal of Experimental Psychology: Applied, 13*(1), 11–21.

Weinstein, N. D., Atwood, K., Puleo, E., Fletcher, R., Colditz, G., & Emmons, K. M. (2004). Colon cancer: Risk perceptions and risk communication. *Journal of Health Communication., 9*, 53–65.

Weinstein, N. D., Sandman, P. M., & Roberts, N. E. (1989). *Communicating effectively about risk magnitudes, phase one.* Washington, DC: United States Environmental Protection Agency.

Willis, G. B. (2004). *Cognitive interviewing: A tool for improving questionnaire design.* Thousand Oaks, CA: Sage Publications.

Windschitl, P. D. (2002). Judging the accuracy of a likelihood judgment: The case of smoking risk. *Journal of Behavioral Decision Making, 15*(1), 19–35.

Windschitl, P. D., Martin, R., & Flugstad, A. R. (2002). Context and the interpretation of likelihood information: The role of intergroup comparisons on perceived vulnerability. *Journal of Personality and Social Psychology, 82*(5), 742–755.

Windschitl, P. D., & Wells, G. L. (1996). Measuring psychological uncertainty: Verbal versus numeric methods. *Journal of Experimental Psychology: Applied, 2*(4), 343–364.

Witteman, H. O., Zikmund-Fisher, B. J., Waters, E. A., Gavaruzzi, T., & Fagerlin, A. (2011). Risk estimates from an online risk calculator are more believable and recalled better when expressed as integers. *Journal of Medical Internet Research, 13*(3), e54. doi:10.2196/jmir.1656.

Woloshin, S., & Schwartz, L. M. (2011). Communicating data about the benefits and harms of treatment: A randomized trial. *Annals of Internal Medicine, 155*(2), 87–96.

Woloshin, S., Schwartz, L. M., & Welch, H. G. (2002). Risk charts: Putting cancer in context. *Journal of the National Cancer Institute, 94*(11), 799–804.

Zajonc, R. B. (1980). Feeling and thinking: Preferences need no inferences. *American Psychologist, 35*(2), 151–175.

Zikmund-Fisher, B. J. (2011). Time to retire the 1-in-X risk format. *Medical Decision Making, 31*(5), 703–704.

Zikmund-Fisher, B. J. (in press). The right tool is what they need, not what we have: A taxonomy of appropriate levels of precision in patient risk communication. *Medical Care Research and Review.*

Zikmund-Fisher, B. J., Angott, A. M., & Ubel, P. A. (2011). The benefits of discussing adjuvant therapies one at a time instead of all at once. *Breast Cancer Research and Treatment, 129*(1), 79–87.

Zikmund-Fisher, B. J., Fagerlin, A., Keeton, K., & Ubel, P. A. (2007a). Does labeling prenatal screening test results as negative or positive affect a woman's responses? *American Journal of Obstetrics and Gynecology, 197*(5), 528 e521–e526. doi:10.1016/j.ajog.2007.03.076

Zikmund-Fisher, B. J., Fagerlin, A., Roberts, T. R., Derry, H. A., & Ubel, P. A. (2008a). Alternate methods of framing information about medication side effects: Incremental risk versus total risk of occurrence. *Journal of Health Communication, 13*, 107–124.

Zikmund-Fisher, B. J., Fagerlin, A., & Ubel, P. A. (2007b). Mortality versus survival graphs: Improving temporal consistency in perceptions of treatment effectiveness. *Patient Education and Counseling, 66*(1), 100–107.

Zikmund-Fisher, B. J., Fagerlin, A., & Ubel, P. A. (2010). A demonstration of "less can be more" in risk graphics. *Medical Decision Making, 30*(6), 661–671.

Zikmund-Fisher, B. J., Ubel, P. A., Smith, D. M., Derry, H. A., McClure, J. B., Stark, A. ... Fagerlin, A. (2008b). Communicating side effect risks in a tamoxifen prophylaxis decision aid: The debiasing influence of pictographs. *Patient Education & Counseling, 73*(2), 209–214.

Decision Aids: Do They Work?

20

Nananda F. Col and Vicky Springmann

Practical Implications

- Decision Aids (DAs) are educational tools designed to help patients make better decisions about their health that reflect their personal health history, circumstances, values, goals and preferences.
- Well-designed DAs have been shown to improve patients' knowledge and risk perceptions, reduce decisional conflict and passivity in decision-making, and change decisions about treatment.
- The impact of DAs depends on characteristics of the DA itself, the context in which it is used (which decision, which population), how it is introduced, and the outcome measures used to assess effectiveness.

Background

DAs are a type of decision support tool that are designed to help patients make healthcare choices that reflect their preferences, values, and risks. They are especially helpful when there is no clear best choice because of uncertain evidence or toss-ups between the benefits and harms of treatment (O'Connor et al. 1999; Kassirer 1983). Thus patient DAs often focus on so-called "preference-based" decisions, where the best strategy for an individual depends on their preferences for the benefit/harm tradeoffs inherent in a particular choice. However, DAs can be applied to a broad range of clinical decisions, helping patients organize complex clinical information and predicting future outcomes given their baseline characteristics and under different treatment scenarios. Some DAs are intended to promote informed decision-making (without involving the clinician), others to promote the process of shared decision making between the patient and clinician (Harris et al. 2001; O'Connor and Edwards 2001; Charles et al. 1997). Some decision support tools advocate a particular choice (i.e., smoking cessation) or help manage at-risk patients with 'best practices'. DAs thus represent a heterogeneous group of decision support tools, complicating any global statement about their effectiveness using any single metric.

Defining what works: Determining whether DAs "work" is a messy enterprise because there is no consensus on which measures should be used to assess their effectiveness, or even on what the aims of DAs should be.

The International Patient Decision Aids Standards (IPDAS) Collaboration (2005), a multidisciplinary effort to establish an internationally approved set of criteria for evaluating the

N.F. Col (✉) · V. Springmann
Shared Decision Making Resources, Georgetown, ME, USA
e-mail: nanfcol@gmail.com

V. Springmann
e-mail: Vicky.springmann@gmail.com

© Springer Science+Business Media New York 2016
M.A. Diefenbach et al. (eds.), *Handbook of Health Decision Science*,
DOI 10.1007/978-1-4939-3486-7_20

quality of DAs, concluded that the ultimate goal of DAs is to improve the quality of decision making, and that high-quality decisions are those that result in individuals choosing and/or receiving the health care interventions that are most consistent with their informed and considered values. However, there is as yet no metric for measuring the congruence between an individual's values and the health care options they choose and/or receive (Sepucha and Ozanne 2010). Scores of different measures of effectiveness have been used to gauge the effectiveness of DAs (Stacey et al. 2011). Many of these measures were adopted from other fields or hastily derived with limited or no formal validation. The most commonly used measures sought to address the impact of DAs on treatment decisions, patient knowledge, and the decision-making process (Kennedy 2003).

Evolving concepts of effectiveness: Ideally, we would like to know *whether people are better off if they use a DA as part of clinical care*. But our conception of what it means to be 'better off' has evolved, as has the context in which clinical care is delivered. The steady rise in consumerism, with patients desiring more involvement in decisions about their health, has gradually shifted the balance of power in clinical decision-making away from physician autonomy and towards a more shared model. Many DAs were designed with the goal of helping patients participate in decisions about their health by giving patients unbiased, evidence-based information about their treatment options. These DAs promoted 'informed decision making' and typically targeted the patient, not the health care provider.

Outcome measures commonly used to determine their effectiveness focused on whether patients had enough information about their options (knowledge measures), had realistic expectations (risk perceptions), and were satisfied with the process of making a decision (satisfaction measures). A variety of other short-term measures were used to examine the processes of decision making, most of which were obtained shortly after making a decision. DAs were deemed effective if they improved knowledge, more closely aligned patient expectations with reality, improved

satisfaction with the process of decision making, or reduced passivity in decision making. However, these outcomes are not without controversy. Changes in knowledge do not necessarily correspond to a change in understanding or behavior (Helweg-Larsen and Collins 1997; Krahe and Reiss 1995). Knowledge (e.g. recall of risk information) does not mean the patient understands the meaning of probability statements nor their relevance to decision making (Charles et al. 2005).

Another frequently used process measure is the 'decisional conflict scale,' which captures "uncertainty about which course of action to take when choice among competing actions involves risk, loss, regret, or challenge to personal life values." A DA was thought to be effective if it lowered decisional conflict, based on the assumption that decisional conflict is an undesirable state that is detrimental to decision-making. This measure was also called into question. For some difficult decisions, decision conflict might promote appropriate deliberation about alternative outcomes and personal goals and ongoing engagement in the decision-making process (Charles et al. 2005).

Tension between two powerful movements within clinical medicine further shaped the context in which DAs were evaluated (Shortell et al. 2007). One is evidence-based medicine (EBM), which identifies 'best evidence' to guide clinical practice. The other is the shift from *disease-centered* care to *patient-centered* care. The latter encourages patients to select the treatment that is best for their particular circumstances and preferences, rather than the treatment that is most effective in eradicating or preventing a disease. Patient-centered care focuses on the differences between individuals, such as personal circumstances, race/ethnicity, treatment goals, preferences and values (Kupfer and Bond 2012), which can affect health care decisions and outcomes. On the other hand, EBM focuses on commonalities among patients and blurs individual differences (Entwistle and O'Donnell 2001). Unfortunately, the 'best evidence,' typically derived from large randomized controlled trials, rarely supports or informs patient-centered decision-making. This is because it focuses on the experiences of large cohorts, blurring differences in many individual characteristics. Furthermore, EBM focuses on effectiveness, not side effects, rarely accounts for patient preferences, focuses on prevention of a disease (using a narrow conception of health), not health or quality of life (using a broad conception of health), and application of EBM guidelines is often paternalistic. Ideally, DAs would bridge both EBM and patient-centered care (Healy 2006; Elstein 2004), though tension arises when DAs are used in situations where there is a health advantages to one treatment over another, such as in decisions about managing chronic diseases. Informed patients may elect to pursue a course of action that improves their perceived quality of life, but possibly at the expense of worsening indicators of their chronic disease.

Rising healthcare costs coupled with an aging population and an economic downturn have increased pressure to make the best use of limited health care resources, catalyzing changes in the perceived goals of DAs. Recognizing that healthcare utilization is largely driven by clinical decisions made by providers and patients, attention has increasingly been focused on how these decisions are made and how to influence them. When clinical decisions were primarily made by physicians with little input by patients, attention was focused on changing providers' clinical decisions by applying EBM clinical practice guidelines, preauthorization requirements (Park et al. 1986), academic drug detailing (Avorn and Soumerai 1983), and other programs. With more patient involvement in decision-making came more interest in using DA to influence those decisions. Simultaneously, practice variations were reported for many conditions, leading to the conclusion that the utilization of common treatments can be driven by specialist supply, which can result in ineffective, harmful treatments that are not in the best interests of patients. DA were seen as instruments to combat unwarranted practice variations, assuming that an informed patient would not want or accept a treatment that was unnecessary or harmful (Kuehn 2009). Many DAs were developed specifically targeting treatments or tests that had been identified as being overused (e.g.,

prostatectomy for benign prostatic hypertrophy, hysterectomy for menorrhagia, prostate specific antigen to screen for prostate cancer). When a few studies reported a trend towards decreased utilization of invasive procedures (O'Connor et al. 2003), DAs received considerable attention from third party payers and policy makers as a tool to drive down demand for health care services. The clear expectation was that patients who use a DA will opt for less aggressive and less costly treatment, resulting in lower use and lower costs (Kuehn 2009). Many DAs were developed and tested by an insurance company-supported foundation (Reuters press release 2007).

Evidence exploring the impact of DAs: The impact of DAs has been the subject of considerable research since the 1980s (Chaudhry et al. 2006), when the first randomized controlled trial of a DA was published (Herrera et al. 1983). The most comprehensive source of evidence is the Cochrane Collaborative Review, a meta-analysis of 86 published randomized controlled trials involving 20,209 participants comparing DAs to usual care and/or alternative interventions. This evidence, supplemented with other sources, is summarized below. Most DA trials tracked a number of endpoints, but were powered on short-term decision-making process measures. Typically other endpoints (such as treatment choice or adherence) were included as secondary or tertiary endpoints. For this reason, the most robust findings describe the impact of DAs on short-term process measures; few were adequately powered to assess the impact of DA on long-term outcome measures such as treatment choice. None were designed to measure the cost-effectiveness of DAs. It is important to note that the findings reported here pertain exclusively to the impact of patient DAs, not to other approaches to introducing SDM into clinical practice.

Impact of DAs on Patient's State of Mind and Health

Knowledge: Knowledge typically was assessed through the use of unvalidated ad hoc questions asking patients to recall information presented in the DA. The proportion of accurate responses was then calculated. DAs consistently increased patient's knowledge. More detailed DAs were more effective than simpler DAs. Some studies found that knowledge scores were higher only when the DA was administered during (as compared to prior to) the consultation (Partin et al. 2004; Hamann et al. 2006; Trevena et al. 2008; Watson et al. 2006; Weymiller et al. 2007).

Accurate risk perceptions: Risk perceptions and expectations about treatment effects were measured in 16 studies using unvalidated ad hoc scales asking patients to estimate their perceived probabilities of outcomes, before and after exposed to a DA. Correct responses were those that corresponded to the scientific evidence reported in that DA. DAs that described outcomes and probabilities were more likely to result in more accurate risk perceptions. Exposure to a DA with expressed probabilities resulted in a higher proportion of people with accurate risk perceptions, as did administering the DA during (versus before) the consultation (Weymiller et al. 2007).

Decisional Conflict measures self-reported effective decision-making, overall uncertainty, and the factors contributing to uncertainty, including feeling uninformed, feeling unclear about values, or feeling unsupported in decision-making. DAs fairly consistently reduced their overall decisional conflict and feeling uninformed, unclear about personal values, or unsupported. DAs had no impact on the uncertainty subscale. One study found a greater impact among lower literacy subjects.

Anxiety: DA may lower anxiety related to a treatment decision, but the impact is very short lived (less than one month). Most (19 of 20 studies) used the State Anxiety Inventory (Spielberger 1970). Some trials found DA users to have significantly lower anxiety within 1 month (Montgomery et al. 2007; Protheroe et al. 2007; Green et al. 2004), but no differences were found at one, 3, 6, or 12 months.

Health outcomes: Using scales such as the Medical Outcomes Study 36-item Short-Form Health Survey (SF-36), the 12-item Short-form,

or the Euroqol EQ-5D, DA did not have any impact on mental health or social health ($n = 7$). No impact was reported for condition-specific health outcomes ($n = 9$). Two studies reported improvements in emotional (Vuorma 2003) or physical (Kennedy et al. 2002) role functioning for abnormal uterine bleeding, and improvements in general health and physical function for benign prostatic disease (Barry et al. 1997).

Patient behavior:

Passivity: Passivity in making decisions is one of the few behaviors targeted by DA.

The Control Preference Scale (Degner and Sloan 1992) measures preferred or actual participation in decision-making. DAs reduced the proportion of people who were passive in decision-making.

However, patient self-report of the interaction can be inaccurate if respondents do not know what a meaningful shared decision process entails. For example, patients who simply agreed to follow their physician's recommendation may erroneously report this as sharing decision-making responsibility with their provider.

Feeling undecided: DAs resulted in a lower proportion of people remaining undecided.

Adherence: DAs could potentially improve adherence because a patient may be more likely to adhere to a treatment that they were involved in choosing. However, measuring the impact of DA on adherence is problematic because adherence is variably defined, variably ascertained (e.g., patient self-report versus physician report), and assessed at different time points after initiating treatment (ranging from 6 weeks to 3 years). No difference in adherence was seen in 7 out of 8 trials (warfarin vs. aspirin for atrial fibrillation (Man-Son-Hing et al. 1999), oral bisphosphonates for osteoporosis (Oakley and Walley 2006), blood pressure medications (Montgomery et al. 2003), antidepressants (Loh et al. 2007), statins (Weymiller et al. 2007), or menopausal hormone replacement) (Rothert et al. 1997). One trial found lower adherence to diabetes medication among DA users (97.5 vs. 100 %) (Mullan et al. 2009).

Patient-Provider Communication

Shared decision-making processes: DAs are intended to promote SDM, but few trials examined SDM as an outcome. The OPTION scale assesses the extent to which clinicians actively involve patients in decision making, based on audio-recordings.[1] Two trials found that DAs resulted in more SDM, using the OPTION scale (Weymiller et al. 2007; Mullan et al. 2009). The effect was higher with the DA if it was used within the clinical encounter. Another study found that more patients with coronary heart disease discussed their condition and a plan to reduce their risk with their provider after using a DA (Sheridan et al. 2006).

Patient-provider communication: The COM-RADE (Edwards et al. 2003) scale includes subscales for patient-reported satisfaction with physician communication and confidence in the decision made. No trials included in the Cochrane Review used the COMRADE scale or other patient-provider communication measures.

Patient-centered care: While there are strong moral justifications for more patient-centered care (McWhinney 1995; Grol et al. 1990), there is no empirical evidence that patient-centeredness affects outcomes. Different measures have been developed to assess patient-centeredness but they have low levels of agreement with one another, have relatively low concurrent validity, and variable construct validity (Mead and Bower 2000). No DA trials have assessed their impact on patient-centered care.

Decision-Making Processes

Values-congruent choice: No measures exist for this construct Sepucha and Ozanne (2010). Thirteen studies that were described as reporting on this outcome in the Cochrane Review in fact measured concepts somewhat related to but not equivalent to values-congruent choice. Five of the eight studies that were pooled in the meta-analysis under this label used the multidimensional measure of informed choice (Michie et al. 2002), which measures knowledge and behavioral intent, but not values. The remaining three studies

assessed the extent to which treatment choice was consistent with a single identified preference (Frosch and Bhatnagar 2008) (e.g., 'general concern about prostate cancer,' not specific concerns about sexual and urinary function). This approach does not appear appropriate for treatment decisions with several important attributes, or when these attributes change as patients learn about the condition (78 % of patients with prostate cancer changed the attributes they considered important as they learned more about their condition) (Feldman-Stewart et al. 2004). Additionally, these trials addressed a narrow range of decisions—6 addressed screening decisions, two addressed menopausal hormone replacement. Several studies (5) did not present quantitative data that could be pooled. The Cochrane Review reported that DAs with explicit values clarification compared to those without explicit values clarification resulted in a higher proportion of patients achieving decisions that were informed and consistent with their values (RR 1.25; 95 % CI 1.03–1.52; $n = 8$). Arguably, this evidence could have been more accurately described by saying that DAs with explicit values clarification compared to those without explicit values clarification resulted in a higher proportion of patients achieving decisions that were informed and consistent with their intended behaviors.

Satisfaction with the decision or decision-making process: Using scales such as the satisfaction with the decision scale (Holmes-Rovner et al. 1996), DAs either had no impact on or improved satisfaction or ($n = 12$). However, satisfaction has been found to be driven by expectations, with high satisfaction often reflecting lower expectations rather than high performance (Cleary 1998).

Decision regret: Five trials measured regret about the decision made using the self-reported decisional regret scale (Brehaut et al. 2003), with none finding a statistically significant difference in regret. However, regret could confound the decision process with probabilistic outcomes occurring following the decision. Additionally, responses may vary over time, especially when side effects for different treatments develop over different time horizons.

---

[1]http://www.optioninstrument.com/

Confidence: Three out of five trials found that DAs improved patient confidence in making a decision or engaging in a discussion with their practitioner found.

Healthcare system

Treatment choice: Treatment choice has been measured using patient self-report of the treatment chosen (42 trials) or their preferred or intended treatment option (23 trials), if they had not yet made the decision. DAs have greater influence among patients who have not already made up their mind. DAs have a variable effect on decisions about surgery. No impact was observed for minor elective surgery (circumcision, surgical abortion, or dental orthognathic surgery). The combined overall impact of DAs on major elective surgery (11 trials) found a nonsignificant trend toward fewer choosing surgery (RR 0.80, 95 % CI 0.64–1.00) (Stacey et al. 2011). Only four studies reported statistically significant results. One found higher rates of surgery (114 % more surgery for prophylactic mastectomy), three found lower rates (for cardiac revascularization, mastectomy, and orchiectomy). One study found DA users had a fivefold higher rate of prostatectomy (nonsignificant) (Murray et al. 2001). Another trial, using a nearly identical study design and the exact same DA, found it decreased in the rate of prostatectomy by 44 % (nonsignificant) (Barry et al. 1997). One explanation could be that DA helped to shift utilization rates closer to the 'appropriate' rate, given that the first trial was conducted in the UK, where baseline rates may likely have reflected underutilization, while the second trial was conducted in the US, where baseline rates likely reflected overutilization. The hypothesis that DA can potentially move utilization rates toward the' appropriate' rate is also supported by a study of elective spine surgery. The DA increased rates of surgery among patients with underlying spinal stenosis (39 vs. 29 %, $p = 0.4$), a condition where surgery may be underutilized, but decreased surgery rates among those with herniated disks (32 vs. 47 %, p 0.05 %), a condition where surgery may be over-utilized. The net effect (26 vs. 33 %, $p = 0.08$) combines both of

these rates and conveys little clinical meaning given the disparate events being pooled. To estimate whether DA can affect decisions about surgery, the absolute value of the difference would be a more meaningful estimate. The expectation that DA will drive patients consistently toward one treatment path or away from another stands in stark conflict with the recognition that there is no 'right' decision for preference-based decisions, but rather that these decisions depend on one's personal risk factors, circumstances, values, goals, and preferences. The validity of pooling these utilization rates, as was reported in the Cochrane Review, has not been established.

The impact of DA on uptake of prostate cancer screening (PSA) was similarly variable, ranging from increasing rates by 14 % to decreasing rates by 47 %. The net impact was modest (8 %), with only two trials reporting statistically significant results. The impact of DA on colorectal cancer screening was similarly variable. 2 of 5 studies reported a statistical increase in uptake, 2 found no significant decreases in uptake (Stacey et al. 2011).

Individual studies found that DAs increased choice of hepatitis B vaccination and psycho-educational therapies for schizophrenia (Stacey et al. 2011).

DAs can affect decisions about managing chronic disease. One study found a slightly higher proportion of people with type II diabetes choosing a new type of medication after reviewing a DA, but lower adherence and no significant impact on biomarkers (HgA1c) (Mullan et al. 2009).

Medical Litigation: DAs could potentially improve medical liability and reduce waste associated with defensive medicine. However, no studies have examined this.

Cost: The cost impact of DA remains speculative. No cost-effectiveness study has been done on DAs, and no DA trial has rigorously captured the impact of DAs on cost. Simply decreasing rates of elective surgery will not necessarily lead to lower healthcare costs. The net impact of DAs on costs depends on how DAs impact technical efficiency ("doing things right," or being able to derive more of the same service from the same resource) and allocative efficiency ("doing the right things," or moving toward a more optimal choice of services). DAs may <u>decrease</u> technical efficiency by lengthening the consult time (on average, 2.5 min) (Stacey et al. 2011). The costs of identifying patients appropriate for DAs and of distributing DAs to those patients will also decrease technical efficiency. These costs could potentially be offset by improvements in allocative efficiency, by avoiding unnecessary or unwarranted treatments, or by promoting necessary treatments. Many factors would affect the net cost impact, including characteristics of the DA (e.g., their effectiveness, costs of development, updating, and distribution), and the time horizon of the analysis. Substitution effects, cost shifting, and other downstream effects of the decision also need to be considered. Avoiding an 'unnecessary' surgery does not cure the condition but rather typically results in patients pursuing other approaches to treatment, and in some cases, the delayed surgery. Depending on the condition, scope, and time horizon of the study, avoiding immediate surgery (which would lower short-term costs) may result in higher overall utilization and costs in the long-term costs). Surgeries that are appropriate would presumably be cost-saving in the long-term, but not necessarily in the short-term.

Potential risks associated with DAs: Evaluating the effectiveness of any medical intervention would be incomplete without a thorough assessment of its potential for harm.

<u>Potential for misinformation</u>: It is possible that DAs may provide inaccurate information about the condition or its treatment options. Because DAs typically target decisions where there is substantial uncertainty and much emerging research, their content may need frequent updating to reflect emerging evidence. DAs that are developed as videos or pamphlets are more costly to update than DAs without such features, increasing the likelihood that they may present out of date information.

Sending DAs to patients for whom they are inappropriate may misinform those patients. For example, a patient who is not a candidate for a specific treatment but who receives a DA stating that this treatment is an option could be misinformed by the DA. This possibility has not been examined in clinical trials of DAs because of human subjects protections which results in careful subject selection and screening. When DAs are used in the real world, such safe guards would not be present, especially for web-based DAs.

<u>Potential for introducing bias</u>: Because there are no explicit criteria for what constitutes the most important pieces of evidence to present to patients about their condition or its treatment, DAs could be created that are misleading or biased toward or against certain treatment choices. This bias could be unintentional or intentional. Framing effects, the order in which treatments are presented, and the use of salient terms could subtly influence patient choices in an inappropriate manner. The use of patient testimonials, common in many video-based DAs, have been shown to introduce strong biases and to distort people's perceptions of risks (Ubel et al. 2001). DAs could be used by insurers as a tool to reduce utilization by making more expensive treatments appear less desirable, or conversely, by drug or device manufacturers to make their treatments appear more desirable (Report of the Council on Medical Service).

<u>Emotional distress</u>: Some patients may experience anxiety or depression as a result of information in the DA. Some may feel overwhelmed or confused by the process of clarifying their values or making tradeoffs. To date, there is no evidence that DAs induce anxiety. However, DAs tested in clinical trials were subjected to careful scrutiny, which would not necessarily transpire outside of clinical trials, and DAs were only studied in a small number of clinical situations.

<u>Implementation</u>: Implementing rigid decision-making protocols could create administrative burden for physicians and a potential barrier to patient-centered care.

<u>Loss of Privacy</u>: Protocols for identifying patients who might need a DA through clinical or claims databases might result in loss of patient privacy. Sending a DA to a patient could potentially reveal a diagnosis that they might not

want disclosed; those DAs that require online interaction risk loss of confidential information.

Opportunity cost: If DAs result in physicians spending more time leading them through the decision process for one treatment decision, the opportunity cost of that time would need to be considered. Are they spending less time on other health matters?

Limitations of the evidence from randomized, controlled trials:

The evidence from DA trials presented above is limited in several regards. The patients, physicians, and practices included in these studies were not necessarily representative of those in the general population. Participating physicians and clinics were receptive to introducing DAs into their practices. Similarly, the clinical conditions and decision points that DAs addressed were carefully selected, typically representing settings in which a treatment or test was overused. DA trials lacked standardization according to the type of DA, the setting in which it was used, and the timing in which it was introduced. Some DA trials evaluated the impact of simpler versus more detailed DA, but none examined the impact of the quality of the DA or specific features of the DA on its effectiveness. Standards for measuring the quality of DAs were not developed until 2009 (Elwyn et al. 2009).

DA trials have focused on video DAs, with scant attention to other types of DAs or other approaches to SDM, such as training practitioners in SDM, incentivizing practitioners and/or patients to engage in SDM, or restructuring care.

Many DA trials were too short or too narrowly defined to examine their effect on long-term health outcomes or on overall utilization or cost.

Do DA work in the 'Real World'?

Uptake of DA in clinical practice has remained low. There are no examples of sustained wide-scale adoption of DAs. This failure in adoption of DA in real-world setting severely hinders the effectiveness of DA. The impact of DA in the real world is largely unknown at this time, though it is often incorrectly assumed to equal the impact observed in clinical trials. For example, a study with typical participation rates (Deyo et al. 2000) reported 11 % of subjects participated (most were excluded for clinical reasons; many refused). The 22 % reduction in surgery reported in the DA group corresponds to a 2.4 % reduction (22 % × 11 %) among the referred population. Accounting for subject eligibility and interest dilutes impact by an order of magnitude.

But even after adjusting for rates of participation, the impact of DAs may be exaggerated. Typically, after clinical trials of DAs are completed, the DAs are no longer used, even in trials where physicians and patients reported high levels of satisfaction with the DA. This phenomenon is partly due to the relatively high costs of identifying appropriate candidates for SDM and distributing the DA to patients at the time and place of decision making, and the perceived negative impact of DA on patient flow and physician time (Legare et al. 2008). DA trials used a variety of incentives for patients, providers, and clinical systems, and typically funded staff to support the infrastructure needed for identifying appropriate patients, distributing the DA, and sometimes coaching patients. These incentives likely influenced participation in trials and possibly outcomes.

Previous research has identified features associated with successful clinical decision support (Osheroff et al. 2007; Mollon et al. 2009; Bates et al. 2003). These include integration with workflow, giving recommendations rather than assessments, delivering the tool at the time and place of decision-making, and using computer-based decision support (Kawamoto et al. 2005).

Areas for further investigation: Areas needing further inquiry include:

What constitutes a good decision, and how to measure a values-consistent decision?

Practical approaches to help patients integrate their personal preferences with quantitative evidence, especially when they face many treatments that affect many outcomes.

How do DAs compare to other SDM interventions in terms of health care delivery, resource use, unwarranted variation, and clinical outcomes?

What is the cost-effectiveness of different approaches to SDM?

How to involve the patient's family and other healthcare professionals in decision-making, recognizing the interprofessional context in which decisions are made.

How are effective approaches for integrating and sustaining SDM in routine clinical care?

Are we giving patients the right kind of information to help them with decisions?

How do we ensure quality control of DAs, which could be created as marketing tools to encourage patients to choose more (or less) expensive options? Measures of bias and disclosure of conflicts of interests of groups creating SDM tools are needed.

What are the 'active ingredients' of DAs that account for their effectiveness?

References

Avorn, J., & Soumerai, S. B. (1983). Improving drug-therapy decisions through educational outreach. A randomized controlled trial of academically based "detailing". *New England Journal of Medicine, 308* (24), 1457–1463.

Barry, M. J., Cherkin, D. C., Chang, Y., Fowler, F. J., & Skates, S. (1997). A randomized trial of a multimedia shared decision-making program for men facing a treatment decision for benign prostatic hyperplasia. *Disease Management & Clinical Outcomes, 1*, 5–14.

Bates, D., Kuperman, G., Wang, S., Gandhi, T., Kittler, A., Volk, L., et al. (2003). Ten commandments for effective clinical decision support: Making the practice of evidence-based medicine a reality. *Journal of the American Medical Informatics Association, 10*(6), 523–530.

Brehaut, J. C., O'Connor, A. M., Wood, T. J., Hack, T. F., Siminoff, L., Gordon, E., & Feldman-Stewart, D. (2003). Validation of a decision regret scale. *Medical Decision Making, 23*, 281.

Charles, C., Gafni, A., & Whelan, T. (1997). Shared decision-making in the medical encounter: What does it mean? (or it takes at least two to tango). *Social Science and Medicine, 44*(5), 681–692.

Charles, C., Gafni, A., Whelan, T., & Obrien, M. (2005). Treatment decision aids: conceptual issues and future directions. *Health Expectations, 8*, 114–125.

Chaudhry, B., Wang, J., Wu, S., et al. (2006). Systematic review: Impact of health information technology on quality, efficiency, and costs of medical care. *Annals of Internal Medicine, 144*, 742–752.

Cleary, P. (1998). Satisfaction may not suffice! A commentary on 'a patient's perspective'. *International Journal of Technology Assessment in Health Care, 14* (1), 35–37.

Degner, L. F., & Sloan, J. A. (1992). Decision making during serious illness: What role do patients really want to play. *Journal of Clinical Epidemiology, 45*, 941–950.

Deyo, R. A., Cherkin, D. C., Weinstein, J., Howe, J., Ciol, M., & Mulley, A. G. (2000). Involving patients in clinical decisions: Impact of an interactive video program on use of back surgery. *Medical Care, 38*, 959–969.

Edwards, A., Elwyn, G., Hood, K., et al. (2003). The development of COMRADE—A patient-based outcome measure to evaluate the effectiveness of risk communication and treatment decision-making in consultations. *Patient Education Counsel, 50*, 311–322.

Elstein, A. S. (2004). On the origins and development of evidence-based medicine and medical decision making. *Inflammation Research, 53*(Supplement 2), S184–S189.

Elwyn, G., O'Connor, A. M., Bennett, C., Newcombe, R. G., Politi, M., Durand, M. A., et al. (2009). Assessing the quality of decision support technologies using the international patient decision aid standards instrument (IPDASi). *PLoS ONE, 4*(3): e4705. http://www.plosone.org/article/info%3Adoi%2F10.1371%2Fjournal.pone.0004705 (PMCID: 2649534).

Entwistle, V., & O'Donnell, M. (2001). Evidence-based health care: What roles for patients? In A. Edwards & G. Elwyn (Eds.), *Evidence-based Patient Choice: Inevitable of Impossible?* (pp. 34–40). Oxford: Oxford University Press.

Feldman-Stewart, D., Brundage, M. D., Van Manen, L., & Svenson, O. (2004). Patient-focussed decision-making in early-stage prostate cancer: Insights from a cognitively based decision aid. *Health Expectations, 7*, 126–141.

Frosch, D. L., & Bhatnagar, V. (2008). Internet patient decision support: A randomized controlled trial comparing alternative approaches for men considering prostate cancer screening. *Archives of Internal Medicine, 168*(4), 363–369.

Green, M. J., Peterson, S. K., Baker, M. W., Harper, G. R., Friedman, L. C., Rubinstein, W. S., et al. (2004). Effect of a computer-based decision aid on knowledge, perceptions, and intentions about genetic testing for breast cancer susceptibility: A randomized controlled trial. *JAMA, 292*(4), 442–452.

Grol, R., de Maeseneer, J., Whitfield, M., & Mokkink, H. (1990). Disease-centred versus patient-centred attitudes: Comparison of general practitioners in Belgium Britain and the Netherlands. *Family Practice, 7*, 100.

Hamann, J., Langer, B., Winkler, V., Busch, R., Cohen, R., Leucht, S., et al. (2006). Shared decision making for in-patients with schizophrenia. *Acta Psychiatrica Scandinavica, 114*(4), 265–273.

Harris, R. P., et al. (2001). Current methods of the U.S. preventive services task force: A review of the process. *American Journal of Preventive Medicine,* *20,* 21–35.

Health Dialog $775 Million Sale to BUPA Yields 15-Fold Return to Spencer Trask Investors. Reuters press release Dec 18, 2007. http://www.businesswire.com/news/home/20071218006054/en/Health-Dialog-775-Million-Sale-BUPA-Yields. Accessed June 7, 2016.

Healy, B. (2006). Who says what's best? U.S. News and World Report 9/ 11/2006, 75.

Helweg-Larsen, M., & Collins, B. E. (1997). A social psychological perspective on the role of knowledge about AIDS in AIDS prevention. *Current Directions in Psychological Science, 6,* 23–26.

Herrera, A. J., Cochran, B., Herrera, A., & Wallace, B. (1983). Parental information and circumcision in highly motivated couples with higher education. *Pediatrics, 71,* 233–234.

Holmes-Rovner, M., Kroll, J., Schmitt, N., et al. (1996). Patient satisfaction with health care decisions: The satisfaction with decision scale. *Medical Decision Making, 16,* 58–64.

International Patient Decision Aid Standards (IPDAS) Collaboration. (2012). IPDAS collaboration background document. February 17, 2005. In A. O'Connor, H. Llewellyn-Thomas & D. Stacey (Eds.). http://ipdas.ohri.ca/IPDAS_Background.pdf. Accessed August 23, 2012.

Kassirer, J. P. (1983). Adding insult to injury—Usurping patients' prerogatives. *New England Journal of Medicine, 308*(15), 898–901.

Kawamoto, K., Houlihan, C., Balas, E., & Lobach, D. (2005). Improving clinical practice using clinical decision support systems: A systematic review of trials to identify features critical to success. *British Medical Journal, 330*(7494), 765–768.

Kennedy, A. (2003). On what basis should the effectiveness of decision aids be judged? *Health Expectations, 6*(3), 255–268.

Kennedy, A. D., Sculpher, M. J., Coulter, A., Dwyer, N., Rees, M., Abrams, K. R., et al. (2002). Effects of decision aids for menorrhagia on treatment choices, health outcomes, and costs: A randomized controlled trial. *JAMA, 288*(21), 2701–2708.

Krahe, B., & Reiss, C. (1995). Predicting intentions of AIDS preventive behavior among adolescents. *Journal of Applied Social Psychology, 25,* 2118–2140.

Kuehn, B. M. (2009). States explore shared decision making. *JAMA, 301*(240), 2539–2541.

Kupfer, J. M., & Bond, E. U. (2012). Patient satisfaction and patient-centered care: necessary but not equal. *JAMA, 308*(2), 139–140.

Legare, F., Ratte, S., Gravel, K., & Graham, I. D. (2008). Barriers and facilitators to implementing shared decision-making in clinical practice: Update of a systematic review of health professionals' perceptions. *Patient Education and Counseling, 73*(3), 526–535.

Loh, A., Simon, D., Wills, C. E., Kriston, L., Niebling, W., & Harter, M. (2007). The effects of a shared decision-making intervention in primary care of depression: A cluster-randomized controlled trial. *Patient Education and Counseling, 67*(3), 324–332.

Man-Son-Hing, M., Laupacis, A., O'Connor, A. M., Biggs, J., Drake, E., Yetisir, E., et al. (1999). A patient decision aid regarding antithrombotic therapy for stroke prevention in atrial fibrillation: A randomized controlled trial. *JAMA, 282*(8), 737–743.

McWhinney, I. R. (1995). Why we need a new clinical method. In M. Stewart, J. B. Brown, W. W. Weston, I. R. McWhinney, C. L. McWiliam, & T. R. Freeman (Eds.), *Patient-centred medicine: Transforming the clinical method.* Thousand Oaks: Sage.

Mead, N., & Bower, P. (2000). Measuring patient-centredness: A comparison of three observation-based instruments. *Patient Education and Counseling, 39,* 71–80.

Michie, S., Dormandy, E., & Marteau, T. M. (2002). The multidimensional measure of informed choice: A validation study. *Patient Education and Counseling, 48,* 87–91.

Mollon, B., Chong, J., Holbrook, A., Sung, M., Thabane, L., & Foster, G. (2009). Features predicting the success of computerized decision support for prescribing: A systematic review of randomized controlled trials. *BMC Medical Informatics and Decision Making, 9,* 11.

Montgomery, A. A., Emmett, C. L., Fahey, T., Jones, C., Ricketts, I., Patel, R. R., et al. (2007). Two decision aids for mode of delivery among women with previous caesarean section: Randomised controlled trial. *BMJ, 334*(7607), 1305.

Montgomery, A. A., Fahey, T., & Peters, T. J. (2003). A factorial randomised controlled trial of decision analysis and an information video plus leaflet for newly diagnosed hypertensive patients. *British Journal of General Practice, 53*(491), 446–453.

Mullan, R. J., Montori, V. M., Shah, N. D., Christianson, T. J., Bryant, S. C., Guyatt, G. H., et al. (2009). The diabetes mellitus medication choice decision aid: A randomized trial. *Archives of Internal Medicine, 169* (17), 1560–1568.

Murray, E., Davis, H., Tai, S. S., Coulter, A., Gray, A., et al. (2001). Randomised controlled trial of an interactive multimedia decision aid on benign prostatic hypertrophy in primary care. *British Medical Journal, 323,* 493–496.

O'Connor, A., & Edwards, A. (2001). The role of decision aids in promoting evidence-based patient choice. In A. Edwards & G. Elwyn (Eds.), *Evidence-based patient choice: Inevitable or impossible?* (pp. 220–242). Oxford: Oxford University Press.

O'Connor, A. M., Stacey, D., Entwistle, V., Llewellyn-Thomas, H., Rovner, D., Holmes-Rovner, M., et al. (2003). Decision aids for people facing health treatment or screening decisions (Cochrane Review). In: *The cochrane library,* Issue 2. Oxford: Update Software.

O'Connor, A. M., et al. (1999). Decision aids for patients considering options affecting cancer outcomes:

Evidence of efficacy and policy implications. *Journal of the National Cancer Institute. Monographs, 25,* 67–80.

Oakley, S., & Walley, T. (2006). A pilot study assessing the effectiveness of a decision aid on patient adherence with oral bisphosphonate medication. *Pharmaceutical Journal, 276*(7399), 536–538.

Osheroff, J. A., Teich, J. M., Middleton, B., Steen, E. B., Wright, A., & Detmer, D. E. (2007). A roadmap for national action on clinical decision support. *Journal of the American Medical Informatics Association, 14*(2), 141.

Park, R. E., et al. (1986). Physician Ratings of Appropriate Indications for Six Medical and Surgical Procedures. *American Journal of Public Health, 76* (7), 766–772.

Partin, M. R., Nelson, D., Radosevich, D., Nugent, S., Flood, A. B., Dillon, N., et al. (2004). Randomized trial examining the effect of two prostate cancer screening educational interventions on patient knowledge, preferences, and behaviors. *The Journal of General Internal Medicine, 19*(8), 835–842.

Protheroe, J., Bower, P., Chew-Graham, C., Peters, T. J., & Fahey, T. (2007). Effectiveness of a computerized decision aid in primary care on decision making and quality of life in menorrhagia: Results of the MENTIP randomized controlled trial. *Medical Decision Making, 27*(5), 575–584.

Report of the Council on Medical Service. CMS Report 7-A-10. Subject: Shared Decision Making, Presented by Barbara L. McAnemy, Reference Committee A, Glenn A. Loomis: Chair).

Rothert, M. L., Holmes-Rovner, M., Rovner, D., Kroll, J., Breer, L., Talarczyk, G., et al. (1997). An educational intervention as decision support for menopausal women. *Research in Nursing & Health, 20*(5), 377–387.

Sepucha, K., & Ozanne, E. M. (2010). How to define and measure concordance between patients' preferences and medical treatments: A systematic review of approaches and recommendations for standardization. *Patient Education and Counseling, 78*(1), 12–23.

Sheridan, S. L., Shadle, J., Simpson, R. J, Jr., & Pignone, M. P. (2006). The impact of a decision aid about heart disease prevention on patients' discussions with their doctor and their plans for prevention: A pilot randomized trial. *BMC Health Services Research, 6,* 121.

Shortell, S. M., Rundall, T. G., & Hsu, J. (2007). Improving patient care by linking evidence-based medicine and evidence-based management. *JAMA, 298,* 673–676.

Spielberger, C. D., Gorsuch, R. L., Lushene, R. E. (1970). *Manual for the state-trait anxiety inventory (self-evaluations questionnaire).* Palo Alto, CA: Consulting Psychologists Press.

Stacey, D., O'Connor, A. M., Bennett, C. L., Barry, M., Col, N. F., Eden, K. B., et al. (2011). Cochrane review of decision aids for people facing health treatment or screening decisions; Cochrane Consumers and Communication Review Group. http://decisionaid.ohri.ca/cochsystem.html

Trevena, L. J., Irwig, L., & Barratt, A. (2008). Randomized trial of a self- administered decision aid for colorectal cancer screening. *Journal of Medical Screening, 15*(2), 76–82.

Ubel, P., Jepson, C., & Baron, J. (2001). the inclusion of patient testimonials in decision aids: Effects on treatment choices. *Medical Decision Making, 21*(1), 60–68.

Vuorma, S., Rissanen, P., Aalto, A. M., Hurskainen, R., Kujansuu, E., & Teperi, J. (2003). Impact of patient information booklet on treatment decision—A randomized trial among women with heavy menstruation. *Health Expectations, 6*(4):290–297.

Watson, E., Hewitson, P., Brett, J., Bukach, C., Evans, R., Edwards, A., et al. (2006). Informed decision making and prostate specific antigen (PSA) testing for prostate cancer: A randomised controlled trial exploring the impact of a brief patient decision aid on men's knowledge, attitudes and intention to be tested. *Patient Education and Counseling, 63*(3), 367–379.

Weymiller, A. J., Montori, V. M., Jones, L. A., Gafni, A., Guyatt, G. H., Bryant, S. C., et al. (2007). Helping patients with type 2 diabetes mellitus make treatment decisions: statin choice randomized trial. *Archives of Internal Medicine, 167*(10), 1076–1082.

Part V

Decision Making on the Organizational, State and National Level

The Promise and Perils of Shared Decision-Making in Clinical Practice

21

Rachel A. Greenup and Jeffrey Peppercorn

- Shared decision-making, a fundamental component of "patient-centered care," should include a two-way exchange of information between the doctor and patient in which both parties have the opportunity to express treatment p and arrive at treatment decisions that are both medically sound and consistent with the goals and preferences of a well-informed patient.
- Shared decision-making is meant to respect patient autonomy, consider patient comfort and satisfaction with medical care, and honestly convey information about the costs and trade-offs of treatment decisions for patients and their families.
- Patients retaining autonomy over their healthcare decisions has been shown to have several benefits including improved patient satisfaction with medical decisions, improved patient satisfaction with consequences related to those decisions, greater adherence to medical therapy, and improved long-term clinical outcomes

- Issues such as the patient's desire to delegate decision-making back to the provider, the provider's unwillingness to share treatment decisions, the complex nature of a medical condition, an overwhelming volume of potentially relevant medical information, demographic characteristics of the patient, and time constraints associated with a busy clinical practice may complicate the process of shared decision-making.
- In situations where there is a clear "best" clinical practice for a given scenario, patients may benefit from learning information about their diagnosis, making a choice as to whether or not to participate in the decision to undergo therapy, but ultimately delegate the specific treatment decision and planning to their physician. However, in more complex medical situations, where two treatment options have relatively equal clinical value, shared decision-making may be most useful.

R.A. Greenup (✉) · J. Peppercorn
Duke University Medical Center, Durham, NC, USA
e-mail: rachel.greenup@duke.edu

J. Peppercorn
e-mail: jpeppercorn@mgh.harvard.edu

© Springer Science+Business Media New York 2016
M.A. Diefenbach et al. (eds.), *Handbook of Health Decision Science*,
DOI 10.1007/978-1-4939-3486-7_21

Background

Shared decision-making is defined as the process in which patients act in partnership with their healthcare providers to make treatment decisions

(Emanuel and Emanuel 1992). In its optimal form, it involves a collaborative relationship between patient and provider, through which available evidence-based healthcare recommendations offered by providers are considered and pursued in the context of patient preferences and values (Edwards and Elwyn 2009).

The concept of shared decision-making is a fundamental component of "patient-centered care," which focuses on the goals and values of individual patients, as opposed to care based mainly on consideration of the pathophysiology of disease and clinical data, with a view to optimizing standard clinical outcomes such as survival, response to therapy, and tolerability. Implicit in this model is the recognition that individual patients will have different preferences for the outcomes of medical care, differing expectations and tolerance for the components of care, and different risk/benefit thresholds that will impact decision-making. This concept gained traction in 2001, when the U.S. Institute of Medicine officially endorsed and promoted a culture of "patient-centered care" and included it as a quality metric in its landmark report "Crossing the Quality Chasm." Since that time, the importance of incorporating the patient's perspective into medical decision-making, and supporting the process of shared decision-making, has been recognized as a component of quality health care (Woolf et al. 2005; Epstein et al. 2004). In an era of decreasing medical paternalism, increasing patient autonomy, and ready access to medical information, shared decision-making has become both more important and more complex. This chapter outlines the promise of shared decision-making and the challenges in implementing this process in clinical practice, including issues facing patients, providers, and the medical system as a whole.

The Promise of Shared Decision-Making

The ultimate promise of shared decision-making is that doctors and patients together will discuss and arrive at treatment decisions that are both medically sound and consistent with the goals and preferences of a well-informed patient. The "right" decision should include treatment plans that are acceptable to the patient, a risk/benefit ratio that matches the patient's risk tolerance and considers their satisfaction with their current state of health and the potential consequences of receiving or forgoing a given test, intervention, or plan of care. The underlying assumption is that shared decision-making includes a two-way exchange of information between the doctor and patient in which both players have the opportunity to express treatment preferences and to be involved in the decision-making process (Charles et al. 1999; Sheridan et al. 2004). Physicians are expected to communicate comprehensive medical information regarding diagnosis and treatment options. In turn, patients are expected to communicate their informed preferences, values, and goals. This exchange presumably reviews standard medical approaches and alternatives, risks and benefits, and costs of pursuing or failing to pursue a given care plan. Ideally, the patient and provider will then concur on the plan of action (Barratt 2008; Barry and Edgman-Levitan 2012).

The conversation may starts with a review of multiple evidence-based options and concludes with identification of the choice that best matches the patient's goals and preferences. From the provider perspective, shared decision-making is meant to respect patient autonomy, consider patient comfort, and satisfaction with medical care, and honestly convey information about the costs and trade-offs of treatment decisions for patients and their families. Additionally, patients and physicians should jointly consider the severity of disease, the morbidity associated with treatments, and the barriers to patient adherence to medical recommendations (Charles et al. 1997). According to this model, then, the appropriate medical decision will be the one that is right for the individual patient and his or her circumstances, rather than one that is based on consideration of clinical factors alone. For example, in the treatment of many cancers the benefit of postoperative (adjuvant) radiation therapy may be considered differently by different patients. A 5-10 % reduction in the risk of breast cancer recurrence may be deemed worth-while by a patient who lives in close geographic proximity to a radiation treatment facility where daily, short treatment sessions add minimal interference to daily life. In contrast, for a patient who is required to temporarily relocate to a new city or to drive an hour each day for 6 weeks of radiation therapy, this real but small reduction in recurrence risk may be deemed insufficient to justify the substantial investment of time and finances required for daily radiation treatments. Similarly, in the same clinical scenario, some patients may be unwilling to undergo the dis-comfort of radiation (which while transient, can be severe) or to accept the rare risks of compli-cations such as lung injury in exchange for modest absolute risk reduction, particularly, if it is in the setting of a relatively low baseline risk of cancer recurrence. The physician may feel that the benefits outweigh the risks and recommend radiation as the starting point for conversation, but based on discussion of the patient's prefer-ences the doctor and patient may reach an informed decision to forgo this intervention.

Although this model is compelling, it raises a number of issues. First and foremost, there is the issue of how much information should be dis-cussed, what level of detail is appropriate, what form the information should take, and whether the goal is simply to present information and/or to ensure that patients understand the information provided. Charles et al. define the process for shared decision making as follows: "At a mini-mum, the physician must inform the patient of all information that is *relevant* to making the deci-sion," while the patient "needs to provide infor-mation to the physician on issues raised…values, preferences, lifestyles, beliefs" (Charles et al. 1999). This definition helps to focus the inter-change on what constitutes relevant information, and provides some boundaries on what can and should be discussed. Ideally, all relevant treat-ment options are communicated to the patient, and treatment decisions are then considered in the context of that individual. However, as we

explore in greater detail below, physicians and patients may have different standards and goals for what level of evidence should be considered regarding options for treatment.

Benefits of Shared Decision-Making

Most patients express a desire to obtain more information about their diagnoses and treatment options, and wish to participate in medical decisions affecting them or their family members (Tariman et al. 2010). A growing body of the literature suggests that patients informed of their treatment options have greater knowledge of their medical condition, gain improved under-standing of potential treatment risks and benefits, and express increased satisfaction with care (Woolf et al. 2005).

Shared decision making has been shown to have several benefits including improved patient satisfaction with medical decisions, improved patient satisfaction with consequences related to those decisions, and improved long-term clinical outcomes. Woolf et al. demonstrated that patients informed of their treatment choices demonstrated greater adherence to medical therapy. Improved adherence can in turn lead to improved disease outcomes.

The process of shared decision-making is particularly relevant to what are termed "preference-based" decisions, where medical treatment options lead to equivalent clinical outcomes, and patients truly have a choice that does not compromise survival or disease control. For example, among patients with early stage breast cancer, treatment decisions depend largely on the patient's decision-making metrics related to personal preferences, values, and goals when choosing between breast-conserving surgeries followed by radiation therapy versus mastectomy alone. While scientific data suggests the two options are equivalent in terms of overall survival (Hwang et al. 2013; Fisher et al. 2002), numer-ous medical details and personal implications influence choice of therapy for any individual patient. The majority of patients with early stage breast cancer will survive the disease and live for decades with the consequences of initial treatment decisions. Keating and colleagues found that among 1000 women with breast cancer, roughly half reported that their actual level of participation in surgical decision-making matched their preferred involvement in the decision-making process. Among these individuals, patients who were able to participate in decision-making at a level that matched their preference demonstrated greater satisfaction with the type of breast surgery they received (Keating et al. 2002). Additional research in this area suggests that providing patients with more treatment choices and promoting patient involvement in treatment decisions reduces the risk of regret they might experience later about healthcare choices (Caldon et al. 2008).

In addition to improving satisfaction, the process of shared decision making may also serve to remind patients that although providers navigate patients and their families through complex medical decisions, patients ultimately retain autonomy over their healthcare decisions (Charles et al. 1997). Increasing knowledge and sense of control can translate into improved health behaviors and outcomes. Further benefits may include improvement in patient's ability to cope with illness. In a study of 256 cancer patients, Cassileth et al. reported that patients who were actively involved in decision-making remained more hopeful during treatment, and less likely to experience unrealistic fears about their health outcomes (Cassileth et al. 1980). Schroy et al. (2012) found that a shared decision making model increased colorectal cancer screening, albeit modestly, at an urban academic medical center. In their randomized trial involving 825 patients, a decision-aid based intervention in which patients were informed of their individual risks and asked their preferences for screening was deployed, resulted in a 10 % higher rate of completing colorectal cancer screening compared to a control arm in which patients received general information about colon

cancer and routine referral for screening from their doctor alone.

The promise of shared decision-making requires that patients and their providers engage in an equal exchange that meets the needs of both invested parties. Though shared decision-making is desired by patients and doctors alike, implementing this process can be difficult in a real-time clinical setting. Issues related to the patient, the provider, or the clinical situation may complicate the process of shared decision-making. These include the patient's desire to delegate decision-making back to the provider, the provider's unwillingness to share treatment decisions, the complex nature of a medical condition, an overwhelming volume of potentially relevant medical information, and time constraints associated with a busy clinical practice. In addition, there may not always be consensus among clinicians, let alone between a patient and their physician, on what constitutes relevant evidence or reasonable treatment options to consider. (Peppercorn et al. 2008)

Challenges of Shared Decision-Making

The potential promise of shared decision making is clear; promoting improved medical decisions that match patient values and preferences, leading to greater patient satisfaction, improving treatment compliance, and clinical outcomes. The challenges to this process are considerable. As noted above, patients vary in their preferences for information, desired involvement in decision-making, and in their ability to clearly elicit these preferences. In addition, many clinical encounters occur in a narrow time frame with multiple components competing for patient and physician attention. In this context, shared decision-making can easily become a neglected priority. Furthermore, in some settings, important decisions need to be made quickly and both conveying information and allowing time for an informed decision can be challenging. Cost can also be a factor both in terms of reimbursement for the shared decision-making process, and in terms of the financial impact of resulting medical decisions. Implicit and explicit costs resulting from the shared decision-making process may not be recognized by doctors and patients at the time of decision making.

While shared decision-making ideally leads to care that matches patient's informed preferences, doctors and patients may disagree about what constitutes an acceptable option for a given clinical scenario. Ethical conflicts may emerge between the physicians obligation to respect patient autonomy and their obligation to the principle of beneficence which requires the physicians to try to improve the patients health (Peppercorn 2012). We explore some of these challenges and available data on the complexity of shared decision-making below.

Challenges that Affect Patient Preferences

Though current medical culture encourages physicians and patients to engage in shared decision-making, it is not clear that a given patient actually wants to participate in their care and if so, to what degree. Patient-related factors correlates with desired involvement in shared decision-making. Arora and McHorney surveyed 2197 patients with chronic medical illnesses, including cardiovascular disease, diabetes, and depression, and found that 69 % preferred to leave medical decision-making to their physicians (Arora and McHorney 2000). Desired level of participation varied with patient characteristics. Female gender, younger age, and increased level of education were associated with an increased desire to actively participate in clinical decisions. Among advanced cancer patients, high levels of information were more likely preferred by younger, more educated, and more hopeful patients (Cassileth et al. 1980). Younger age also predicted an increased level of desired participation in decision-making among healthy volunteers surveyed to determine predictors of shared decision-making (Swenson et al. 2004). While demographic characteristics, such as

income, social support, marital status, and health distress seem to correlate reliably with interest in shared decision making, it is important to identify the individual patient's preferences for information and involvement in decisions (Barry and Edgman-Levitan 2012). As Miller has documented, patients with cancer do best from a psychological and behavioral perspective when there is a match between their personal coping style, which may call for more or less information and more or less involvement, and way shared decision making is approached by the clinician (Miller 1995).

Degner et al. surveyed breast cancer patients to determine whether patients' desired level of participation in shared decision-making matched their perceived level of participation (Degner et al. 1997). Results reflected that patients vary in terms of their preferences: 22 % of women expressed a preference for an active role in shared decision-making, while 44 % preferred a collaborative role (sharing the responsibility of decision-making with their physicians), and 34 % expressed interest in entirely delegating decision-making to their providers. Further, only 42 % of patients believed they had achieved their desired level of participation in treatment decisions (Degner et al. 1997). This study highlights the common discrepancy between attained and desired level of participation in medical decisions.

Since patients vary in terms of the level, type, and role they desire to play in medical decision-making, it is important that providers be able to assess and address these subtypes of patient preferences. At one extreme, the data suggest that few patients desire complete autonomy. For these individuals, efforts at shared decision-making can devolve to presenting patients with a menu of options without providing sufficient clinical guidance.

In a study involving outpatients with varied diagnoses (breast cancer, prostate disease, orthopedic injuries, multiple sclerosis to name a few), patients were surveyed regarding their preferred participation in treatment decisions. The investigators used the problem-solving decision-making scale based on patient scenarios describing options for making treatment decisions (Deber et al. 2007). Participants were queried regarding their beliefs on who should lead different aspects of the patient–doctor encounter including diagnosis, treatment options, prediction of risks and benefits, and ultimately treatment decisions. Over 2500 outpatients with chronic and acute medical issues, only 1 % of patients expressed interest in independently making healthcare treatment decisions without input from their providers (Deber et al. 2007). 77.8 % of patients in this study preferred a shared decision-making approach, and only 20 % preferred a passive role, delegating decision-making entirely to their physicians. Greater familiarity with the diagnosis, increased education, and younger age correlated with a desire for increased participation in shared decision-making (Deber et al. 2007).

A further challenge is that physicians may not be able to accurately estimate their patients' desired level of participation in sharing medical decisions. Strull et al. revealed this discrepancy through a survey of 200 hypertensive patients and their caring providers (Strull et al. 1984). In this study, after consultation with their physician, 41 % of patients still wanted more information about their diagnosis. However, only 53 % of patients preferred to participate in shared decision-making as opposed to being given a clear medical recommendation. In contrast, clinicians estimated that 78 % of patients desired to participate in treatment decisions. The authors concluded that physicians generally underestimate a patient's desire for medical information, but overestimate their desire to participate in shared decision-making. As a result, physicians may expect patients and their families to make independent medical decisions in the face of limited presented medical information.

It is challenging to identify an individual patient's preferences for the amount and type of medical information, and the patient's desired level of participation in decision-making. Though few patients want to entirely delegate treatment decisions to their doctors, even fewer appear to want to make decisions independently. Specifically, fewer patients may wish to participate in medical decision-making less often than expected. Although the literature suggests subsets of patients who may be more likely to prefer shared decision-making, there may be patients that fail to fit the mold: a younger well-educated patient who wants a clear treatment decision directed by the clinician and an older less well-educated patient for whom participation in decision-making is both desired and critical for treatment satisfaction and compliance.

Patient preferences for involvement in shared decision-making have consistently demonstrated generational differences ("older versus younger") across several studies. It remains unclear whether these patterns hold true due to temporal changes in the way medical care is approached (i.e., we have moved from a period of greater emphasis on paternalism to a period of greater emphasis on autonomy), or whether they reflect something relatively constant in the way age cohorts of patients approach medical decisions. Older patients may be more likely to defer to the physicians medical authority or believe that they are not qualified to make treatment decisions. In contrast, younger patients consistently express interest in taking ownership of their health care, and participating in shared decision-making (Cassileth et al. 1980). It is unclear whether these patterns will persist over time, with today's young patients developing less of a preference for shared decision making as they get older, or if this reflects cultural changes such that soon all patients, of any age, will be interested in (or feel compelled to exert) shared decision making. Given changes of the role of medicine in society over time, it seems likely that older patients will be increasingly be interested in shared decision-making. Clinicians and research must be aware of large variation in this area and account for individual preferences in clinical practice and future studies.

Challenges Based on Disease Chronicity and Setting

Although the theoretical benefits and importance of shared decision-making are equally relevant to the acute and chronic disease settings, there are principled distinctions that mediate the effects of patient-provider interactions. In chronic diseases such as hypertension, diabetes, and cardiovascular disease, patient input into managing their long-term medical conditions is critical. On a day-to-day basis, the patient either may or may not choose to take their medication or adhere to their diet and other aspects of self-care. Patient participation in the treatment decision-making process can encourage compliance, communication about treatment failures and successes, and support an open long-term relationship between patients and providers. In this setting, shared decision-making often consists of many nonurgent but ultimately important decisions made between patients and their physicians over time.

One potential challenge in chronic care management of patients is the increasingly fragmented nature or the healthcare system, where patients may switch providers frequently due to insurance and other issues. In addition, multiple providers caring for patients complicate both coordination of care and communication as patients move from clinic to clinic and between the inpatient and outpatient setting. Decisions to pursue therapy for chronic conditions may be made or medications may be adjusted with little communication among providers. While theoretically, there is potential for a long-term relationship between a patient and a physician and time to make nonurgent decisions within a shared decision-making framework for chronic conditions, actual management of chronic conditions occurs over many encounters and fidelity to this process may be variable based on the setting and the clinicians involved.

In contrast, in the acute context, certain illnesses require that treatment decisions be made urgently between patients and physicians, often without a prior relationship. Decisions in the setting of the emergency department, intensive care unit, or in any setting where acute symptoms and rapidly evolving disease conditions are managed can have both acute life and death consequences and dramatic long-term impact on the patients' health and morbidity. (Sheridan et al. 2004). Need for rapid establishment of trust, high volumes of information delivered to overwhelmed patients, and pressured decision-making can complicate the process of shared decision making in the acute setting. Patients' preference for knowledge of their disease and preferences for decision-making will not necessarily translate into an ability to make an informed decision under these conditions. Coping with the shock of a recent diagnosis may also render patients less able or even unable to participate in treatment decisions. Challenges in these settings do not diminish the importance of considering shared decision-making, but these limitations and challenges must be acknowledged and more research is needed to develop better methods for decision making in urgent and high-risk settings.

Cost Implications of Shared Decision-Making

It is difficult to adequately discuss models for decision-making without considering the resources required to support these models or the impact of medical decisions on both the patient's expenses and societal costs of care. Health care spending is increasingly becoming unsustainable, leading to pressure to explicitly consider the costs of care involved in medical decision-making. The US currently spends roughly 18 % of the gross domestic product on health care, and without changes to the system it is projected that health care spending will soon account for 1/5 of every dollar spent in the US economy. Given these circumstances, physicians are required to consider the costs of care in decision-making and to review costs with patients. The American Society of Clinical Oncology has suggested that discussions of costs of cancer care should be considered a component of high quality care delivery (Meropol et al. 2009).

Physicians view costs as an important part of medical decisions, but are frequently unsure of the costs of care or how to address this with patients (Neumann et al. 2010). For their part, patients express a high degree of interest in being informed of costs of care, but differ in their belief that costs should influence decision-making and as to whether discussions of cost should include only direct costs to the patient, or also societal/payer costs of care (Irwin et al. 2013).

Shared decision-making has potential to add costs to the increasingly burdened healthcare system, and is most cost-effective for decisions that are highly sensitive to patient values (Ubel and Arnold 1995). Timely exchanges of information, expressed need for additional work-up and return visits to fully communicate risks and benefits of treatment can add to the cost of this process. On the other hand, decisions that better match patient preferences can lead to better adherence and improved outcomes (such as preventing disease recurrence in the setting of cancer, or stroke in the setting of hypertension) as noted above, which can translate into downstream cost savings for both the patient and society. In addition, literature on end-of-life care suggests that many patients will forgo expensive futile care when physicians provide them with adequate information about their prognosis and discuss their preferences for care (Peppercorn et al. 2011).

Challenges of Shared Decision-Making for Patients

Ideally anyone making a complex decision would be poised to gather and process information they need and would be able to consider their options without time pressure or coercion from any source. The actual experience of patients faced with medical decisions falls far short of this ideal. Physical strain of illness may be anticipated to impact patient's desire or ability to be involved in their treatment decisions.

In addition, active participation in medical decision-making may impose a greater burden and responsibility on patients than the process of delegating decision-making to the provider. Specifically, when unexpected negative outcomes occur, it may be that having engaged in shared decision making increases the burden experienced by patients. Complications from treatments, treatment failures or side effects may prompt some patients to reflect on and question treatment decisions. Struggling through medical

failures takes a significant emotional and physical toll on both patients and providers. Patients who are directly suffering the adverse consequences of treatment (i.e. side effects of chemotherapy, surgical complications like poor wound healing, prolonged hospital stays, time off of work, etc.) may not always find that participating in the treatment decision makes these burdens easier to bear.

While above we have highlighted the potentially beneficial effects of shared decision-making in terms of greater patient satisfaction and adherence with a plan of care, there is also potential for exaggerated negative consequences if undesired outcomes occur. Little attention has been given to this issue in the literature. Consequences resulting from shared decisions, including morbidity and mortality, may not be shared with equal responsibility between doctor and patient. In addition, adverse outcomes resulting from shared decision-making often lead to psychological, as well as physical consequences from treatment decisions. Though the medical decision was "shared" the patient carries the majority of the physical burden related to treatment decisions, and providers can carry significant psychological burden related to treatment consequences. There has been little exploration in the literature of the consequences of poor outcomes and whether they differ based on decision-making process. Physicians should evaluate for additional burdens experienced as a result of treatment decision-making and address both the physical and psychological consequences of adverse events, regardless of whether the patient participated in decision making or not.

Challenges of Shared Decision-Making for Providers

While modern medicine is characterized by greater respect for patient autonomy and less paternalism than was the norm 50 years earlier, many practitioners work under the assumption that medical training teaches us to "know what is best" for patients and their families. Even though providers may be less likely to dictate a care plan and expect that patients will accept their recommendations unquestionably, physicians still hold tremendous influence over medical decisions based both on the power of their recommendations and their ability to bias the presentation of information, intentionally or not. Patients can be biased toward medical treatments that the physician has predetermined to be in their best interest. There is not consensus among physicians regarding how and when shared decision making should occur, and differences in practice and skills in this areas have been inadequately evaluated to date. Additionally, physician bias against shared decision-making may negatively impact engaging patients in this process. Even when providers are motivated to involve patients in treatment decisions, barriers to realizing this balance exist.

Identification of patient preferences for shared decision making and the skills of using preferences to guide treatment decision-making is a distinct skill set from the core competencies that are typically the focus of medical training and practice. Not all providers are equally skilled in the art of medicine, such that they can balance medical recommendations with facilitation of shared decisionmaking. Physicians may lack training to facilitate shared decision-making or be unable to provide information that is accessible and comprehensible to a given patient (Sheridan et al. 2004). Consistent with this attitude, physicians may expect patients to understand complex and sophisticated medical evidence and to have the skills to make individual treatment decisions based on the population-based data that are presented to them (McNutt 2004). When clear and well-organized evidence is unavailable, the process of shared decision-making becomes complex, confusing and may be ultimately detrimental to patients.

In situations where there is a clear "best" clinical practice for a given scenario, patients may benefit from learning information about their diagnosis, making a choice as to whether or not to participate in the decision to undergo therapy, but ultimately delegate the specific treatment decision and planning to their physician. However, in more complex medical situations, where two treatment options have

relatively equal clinical value, or clinical "equipoise," shared decision-making may be most useful (De Haes 2006). Determining how to apply shared decision making under different medical conditions, in addition to accounting for different preferences among patients is a distinct medical skill. There is a clear need clinical training to focus on development of this skill and a need for research to define optimal patients communication techniques.

Deliberation is an integral part of shared decision-making. As described by Charles et al., deliberation is a two-way exchange of information between patient and physician that requires an often time-consuming exchange of information to build trust and reach conclusions (Sheridan et al. 2004). In attempts to minimize unrealistic time investments by busy practitioners, and to eliminate decision-making in a pressured setting, shared decision-making tools have been developed and advocated. Shared decision-making tools offer treatment choices to patients, presenting equal treatment efficacy with different side effect, quality of life, and risk profiles. These tools describe the patient experience from the patient perspective, including convenience, recovery time, and treatment side effects.

Despite the potential advantages of these adjunct clinical tools, Holmes-Rovner et al. demonstrated low patient referral to shared decision-making programs by physicians due to perceived time and productivity pressures (Holmes-Rovner et al. 2000). Physicians in this study were reluctant to introduce a process that could slow the time to decision and treatment intervention. In a literature review by Gravel et al., including 31 publications on physician perception of shared decision-making, the most commonly cited physician-perceived barriers to sharing treatment decisions included time constraints, lack of applicability based on patient characteristics, and lack of applicability to the clinical situation (Gravel et al. 2006). Physicians in this study cited additional barriers to shared decision-making including the perception that some patients did not want to participate in treatment decisions, and not agreeing with asking patients about their preferred role in decision-making.

Physicians wishing to engage patients in shared decision-making require fundamental interpersonal skills, knowledge, and communication skills. Elwyn et al. reviewed the complex set of competencies required by providers in preparation for shared decision-making. These include: developing a partnerships with patients, establishing and reviewing patient preferences for information, reviewing patient preferences for their role in decision-making, responding to patient expectations, identifying choices, presenting evidence-based treatment options, helping the patient reflect upon the anticipated impact of treatment decisions, negotiating a decision in partnership, and agreeing upon an action plan (Elwyn et al. 2000). Though acquiring these skills and utilizing them with patients is medically appropriate, it is labor-intensive in the context of most clinical practices.

The authors surveyed general practitioners through focus group interviews to review opinions about shared decision-making, and to determine challenges to implementation as key informants. Despite positive attitudes about shared decision-making, and an overall desire to include patients in treatment decisions, physicians relayed that interpersonal skills and knowledge about all treatment choices remained practical barriers to implementing shared decision-making (Elwyn et al. 2000). Risk communication, managing a difference of opinion between patient and doctor, conflict resolution, and difficulty in eliciting patient preferences have been previously described as critical interpersonal skills for doctors participating in shared decision-making (Say and Thomson 2003; Godolphin et al. 2001). Although physicians typically strive to engage patients in the process of shared decision-making, providers continue to perceive clinical barriers that prevent them to make this a clinical reality for every patient.

Challenges When Patients and Physicians Disagree About Shared Decision-Making

A premise of shared decision making is that physicians should not pursue what on strict clinical terms they deem the "best" treatment, and instead pursue what they deem an "adequate" care plan that best matches the patient's preferences, after careful exchange of the pros and cons of different treatment options. An inherent risk of not relying on medical judgment alone is that patients who hold strong but nonevidence-based opinions may be more likely to experience negative medical outcomes when judged by conventional standards. It is therefore critically important to distinguish between patient preferences for outcomes and patient preferences for treatments. For example, a patient with early stage breast cancer may have a weak preference to avoid mastectomy as a treatment but a strong preference for the outcome of a good cosmetic result from surgery. In some cases, the best cosmetic outcome might be achieved by mastectomy with reconstruction, and the patient will be best served by a decision-making process that identifies the cosmetic outcome as a priority and then discusses which treatment will be most likely to achieve that outcome, instead of focusing on the preferences for type of treatment alone. Patient preferences for outcomes may be different from the physicians preferences and as a result lead to changes in treatment plan (for example, a patient with advanced cancer who prefers to focus on palliative care alone vs. a physicians desire for further disease directed therapy, or vice versa). If the patients has a strong preference to die at home and/or to forgo an intervention and its immediate side effects and chooses a path that shortens their survival but allows them to meet their quality of life goals, this decision should not be deemed a "bad outcome" by the clinician, even if the patient foregoes prolonged survival.

In contrast, if the physician and the patients both wish to prioritize the same outcome, such as cure of early stage breast cancer, but the patient has a strong belief in the power of diet alone to prevent cancer recurrence and/or believes that evidence-based options such as chemotherapy or radiation therapy are harmful, it may not be possible to arrive at true consensus for a shared treatment decision. Clinicians need to consider the potential for patients to make decisions that are viewed as medically unwise, or even dangerous {Peppercorn 2012). In such cases, evidence may suggest that the option preferred by the patient will actually increase the likelihood of an outcome that the patient wishes to avoid. For example, a patient with bulky lymph node involvement of breast cancer may wish to forgo radiation out of fear of the potential risk of nerve damage and resulting loss of arm function, but in doing so, place herself at greater risk of loss function due to cancer recurrence. It is important for clinicians to identify the patients goals and to make an evidence-based recommendation on how they can best achieve those goals, but this will not always change the patients preferred treatment plan. In some cases, even an adequately informed patient will still wish to pursue a plan that matches their preferences (for example, avoiding radiation therapy) but that the clinician believes is inconsistent with their expressed goals (such as survival).

These circumstances highlight an important limitation of the shared decision making model. Physician support for shared decision making requires an assessment of the patients goals and preferences but does not mean that the physician must ultimately defer all medical judgment or agree to participate in a plan that they believe is harmful or nonevidence based. Good communication regarding the reasons for strong differences in opinion between patients and physicians is essential. In some, but not all cases, efforts to understand the basis for differences in opinion or care preferences may result in better outcomes for the patient.[1]

Conclusion

Despite the ideal of shared decision-making in which physician and patient act in partnership through evidence-based and informed decisions, challenges to realizing this ideal remain in the clinical setting. The U.S. Preventive Services Task Force encourages clinicians to participate in shared decision-making [D]. The recommendation for physicians is to provide patients with "balanced, evidence-based information" when clear benefit exists, and to discuss other options of high-visibility of particular importance to the individual patient's clinical situation [D]. Patients should be informed of their opportunity to participate in medical treatment decisions, and directed toward decision-making tools and resources. Physicians should be trained to assess a patient's level of interest in participating in treatment decisions, and be provided with the resources to engage patients in this process. Considerable challenges will likely remain, but awareness of such challenges, and of the desire for shared decision-making on the part of many patients, should make it more likely for the potential benefits of shared decision-making to be achieved in clinical practice.

References

Arora, N., & McHorney, C. (2000). Preferences for medical decision making: Who really wants to participate? *Medical Care, 38*(3), 335–341.

Barratt, A. (2008). *Evidence based medicine and shared decision making: The challenge of getting both evidence and preferences into health care.* Elsevier Ireland Ltd: Patient education and counseling.

Barry, M., & Edgman-Levitan, S. (2012). Shared decision making-the pinnacle of patient-centered care. *NEJM, 366*(9), 780–781.

Caldon, L., Walters, S., & Reed, W. (2008). Changing trends in the decision-making preferences of women with early breast cancer. *British Journal of Surgery, 95*, 312–318.

Cassileth, B., Zupkis, R., Sutton-Smith, K., & March, V. (1980). Information and participation preferences among cancer patients. *Annals of Internal Medicine, 92*(6), 832–836.

Charles, C., Gafni, A., & Whelan, T. (1997). Shared decision-making in the medical encounter: What does it mean? (or it takes at least two to tango). *Social Science and Medicine, 44*(5), 681–692.

Charles, C., Gafni, A., & Whelan, T. (1999). Decision-making in the physician-patient encounter: Revisiting the shared treatment decision-making model. *Social Sciences & Medicine., 49,* 651–661.

De Haes, H. (2006). Dilemmas in patient centeredness and shared decision making: A case for vulnerability. *Patients Education and Counseling., 62,* 291–298.

Deber, R., Kraetschmer, N., Urowitz, S., & Sharpe, N. (2007). Do people want to be autonomous patients? Preferred roles in treatment decision-making in several patient populations. *Health Expectations, 10,* 248–258.

Degner, L., Kristjanson, L., Bowman, D., Sloan, J., et al. (1997). Information needs and decisional preferences in women with breast cancer. *JAMA, 277,* 1485–1492.

Edwards, A., & Elwyn, G. (2009). Shared decision-making in health care: Achieving evidence-based patient choice. *Shared decision-making in health care.*

Elwyn, G., Edwards, A., Kinnersley, P., & Grol, R. (2000). Shared decision making and the concept of equipoise: The competences of involving patients in health care choices. *British Journal of General Practice, 50,* 892–897.

Emanuel, E., & Emanuel, L. (1992). Four models of the physician-patient relationship. *JAMA, 267*(16), 2221–2226.

Epstein, R., Alper, B., & Quill, T. (2004). Communicating evidence for participatory decision making. *JAMA, 291*(19), 2359–2366.

Fisher, B., Anderson, S., Bryant, J., et al. (2002). Twenty-year follow-up of a randomized trial comparing total mastectomy, lumpectomy and lumpectomy plus irradiation for the treatment of invasive breast cancer. *New England Journal of Medicine, 347*(16), 1233–1241.

Godolphin, W., Towle, A., & McKendry, R. (2001). Challenges in family practice related to informed and shared decision-making: Survey of preceptors of medical students. *JAMC, 165*(4), 434–435.

Gravel, K., Legare, F., & Graham, I. (2006). Barriers and facilitators to implementing shared decision-making in clinical practice: a systematic review of health professionals' perceptions. *Implementation Science, 1,* 16.

Holmes-Rovner, M., Valade, D., Orlowski, C., et al. (2000). Implementing shared decision-making in routine practice: Barriers and opportunities. *Health Expectations, 3,* 182–191.

Hwang, E. S., Lichtensztajn, D. Y., Gomez, S. L., Fowble, B., & Clarke, C. A. (2013). Survival after lumpectomy and mastectomy for early stage invasive breast cancer: The effect of age and hormone receptor status. *Cancer, 119*(7), 1402–1411.

Irwin, B., Zafar, S., Marcom, P.K., Kimmick, G., Houck, K.,Peppercorn, J. (2013). Patient experience and attitudes towards addressing the cost of breast cancer care. In *American Society of Clinical Oncology Annual Meeting.* Chicago.

Keating, N., Guadagnoli, E., Borbas, C., & Weeks, J. (2002). Treatment decision making in early-stage breast cancer: Should surgeons match patients' desired level of involvement? *Journal of Clinical Oncology, 20,* 1473–1479.

McNutt, R. (2004). Shared medical decision making: Problems, process, progress. *JAMA, 292*(20), 2516–2518.

Meropol, N. J., Schrag, D., Smith, T. J., Mulvey, T. M., Langdon, R. M, Jr., Blum, D., et al. (2009). American Society of Clinical Oncology guidance statement: The cost of cancer care. *Journal of Clinical Oncology, 27* (23), 3868–3874.

Miller, S. M. (1995). Monitoring versus blunting styles of coping with cancer influence the information patients want and need about their disease. Implications for cancer screening and management. *Cancer, 76*(2), 167–177.

Neumann, P. J., Palmer, J. A., Nadler, E., Fang, C., & Ubel, P. (Jan–Feb, 2010). Cancer therapy costs influence treatment: A national survey of oncologists. *Health Affairs (Millwood) 29*(1), 196–202. doi:10. 1377/hlthaff.2009.0077

Peppercorn, J. (2012). Ethics of ongoing cancer care for patients making risky decisions. *Journal of Oncology Practice, 8*(5), e111–e113.

Peppercorn, J., Burstein, H. J., Miller, F. G., Winer, E. P., & Joffe, S. (2008). Self Reported Practices and Attitudes of U.S. Oncologists Regarding Off-Protocol Therapy. *Journal of Oncology Practice 26,* 5994–6000.

Peppercorn, J. M., Smith, T. J., Helft, P. R., Debono, D. J., Berry, S. R., Wollins, D. S., et al. (2011). American society of clinical oncology statement: toward individualized care for patients with advanced cancer. *Journal of Oncology Practice.*

Say, R., & Thomson, R. (2003). The importance of patient preferences in treatment decisions-challenges for doctors. *BMJ.*

Schroy, P. C, 3rd, Emmons, K. M., Peters, E., Glick, J. T., Robinson, P. A., Lydotes, M. A., et al. (2012). Aid-assisted decision making and colorectal cancer screening: A randomized controlled trial. *American Journal of Preventive Medicine, 43*(6), 573–583.

Sheridan, S., Harris, R., & Woolf, S. (2004). Shared decision making about screening and chemoprevention: A suggested approach from the U.S. preventive services task forces. *American Journal of Preventive Medicine, 26*(1), 56–66.

Strull, W., Lo, B., & Charles, G. (1984). Do patients want to participate in medical decision making? *JAMA, 252* (21), 2990–2994.

Swenson, S., Buell, S., Zettler, P., White, M., et al. (2004). Patient-centered communications: Do patients really prefer it? *Journal of General Internal Medicine, 19,* 1069–1079.

Tariman, J., Berry, D., Cochrane, B., Doorenbos, A., & Schepp, K. (2010). Preferred and actual participation roles during health care decision making in persons with cancer: A systematic review. *Annals of Oncology, 21,* 1145–1151.

Ubel, P., & Arnold, R. (1995). The unbearable rightness of bedside rationing: Physician duties in a climate of cost containment. *Archives of Internal Medicine, 155*, 1837–1842.

Woolf, S., Chan, E., Harris, R., et al. (2005). Promoting informed choice: Transforming health care to dispense knowledge for decision making. *Annals of Internal Medicine, 143*, 293–300.

Evidence-Based Medicine and Decision-Making Policy

George Cheely and David Zaas

- Population health creates impetus for organizations to generate, deploy, and sustain policies integrating evidence-based medicine into clinical decisions
- Factors enabling policy generation include: centralization of provider organizations, integration of evidence-based medicine into quality measurement, availability of high-quality evidence
- Deployment of policies has been feasible with: acceptance among providers of the need for evidence to inform decisions, Information Technology infrastructure to integrate policies into workflows, and financial incentives to encourage deployment
- Successful sustainment of policies hinges on: forethought about policy governance structures, incorporation of mechanisms to update policies with new evidence, and development of tools to feedback performance to individual providers

- Pressures driving further evolution of policies will include: production pressures as insured populations expand with the ACA, scrutiny of cost relative to benefit, and emphasis on patient preferences

Introduction

Picture the Rockwellian physician of 1958. He was the quintessence of yesteryear's medical practitioner—a silver-haired man, clad in white coat, ministering to his patients in solo practice. Oral penicillin may have only recently reached his small but growing armament of therapeutics. The New England Journals on his desk would have described such findings as case series of bronchodilator and steroid use in COPD and sulfa drugs in pyelonephritis (Franklin et al. 1958; Grieble et al. 1958). How would that wizened veteran of experiential medicine react to today's practice? The New England Journals of 2014 include such topics as randomized controlled trials of co-trimoxazole in HIV-positive children in Africa and combined medical and interventional therapies for renal artery stenosis (Bwakura-Dangarembizi et al. 2014; Cooper et al. 2014).

He might be, on the one hand, overwhelmed by the sheer volume of information to read, digest, trial, and integrate into his practice. On

G. Cheely (✉)
Department of Medicine, Duke University Medical Center, Duke University School of Medicine, #100800, 2301 Erwin Rd, Durham, NC 27707, USA
e-mail: george.cheely@duke.edu

D. Zaas
Department of Medicine, Duke University School of Medicine, 3400 Wake Forest Rd, Raleigh, NC 27609, USA
e-mail: david.zaas@duke.edu

© Springer Science+Business Media New York 2016
M.A. Diefenbach et al. (eds.), *Handbook of Health Decision Science*,
DOI 10.1007/978-1-4939-3486-7_22

the other, he would undoubtedly be glad for society guidelines to distil down the most salient standards of care, for information technology to support readier access to higher quality information, and maybe even for the integration of his private practice into the fabric of the local health system to spread the hours needed to align on evidence-based practice patterns and the cost of technological solutions to standardize those patterns over a growing number of providers.

This chapter begins by reviewing how an awareness and understanding of medical science underpins sound decisions at the bedside. This discussion provides context for subsequent remarks describing how policies to integrate the use of medical science into decisions are generated, deployed, and sustained at the organizational level.

The Intersection Between Evidence-Based Medicine and Clinical Decision-Making

While some uphold that the fundamental tenets of Evidence-Based Medicine (EBM) have their roots in ancient history, our current understanding of EBM rests squarely upon the foundations of the science underpinning clinical decisions. Indeed, authors have made reference to biblical and ancient Chinese texts describing early "controlled stud[ies]" in which outcomes among populations receiving a special treatment were compared against outcomes among populations receiving standard treatment (Claridge et al. 2005). In 1972, Archie Cochrane extolled the virtues of the modern-day Randomized Controlled Trial, disseminating the importance of study design as tantamount to using data to inform clinical decisions (Cochrane 2004). The modern definition of EBM is often credited to David Sackett when he, in 1996, described EBM as the application of the most current and highest quality evidence to the clinical decision-making for an individual patient (Sackett 1996). Since the 1990s, EBM has received steadily growing attention in the literature with growth from some 100 articles indexed on MEDLINE in 1990 to several thousand in 2006

(Kohn 2011). As such, the field has continued to mature along with the proliferation of available evidence to inform decisions. At its core, today's optimal translation of the evidence base to inform clinical practice decisions involves a careful interpretation of not just the primary outcomes of an individual study, but also the study design, the characteristics of the population studied, and the context of the outcomes for related studies addressing similar questions. This decision-making process of combing the vast array of available evidence and imposing multiple levels of interpretation introduces the potential for a high degree of variability in those decisions.

While the scientific methodology for generating sound evidence continues to have reasonable consensus, a variety of factors have contributed to the perpetuation of variability in the application of that evidence. First, while the merits of EBM have been widely acknowledged, the best practice for disseminating the skills required to interpret studies and to incorporate those interpretations into decisions remains less clear (Ahmadi et al. 2012). As such, even the approach to establishing the knowledge base to translate evidence into decisions is varied. Second, the nature of study design limits the generalizability of findings to many real-world situations, increasing the variability with which those results are applied. As the baby boomers continue to accumulate years and medical comorbidities, it becomes more difficult to apply the results of the majority of clinical trials which examine relatively younger and less medically complicated patients (Stewart et al. 2007). Furthermore, as our knowledge of rare diseases grows, traditionally trusted study designs fall short in their abilities to address clinical questions pertinent to those diseases (Frankovich et al. 2011). Third, as providers face growing pressures to increase productivity, combing the burgeoning canon of evidence for the study best suited to inform a decision for a particular patient is not practical. If providers have difficulty keeping pace with medical literature, it is not surprising that significant variability exists in the proportion of provider decisions enacting current evidence-based care (Grol and Grimshaw 2003). Finally, chief among these factors has been the traditional model of care delivery emphasizing the supremacy of individual provider decisions. The traditional solo practitioner functioned in relative isolation from his or her colleagues, relying on the accumulation of individual experience to inform clinical decisions (Eddy 2005). While recent practice trends have veered away from this solo model, the foundations of the profession have been built upon the power of the individual decision-maker. In an environment emphasizing individual autonomy, there is no broader organizational framework to standardize variation in individuals' decisions in applying the evidence base.

While the historical provider model emphasized individualism, changes in the current health care landscape are culminating to increase the sphere of influence of organizations to generate, to deploy, and to sustain policies governing the integration of evidence-based medicine into decision-making. We depict our view of the historical process of provider decision-making where individuals used evidence variably and did not have means to systematically monitor outcomes. This process stands in distinction to the future state we will develop over the chapter where, increasingly, provider organizations will oversee application of a standardized base of evidence through policies targeting provider groups and deployed through electronic tools with a systematic means to both track and improve outcomes (Fig. 1). The growth of Accountable Care Organizations, the standardization of electronic tools

Fig. 1 Historical and future state processes for provider decisions

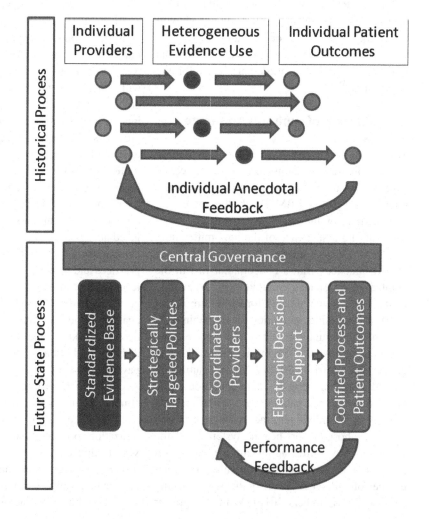

for documentation and care delivery, and the emphasis on getting value for health care dollars, all signal an increase in capability and momentum for population management. These broader trends underline the integral role organizational policy will play in driving toward this future state.

Policies Governing Evidence-Based Medicine at the Organizational Level

Policy Generation

For organizations to be able to generate policies governing evidence-based medicine, organizations must be centralized and coordinated with sufficient authority to create policies. The application of EBM to everyday practice must therefore be normalized among and integrated with the workflows of the organization's provider base. Further, sufficient impetus to devote resources to policy creation must exist for the organization.

Centralization of Authority to Create Policies

The trend toward centralization and coordination of provider organizations has begun to create entities with the authority necessary to generate policies governing EBM. With the increasing complexities of the healthcare regulatory environment, the first decade of the new millennium has seen a steady decline in small, physician-owned, practices with a concomitant rise in the number of physicians employed by larger hospitals. The passage of the Affordable Care Act in 2010 has intensified penalties for remaining out of step with regulations and is expected to drive hospital employment of physicians at an even greater rate (Harrison 2012). This reorganization around a central point for administration shifts the oversight of patient care from resting squarely with individual practices to one shared with the hospital or health system. As the employer, the central administrative entity has not just a greater stake in, but also a greater degree of influence over, policies governing patient care (Lammers 2012). With this greater

degree of influence, hospitals and health systems are better positioned to ensure that the care delivered by their physicians is in accord with national quality standards. The Affordable Care Act establishes a clear message that these quality standards must be rooted in the evidence base (Long and Brewer 2011). As such, recent national policy changes reinforce the authority of centralized provider organizations to put policies into place to more systematically deliver high-quality, evidence-based patient care.

While concerns about the difficulty of keeping pace with the changing regulatory landscape have motivated much of this trend toward centralization to date, alternative payment structures designed to better coordinate care also provide a shared incentive to drive centralization in the name of improving patient care. The Center for Medicare and Medicaid Innovations pilot program for Bundled Payments reflects a strong interest on the part of CMS to develop alternative payment structures aligning financial incentives with efficient provision of care in the acute and post-acute setting. The bundled payment models include provisions for shared savings in which providers and hospitals may divide financial gains resultant from the provision of more efficient care rooted in the evidence base—provisions that give hospitals a greater stake in the care provided on their wards (Delisle 2012). Private payers have also been deploying payments for conditions targeted at standardizing physician practices around evidence-based care. These efforts target larger practices and provide a financial incentive for the leadership of those practices to establish policies governing the provision of evidence-based care, again providing financial impetus to shift decision-making authority centrally (Goozner 2011). In addition to public and private efforts paying for episodes of care, the creation of Accountable Care Organizations, with payment structures bundling care for populations, provides additional illustration of incentives driving centralization to create policies governing care provision. Indeed, in the wake of legislation promoting ACOs, there has been an increase in physician–hospital relationships in an attempt to better coordinate care across the spectrum of care settings (Matthews 2010). As these relationships have solidified, experience with performance-based compensation and performance measurement overall was deemed an "essential" factor in ensuring that quality of care was maintained while realizing financial savings during the shift to population-based care (Larson et al. 2012). Some degree of skepticism exists about the extent to which bundled payments or ACOs will pervade as a future payment model (Ginsburg 2012). While we believe a population-based delivery model more appropriately aligns incentives with longitudinal outcomes than a bundled payment model, both reflect a broader trend toward aligning incentives with a greater degree of centralization and organizational authority for creating policies focused on quality of care.

Impetus to Integrate Evidence Based Medicine into Organizational Policies

As broader national trends have driven a centralization of authority over policies governing the provision of care, they have also provided financial impetus to focus that power—at least in part—on creating policies aimed specifically at providing evidence-based medicine. Unitedhealth's bundled payments for cancer care focus on developing specific algorithms, based on the best available evidence, to guide the chemotherapeutic decisions of individual practitioners (Goozner 2011). Geisinger's ProvenCare—the system largely informing the shape of the Center for Medicare and Medicaid Innovation (CMMI) pilot bundled payments program—emphasizes the importance of integrating evidence-based medicine into clinical practice processes (Berry et al. 2009). Our own experience in the CMMI pilot program has emphasized the importance of an evidence-based care path to serve as a roadmap to outline the expected care for a particular condition thereby decreasing variability, improving quality, and lowering costs. Similarly, the value proposition of the Accountable Care Organization relies on its ability to leverage performance and quality measures to better deliver evidence-based care and greater value (O'Halloran et al. 2012). As organizations gain authority to create policies

governing patient care, financial incentives align the generation of those policies with evidence-based medicine.

In addition to the trends driven by payment structures, the expansion of the provider pool to increasingly integrate advanced practice providers (APP) has compelled many provider organizations to integrate evidence-based medicine into their organizational policy. As the expanding need for providers has outpaced the growth in physician supply, many have suggested integrating APPs into practices as a strategy to improve access to care (Newhouse et al. 2011). In so doing, many organizations have sought to standardize care delivery to ensure maintenance of quality standards and evidence-based practice patterns. As APPs have demonstrated a greater ability than some physician groups to adhere to evidence-based guidelines, they are a growing provider group well suited to deliver evidence-based care (Wilson et al. 2005). The integration of the most current evidence-based practices into treatment protocols was felt to be among the factors most important to the successful implementation of a Nurse Practitioner heart failure disease management program (Whellan et al. 2001). By clearly outlining medications shown to benefit patients with heart failure and systematically ensuring patients were prescribed those medicines, nurse practitioners drove a reduction in hospitalizations. Similarly, in the inpatient ICU setting, computer-based platforms have proved effective in facilitating the delivery of evidence-based care for sepsis with the integration of APPs into the provider mix (McKinley et al. 2011). As evidence-based medicine becomes increasingly synonymous with quality, organizations seeking to maintain quality while growing their provider pool do so through the implementation of protocols and decision support tools facilitating the delivery of evidence-based medicine regardless of the provider type delivering care. The demands to grow the provider base with APPs while maintaining quality have primed organizations' pumps to shape policies guiding the delivery of larger scale evidence-based care paths to which all providers will be expected to adhere.

Evidence-Based Substrate to Generate Policies

To generate policies based on evidence, sufficient evidence must exist to guide decisions for the conditions organizations have prioritized as having the biggest impact on the systems and populations they govern. As the available evidence to guide clinical decisions has grown, professional organizations have increasingly embraced the opportunity to assimilate evidence into guideline recommendations governing the major clinical decisions facing their providers. While some argue that guidelines have proliferated to an unwieldy extent, the role of professional societies in advancing evidence-based medicine cannot be understated (Stewart et al. 2007). These guidelines—along with protocols and best practices—have been the primary modalities through which the evidence base has been translated to clinical practice (Xiao 2009). Some argue that guidelines are too blunt of an instrument to apply universally to clinical decision-making—that they do not afford the clinician the opportunity to tailor decisions to individual patient situations (Barrett 2008). Others maintain that guidelines will be most efficacious in shaping clinical decisions if they can be written and disseminated in a way that integrates with workflows and decision support systems (Kastner et al. 2011). In spite of some shortcomings related to their current deployment, guidelines represent a distillation of evidence often targeting the most common conditions encountered by a specialty and, consequently, the conditions more commonly affecting the patients of an organization. As such, guidelines represent an important starting point for organizations beginning to generate evidence-based policies.

As organizations prioritize conditions to target with policies based upon the magnitude of impact a policy might have on their patient populations, guidelines likely will not provide sufficient guidance as rarer conditions or more unique populations are targeted. As clinicians find value in systematic reviews and meta-analyses, organizations can turn to these studies as more summative accounts of trends in the literature as well as aggregates of studies among several populations

to guide policymaking (Sauerland and Seiler 2005). Not surprisingly, systematic reviews are also subject to limitations related to both the populations studied as well as the difficulty with which results can be translated into clinical practice (Murthy et al. 2012). To develop policies employing evidence-based practices, organizations will also require expertise in identifying the highest quality studies most pertinent to their populations—whether those are randomized controlled trials or case series. Whether bought or built, this expertise may not be sufficient in all cases. For certain rare conditions, providers have begun to leverage the data existent in their own organization's electronic health record to compile case series for conditions about which little published literature exists (Frankovich et al. 2011). As the policies governing evidence-based medicine expand within an organization and as rarer conditions are targeted, one can imagine the integration of an electronic health record query along with a literature query to set the pace for care for that rare condition. As such, an approach to identifying evidence for policymaking should focus on a systematic methodology to investigate literature as well as institutional evidence to inform decisions.

As care delivery becomes centralized and the organizations governing that delivery face increasing pressures to integrate the evidence base with that care, a system to prioritize conditions for policymaking and to identify the evidence guiding care for those conditions provides the backbone for effective policy deployment. With alignment on what evidence should be incorporated into policies, organizations must then turn to the operational considerations for implementing policies—the people, the infrastructure, and the push needed to get it done.

Policy Deployment

A Receptive Provider Pool

While the solo practitioner model introduced few elements to motivate providers to keep pace with the changing landscape of care, in the modern day, board licensure has underlined the importance of staying up to date by mandating continuing medical education as an essential component to maintaining a license. In 2012, sixty-two boards require continuing medical education (CME) for licensure, with some requiring a proportion of CME hours devoted to specific topics (AMA 2012). While no clear consensus exists regarding the optimum content, modality, or frequency for CME, the emphasis on staying current with evidence cuts across states and across professions. CME has been viewed as an appropriate vehicle to translate guidelines into practice and, more broadly, to deploy quality improvement efforts centered on improving patient outcomes (Mazmanian et al. 2009). While heterogeneity exists in the content of CME, the American Academy of Family Physicians has placed particular emphasis on evidence based CME by awarding double hours for so-called EB-CME sessions. As the central tenet of continuing medical education is remaining abreast of current evidence, it is no surprise that participants found these EB-CME sessions to offer information more readily applicable to clinical practice (Davis et al. 2009). Thus, this requirement of staying current with evidence for licensure has already established an evidence-based medicine imperative in the minds of providers upon which organizations may build when preparing providers for policies governing evidence-based medicine.

Although CME has rooted the idea of staying current with evidence in physician minds, it is the application of quality improvement principles to healthcare delivery that has provided both a conceptual framework and a toolkit for providers to translate this evidence into practice. While the integration of evidence-based medicine into QI interventions is not systematic, a natural synergy exists between the two movements and, in fact, early applications of QI to health care included very explicit methodologies to survey and integrate salient evidence (Glasziou et al. 2011). While significant institutional gaps must be bridged before implementation of QI efforts can be maximally effective, the efforts of the Institute of Medicine to increase understanding about what QI is and what impact it might have on the shape of

medical practice cannot be understated (Alexander and Herald 2011). The fundamental concept of continuous improvement aligns closely with the concept of revising practice patterns to keep pace with evolving medical science. A recent systematic review of the surgical literature identified 903 unique citations describing surgical quality improvement endeavors, evidence of the growing traction for QI as a discipline in the literature. While the interventions varied in the extent to which they focused on the integration of care improvement with clinical processes, interventions seeking to improve infection control, antibiotic use, and complication rates underline the engagement of providers in the implementation of processes to improve quality (Nicolay et al. 2012). It is this increased awareness among and engagement of providers in continuous process improvements in medicine that facilitates the deployment of policies designed to standardize implementation of evidence-based medicine. In this era of increasing financial pressure in medicine, leveraging QI and EBM with an added focus on cost to hone processes for antibiotic selection, appropriate diagnostic and therapeutic ordering patterns, and even operating room supplies seems a natural next-stop for provider institutions.

Necessary Infrastructure

While centralization, focus on quality, and growth of available evidence have positioned organizations to be able to generate policies prioritized for impact, and an emphasis on CME and a need to improve quality have helped to increase traction among providers for policy deployment, the implementation of policies would be an order of magnitude more difficult without the rise of the electronic health record. Even with appropriate motivation, receptivity, and training, the implementation challenges of applying evidence at the point of medical decision-making have been difficult hurdles to overcome (Barratt 2012). Deploying policies governing decisions has been that much more challenging given the difficulty of enacting real-time decision support. Electronic Health Records and Computerized Physician Order Entry have been oft touted as the optimum tools for integrating guidelines and evidence-based medicine into the daily workflows of providers since they are the tools by which providers enact decisions (Stewart et al. 2007). Despite these noted advantages, the financial investment and learning investment required remained barriers to widespread adoption.

The passage of the HITECH Act in 2009 provided federal funding to speed this adoption, paving the way for organizations to construct the framework necessary for policy deployment. The stipulations governing meaningful use seek to establish broad standards outlining the ways in which this technology should be used to support clinical processes. Specifically, to qualify for funding, providers will be required to leverage EHRs as tools to improve care rather than simply as modalities for documentation. Stage 1 of this meaningful use focuses on basic functionality but also the incorporation of electronic decision support elements into the EHR (Marcotte et al. 2012). This mandate illustrates an evolution in the process of clinical decision-making. What historically has been a provider leveraging his or her own individual knowledge to make clinical decisions is evolving to a more standardized armament of resources to support those decisions. Indeed, thought leaders espouse that attention to clinical thought processes along with clinical workflows will maximize the potential improvements resultant from the implementation of technology (Amatayakul 2011). By many accounts, the establishment of the meaningful use criteria marks a step forward in facilitating organizations' abilities to deploy policies governing evidence-based medicine at a level of granularity that was previously far less tenable.

While HITECH and Meaningful Use have fostered the spread of EHRs and their use as decision support tools, readying EHRs to deploy policies represents an additional barrier to implementation. That is, the expertise and time required to distill available literature and guidelines into policies and to integrate those policies into the IT infrastructure represent a material organizational investment. To be able to bring the evidence base to the point of decisions across different decision points and provider types, IT systems require standardization of methodologies to store and deploy data as well as a high degree of interoperability (Davis 2010). As industry has realized economies in both generating tools to deploy evidence as well as integrating those tools with institutions' IT infrastructure, organizations have increasing options beyond organically combing literature to create policies and integrating those policies with their EHRs individually (Hagland 2011). The growth of companies dedicated to easing the deployment of evidence-based policies serves to more seamlessly integrate those policies and to position organizations to more easily capitalize on EHR meaningful use dollars. Deciding on an appropriate vendor, allocating funds for initial purchase and updating, and planning for periodic survey of additional vendor options all represent additional resources that organizations must anticipate to take maximal advantage of EHRs as tools to deploy appropriate evidence at the time medical decisions are made.

Impetus to Deploy Policies

The Affordable Care Act has ushered in an era of heightened focus upon, and unprecedented access to, data around organizational performance. Value-Based Purchasing, one component of the Affordable Care Act, offers a program of national scope and nearly universal applicability which allows the Center for Medicare and Medicaid Services to align financial incentives with specific care improvement priorities, tying an organization's revenues to its performance relative to its peers (VanLare et al. 2012). Since adherence to evidence-based recommendations has been incorporated into the VBP measures, the program signals a commitment on the part of CMS to improve the integration of clinical processes and evidence-based medicine. While the expected changes in payments are small in the first year of the program, the magnitudes of the penalties and rewards is slated to grow year over year (Werner and Dudley 2012). Regardless of the magnitude of initial rewards and penalties, in its willingness to modify the program in response to feedback from organizations, CMS has signaled its investment in the success of VBP (Selvam 2011). As has historically been the case, private payers have begun to follow suit in developing their own VBP programs (Bush 2011). The financial impact of the CMS program thus has the potential to magnify the risks and rewards around specific performance measures if private payers choose to align their measures with CMS. For organizations seeking to maintain financial viability, the deployment of policies targeted at improving performance in accord with the evidence base will be critical, particularly as patients gain increasing access to performance data and incorporate those data into hospital and provider selection.

In addition to payment structures comparing organizational performance, the growth in transparency for patients has intensified the focus on performance measures and the need for such measures to drive improvement. CMS has developed a user-friendly interface to compare hospitals against each other across performance and quality measures (U.S. Department of Health and Human Services 2012). A number of the quality of care measures center around delivery of evidence-based care. Though the measures have been criticized in some cases because they are not directly tied to patient outcomes, they have been generally well received because of their sound evidence base (Stefan et al. 2012). Hospital Compare is only one among a growing number of websites allowing patients to compare hospital performance. Criticisms of the websites have included wide variations in the quality of data, variations in the level of detail, and a lack of standardization of quality measures (Leonardi et al. 2007). As patients find a growing number of sources for information about quality of care, each source may focus on different measures of quality. Organizations will likely need to understand those measures felt to be most relevant in their local markets to be able to integrate healthcare consumerism into the calculus used to prioritize policies.

Policy Sustainment and Management

With sufficient impetus and tools for generation and deployment of policies, organizations must also consider factors critical for the sustainment and management of such policies. Those factors include policy ownership and governance, methodologies for updating policies, and tools to track performance and drive improvement.

Policy Ownership and Governance

Forethought about who will own policies and who will govern their deployment and modification are important considerations as organizations prepare to enact policies. Delegating policymaking authority to the groups of providers for whom policies would most closely pertain might foster increased buy-in among those providers and might ease the maintenance of individual policies. Among the biggest drawbacks to a tactic of decentralization would be increasing the difficulty with which the organization can direct policies to suit its overall priorities compared to the possibly competing priorities of its constituents. Bodies governing infection control provide a useful case study in the benefits of centralized ownership of a process focusing on integrating evidence-based medicine with clinical processes. In this context, centralization has the benefit of reducing sources of ambiguity and augmenting the ability to achieve consensus around strategic priorities and tactics for implementation (Chou et al. 2008). That is, organizations that established a central body to decide which antibiotics would be used for which indications were more likely to use antibiotics appropriately and to minimize the likelihood of resistance. As the scope of policies extends beyond the realm of infection control, the benefits of centralization to decrease provider variability in the deployment of evidence-based medicine are likely magnified. Centralization of policy governance does not disaggregate providers from policies—in fact, providers have an imperative to stay abreast of evidence and to make cases for policy change (Muir Gray 2004). The clearer authority lines of a centralized structure for policy governance, while taking steps to maintain provider engagement, is important for maintaining the strategic direction of targeted policies.

Consideration of the specifics of that centralized structure will position organizations to maintain provider engagement with policies governing EBM. The shape of that structure should take into consideration the need to integrate providers with leadership to prioritize policies as well as to involve experts in policymaking. Leveraging existing governance structures will allow for efficient assimilation of a centralized body providing evidence-based medicine policy oversight into the organization. As many healthcare organizations utilize committees for governance, assembling a multidisciplinary committee comprised of administrative, physician, nursing, pharmacy, and information technology leadership will begin to convene the key stakeholders integral to policy management. Vesting this committee with the authority to prioritize, critique, deploy, and update policies offers an appropriate scope of responsibility for policy management. Simultaneously creating clinician councils to research and develop specific policies through an algorithmic approach has allowed for an efficient means to standardize policy development (Oman et al. 2008). It would also be prudent for the committee to establish and monitor quality measures related to the care governed by the policy to allow for course correction in the event of unintended consequences resultant from policy deployment (Ghafoor and Silus 2011). Finally, developing an approach to ensure regular literature surveys and policy updates will keep the evidence upon which policies are developed current. While warfarin was the one-time standard of care for recurrent venous thromboembolism prophylaxis, without a mechanism to ensure regular updating, institutions would likely have been slower to integrate the accumulating evidence supporting enoxaparin as the drug of choice (Noble et al. 2008).

Policy Updating

In order to maintain policies governing the provision of current evidence-based medicine, organizations will require standards for updating policies. The process of updating policies organically will likely involve revisiting the literature review utilized to generate the initial policy to identify studies that alter the management governed by the policy. The policy itself can then be revised to reflect these changes, vetted through the appropriate governing structure, and integrated into the current delivery mechanism. Additionally, organizations may consider standardizing methodologies to mine the data repositories from their own electronic health records to generate evidence based upon outcomes among the specific populations they serve to further inform the modification of policies (Stewart et al. 2007). As organizations scale their policies, the resource investment required to update policies will grow. As such, anticipating the frequency and extent of updates required will allow for planning appropriate capacity to maintain current policies. However, anticipating the appropriate frequency with which to revisit reviews can be challenging as a great degree of variability exists in the timing of publication of studies that would likely drive changes in policies (Shojania et al. 2007). Given this degree of variability, some have found success in a hybrid approach employing the combination of periodic reviews and discussions with clinical experts to determine whether policies reflect current practices supported by the literature (Lyratzopoulos et al. 2012). This hybrid approach is possible for organizations possessing adequate clinical expertise across the spectrum of their policy-driven decisions. While the availability of expertise may influence the prioritization of some policies over others, organizations without adequate clinical expertise will need to employ alternative mechanisms to ensure policies are up to date, such as collaborating with expert institutions or considering commercial products developed by experts.

For many organizations, the level of customization and ownership gained from dedicating scarce resources to undertake literature reviews and involving appropriate clinical experts may not be worth the investment. Larger organizations with higher degrees of sub specialization or extensive academic enterprises already undertaking literature reviews for research purposes may be able to leverage these existing resources for policy updating. Many organizations are, however, turning to industry to facilitate their policy updating. Several companies have realized a value proposition not just in standardizing order sets and decision support tools for clinicians, but also in offering periodic updates to those sets and tools in accord with advances in the literature (Hagland 2011). In addition, the Agency for Healthcare Research and Quality has been exploring alternative means of updating evidence briefs and reviews. They have recently studied the feasibility of a wiki platform for generating and disseminating such updates (Erinoff 2012). While such a platform might offer free updates that organizations could leverage, the quality of those updates would be subject to concerns about update frequency as well as the individual updater's expertise. If the governance of such a wiki site could address quality control, it might present another viable alternative for organizations looking outside their own personnel for updates. Regardless of the modalities chosen for updating, the value of updating policies can only be realized if providers adhere to changing policies, underlining the importance of systems to monitor and feed back performance.

Performance Tracking and Improvement

Organizations may invest extensively in mechanisms to govern and update policies, but without mechanisms to monitor adherence to policies and to improve adherence, organizations will limit their return on those investments. Establishing both process measures to determine adherence to policies and outcome measures to monitor the impact of those policies on patients are important to understanding the success of policies and developing mechanisms to improve policies. On first pass, it might seem appropriate for providers themselves to establish measures to increase provider engagement. Leveraging the multidisciplinary governing body to determine measures will bring to bear the expertise of all stakeholders with authority over policies—providers as well as administrators (Hagland 2011). The ease with which data can be obtained may also influence measures available to promote provider adherence. Electronic health records have previously been described as critical tools for policy deployment, but they are also recognized as important means to both measure and improve provider performance (Liang 2011). EHRs may thus serve as the sources for data underpinning performance measurement. Furthermore, the

extent to which EHRs have been integrated into workflows may also position them as means to feed back performance. In particular, decision support tools may be deployed as a means to provide real-time feedback about individual provider performance at the point of decision-making (Doran et al. 2007). One might imagine an alert notifying a provider at the time of discharge that his or her patient was known to have heart failure but was not prescribed appropriate medications for heart failure. Additionally, leveraging existing institutional mechanisms for performance feedback, such as balanced scorecards or report cards, may offer synergies obviating the need to create entirely new feedback mechanisms. Once measures and data sources have been identified and an infrastructure to share data developed, target selection and incentive development should follow as tools to improve performance.

While sharing provider-level performance data may bring about some improvement in policy adherence, developing additional tools will likely enhance that improvement. Auditing adherence to policies and feeding back the degree of adherence to individual providers without additional incentive structures has led to improvement (Ivers et al. 2012). However, developing performance targets can provide more tangible goals for individual providers. If those targets are developed based on national benchmarks, targets can also serve as a broader frame of reference for individual or even organizational performance. Additionally, openly sharing performance data among providers is an important tool for high performing work practices to bring performance in line with peers (Robbins et al. 2012). Creating incentive structures to reward target achievement or to penalize underperformance can further magnify the impact of such data transparency. Tying financial incentives to the delivery of evidence-based care, such as the proportion of a primary care physician's eligible patients receiving appropriate colorectal cancer screening, has been associated with a larger proportion of patients receiving evidence-based care compared to a conventional setting without incentives (Gilmore et al. 2007). Finally, individual providers may feel removed from the impact of

Value-Based Purchasing on the organizations with which they are affiliated though their actions influence organizational compensation. Aligning incentives with policies tied to the evidence-based medicine components of VBP can position organizations to better translate the financial impact of provider behavior to those providers. As increasing numbers of payers tie compensation to the delivery of evidence-based medicine, the ability to feedback and improve provider behaviors by identifying patients experiencing inappropriate practice patterns and the dollars associated with those patterns will be important for physician financial viability as well as the quality of patient care. There is some concern about the development of dissatisfaction among providers resulting from a diminished perception of autonomy as an increasing proportion of their income becomes tied to prescribed behaviors.

Increasingly, organizations' ability to deliver quality care rests on their ability to translate the evidence base into policies integrated with provider workflows. Mechanisms to govern policy generation, deployment, and management as well as the ability to update policies and to measure and improve performance impacted by those policies are critical for organizations' success in more uniformly practicing evidence-based medicine.

Looking Ahead

As organizations develop their own infrastructures for policy generation, deployment, and management, an overarching focus on the management of the individual patient persists. Perhaps this focus has roots in the traditional fee-for-service environment as well as the evolution of the doctor–patient relationship. We anticipate, however, that as the traditional fee-for-service compensation structure continues to dissipate and as care delivery models continue to evolve to meet increasing needs for access to providers, the management of populations will continue to grow in emphasis and importance. While hospitals have acted as centralizing organizations in recent years, the ability to integrate with outpatient providers and to deliver care in more diverse settings will be

tantamount to organizational survival. Organizations' ability to manage policies governing the delivery of evidence-based medicine will be vital for ensuring the provision of quality care in this changing landscape. Future directions for investigation should include: how to further streamline the deployment of policies through EHRs as the growth in insured patients through the Affordable Care Act further stresses a constrained provider pool; how organizations should approach policies governing the benefits and costs of therapies supported by strong evidence as the cost of US healthcare continues to grow; and how EHRs can integrate patient preferences into provider workflows at the point of decision-making to accommodate growing patient consumerism.

Acknowledgements We would like to thank Connie Schardt for her assistance with the literature search that has informed this work.

References

Ahmadi, N., et al. (2012). Teaching evidence based medicine to surgery residents-is journal club the best format? A systematic review of the literature. *Journal of Surgical Education,* 91–100.

Alexander, J. A. & Herald, L. R. (2011). The science of quality improvement implementation: Developing capacity to make a difference. *Medical Care,* S6–S20.

American Medical Association (AMA) (2012). Continuing medical education for licensure registration. *State Medical Licensure Requirements and Statistics,* 65–68.

Amatayakul, M. (2011). Why workflow redesign alone is not enough for EHR success. *Healthcare Financial Management,* 130–132.

Barratt, A. (2008). Evidence based medicine and shared decision making: The challenge of getting both evidence and preferences into health care. *Patient Education and Counseling,* 407–412.

Barrett, B. (2012). Evidence, values, guidelines and rational decision-making. *Journal of General Internal Medicine,* 238–240.

Berry, S. A., et al. (2009). ProvenCare: Quality improvement model for designing highly reliable care in cardiac surgery. *Quality Safety Health Care,* 360–368.

Bush, H. (2011, June) Hospitals partner with blue cross blue shield on value-based purchasing. *Hospitals & Health Networks,* 16.

Bwakura-Dangarembizi, M., et al. (2014). A randomized trial of prolonged co-trimoxazole in HIV-infected children in Africa. *The New England Journal of Medicine,* 41–53.

Chou, A. F., et al. (2008). Structural and process factors affecting the implementation of antimicrobial resistance prevention and control strategies in US hospitals. *Health Care Management Review*, 308–322.

Claridge, J. A., et al. (2005). History and development of evidence-based medicine. *World Journal of Surgery*, 547–553.

Cochrane, A. L. (2004). *Effectiveness & efficiency: Random reflections on health services*. London: Royal Society of Medicine Press Limited.

Cooper, C., et al. (2014). Stenting and medical therapy for atherosclerotic renal-artery stenosis. *The New England Journal of Medicine*, 13–22.

Davis, B. J. (2010). Improving healthcare outcomes through EBM. *Health Management Technology*, 24–25.

Davis, N. L., et al. (2009). Improving the value of CME: Impact of an evidence-based CME credit designation on faculty and lecturers. *Family Medicine*, 735–740.

Delisle, D. R. (2012). Big things come in bundled packages: Implications of bundled payment systems in health care reimbursement reform. *American Journal of Medical Quality* (ePub ahead of print).

Doran, D. M., et al. (2007). Outcomes-focused knowledge translation: A framework for knowledge translation and patient outcomes improvement. *Worldviews on Evidence-Based Nursing*, 3–13.

Eddy, D. M. (2005). Evidence-based medicine: A unified approach. *Health Affairs*, 9–17.

Erinoff, E. G. (2012). *Feasibility study for a wiki collaboration platform for systematic reviews*. Rockville: Agency for Healthcare Research and Quality, 2011 September 02–12. http://www.ncbi.nlm.nih.gov/books/NBK82273/

Franklin, W., et al. (1958). Bronchodilators and corticosteroids in the treatment of obstructive pulmonary emphysema. *The New England Journal of Medicine*, 774–778.

Frankovich, J., et al. (2011). Evidence-based medicine in the EMR era. *New England Journal of Medicine*, 1758–1759.

Ghafoor, V. L., & Silus, L. S. (2011). Developing policy, standard orders, and quality-assurance monitoring for palliative sedation therapy. *American Journal of Health System Pharmacy*, 523–527.

Gilmore, A. S., et al. (2007). Quality and outcomes: Patient outcomes and evidence-based medicine in a preferred provider organization setting: A six-year evaluation of a pay-for-performance program. *Health Services Research*, 2140–2159.

Ginsburg, P. B. (2012). Fee-for-service will remain a feature of major payment reforms, requiring more changes in medicare physician payment. *Health Affairs*, 1977–1983.

Glasziou, P., et al. (2011). Can evidence-based medicine and clinical quality improvement learn from each other? *British Medical Journal of Quality and Safety*, i13–i17.

Goozner, M. (2011). United healthcare, five oncology practices try bundled payments. *Journal of the National Cancer Institute*, 8–10.

Grieble, H., et al. (1958). Prolonged treatment of urinary-tract infections with sulfamethoxypyridazine. *The New England Journal of Medicine*, 1–7.

Grol, R., & Grimshaw, J. (2003). From best evidence to best practice: Effective implementation of change in patients' care. *Lancet*, 1225–1230.

Hagland, M. (2011). Gold from the mine: Helathcare IT and clinician leaders make evidence-based care a reality. *Healthcare Informatics*, 10–17.

Harrison, J. D. (2012, July 20). Health-care law driving doctors away from small practices, toward hospital employment. *The Washington Post*.

Ivers, N., et al. (2012). Audit and feedback: Effects on professional practice and healthcare outcomes. *Cochrane Database Systematic Review*, 1–229.

Kastner, M., et al. (2011). Better guidelines for better care: enhancing the implementability of clinical practice guidelines. *Expert Review of Pharmacoeconomics & Outcomes Research*, 315–324.

Kohn, M. K. (2011). Evidence-based decision making in health care settings: From theory to practice. *Biennial Review of Health Care Management (Advances in Health Care Management)*, 215–234.

Lammers, E. (2012). The effect of hospital-physician integration on health information technology adoption. *Health Economics* (Epub ahead of print).

Larson, B. K., et al. (2012). Insight from transformations under way at four Brookings-Dartmouth accountable care organization pilot sites. *Health Affairs*, 2395–2406.

Leonardi, M. J., et al. (2007). Publicly available hospital comparison websites. *Archives of Surgery*, 863–869.

Liang, L. (2011). The gap between evidence and practice. *Health Affairs*, w119-w121.

Long, L. E., & Brewer, T. (2011). Evidence-based policy in the new organizational paradigm part 1. *Journal of Pediatric Nursing*, 385–387.

Lyratzopoulos, G., et al. (2012). Updating clinical practice recommendations: Is it worthwhile and when? *International Journal of Technology Assessment in Health Care*, 29–35.

Marcotte, L., et al. (2012). Achieving meaningful use of health information technology: A guide for physicians to the EHR incentive programs. *Archives of Internal Medicine*, 731–736.

Matthews, A. W. (2010, November 29). Embracing incentives for efficient health care. *Wall Street Journal*, B1.

Mazmanian, P. E., et al. (2009). Continuing medical education effect on clinical outcomes. *Chest*, 49S–55S.

McKinley, B. A., et al. (2011). Computer protocol facilitates evidence-based care of sepsis in the surgical intensive care unit. *Journal of Trauma*, 1153–1167.

Muir Gray, J. A. (2004). Evidence based policy making. *British Medical Journal*, 988–989.

Murthy, L., et al. (2012). Interventions to improve the use of systematic reviews in decision-making by health system managers, policy makers and clinicians. *Cochrane Database Systematic Review*, 1–62.

Newhouse, R. P., et al. (2011). Advanced practice nurse outcomes 1990–2008: A systematic review. *Nursing Economics*, 230-250.

Nicolay, C. R., et al. (2012). Systematic review of the application of quality improvement methodologies from the manufacturing industry to surgical healthcare. *British Journal of Surgery*, 324–335.

Noble, S. I., et al. (2008). Management of venous thromboembolism in patients with advanced cancer: A systematic review and meta-analysis. *Lancet Oncology*, 577–84.

O'Halloran, K., et al. (2012). The role of accountable care organizations in delivering value. *Current Reviews in Musculoskeletal Medicine*, 283–289.

Oman, K. S., et al. (2008). Evidence-based policy and procedures. *The Journal of Nursing Administration*, 47–51.

Robbins, J., et al. (2012). How high-performance work systems drive health care value: An examination of leading process improvement strategies. *Quality Management in Health Care*, 188–202.

Sackett, D. L., et al. (1996). Evidence based medicine: What it is and what it isn't. *British Medical Journal*, 71–72.

Sauerland, S. & Seiler, C. M. (2005). Role of systematic reviews and meta-analysis in evidence-based medicine. *World Journal of Surgery*, 582–587.

Selvam, A. (2011). Moving in the right direction: Value-based purchasing changes meet approval. *Modern Healthcare*, 8–9.

Shojania, K. G., et al. (2007). How quickly do systematic reviews go out of date? A survival analysis. *Annals of Internal Medicine*, 224–233.

Stefan, M. S., et al. (2012). Hospital performance measures and 30-day readmission rates. *Journal of General Internal Medicine* (Epub ahead of print).

Stewart, W. F., et al. (2007). Bridging the inferential gap: The electronic health record and clinical evidence. *Health Affairs*, w181–w191.

U.S. Department of Health and Human Services (HHS) (2012, October 11). *Hospital Compare*. http://www.hospitalcompare.hhs.gov/. 2012, October 11

VanLare, J. M., et al. (2012). Value-based purchasing–National programs to move from volume to value. *New England Journal of Medicine*, 292–295.

Werner, R. M. & Dudley, R. A. (2012). Medicare's new hospital value-based purchasing program is likely to have only a small impact on hospital payments. *Health Affairs*, 1932–1940.

Whellan, D. J., et al. (2001). The benefit of implementing a heart failure disease management program. *Archives of Internal Medicine*, 2223–2228.

Wilson, I. B., et al. (2005). Quality of HIV care provided by nurse practitioners, physician assistants, and physicians. *Annals of Internal Medicine*, 729–736.

Xiao, Q., et al. (2009). An exploratory study of institutional effects on the practice of evidence-based medicine in acute care hospitals. *Academy of Health Care Management Journal*, 1–29.

Introduction: Transformations in Health Care Delivery and Financing

23

Stephen M. Weiner

Clinical decision-making ideally should be a partnership of caregiver and patient, and, where applicable, the patient's family members or other representatives, engaged in a robust exchange of information about the individual's specific health care needs and how they relate to, or are affected by, other aspects of the patient's life situation and overall well-being. The reality in the United States is far from the ideal. To begin to grasp the challenges facing both patient and caregiver in structuring a productive relationship requires an understanding of the complexity of the context in which such decision-making occurs in this country.

While the United States health care system appears to be an ever-changing organism, especially with the implementation of the 2010 Affordable Care Act (ACA), some trends can be discerned and some generalizations made that have some validity for framing the current context and how it may evolve. But setting out trends and generalizations in this field must be conditioned on one important caveat: predictions are notoriously unreliable, and any effort to state with certainty what the future of health care will look like in the United States should be met with substantial skepticism. Nonetheless it is appropriate

to identify some key trends and their underlying dynamics relating to clinical decision-making and progress toward the ideal of the patient–caregiver partnership.

From a very broad perspective one can see the core tension within the United States health care delivery system as that between access and cost, or, more precisely, access and cost containment. On one end of a theoretical continuum is the goal of assuring unlimited access to high quality care. There are a number of ways to achieve this goal, but, whatever approach is used, the resulting increase in the cost of health care and stress on available resources would be potentially catastrophic. On the other end of the theoretical continuum is the goal of cost containment, which in its most extreme form would be true rationing of health care to constrain cost within preestablished limitations. The social and political costs of rationing would be incalculable, especially in light of the virtual impossibility of making a rational, and equitable, determination of how it would work. Between these two theoretically possible but implausible extremes, the tension between access and cost containment oscillates around an ever-moving, and sometimes not entirely evident, equilibrium point. At any point in time one goal is favored over the other. But over the past few years, especially in the context of the efforts to enact, and then implement, the ACA, and with the intense political focus on deficit reduction at the federal and many State levels, the tension between improving access and

S.M. Weiner (✉)
Chair, Health Law Practice, Mintz, Levin, Cohn, Ferris, Glovsky and Popeo, P.C, One Financial Center, Boston, MA 02111, USA
e-mail: sweiner@mintz.com

© Springer Science+Business Media New York 2016
M.A. Diefenbach et al. (eds.), *Handbook of Health Decision Science*,
DOI 10.1007/978-1-4939-3486-7_23

the costs associated with doing so has taken on a tangible political reality.

Two examples of how access and cost have been balanced as matters of public policy may be seen in the different approaches to access reform and its attendant costs adopted in Massachusetts in 2006 and by the federal government in 2010 with the ACA. In both cases the policy and political motivations were to address the large numbers of residents who had no or wholly inadequate insurance coverage.

In Massachusetts a bipartisan and broad-based political consensus developed to seek access reform, with the goal of covering as many legal residents of the Commonwealth as feasible. But there was also recognition that the consensus would not be sustainable if cost containment were to be addressed simultaneously. Decisions as to who would bear the financial burden of reform are always the hardest of issues to resolve. The consensus called for deferring the issue, recognizing that access reform would increase the cost of care—whether because of greater demand for services by newly insured individuals or because of the need to provide government subsidies in support of purchasing affordable health insurance—but that access could not be achieved simultaneously with instituting cost containment policies. Massachusetts' subsequent initiatives to address cost containment—the issue was deferred but not forgotten—will provide useful illustrations of changes taking place that are directly relevant to the patient–caregiver partnership.

At the federal level, because of "scoring" as part of the federal budget process, dealing with the costs to the federal government expected to be generated because of the ACA's access reform, through for example subsidies for obtaining insurance coverage, could not be deferred. "Scoring" required balancing projected additional costs with savings in the form of revenue increases or cost reductions. The ACA used short-term offsets but also held out the possibility that long-term structural changes could reduce federal budgetary costs overall. Examples of the short-term approach included reductions in Medicare's payment rates to hospitals, including disproportionate share hospitals (justified on the basis that more insured patients would generate more revenue for those institutions) and tax increases such as the medical device tax. Examples of the longer term approach included the efforts at undertaking delivery system and payment reforms on a demonstration basis, such as the Medicare Shared Savings Program (promoting accountable care organizations or ACOs), patient-centered medical home programs and bundled payment initiatives.

The longer term approaches identified in the ACA are relevant to the discussion of decision-making because they pointed to the linkage between cost containment and broader reforms of the health care delivery system. The MSSP pilot, at the conceptual level, identified the importance of the organized delivery of care, the associated management of that care, and the incentives created by having providers share with Medicare in resulting savings as vehicles for achieving reductions in the inefficiency with which care is provided in the United States. Equally important, the MSSP incorporated the use of quality measures in assessing the availability of financial benefits from MSSP participation. Incentives based on the quality of care had already been introduced into the payment methodologies of both private and public payers, often with penalties for not meeting quality benchmarks. MSSP was an example of moving beyond penalties to rewards for good quality care.

The post-2006 developments in Massachusetts show a consistent but even more refined and comprehensive approach to seeking cost containment through delivery and payment system reform. Through a series of enactments in 2008, 2010 and 2012, Massachusetts set in place mechanisms for extensive data gathering about the cost and quality of care; instituted processes to establish uniform metrics for cost and quality to allow greater comparative analysis of provider behavior; and created commissions to explore payment reform as a means of changing incentives for overutilization of care and to understand the market impact of provider–payer negotiations and provider system consolidations.

Building on much of the learning initiated under the 2006, 2008 and 2010 legislation, in 2012 Massachusetts enacted Chapter 224 of the Acts of 2012 (Chapter 224), which sets annual benchmarks for the overall growth in aggregate health care expenditures in the Commonwealth and establishes mechanisms for monitoring performance against these benchmarks to hold providers and payers accountable if the benchmarks are not met. It also encourages or, in the case of government payers, especially Medicaid, mandates the use of alternative payment methodologies as alternatives to fee-for-service payment, and encourages the restructuring of care into more coordinated models such as ACOs and patient-centered medical homes.

The ACA and, in many respects even more immediately, Chapter 224 recognize that access reform requires the creation of efficiencies in the health care system, or at least serious efforts to create those efficiencies. For providers of care such efforts pose both major opportunities and major challenges. Some ways of doing business will inevitably change, and a key question is how adapting to these changes will affect the way in which providers, especially physicians, will interact with their patients. The "new world"— not so new really, but becoming much more extensive than has been the case in the US historically—will require collaboration and coordination with peers; acceptance of increasingly standardized means of providing care, such as through guidelines and protocols; and a willingness to share caregiving responsibilities with those who traditionally were not peers.

Under the emerging forms of care delivery and payment the balance between too much care and too little care will need to be recalibrated. Under the traditional fee-for-service world there were no significant penalties for providing or ordering too much care as long as there was a credible argument that the care was medically necessary. Now the penalties for too much care may be self-imposed or may be externally imposed by payers, but they are likely to be real. If providers are taking risk together, or have the opportunity to benefit from savings they collectively achieve, greater scrutiny will be paid to the

outliers who practice "too expensive" a brand of care. Analytics of practice patterns and the increased reliance on protocols or guidelines will have the effect of bringing all participants in the care coordination arrangement into line with a normative practice model. For physicians used to practicing their own individualized style of medicine, this could be quite traumatic, leading to potentially serious loss of income or early retirement from practice.

At the same time—in health care for every yin there is a yang—concern will focus on whether the new financial incentives are resulting in too little care being provided. This was one of the concerns that led to the so-called "managed care revolution" in the late 1990s. While metrics are improving regarding when there may be too much care, it is not at all evident what measures allow for determining when, from a clinical perspective, the care is not enough (except when it may trigger a malpractice action—see below). It will be instructive to ascertain if the collective approaches to monitoring clinical activities that are arising from the evolving models of care delivery and payment can assess insufficient care as well as they may be able to assess overabundant care.

One of the arguments made for why it was appropriate for clinicians to err toward too much care arose from medical malpractice concerns and the perceived attendant need to practice defensive medicine. It is not entirely surprising that efforts at delivery and payment reform are now, to a certain extent, being accompanied by efforts at malpractice reform. Utah began its reform efforts by focusing on malpractice reform. Chapter 224 took some steps toward malpractice reform, most notably by promoting and protecting the use of "apology" as a means of reducing the likelihood of a patient suing a physician. Efforts to support more effective patient–caregiver relationships, addressed later in this chapter, build upon a history demonstrating that improving these relationships reduces the likelihood of malpractice claims.

In addition to incentives to reduce presumably unnecessary care, other elements of creating an efficient delivery system are emerging that have readily perceived benefits, but may nonetheless create tension, if not outright hostility, within the medical profession. One such highly visible element that is directly driven by access reform relates to initiatives promoting the use of primary care resources in addition to primary care physicians.

One of the first effects of the 2006 Massachusetts access reform legislation was too many newly insured people seeking resources that were insufficient to meet the new demand, specifically for primary care physicians. Prior to enactment of the reform Massachusetts had a shortage of primary care physicians. The reform exacerbated that shortage. A 2011 Massachusetts Medical Society study found that, from 2007 to 2011, while approximately 400,000 residents became newly insured, the number of family physicians accepting new patients decreased consistently, with only 47 % doing so in 2011. In parallel, wait time to see internal medicine physicians was high, averaging 49 days, an increase of 9 days from the enactment of the reform. The result, as could have been expected, was continued and increasing reliance on hospital emergency departments. While it is too early to tell, it is likely that similar effects will be experienced now that the individual mandate and the exchanges under the ACA are being implemented.

Increasing the supply of primary care physicians is challenging. First there is a pipe line issue: creating incentives now will likely not be felt until after current medical school students finish both undergraduate and some graduate medical training. Second, physician payment structures, including Medicare's, favor specialty physicians over primary care. Third, medical school debt supports the need for pursuing well-reimbursed specialties. Certainly there have been initiatives to address some of these disincentives, including loan forgiveness programs or other forms of support for physicians seeking a career in primary care. Changes in the payment system may help move away from fee-for-service and provide financial incentives for the primary care physician's care management role. But these efforts will not necessarily have an immediate effect on increasing the primary care physician supply, while public policy promoting access will have a much more immediate effect on people seeking care from such physicians.

One approach has been to extend the scope of primary care resources by expanding beyond primary care physicians. Turning again to Massachusetts for an example, to address the primary care physician shortage, in addition to authorizing loan programs and the like to support physician choice of a primary care practice, legislation expanded the ability of both nurse practitioners and physicians' assistants to assume a greater role in care delivery.

In addition, entrepreneurial efforts have gained significant ground in filling the space between primary care physician offices and the hospital emergency room. MinuteClinic, a retail affiliate of CVS Health, provides care that is characterized as limited and does so in a convenient retail setting. Care is provided by nurse practitioners and physicians' assistants, but not directly by physicians, who are available for consultation and supervision. While the specific scope of a retail clinic's services may be somewhat amorphous, internal guidelines, and in some cases regulations, seek to assure that what is done in that setting is not a substitution for the range of services that can be provided in more intense settings, including physician offices. For example, while a nurse practitioner working within a retail clinic setting can function within her or his legally permitted scope of practice, the limited resources available to the nurse practitioner in that setting act as constraints on the level of complex services that she or he can provide.

As an historical and political matter, expansion of the roles of nurse practitioners, physician assistants, and nontraditional care settings such as urgent care centers and retail clinics, may present threats to traditional physician practices. Nonetheless, with the demand for physician services resulting from access reform, physicians will need to reassess their role within the health care continuum and assume responsibility for a higher level of complexity of care while allowing, voluntarily or not, personnel that had been considered "ancillary" to move to a position more like that of peers. The pressures on primary care physicians, initiatives to create teams of collaborating practitioners through models such as that of ACOs, and the resurgence of financial risk arrangements for payment of care reinforce the trend toward increased reliance on non-physician resources in the direct provision of care to patients. And, interestingly, it appears that, in light of the pressures faced by primary care physicians, traditional resistance by organized medicine to such scope of practice expansion may be waning.

While these developments may cause tension between physicians and other providers of primary care as physicians adapt to collaborative models of care, it is also important to consider the effect on the patient. Because of the historical dominance of the role of physicians in the delivery system, patients have become acculturated to relying on physicians even when, for example, nurse practitioners perfectly competent to address the patient's need are readily available. The evolution of roles in the primary care arena poses another challenge to the patient–caregiver relationship and impacts on how that partnership makes treatment decisions.

Technology of course represents one of the major sources of change in the health care environment. It is impacting every aspect of care and is changing how caregivers practice and how patients themselves define their role. Two types technological development, and their impact in decision-making, will be briefly discussed: electronic medical records, including personal health records; and telehealth, including both in direct care and for gathering data for clinical analysis.

The transition to nationwide electronic health records is a key objective of government health care policy. The American Recovery and Reinvestment Act of 2009 included what is known as the HITECH Act, establishing a framework and incentive funding for achieving a national distribution of interoperable electronic health record systems. The rationale for the importance of EHR has variously been indicated to be improvement in quality, more effective coordination of care, and cost savings. These tend to be interrelated objectives and, in fact, none can adequately be achieved without all three being addressed together. The information available through an EHR system should allow a caregiver to derive and analyze more data points more efficiently in making any individual care decision. Depending on how the information is used, data sharing can result in better coordination of care. The cost containment objectives are somewhat more speculative: proper use of EHR systems should reduce the amount of duplicative services that are provided since information about prior diagnostic tests, for example, will be available as care decisions are made and will not need to be repeated. In an alternative payment world, the benefits of being able to manage information are compatible with the financial incentives built into payment systems.

However, since nothing is simple in the health care world, successful deployment of EHR systems to improve health care decision-making and create more efficient care delivery must identify and address sources of resistance. The first is the importance of interoperability. While many large practices and hospital systems have adopted EHR systems that work within their own institutions and among their employed physicians or affiliated physicians (see below) these systems can achieve the anticipated benefits only if they capture all the clinical data about their patients. This assumes that patients will be willing to stay within a closed system of care. That seems unlikely, and may in fact be even less the case in the future. While clinicians in one system may transmit patient information to another system in which the same patient is receiving care, compatibility of systems may pose a problem.

Therefore, for EHR to have its most efficacious impact it must be connected to other systems through a heath information exchange (HIE). Absent the ability to force patients to stay within a closed care delivery system the benefits of EHR become more limited without adoption of an effective HIE. Interoperability, however, requires provider systems to be willing to collaborate with each other, even when they have already developed their own EHR capabilities. Given that one of the motivations for provider systems to be early adopters of EHR was gaining a competitive edge in their markets, the benefits of interoperability need to be tangible, or mandated. The HITECH Act encourages the development of a nationwide HIE and provides funding in support of this objective. Some States have mandated the adoption of interoperable EHR systems.

At the same time, the dissemination of personal health information (PHI) among EHR systems poses additional privacy and security challenges. HIPAA was enacted as electronic transmission of PHI was first developing. As usually happens in health care, the law follows, not leads, developments on the ground. The increasing reliance on electronic data and the increasing likelihood that this data will be transmitted between systems poses challenges to both HIPAA and traditional privacy law. What additional security systems will be needed to protect the data? How will concepts such as opt-in/opt-out rights, or the segregation of certain PHI, such as that relating to mental illness of HIV/AIDS, be handled when data is transmitted electronically and the protections that could be incorporated into paper records may not be as readily available? These issues require the evolution of law to be sure they are addressed fairly and effectively, as well as the evolution of the technology itself to assure that the values underlying established legal doctrine, such as those inherent in HIPAA, are respected.

Notwithstanding the public policy goal of achieving nationwide dissemination of interoperable EHR, there are sources of resistance, and how resistance is resolved has significant implications for the delivery of health care and the patient/caregiver relationship.

One source of resistance is cultural. Many older practitioners are not readily prepared to adapt to the new technology. In part this may be due to a discomfort with technology generally, especially on the part of older primary care physicians. These practitioners may be reluctant to learn new ways of doing business. Some, though, may genuinely fear that use of EHR may impact their practice by requiring them to cease using their experience and intuition in making clinical judgments and instead to follow preset algorithms of analysis. These feelings about the introduction of the new technology may lead practitioners to leave medicine entirely rather than to adapt. An unintended effect of the desire to promote more access and a more efficient delivery system may very well be to limit access to the more seasoned primary care physicians.

A second source of resistance to EHR dissemination is cost. While deployment of interoperable EHR is seen as serving cost containment objectives, the direct and immediate cost of deployment is quite substantial, while eventual savings seem somewhat more diffuse. That is, the longer term savings may redound to the benefit of the system as a whole, or the payers for health care services, but the immediate investment must be made by the practitioners who will be using the EHR systems at the outset. The costs include direct expenditure for the hardware and software systems needed to support interoperable EHR. But in addition there are opportunity costs associated with time spent away from seeing patients in order to learn the use of and deploy these new systems in office settings. How practitioners are able to underwrite the cost of deployment is being addressed through a combination of legal and business strategies.

Two examples of the legal strategies are the HITECH Act and the adoption of applicable safe harbors and exceptions under the federal Anti-Kickback Statute (AKS) and Stark Law (Stark).

The HITECH Act authorizes incentive payments for certain categories of Medicare and Medicaid provider participants to adopt interoperable EHR systems that satisfy federal standards regarding their capabilities, generally referred to as "meaningful use" standards. While the dollars appropriated for this purpose overall are substantial, the amount available to individual provider groups or institutions is likely to be insufficient to underwrite the entire cost of deployment of systems that meet the meaningful use standards. In addition after 2015 the Medicare participating providers in the categories eligible to receive these incentive payments are subject to penalties for failing to meet meaningful use standards. It will be interesting to determine whether some of them do a cost/benefit calculation to determine if the penalties are greater or less than the costs of deployment not covered by the incentive payments.

Further, the cost associated with adoption of interoperable EHR systems has meant that, to a large extent, hospital systems or large physician group practices with greater resources have been earlier adopters. But these greater resources also make them an attractive alternative source to fund the less resourced providers who are nonetheless obliged to meet federal requirements. The business need of physicians to turn to hospital systems, however, poses a problem under the AKS and Stark, two federal statutory schemes applicable to Medicare payment (and Medicaid in the case of the AKS) that criminalized (AKS) or otherwise penalized (Stark) certain financial relationships between hospital systems and physicians who are not their employees. The agencies responsible for these statutory schemes ultimately issued safe harbors or exceptions that permitted some level of subsidy by hospital systems for non-employed physicians to assist in their acquisition of EHR capacity. These exceptions are quite technical and somewhat crimped in the freedom they provide for the subsidies to be forthcoming, but they do represent an effort to accommodate the law to the practical realities being faced by private practitioners in implementing a program of public policy importance.

As might be inferred from the preceding paragraph, the legal issues associated with funding EHR deployment lead directly to a business strategy. Independent practicing physicians struggling to afford the costs of EHR deployment may see that a safer course to follow to access funds is to become employed by hospital systems or larger physician group practices or systems to which they send their referrals. Bona fide employment relationships are not subject to the AKS, and can be structured with some ease to avoid violating Stark There has been, then, an increasing interest on the part of private practitioners to enter into employment arrangements with hospital systems, or to become employed by large multi-specialty group practices. With hospital systems, the employment relationship will not only insulate financial support for EHR but also allow for other forms of financial support, including for practice management and recruitment.

When previously independent private practitioners become employees of either a hospital system or a much larger private practice group, careful assessment is needed to determine what impact, if any, there may be on physician clinical decision-making. While generally employment arrangements between hospital systems include the express understanding that the physician is to exercise independent clinical judgment, some concern has been raised as to the extent that employed physicians may be incentivized, directly or more likely indirectly, to make decisions that are more in the interest of the employer than of the patient. Notwithstanding the concern, employment arrangements enhance the resources available to the physicians and drive expectations that they will work within a larger collaborative environment. These effects support and are to an extent driven by the direction the health care system seems to be taking, and has potentially significant benefits for the caregiver/patient relationship. The increasing prevalence of the employment model is one manifestation that the public policy objective to create a more efficient health care delivery system is itself having a major impact on the design of that system.

Telehealth is a technology that seems thoroughly consistent with creating efficiencies in the delivery of care and at the same time enhancing communications between patients and caregivers. But it raises a host of practical, policy and legal concerns that must be addressed. The efficiencies seem evident. Telehealth can replace the often great inconvenience of a patient coming to a hospital or a physician's office, especially soon after discharge for inpatient services. It is an exemplar of the paradigm of bringing care to where the patient is, rather than organizing care around the convenience of the caregiver. It allows more frequent, brief interactions to determine status and compliance with treatment regimens, including medications. It addresses the inadequacy of primary care resources noted above by allowing more efficient use of the resources that are available, especially in rural areas.

As the technology has become more sophisticated, telehealth involves not only direct internet interaction between patient and caregiver but also the ability to monitor a patient in real time and to measure various key indicators of health status, including increasingly through mobile applications. The information can then flow into an electronic health record and provide not only a better basis for diagnosis and treatment but also the ability to intervene more rapidly when indications of a decline in condition become evident.

For purposes of considering the resistances to the further deployment of telehealth technology, it is helpful to divide the technology between that which involves direct interaction between patient and caregiver and that which supports ongoing monitoring and compliance but not direct personal interaction. The latter raises "traditional" issues about regulation of medical devices by the Food and Drug Administration (FDA), but also new issues about the interaction between the Federal Communications Commission and the FDA regulatory structure because of the often wireless nature of mobile health applications. The need for blending two regulatory schemes adds complexity to the dissemination of this form of telehealth technology, and is an example of how the law needs to adapt to changes taking place "on the ground."

The former—the use of telehealth technology for direct communications between patients and caregivers, especially physicians—is an even better example of the tension between new developments in care delivery and laws developed based on older paradigms. While deploying telehealth for direct care purposes seems like a "natural" in light of the trends seen in the broader health care system, the legal issues associated with its dissemination are thorny. The key legal issues that pose obstacles to increased use of telehealth fall within the traditional domains of the individual States. The practice of medicine is regulated by boards of registration in medicine in each State. Telehealth could accommodate itself to the current state of the law if each physician who engages in a patient encounter through remote means is licensed both in the State in which she or he is located and in the State in which the patient is located. But telehealth can be and is employed across a broad geographic span, especially now that it is being used, for example, by national insurers as a means of managing the care of their enrollees more effectively and thereby presumably reducing premium costs. It is simply impractical to have physicians providing services in such a context be licensed wherever a patient may be located.

Whether a physician can interact with a patient located in a State in which she or he is not licensed turns, first, on whether or not the service is defined as being within the scope of the "practice of medicine" in the patient's State of residence. Generally the practice of medicine involves diagnosis and treatment, but the boundaries are more nuanced. Is a consultation with the patient, during which no particular course of treatment is provided, within or outside the scope of the practice of medicine? Can a consult with the patient and the patient's local physician be considered outside the scope since there is a physician duly licensed in the State involved in the matter? The issue of this boundary is important especially if the physician does not in fact intend to establish a patient–physician relationship with the patient. But absent certainty that the services being provided are not within the scope of "the practice of medicine"—a definition that varies from State to State—the requirements of the boards of registration in each of the States in which the patients are located must be examined.

Even if telehealth is undertaken where the physician and the patient are in the same jurisdiction, the "practice of medicine" requires that a patient–physician relationship be established. Such a relationship is needed, for example, for the physician to prescribe medications for the patient, an act clearly within the scope of the typical definition of medical practice. In some States that relationship can be established without an in-person visit, so that telehealth alone is sufficient to create the bond. In most States, though, at least an initial in-person visit is required, so that telehealth may be employed only in situations in which there has been that initial encounter. This requirement may limit the ability to disseminate telehealth techniques across broad geographic areas, even within the same State.

Once the patient–physician relationship has been established there is no differentiation—nor should there be—with regard to the physician's responsibilities to the patient. That is, the same standards of professional responsibility and accountability should apply regardless of whether the encounter is in-person or electronic. However, the use of electronic communications with no opportunity for in-person observation may increase the risk of misdiagnosis or prescribing of inapt treatments. From a patient perspective this requires assurances that the diagnostic and treatment training for persons seeing patients via telehealth modalities is the same as for in-person encounters and that the understandable expectation that there will be no difference in the standards of care will not be frustrated. From the perspective of a physician providing services via telehealth that fall within the definition of "practice of medicine" in the particular jurisdiction requires understanding what additional potential liability is being assumed, and whether malpractice coverage will be available to the same extent it is for the more "traditional" care model.

Because of the thorny State law issues raised by the dissemination of telehealth modalities, some States have made attempts to codify the role of telehealth under State law in a way purportedly intended to be supportive (although not always entirely successfully). Ultimately, though, it appears that the issues that pose obstacles to the further expansion of telehealth nationally may need a federal resolution. Such an approach would presumably be a valid exercise of federal jurisdiction because of the extent to which telehealth interacts in interstate commerce, but such an initiative would entail federal encroachment on an area that has historically been virtually entirely within the jurisdiction of State law.

Telehealth is an excellent paradigm for understanding some of the complex dynamics in the American health care system. In and of itself it would seem to be consistent with furthering a number of important policy objectives, as long as there is some certainty that the standards of care exercised by physicians in providing medical services via telehealth will be no less than what is expected in the context of in-person encounters. But for it to be used most effectively requires threading one's way through a myriad of State law requirements and peculiarities, therefore strongly supporting the need for either federalization or adoption of a uniform code to be enacted by the States, The balance between system-wide policy objectives, physician-specific interests, patient interests and federal and State interests all come into play in seeking an orderly approach to promoting the further use of telehealth modalities.

Technology promotes more efficient use of health care resources and a greater ability to assemble and integrate a variety of data sources for providing information about the individual patient. While developed principally as better aids to diagnosis and treatment, and therefore to make the practice of medicine more accurate and effective, the proliferation of sources of patient-specific information also has a democratizing effect. This may be seen, for example, with the growth of personal health records, which individuals can assemble themselves from the multiple sources of data available about them in different EHR systems.

The increased data available to the individual is occurring at the same time that individuals are being encouraged to take greater personal responsibility for their care decisions. This is true not only with respect to "lifestyle" choices, such as weight reduction and greater exercise, but also with respect to clinical decision-making. The image of a person arriving in a physician's office with reams of data culled from the Internet and announcing both the diagnosis and the course of treatment to the physician, who must then explain why at least 95 % of the information is irrelevant, will likely eventually be replaced with an image of the individual arriving in that physician office (or connecting with the physician remotely) with a diversity of information about his or her own circumstances culled from personal health records, mobile health applications, genomic data, etc., and prepared to discuss the meaning of the data.

This emerging image is changing the paradigm of the patient/physician relationship. While sometimes described as "patient empowerment," that term is not helpful since it perpetuates the definition of the relationship as a fundamentally political one. Historically the physician was seen as having "power" over the patient because of his or her access to information and expertise not available to the patient. Seeing the relationship in such terms has had some benefits, including doctrines regarding patient–physician privilege; imposition of fiduciary-type responsibilities to the patient on the part of the physician; and disclosure obligations requiring physicians to report external financial relationships, such as with drug companies, that might be seen as improperly influencing the physician's clinical judgment.

The patient–physician relationship is changing, however, in part because the patient may now have greater access to relevant and useful information. What has not changed is the expertise to analyze and determine appropriate steps to be taken based on the data. And indeed it is the expertise of the physician that argues for the perpetuation of the doctrines identified above even as the relationship changes, or argues, at least, for careful research and understanding of how these doctrines might be modified, if at all, in light of the changes in the relationship. But the democratization of the relationship by enhancing the availability of relevant information available to the patient argues not for thinking in political terms but rather in partnership terms: the two parties reviewing the data and coming to a combined conclusion as to the appropriate course to follow, the patient being able to examine the data with the physician and ask questions derived from the data (either by herself or himself, or through a representative, as appropriate), guided by the physician's expertise.

In this partnership paradigm, since medicine tends to be more an art than a science, the physician alone would no longer make the determination as to the course of treatment and tell the patient what is to be done. Rather, the physician should guide the patient to the most suitable course of action, clinically but also psychologically or sociologically, through an interaction around choices that emerge from the data.

A key concept in the preceding paragraph is that, in the partnership model, decisions on course of treatment are not exclusively clinical ones but involve an understanding of other dimensions of the patient's circumstances. Whether referred to as "patient-centered" care or "compassionate care," the effort to have all caregivers, including physicians, understand and give weight to these other dimensions serves not only to promote respect for the patient but seems also correlated with promoting the cost containment objectives described earlier in this chapter. An analysis of research on "compassionate care" compiled by the Schwartz Center for Compassionate Care, based in Boston, reported in 2012, concluded that compassionate, patient-centered care is associated with, among other effects, improved health outcomes, reduced health care expenditures, increased patient satisfaction, fewer malpractice claims and better adherence to treatment recommendations.

In summary, public policy has moved from a principal focus on access reform to address the cost implications of achieving that objective. Achieving efficiencies in the delivery of care is high on the agenda at both the federal and State levels. Improving efficiency to any significant degree is complicated because of the multiplicity of interests at play in the field of health care and especially its financing. The decentralized structure of health care regulation, oversight and financing frustrates the ease with which efficiency can be achieved. At the same time developments that are promoted by both the public and private sector, such as technological innovations in health care information gathering, processing, use and monitoring, are sometimes frustrated by legal doctrines based on older paradigms. Eventually, if the forward progress of access is to be sustained, these sources of frustration will need to be overcome. And, regardless of how they are overcome, it is clear that, at the point of the interaction between patient and caregiver, at the point data, clinical and otherwise, is gathered and analyzed, at the point that treatment decisions are made, the most effective means of promoting efficiency, and its companion goal of good quality of care, is to have both the caregiver and the patient bring each one's own particular expertise to the relationship, one relating to clinical issues and one relating to the other dimensions of the patient's circumstances that demand weight in making clinical decisions. Adapting to this collaborative approach is a major challenge for clinicians.

- A fundamental tension in the US health care system is between access and cost containment
- As access is improving, cost containment demands require more efficient models of care, such as through technology and restructuring of provider relationships
- New models of care delivery, such as ACOs, and PCMHs, require greater levels of collaboration among providers (not just physicians) an between providers and patients
- To achieve both access and efficiency goals, the emerging models of care require more effective means of communication between patients and providers

Part VI
The Future of Decision Making

The Internet, Social Media, and Health Decision-Making

Amanda L. Graham, Caroline O. Cobb
and Nathan K. Cobb

Introduction

Summary of Key Points

(1) The Internet and social media are important channels through which a growing number of patients and caregivers connect with others with similar health concerns.

(2) "Expert" patients in online communities and social networks can provide health-related information and support that may confer specific advantages compared to what individuals receive from healthcare providers.

(3) There are unique methodological challenges involved in studying the influence of online social networks for health behavior change and health decision making.

(4) Improved understanding of how and for whom online social networks influence behavior change is an important goal for future research efforts.

A.L. Graham (✉) · C.O. Cobb
Schroeder Institute for Tobacco Research and Policy Studies, Truth Initiative, 900 G Street NW, 4th Floor, Washington, DC 20001, USA
e-mail: agraham@truthinitiative.org

C.O. Cobb
e-mail: cobbco@vcu.edu

A.L. Graham
Department of Oncology, Georgetown University Medical Center / Cancer Prevention and Control Program, Lombardi Comprehensive Cancer Center, Washington, DC, USA

N.K. Cobb
Division of Pulmonary, Critical Care, and Sleep Medicine, Department of Medicine, Georgetown University Medical Center, Washington, DC, USA
e-mail: nkc4@georgetown.edu

Scleroderma. The doctor's tone was ominous. The rest of her words rushed by me as she explained the diagnosis. Autoimmune disorder. Fibrosis. Antinuclear antibodies. CREST syndrome. More common in women but still pretty rare. Two types—one which doesn't kill you and one that does—only time would tell which type I had. No known cause. No cure. I walked out of her office in a daze, my new death sentence in tow. At home I went straight to the computer to get online. I read everything medical I could get my hands on and within just a few hours I felt like an expert on all things scleroderma. An expert paralyzed with fear. I read 5 and 10 year survival statistics and wondered which ones applied to me. I saw pictures of skin sores, amputated fingers, deformed facial features. I watched videos of patients describing the progression of their disease, and the miserable side effects of their medications. The saving grace was stumbling into an online support community

© Springer Science+Business Media New York 2016
M.A. Diefenbach et al. (eds.), *Handbook of Health Decision Science*,
DOI 10.1007/978-1-4939-3486-7_24

and reading other people's stories. I found other people who described symptoms that sounded just like mine. Some had been living with the disease for 17 years... coping with a range of symptoms from mildly aggravating to pretty debilitating... but living! I've been a member of this online community for a little over 2 years, and in that time I've gotten some of the most helpful and practical advice. Based on other people's experience, I've decided not to take any medication yet and am managing symptoms on my own. At least for now. The most helpful thing has been connecting with people who really understand what I'm going through. Having an outlet to share my feelings with other people living with disease has quite literally been a lifesaver for me. (—JoAnne, age 61)

Overview

The Internet has fundamentally changed healthcare and health decision-making. For patients like JoAnne struggling to make sense of a new diagnosis, the Internet provides a wealth of information on everything from the etiology of disease to its genetic underpinnings, details on its manifestation and symptom progression, and effective treatments. An encyclopedic amount of information is available literally with just a few clicks of the keyboard. There are thousands of health information websites from hospitals and hospital systems, HMOs, federal and state government agencies, academic institutions, non-profit organizations, pharmaceutical companies and other commercial entities, and research institutes, to name just a few. And it is not just text-based information: there are photos and videos and bar charts and graphs for every possible medical condition one can name. There are interactive symptom checkers, pill identification tools, body mass calculators, quizzes and assessments, and even games for health. With this dizzying array of informational resources, it might be easy to envision personal health decisions being made in isolation, by individuals sitting alone in front of their computer, parsing through a massive amount of information.

However, available data suggests that even with the vast amount of information available online, people appear to make decisions the way they always have—in the context of social relations.

Doctors and other health experts still play a central role in their health care experience, but increasingly, patients like JoAnne are seeking out peer information and support to help them prevent, treat, and cope with illness. Reaching out to friends and family and other close ties is certainly not a new phenomenon; the impact of social connections and the benefits of social support on physical and mental health are well documented. What *is* a relatively new phenomenon is the exchange of health-related personal stories, medical data, emotional support, and practical advice that occurs among complete strangers via the Internet. Online communities and networks have exploded in recent years, in large part due to the ubiquity of social media and Web 2.0 applications that facilitate and encourage the creation and sharing of user-generated content. User-generated blogs, forums, discussion boards, personal profiles, video sharing, and even data sharing sites are an important component of the healthcare landscape. For a rapidly growing proportion of the United States (U.S.) population, these resources play a central role in health decision-making.

Given the ubiquity of the Internet and online social networks, it is critical to understand the implications of their use for both research and practice. Online social processes may be beneficial or iatrogenic from a clinical standpoint; in research, they may represent contamination or additional complexity not readily addressed with traditional research methods. We begin this chapter with a brief review of what is known about the role of social connections in health and health decision-making from decades of research in the "offline" world, including hypothesized mechanisms of how social ties influence health. This literature spans large epidemiological studies documenting the association of social ties to health, pathophysiological inquiries into the biological pathways, and randomized controlled trials of interventions designed to manipulate social ties to improve health. Next, we present the latest data on Internet use in the U.S., with a specific focus on the use of two types of online social networks: (1) virtual communities comprised of people who most likely have no real-world connection but who share an interest or background (in this case a health condition or concern), and (2) social networking sites that mirror an individual's real-world social network (Ellison et al. 2007). We highlight illustrative and current examples of both types of online social networks, and describe the user experience in engaging in each of these applications for health-related concerns. Building on this section, we review the available evidence regarding the impact and effectiveness of online social networks on health behavior change and health decision-making.

Although there is compelling evidence for the benefits of participation in online social networks on health and health behavior change, there are also a number of caveats, challenges, and considerations that are inherent to this setting. We discuss several of these issues including methodological challenges in conducting research in online social networks, concerns about the accuracy of user-generated content, and the challenges in verifying the identity of users and the reliability of information. Finally, we conclude by presenting several areas of inquiry that we believe will be fruitful to advance our understanding of how to harness the power of online social networks for health. We use smoking cessation as an exemplar in describing this work, but believe that these approaches will likely have relevance to other areas of health behavior change.

The overarching aim of this chapter is to familiarize the reader—researchers and practitioners alike—with the theoretical foundations, scientific evidence, and available data that underlie the widespread availability and use of online social networks for health. The influence of social ties in health decision-making cannot be overstated, regardless of whether these ties are formed "offline" in one's immediate network of family, friends, neighbors, and other community members, or "online" in virtual communities and social networking sites. As noted by Lisa Berkman, "…individuals do not live in a vacuum, rather they are enmeshed in a social environment and in a series of social relationships… the extent to which these relationships are strong and supportive and individuals are integrated into their communities is related to the health of the individuals who live within such social contexts" (Berkman 1995, p. 245).

Social Connections and Health

We naturally desire to love other human beings and to be loved by them. A totally loveless life - a life without friends of any sort - is a life deprived of much needed good.
—Aristotle, 350 B.C. (Adler 1997)

It has long been recognized that social networks play an important role in health. Social networks represent the web of social relationships that surround an individual; including both intimate, close relationships with family and friends, and weaker, more extended ties with other individuals and groups (Granovetter 1973; Seeman 1996). Research has consistently demonstrated that people who are more socially integrated—measured as the number of social roles one holds (e.g., spouse, sibling, parent, neighbor, co-worker, etc.) —live longer and are healthier than more socially isolated individuals (reviewed by Berkman 1995; Berkman et al. 2000; Cohen 1988; Holt-Lunstad et al. 2010; House et al. 1988; Seeman 1996).

Social networks are theorized to "get under the skin" and "into the mind" by providing opportunities for social support, social influence, social engagement, and access to resources (Berkman et al. 2000). Each of these social processes, in turn, affects health risk behaviors and health decision-making across the health continuum, from prevention and screening to diagnosis and treatment. Social support—both perceived and actual—can take many forms including informational, instrumental, appraisal, and emotional (House and Kahn 1985). Informational support involves the provision of guidance, advice, or information specific to a particular need or problem. Having a greater number of social ties provides access to more sources of health-related information which may encourage health-promoting behaviors and the use of medical services (Cohen 1988). Social ties may help an individual weigh the risks of testing against the potential benefits of treatment. Personal experiences from family and friends with a medical concern may be more powerful at influencing a decision than aggregate information based on the best available clinical data from a healthcare provider. Instrumental support refers to practical, tangible assistance that may take the form of assistance locating a doctor or traveling to a medical appointment, financial aid, or help with daily life activities when one is sick. Appraisal support comes from the availability of people with whom to talk about one's problems or concerns and involves the provision of information that is useful for self-evaluation and decision-making, including constructive feedback, affirmation, and social comparison. Emotional support refers to the love, caring, sympathy, and understanding provided by others and the feelings of self-esteem and positive effect that come from being valued and accepted.

Social networks may also impact health through social influence, defined in this context as the communication of network values and norms around health behaviors. Research has shown that socially integrated individuals are subject to social controls and peer pressures from their social network for behaviors such as smoking (Christakis and Fowler 2008), healthy eating (Emmons et al. 2007), alcohol consumption (Cohen and Lemay 2007), contraceptive use (Yee and Simon 2010), and cancer screening (Kang and Bloom 1993; Suarez et al. 1994), to name just a few. Finally, social engagement or social participation provides a sense of belonging, companionship, and sociability. Spending time with others helps to establish one's identity and specific role with a network, and often provides meaning to one's life. These aspects of social engagement may enhance motivation for health behaviors and facilitate

health decision-making. Finally, social networks may impact health and well-being by providing access to material resources (e.g., food, clothing, and housing) that prevent disease and limit exposure to risk factors (Cohen 1988).

The robust associations observed between social networks and health behaviors led to intervention studies aimed at improving health outcomes by manipulating various aspects of social networks, most often by attempting to change the availability and/or the effectiveness of perceived support at the dyadic or small group level. Some interventions focused on developing new social ties through peer interventions, "buddy" systems, or support groups that linked people facing similar demands, stressors, or life transitions (Preyde and Ardal 2003). Other interventions focused on enhancing existing social ties by training network members—often a spouse or partner—to develop skills for providing positive social support (Lichtenstein et al. 1986; Mermelstein et al. 1986, 1983). Much to the puzzlement of many researchers across myriad domains of health behavior change, the evidence regarding the effectiveness of these interventions has been mixed (Boothroyd and Fisher 2010; Brownson and Heisler 2009; Cohen and Janicki-Deverts 2009; Dale et al. 2012; Ferri et al. 2006; Groh et al. 2008; Hoey et al. 2008; Kownacki and Shadish 1999; Tang et al. 2011; Webel et al. 2010). For example, several studies have found positive effects of partner involvement in a behavioral weight loss program (Brownell et al. 1978), while others have found such involvement to be ineffective (Wilson and Brownell 1978) and even detrimental to weight loss efforts (Zitter and Fremouw 1978). Buddy systems have shown some short-term benefit in clinic-based smoking cessation interventions (Gruder et al. 1993), but there is little evidence of their effectiveness in community settings (May and West 2000). Interventions designed to enhance partner support for smoking cessation have yielded little benefit over traditional cessation treatment (Park et al. 2004).

There are a number of potential reasons for these mixed findings. As noted by Cohen and Janicki-Deverts, "although the correlational studies have found that characteristics of *natural* [emphasis added] social networks were protective, intervention studies have generally manipulated support by facilitating interactions with strangers facing the same or similar threats" (Cohen and Janicki-Deverts 2009, p. 2). It may also be that having a larger number of people available to provide different kinds of support for a sustained period of time over different phases of life stressors or transitions provides a better match for the changing needs for support. While an individual may naturally be exposed to social support and normative influence from a wide range of sources, a majority of research studies have focused on modifying a small number of existing relationships or adding a small number of new relationships to effect behavior change. Dyadic or small group, time-limited interventions may simply be a mismatch for individuals facing difficult behavior changes or coping with chronic illness. For example, in the case of smoking cessation, exposure to people in various stages of the quitting process may be more helpful than pairing smokers to quit together. Former smokers can model abstinence behaviors and share their insights and strategies for successful cessation, while current smokers who are struggling to quit at the same time can empathize and provide a common shared experience. It may be that a spouse or buddy or partner can each provide some of these support functions, but cannot possibly meet all of the varying needs of someone making a major health change.

In order for social processes like social support or social influence to impact health decision-making, different forms of ties may be necessary. In the diffusion of innovations literature this has been described as a threshold effect, or the number of contacts that an individual must have before making a decision to adopt a new process (Valente 1996); more recently it has been conceptualized as complex contagion (Centola 2010) where individuals become more likely to adopt a new behavior with increasing exposure to it from other members of their social network. Data from the Framingham Heart Study are consistent with these ideas, demonstrating a persistent clustering pattern among smokers within their social networks and significantly less integration, as well

as clusters of smokers quitting together (Christakis and Fowler 2008).

If health behavior change is indeed subject to threshold or complex contagion effects, previous social support interventions may have fallen short because they lacked the necessary scale. Rather than enrolling someone seeking to lose weight into a time-limited treatment group with 15 like-minded overweight people, a more effective approach may be to integrate them into a network of hundreds of people capable of providing a much broader array of support functions over a longer period of time. Rather than focusing on dyads or small, artificially created groups, interventions may need to involve multiple members of an individual's natural social network. Until recently, interventions of this nature were simply not feasible. However, the widespread use of the Internet, the development of social media ("Web 2.0") tools, and public acceptance of interpersonal communications online have all led to a paradigm shift. It is now feasible for an individual to join an online community populated by thousands of people dealing with a similar health issue, or to elicit support from their own network via communications through Facebook, Twitter, or an online blog like CaringBridge. Health decision-making still occurs largely in the context of "offline" social networks (Fox 2011; Fox and Jones 2009). However, an important and growing phenomenon is the use of the Internet—and social media in particular—to find and connect with other people with similar health concerns.

The Internet and Social Media in Health

e-Patients… are equipped, enabled, empowered, and engaged in their health and health care decisions (Ferguson and The e-Patient Scholars Working Group 2007, p I)

The Internet is a major source of health information for a majority of U.S. adults. Countless web pages and health portals serve as repositories for medical articles, encyclopedias, and abstracts about any disease and drug that one can name (Jain and Raut 2011). As of May 2013, 85 % of adults in the United States use the Internet (Pew Internet and American Life Project 2013). Nearly two thirds of adults report using the Internet to search for health information each year (Fox and Duggan 2013). The most common searches by Internet users are for information about a specific disease or medical problem (55 %) followed by information about specific medical treatments or procedures (43 %) (Fox and Duggan 2013). Searches for health information online are more common among caregivers who often outpace other Internet users in their quest for health information by significant margins (Fox and Brenner 2012).

> With the rapid development of software applications deliberately designed to facilitate social interaction, a new era is dawning in which patients and their loved ones can collaboratively build knowledge related to coping with illness, while meeting their mutual supportive care needs in a timely way, regardless of location (Bender et al. 2008, p S42)

While healthcare providers are regarded as reputable sources of medical facts, they are often an inadequate source of emotional support in dealing with a health issue or informational support in identifying a quick remedy for an everyday health issue (Fox 2011). Patients are aware that there is much to learn from others facing similar challenges whether as a patient or caregiver (Ferguson and The e-Patient Scholars Working Group 2007). With the advent of social media tools, users can now also learn from the valuable personal experiences of hundreds or thousands of others coping with a specific diagnosis, undergoing a particular treatment, taking certain medications, or attempting to make a healthy lifestyle change. Social media refers to a group of Internet-based applications that allow the creation and exchange of user-generated content. These applications can take many forms, including electronic mailing lists, chat rooms, forums or message boards, blogs and

microblogs, online social network sites, and picture and video sharing sites (Korda and Itani 2011; Ziebland and Wyke). Typical aspects of social media include the ability to create personal profiles, "friend" or follow other people online, create content in the form of text, photos, audio, or video, and share, tag, rate, comment on, or vote on content created by others.

Social media tools have revolutionized the way people identify and communicate with people and identify information that is relevant to them (Eysenbach 2008). The availability of user-generated content, the experience of a shared community, the rapid distribution of content, and the now-normative open, two-way dialog that happens through social media have changed the nature of online interactions (PricewaterhouseCoopers 2012). Health information obtained through social media can influence satisfaction and trust in health messages (Eysenbach 2008) and health decision-making: 45 % of consumers said information found via social media would affect their decisions to seek a second opinion; more than 40 % said that information found via social media would affect the way they coped with a chronic condition or their approach to diet and exercise; and about a third indicated that it would affect their decisions regarding taking certain medications and undergoing specific procedures or tests (PricewaterhouseCoopers 2012).

These online interactions have the potential to address many of the shortcomings of traditional social networks in providing support (Wright and Bell 2003). First and foremost, the Internet provides easy, round-the-clock access to hundreds if not thousands of "expert" patients—those further ahead on the illness trajectory—that can provide firsthand experience about what might happen and how things feel (Cobb and Graham 2006; Ziebland and Wyke 2012) to demystify and "de-awfulize" a medical condition (Ferguson and The e-Patient Scholars Working Group 2007). The Internet transcends geography to provide access to a global network of people coping with a new diagnosis, taking the same medication, navigating the same difficult behavior change, or struggling with the same chronic condition that is likely much larger than one's personal social network. People coping with rare medical conditions and/or living in rural areas may never come across anyone in their offline network with the same condition, which can lead to feelings of isolation and stigma. Online communities may also represent a major source of medical guidance for individuals with limited access to professional care (Ferguson and The e-Patient Scholars Working Group 2007). Finding and forming interpersonal relationships with similar others can create a powerful sense of belonging, acceptance, empowerment, and comradeship and can reduce the feelings of stigma associated with many illnesses. The availability of a larger, more heterophilous social network through the Internet may also provide better-matched and more sustained support than traditional networks. Whereas a spouse or family members may become burned out over a period of time, the change, flux, and persistence of long-term members in online communities means that there is always someone available for support. The relative anonymity or "pseudonimity" (Wright and Bell 2003) of the Internet may facilitate the exchange of support since respect is determined by one's skill in communicating, the quality of their ideas, their apparent integrity as person, and their ability to achieve the goals or milestones that are valued within the particular community. Everyone starts off on a level playing field regardless of age, race, education, income, or professional status (Barak et al. 2008). The invisibility afforded by the Internet may also foster communications and support since people, do not have to worry how they look or sound in online communications, are unaware of any signs of disapproval such as frowns, eye rolling, or bored expressions, and do not have to avert their eyes as they might in face-to-face interactions with people who are disabled or disfigured (Barak et al. 2008). Indeed, online communities often elicit high levels of self-disclosure due to the online disinhibition

effect brought on by the anonymity and invisibility (Suler 2004).

Virtual "Peer-to-Peer" Communities

One way that people interact online is through virtual communities, defined as social networks formed or facilitated through electronic media where individuals—most often strangers united by a common interest or struggle—share experiences, ask questions, or provide emotional support and self-help (Eysenbach et al. 2004). There are now thousands of these "created networks" (Cobb et al. 2011), ranging from simple email lists, newsgroups, and bulletin boards centered around the exchange of messages related to a single behavior or condition (Barker 2008; Hu et al. 2012; Hwang et al. 2010; Idriss et al. 2009; Leggatt-Cook and Chamberlain 2011; Rimer et al. 2005; Weis et al. 2003), to complex interactive health communication applications (Robinson et al. 1998) that provide some combination of treatment, psychoeducation, and decision support —often across a range of technology platforms (e.g., web, mobile, text messaging, etc.)—but in which peer-to-peer support may be adjunct to the broader intervention (Carlbring et al. 2006; Carlbring et al. 2005; Frost et al. 2008; Gustafson et al. 1999; Schwitzer 2002; Shaw et al. 2000; Tate et al. 2001; Wicks et al. 2010, 2012; Womble et al. 2004; Zabinski et al. 2004). In addition, well-known online health portals like MayoClinic and WebMD that have long been used to locate expert-generated information recently began providing access to user-generated health information through condition-specific, user-created discussion boards (MayoClinic Admin 2011; WebMD Health Corp 2010).

While participation in virtual communities is common—and cuts across education, race, ethnicity, and healthcare access (Chou et al. 2009; Fox and Jones 2009; Kontos et al. 2010)—it is far from universal. Among Internet users, 34 % have read someone else's commentary or experience about health or medical issues on an online news group, website, or blog; 25 % have consulted online reviews of particular drugs or medical treatments; and 18 % have gone online to find others with similar health concerns (Fox 2011). One in four Internet users living with a chronic condition such as high blood pressure, diabetes, heart or lung problems, or cancer reported going online to connect with other people with similar health concerns (Fox 2011). According to a survey by PricewaterhouseCoopers, 25 % of consumers have posted about their own health experience, and 20 % have joined a health forum or community (PricewaterhouseCoopers 2012). Age is an important factor in the use of social media: more than 80 % of individuals' ages 18–24 said they would be likely to share health information compared to 45 % of adults 45–64 (PricewaterhouseCoopers 2012). The use of social media for health is more common among caregivers: 44 % read about others' experience in an online newsgroup or blog and 26 % have gone online to find people with similar health concerns (Fox and Brenner 2012).

Online Social Networks

While the dividing lines are not always clear, online social networks can be differentiated from virtual communities by the fact that they allow an individual to see the friends or contacts of other individuals. Boyd and Ellison (boyd and Ellison 2008) proposed three criteria that online social networks have in common: (1) the ability to construct a public or semi-public profile within a bounded system, (2) the capacity to articulate a list of other users with whom they share a connection, and (3) a function to view and traverse their list of connections and those made by others within the system. This visibility and opportunity for traversal is thought to be one of the factors that led to the rapid growth of second-generation networks such as MySpace, Facebook, and LinkedIn. As of September 2013, 73 % of online adults reported using online social networks such as Facebook, Twitter, MySpace or LinkedIn (Duggan and Smith 2014). This estimate is stark

contrast to the 8 % of online adults who reported use of online social networks in 2005 (Brenner and Smith 2013). The expansion of these networks and their increasing integration into daily life provides a novel set of approaches to reach and educate individuals about health behaviors and to facilitate health behavior change.

Another distinction is between "reflected" networks such as Facebook that allow individuals to interact with their existing network of friends and family, and "created" networks that form by integrating individuals into an existing structure by introducing them to strangers. Offline examples of created networks include Alcoholics Anonymous (AA) or Weight Watchers, while online examples span video gaming communities to health support communities for rare diseases. It is worth noting that few online networks fall purely into the "reflected" or "created" categories. Individuals may join a support network with a friend, or find an existing friend who is already a member using a search function. Alternatively, while Facebook's focus is on existing real-world connections, it also provides multiple opportunities to interact with strangers or individuals with weak ties through additional features (Groups, Networks, or Pages) which allow interaction between individuals who have not formed formal friendship ties and may not know each other.

Research Evidence

There have been dozens of studies of virtual communities, the majority of which describe the nature of online communities and their reach (Chou et al. 2013; Griffiths et al. 2009b). These studies characterize the user experience on specific sites, covering the ways that individuals can interact and the additional features offered on the site (Frost and Massagli 2008; Frost et al. 2008); the number of individuals using online social networks and their demographic and clinical characteristics (Idriss et al. 2009); the nature and quantity of online social network utilization, including both quantitative (Kummervold et al. 2002) and qualitative data (Cunningham et al. 2008; Eichhorn 2008; Johnsen et al. 2002; Meier et al. 2007; Selby et al. 2010); the specific needs, motivations, and reasons that individuals turn to online social networks (Shaw et al. 2000; Smithson et al. 2011); and the advantages and disadvantages of online social networks (White and Dorman 2001). Most studies have demonstrated improvements in various aspects of quality of life and well-being; participants report feeling more informed and empowered, better able to cope, and an improved sense of well-being. For example, in a survey of epilepsy patients participating in an online community on PatientsLikeMe, 30 % did not know anyone else with epilepsy prior to using the site. The perceived benefits of using the site included finding another patient experiencing the same symptoms, gaining a better understanding of seizures, and learning more about symptoms or treatments, with the number of perceived benefits positively associated with the number of relationships formed with other patients (Wicks et al. 2012). Houston and colleagues (Houston et al. 2002) reported a dose-response relationship in their study of Internet-based depression support groups, with heavier users experiencing greater resolution of depression symptoms.

> The old Industrial Age paradigm, in which health professional were viewed as the exclusive source of medical knowledge and wisdom, is gradually giving way to a new Information Age worldview in which patients, family caregivers, and the systems and networks they create are increasingly seen as important healthcare resources (Ferguson and The e-Patient Scholars Working Group 2007, p IX).

Online tools have also allowed patients to become increasingly engaged in collaborative health decision-making, engaging with healthcare providers to devise an optimal plan of action that considers the patient's expertise about their own life issues and experiences (O'Grady and Jadad 2010). As noted by Barak et al., "individual decision-making is enhanced through discussions in an online support group because participants learn more sophisticated ways of gathering information, gain a better understanding of the nature of their distress, develop enhanced

considerations in regard to relevant and important factors in the handling of their condition, and learn from the experiences of others" (Barak et al. 2008, p. 1876). Participation in online support groups and communities has led to patients being better informed, more empowered, and reporting enhanced social well-being (van Uden-Kraan et al. 2009) and have resulted in changing dynamics within the doctor–patient relationship (Berg 2005; Hu et al. 2012; Wald et al. 2007).

In contrast to the numerous descriptive studies, there have been relatively few randomized trials of online peer support interventions. A number of trials have evaluated the effectiveness of the Comprehensive Health Enhancement Support System (CHESS), an interactive, computer-mediated intervention that provides information about health and medical issues, social support through discussion groups and personal stories, decision support through health charts, decision aids and action plans, and problem solving tools (Taylor et al. 1994). Gustafson et al. (2001) reported that women newly diagnosed with breast cancer randomized to the CHESS intervention showed higher levels of perceived social support, better emotional well-being, and greater involvement in their health care than the control group. Another randomized study of a CHESS intervention designed for smokers indicated that higher levels of CHESS use (i.e., logins per week) was significantly related to smoking abstinence at three and six months post quit (Japuntich et al. 2006). Interestingly, out of all the services available within this CHESS intervention, support tools were the most popular with a mean use time of 43 min. A randomized trial of CHESS among lung cancer caregivers demonstrated a beneficial effect of the intervention compared to an Internet control group on measures of bonding and caregiver coping strategies, including active coping, positive reframing, and instrumental support (Namkoong et al. 2012).

Several other lines of research also demonstrate beneficial effects of web-based social network interventions. In a study with arthritis patients, Lorig and colleagues (Lorig et al. 2002) found that participants randomized to a closed, moderated email discussion group (plus book and video) experienced significant improvements in pain, disability, role function, and health distress and made fewer physician visits than participants randomized to a control group that received a non-health-related magazine of their choice. The Women to Women Project involved an online self-help support group and health teaching units for chronically ill women in the rural U.S. (Weinert et al. 2005). Compared to the control group, intervention group ratings of self-esteem, social support, and empowerment significantly improved at three months post randomization (Hill et al. 2006). Another study among breast cancer patients examined the effects of a 12-week moderated web-based support group (Bosom Buddies) as compared to a wait-list control group (Winzelberg et al. 2003). Participants in the intervention group reported reductions in measures of depression, perceived stress, and trauma related to cancer. Although these studies appear to provide promising evidence of the value of online social support for health behavior change and health decision-making, in each of these studies, the social support intervention was offered as part of a complex intervention or involved moderation by a health professional, making it difficult to isolate the effects of the support group in particular (Eysenbach et al. 2004). Indeed, there remains little rigorous research regarding the effectiveness of online peer-to-peer communities (Demiris 2006; Eysenbach et al. 2004; Griffiths et al. 2009a).

There is significantly less research on the impact of large-scale social networks such as Facebook despite the use of this website by almost three-quarters of online adults (71 % in 2013) (Duggan and Smith 2014). To date, most intervention studies have involved the use of Facebook Groups or Pages through which study participants are exposed to intervention content and opportunities to connect with other study participants (Bull et al. 2012; Cavallo et al. 2012; George et al. 2013; Napolitano et al. 2013; Valle et al. 2013; Young et al. 2013). The primary advantage of using Facebook Groups and Pages is the ability to form an ad hoc network since study participants are immediately exposed

to the communications and behaviors of other study participants. However, these approaches are limited by the fact they do not allow access to an individual's personal information or his/her network data, limiting the "networkedness" of what are purported to be social network interventions. Rather, these approaches are more likely to mimic the use of created online networks in which individuals interact primarily with people they do not otherwise know and with whom they may be hesitant to interact. They also likely require an existing, functional, scaled support network prior to participant enrollment to avoid the "empty room" phenomenon (Cobb and Graham 2012). For certain areas of health behavior change and decision-making, the use of online social networks in this manner may be necessary for patient safety and confidentiality. However, in other areas of health behavior change, there may be specific advantages to leveraging the social support, social influence, and norms available through an individual's existing network ties (Cobb and Graham 2012; Cobb et al. Cobb et al. 2013a; Kernot et al. 2013).

Caveats and Considerations

Methodological Challenges to Research in Online Social Networks

To date, research on virtual communities and online social networks has largely focused on describing who uses online communities, the ways in which they engage with various systems, and the associations of participation with improvements in general well-being, improved coping, and perceived social support. Many studies have employed cross-sectional surveys to gather this kind of data. There have been a few ethnographic inquiries in which researchers have embedded themselves into an online community to varying degrees (Barker 2008; Dickerson et al. 2000), but this methodology has its limitations including concerns about ethical issues, observer bias, and confidentiality. Studies that investigate the ways in which online social connections affect health behavior change are needed (Eysenbach et al. 2004). In the "offline" literature, constructs such as social norms, self-efficacy, self-esteem, and coping effectiveness have been identified as key constructs linking perceived support to health outcomes (Berkman et al. 2000). It is not yet known how well theoretical models of social influence translate between offline and online contexts (Cobb et al. 2011). Among many extant questions that have been articulated (Ferguson and The e-Patient Scholars Working Group 2007; Moorhead et al. 2013), future research should also address what specific features of online communications make stories and firsthand accounts of health issues compelling (Cobb et al. 2013b; Selby et al. 2010); whether patients' experiences have more value than facts and figures (Ziebland and Wyke 2012); how narrative storytelling can be used in health decision-making (Hwang et al. 2012, 2013; Schwitzer 2002); and how online social support and information function as active ingredients in fostering health behavior change (Graham et al. 2011a).

There are unique methodological challenges to conducting this kind of research that will likely require non-traditional research designs that move beyond the tightly controlled randomized trial and that reflect the real-world nature of this kind of research. Chief among these challenges is the reality that it may not be feasible (or even prudent) to randomize participants to "social support" or "no social support." Given that individuals self-select into these communities and networks based on unique needs and desires, the issue of self-selection bias will need to be carefully addressed in designing research studies. The goal of this kind of research should not be to "get everyone into online communities" but rather to understand for whom, under what conditions, for which types of outcomes, and through what mechanisms online social networks effect health decision-making and health behavior change. Quasi-experimental and dismantling/factorial designs, careful consideration of ethical and pragmatic issues in selecting a control group (Graham et al. 2011a), development and validation of new measurement instruments (Graham and Papandonatos 2008; Graham et al. 2006b;

Graham et al. 2011b; Hwang et al. 2011), and analyses of meta-data (Graham et al. 2006a) will likely play important roles in future research in this area. Researchers would also be well served to include members of virtual communities and online social networks in these efforts not simply as research subjects, but as experts with unique and valuable knowledge to contribute to the advancement of both science and practice.

Another key consideration in research in online social networks is the challenge of externalities. By virtue of an individual's connections with other people, an intervention delivered to a patient is likely to have unintended health effects (either positive or negative) in the individuals to whom that patient is connected. These effects are known as externalities (Christakis 2004). For example, if an individual enrolls in a weight loss program and their spouse loses weight as a result of changes in household food preparation, the spouse's weight loss would be a positive externality; any associated marital stress would be a negative externality. Largely due to human subject considerations, resource constraints, and methodological challenges, few studies have attempted to measure behavioral externalities and few interventions have sought to deliberately create and evaluate them. Despite little research attention, however, it is important to recognize that externalities are an inherent part of network-based interventions. For example, an online smoking cessation intervention delivered over Facebook designed to leverage friends for social support might fail to effectively change behavior in an individual; however, an individual's public attempts to quit smoking could prompt their friends to quit smoking or cut back. A traditional study focusing only on an identified patient or research participant would fail to account for these collateral effects (Christakis 2004). The emerging availability of large-scale databases, such as medical records or administrative data (Barnett et al. 2011), may facilitate the exploration of interactions beyond the patient level, although access to much of "big data" remains guarded by commercial interests (Lazer et al. 2009). Tackling research at this level will require novel methods and public/private partnerships.

Reliability and Accuracy of Online Health Information

> Over the span of a few years, patients have come to have access to more medical information on their smartphones than late-twentieth century Surgeons General had available to them from all their health information resources. (Ferguson and The e-Patient Scholars Working Group 2007, p. 93)

As noted by Dr. Jessie Gruman, President and Founder of the Center for Advancing Health and author of *After Shock—What To Do When The Doctor Gives You or Someone You Love a Devastating Diagnosis*, "using [the Internet] well requires real skill and attention and actually some knowledge in order to be able to separate the wheat from the chaff" (Heffner 2012). Indeed, dozens of studies have documented the variable quality of online information across numerous health behaviors and health conditions (e.g., Eysenbach et al. 2002; Muthukumarasamy et al. 2012; Joshi et al. 2011; Kaicker et al. 2010; Rao et al. 2012; Shahar et al. 2013; van der Marel et al. 2009; Wasserman et al. 2014). Creating online health information is as easy as updating a status on Facebook, uploading a video to You-Tube, or creating a blog post. User-generated content can be linked to or shared or otherwise promoted in ways that the original creator may have never intended or imagined. As a result, the boundary between health information producers and consumers "produsers" (Bruns 2008) has been blurred, along with "boundaries between fact and fiction, authority and amateurism, individual and group/community, public and private, and reality and virtuality" (Adams 2010, p. 394). For some consumers of online health information, the negative impact of online health information that is inaccurate or misleading, difficult to locate, or contradictory may be stronger than the positive impact of high-quality, accurate, evidence-based information (Graham and Abrams 2005). Misinformation disseminated through social media may result in limited time with a health care provider being used inefficiently or unproductively (Murray et al. 2003), the selection of ineffective therapies or sham products and services over evidence-based treatments (Bock et al. 2004, 2008), reinforcement of negative health behaviors (Moorhead et al. 2013), or even misguided adherence to incorrect recommendations from a healthcare provider (Crocco et al. 2002b). Fortunately, the available data suggest these occurrences are rare (Crocco et al. 2002a): 42 % of all adults—and 60 % of e-patients—say that they or someone they know has been helped by following medical advice or health information found on the Internet, and only 3 % report that they or someone they know has been harmed by following online health information (Fox and Jones 2009).

There are no easy answers to the issues of reliability and accuracy. The nature of the Internet and social media as open information systems ensures that there will always be inaccurate, misleading, self-serving, or confusing information that users must sift through. While "top-down" efforts driven by healthcare professionals to enhance online health literacy (Car et al. 2011; Greenberg et al. 2004; Peterson et al. 2003) or to monitor and enhance the quality and reliability of online health information (Eysenbach et al. 2001; Moorhead et al. 2013) may be fruitful, "bottom-up" contributions from members of virtual communities and online networks may also play a valuable role with regards to the reliability and accuracy of online health information. Patients and caregivers in online communities often have "an impressive and up-to-date knowledge of the best sources, centers, treatments, research, and specialists for [their] condition. Smart, motivated, and experienced self-helpers… may well know more about current research and treatments for their disease than their own primary care practitioner" (Ferguson and The e-Patient Scholars Working Group 2007, p. 23). Fact-checking and triangulation of information from others online may serve a powerful quality control function that enables online health information seekers to more readily identify fact from fiction. The sharing of patient-generated data (Wicks et al. 2010, 2012) may augment information from healthcare professionals to provide the most comprehensive, relevant, and informative online health information landscape.

Verifying the Identity of Users and the Reliability of Information

A well-known New Yorker cartoon stated that "on the Internet no one knows you are a dog" (Wikipedia n.d., 2012). While certain online social networks that are designed to mirror real-world networks (e.g., the career site, LinkedIn) may have a strong bias toward real identities and valid information, virtual communities often allow individuals to create anonymous profiles using a pseudonym (username or handle) to identify themselves. Our own experience suggests that people may not enter valid demographic information (e.g., age, gender, or location) and that relying on such information for research purposes may be counterproductive. The limited research to date on the topic suggests that users of "nonymous" social networks (that require their real name) present themselves differently than those in anonymous networks (Zhao et al. 2008), such as traditional virtual communities. If so, data acquired from networks such as Facebook may be more reliable, in part because users are uncomfortable presenting themselves as something they are not to people that already know them. It may just be that in some types of online social networks it is hard to pretend to your friends that you are a cat.

Future Research

Online social networks provide an exciting opportunity to revisit the decades-old question of whether social ties can be fostered or manipulated to "rewire" networks to drive behavior change (Cobb et al. 2011). Network intervention have been defined as "purposeful efforts to use social networks or social network data to generate social influence, accelerate behavior change, improve performance, and/or achieve desirable outcomes among individuals, communities, organizations, or populations" (Valente 2012, p. 49). Network intervention may work by targeting individuals based on their position within the network, or by modifying the social networking process to alter the structure of the network. In online networks, key players who are able to become effective change agents by virtue of their network position can be identified using network analysis of communications patterns (Cobb et al. 2010).

Our group is currently conducting a randomized controlled trial (ClinicalTrials.gov Identifier: NCT01544153) that leverages key players in an online social network to improve user adherence or engagement to a web-based cessation program with the ultimate goal of improving quit rates (Graham et al. 2013). Low levels of adherence have been observed across web-based programs (Eysenbach 2005) which undermine the potential public health impact of Internet-delivered health behavior change interventions. This trial uses a social network approach to integrate smokers into an online social network for cessation where they may be exposed to social support, social influence, and social norms around cessation which are hypothesized to improve engagement and adherence to the site and—ultimately—to improve cessation outcomes. Using proactive, directed, and personalized outreach from key members within the community ("Integrators"), the goal is to draw new members into an existing online social network and facilitate the formation of ties with other members (boyd and Ellison 2008). It is based on several lines of evidence that indicate the following: (1) participation in an online social network is associated with greater overall website utilization (An et al. 2006; Cobb et al. 2005); (2) proactive outreach from existing members of an online social network is effective in integrating new members into the network (unpublished data); (3) social ties can promote website engagement (Poirier and Cobb 2012); and (4) sustained use of online cessation interventions is predictive of higher rates of abstinence (Richardson et al. 2013; Schwarzer and Satow 2012). If this approach proves effective, it could be scaled to meet the demand of even the largest online health communities and may inform advances in intervention design and implementation, making existing Internet programs more effective across a range of behavioral risk factors.

Small shifts in decision-making and health behavior can have significant population impact if the process is widely distributed. Large-scale networks such as Facebook offer this potential. Working directly with Facebook, Bond and colleagues (Bond et al. 2012) demonstrated that they could manipulate who saw an "I voted" button on Facebook and impact voting rates among friends across a 60 million person Facebook sample. While this single study demonstrated the potential of large-scale interventions to alter decision-making, most research groups will need to disseminate their intervention through a network as a starting point. Most trials emphasize a specific kind of behavior change as their primary outcome, but diffusion and reach may be equally important particularly metrics in the early phases of the development of an intervention. Valente has referred to interventions of this nature as "induction interventions," referring to their potential to induce behavior change and "create cascades of information or behavioral diffusion" (Valente 2012). By carefully seeding an intervention into a network, viral spread may be triggered as the intervention is passed from individual to individual. In these models, a key metric of success of any induction intervention is the efficiency of the diffusion process.

Trials of such interventions are ideally suited to networks such as Facebook, where the diffusion of interventions delivered as "apps" can be tracked. Diffusion can be measured using R, the reproductive rate, which is determined by the duration of use (t), the "contagiousness" of an intervention (β), and a participant's total contacts (z). In another trial underway by our research group (ClinicalTrials.gov Identifier: NCT01746472), we developed an evidence-based Facebook app for smoking cessation that allows us to enable or disable various components designed to impact duration of use (expanded content, proactive contact), contagiousness (active and passive sharing), and number of contacts (use by non-smoker supporters) and measure the resultant impact on R, or the number of new users recruited (on average) by an existing user (Cobb et al. 2013a). For example, most interventions are designed to only be used by the target audience. In this case, we have built a secondary version of the app designed for non-smoking friends of smoker

participants. The use of the app by non-smokers can facilitate social pressure on a smoker to promote abstinence, but may also enable the viral spread of the intervention from clusters of smokers through non-smokers and on to new clusters of smokers. An intervention with an R value that exceeds 1.0 is capable of autonomous propagation through a network without new seeds. Even without exceeding a value of 1, an intervention that demonstrates even modest diffusion can markedly decrease recruitment or promotion costs (Cobb and Graham 2012).

Wrap up

Today, a majority of U.S. adults turn to the Internet when faced with the need for health information. While much of this information may come from healthcare professionals or "experts," there is a wealth of evidence that much of the information and support that patients and caregivers are seeking is best provided by social ties and social networks accessed via the Internet. "Patients know what patients want to know" (deBronkart 2011). Fellow "e-Patients" can provide personal information and details about a health condition, what it feels like, what to expect, and how to cope in ways that healthcare professionals cannot. Indeed, millions of individuals interact in online settings, acquiring and evaluating information and making decisions about their own health in social environments. The steady growth of the use of online social networks for health, health behavior change and health decision-making underscores the potential reach that future interventions using these modalities may hold for the public at large. However, researchers and practitioners continue to struggle with how to translate observational data about the widespread use and reported benefits of the use of social media into effective strategies and interventions to drive improved health decision-making. Moving from observational data to effective intervention approaches that can be rigorously evaluated will require innovative research paradigms that can tease out what aspects of online social interactions contribute to positive change and how those processes can be harnessed. Diffusion of interventions, the use of network analysis strategies to target individuals and strengthen ties, and studies of information transmission are areas of active inquiry but represent only a few examples of research needed in this area. Awareness of challenges and pitfalls will serve both practitioners and researchers as they embark on uncharted territory in this area.

The rapid evolution—and, in some cases, dissolution—of social media and online social networks over the past decade means it is likely that the social ecosystem will again reinvent itself over the coming decade. A fundamental and recurring challenge to researchers and practitioners remains the interpretation of existing data from older online social networks and its application to current social networks. Equally important will be the ability of researchers and funders to keep pace with this ever-evolving dimension of health communication. The use of innovative and alternative research strategies and methodologies will be critical to advancing our understanding of how best to harness the power of "equipped, engaged, empowered, and enabled" (deBronkart 2011) healthcare consumers. The coming years will likely witness a paradigm shift in how we conceptualize communication of information and strategies to drive effective health decision-making. Novel thinking about how best to integrate health information obtained via social media into the traditional fabric of healthcare may offer the potential for real breakthroughs in health and healthcare on a population-wide basis for patients like JoAnne and millions just like her.

References

Adams, S. A. (2010). Revisiting the online health information reliability debate in the wake of "web 2.0": An inter-disciplinary literature and website review. *International Journal of Medical Informatics, 79*(6), 391–400. doi:10.1016/j.ijmedinf.2010.01.006

Adler, M. J. (1997). Aristotle for everybody. *Touchstone.*

An, L. C., Perry, C. L., Lein, E. B., Klatt, C., Farley, D. M., Bliss, R. L. … Ehlinger, E. P. (2006). Strategies for increasing adherence to an online smoking cessation intervention for college students. *Nicotine & Tobacco Research, 8*(Suppl 1), S7–12.

Barak, A., Boniel-Nissim, M., & Suler, J. (2008). Fostering empowerment in online support groups. *Computers in Human Behavior, 24*(5), 1867–1883. doi:10.1016/j.chb.2008.02.004

Barker, K. K. (2008). Electronic support groups, patient-consumers, and medicalization: The case of contested illness. *Journal of Health and Social Behavior, 49*(1), 20–36.

Barnett, M. L., Landon, B. E., O'Malley, A. J., Keating, N. L., & Christakis, N. A. (2011). Mapping physician networks with self-reported and administrative data. *Health Services Research, 46*(5), 1592–1609. doi:10.1111/j.1475-6773.2011.01262.x

Bender, J. L., O'Grady, L., & Jadad, A. R. (2008). Supporting cancer patients through the continuum of care: a view from the age of social networks and computer-mediated communication. *Current Oncology, 15*(Suppl 2), s107–es42.

Berg, S. (2005, July/August). The well-informed patient: A new breed of health care consumer. *Asthma Magazine, 28*–30.

Berkman, L. F. (1995). The role of social relations in health promotion. *Psychosomatic Medicine, 57*(3), 245–254.

Berkman, L. F., Glass, T., Brissette, I., & Seeman, T. E. (2000). From social integration to health: Durkheim in the new millennium. *Social Science and Medicine, 51*(6), 843–857. (S0277953600000654 [pii]).

Bock, B. C., Graham, A. L., Whiteley, J. A., & Stoddard, J. L. (2008). A review of web-assisted tobacco interventions (WATIs). *Journal of Medical Internet Research, 10*(5), e39. doi:10.2196/jmir.989

Bock, B., Graham, A., Sciamanna, C., Krishnamoorthy, J., Whiteley, J., Carmona-Barros, R., et al. (2004). Smoking cessation treatment on the Internet: content, quality, and usability. *Nicotine & Tobacco Research, 6*(2), 207–219. doi:10.1080/14622200410001676332

Bond, R. M., Fariss, C. J., Jones, J. J., Kramer, A. D., Marlow, C., Settle, J. E., et al. (2012). A 61-million-person experiment in social influence and political mobilization. *Nature, 489*(7415), 295–298. doi:10.1038/nature11421

Boothroyd, R. I., & Fisher, E. B. (2010). Peers for progress: promoting peer support for health around the world. *Family Practice, 27*(Suppl 1), i62–68. doi:10.1093/fampra/cmq017

Boyd, D. M., & Ellison, N. B. (2008). Social Network Sites: Definition, History, and Scholarship. *Journal of Computer-Mediated Communication, 13*, 210–230. doi:10.1111/j.1083-6101.2007.00393.x

Brenner, J., & Smith, A. (2013). *72% of online adults are social networking site users.* Washington, D.C.: Pew Research Center's Internet & American Life Project.

Brownell, K. D., Heckerman, C. L., Westlake, R. J., Hayes, S. C., & Monti, P. M. (1978). The effect of couples training and partner co-operativeness in the behavioral treatment of obesity. *Behaviour Research and Therapy, 16*(5), 323–333. (0005-7967(78)90002-5 [pii]).

Brownson, C. A., & Heisler, M. (2009). The role of peer support in diabetes care and self-management. *Patient*, *2*(1), 5–17. doi:10.2165/01312067-200902010-00002

Bruns, A. (2008). *Blogs, wikipedia, second life and beyond: From production to produsage*. New York: Peter Lang.

Bull, S.S., Levine, D.K., Black, S.R., Schmiege, S.J., & Santelli, J. (2012). Social media-delivered sexual health intervention: A cluster randomized controlled trial. *Am J Prev Med, 43*(5).

Car, J., Lang, B., Colledge, A., Ung, C., & Majeed, A. (2011). Interventions for enhancing consumers' online health literacy. *Cochrane Database Syst Rev*(6), CD007092. doi:10.1002/14651858.CD007092.pub2

Carlbring, P., Furmark, T., Steczko, J., Ekselius, L., & Andersson, G. (2006). An open study of Internet-based bibliotherapy with minimal therapist contact via email for social phobia. *Clinical Psychologist, 10*, 30–38.

Carlbring, P., Nilsson-Ihrfelt, E., Waara, J., Kollenstam, C., Buhrman, M., Kaldo, V., et al. (2005). Treatment of panic disorder: live therapy vs. self-help via the Internet. *Behaviour Research and Therapy, 43*(10), 1321–1333. doi:10.1016/j.brat.2004.10.002

Cavallo, D.N., Tate, D.F., Ries, A.V., Brown, J.D., DeVellis, R.F., & Ammerman, A.S. (2012). Efficacy of an online social network based physical activity intervention: A randomized controlled trial. *Am J Prev Med, 43*(5).

Centola, D. (2010). The spread of behavior in an online social network experiment. *Science, 329*(5996), 1194–1197. doi:10.1126/science.1185231

Chou, W. Y., Hunt, Y. M., Beckjord, E. B., Moser, R. P., & Hesse, B. W. (2009). Social media use in the United States: Implications for health communication. Journal of Medical Internet Research, *11*(4), e48. doi:10.2196/jmir.1249

Chou, W. Y., Prestin, A., Lyons, C., & Wen, K. Y. (2013). Web 2.0 for health promotion: Reviewing the current evidence. *American Journal of Public Health, 103*(1), e9–18. doi:10.2105/AJPH.2012.301071

Christakis, N. A. (2004). Social networks and collateral health effects. *BMJ, 329*(7459), 184–185. doi:10.1136/bmj.329.7459.184

Christakis, N. A., & Fowler, J. H. (2008). The collective dynamics of smoking in a large social network. *New England Journal of Medicine, 358*(21), 2249–2258. doi:10.1056/NEJMsa0706154

Cobb, N. K., & Graham, A. L. (2006). Characterizing Internet searchers of smoking cessation information. *Journal of Medical Internet Research, 8*(3), e17.

Cobb, N. K., Graham, A. L., & Abrams, D. B. (2010). Social network structure of a large online community for smoking cessation. *American Journal of Public Health, 100*(7), 1282–1289. doi:10.2105/AJPH.2009.165449

Cobb, N. K., Graham, A. L., Bock, B. C., Papandonatos, G., & Abrams, D. B. (2005). Initial evaluation of a real-world Internet smoking cessation system. *Nicotine & Tobacco Research, 7*(2), 207–216.

Cobb, N. K., Graham, A. L., Byron, M. J., Niaura, R. S., & Abrams, D. B. (2011). Online social networks and smoking cessation: A scientific research agenda. *Journal of Medical Internet Research, 13*(4), e119. doi:10.2196/jmir.1911

Cobb, N. K., & Graham, A. L. (2012). Health behavior interventions in the age of Facebook. *American Journal of Preventive Medicine, 43*(5), 571–572.

Cobb, N. K., Jacobs, M. A., Saul, J., Wileyto, P., & Graham, A. L. (2013a). Diffusion of an evidence-based smoking cessation intervention through facebook: A randomized controlled trial study protocol. *BMJ Open*.

Cobb, N. K., Mays, D., & Graham, A. L. (2013b). Sentiment analysis to determine the impact of online messages on smokers' choices to use varenicline. *Journal of the National Cancer Institute Monographs, 47*, 224–230. doi:10.1093/jncimonographs/lgt020

Cohen, S. (1988). Psychosocial models of the role of social support in the etiology of physical disease. *Health Psychology, 7*(3), 269–297.

Cohen, S., & Janicki-Deverts, D. (2009). Can we improve our physical health by altering our social networks? *Perspectives on Psychological Science, 4*(4), 375–378. doi:10.1111/j.1745-6924.2009.01141.x

Cohen, S., & Lemay, E. P. (2007). Why would social networks be linked to affect and health practices? *Health Psychology, 26*(4), 410–417. doi:10.1037/0278-6133.26.4.410

Crocco, A. G., Villasis-Keever, M., & Jadad, A. R. (2002a). Analysis of cases of harm associated with use of health information on the internet. *JAMA, 287*(21), 2869–2871.

Crocco, A. G., Villasis-Keever, M., & Jadad, A. R. (2002b). Two wrongs don't make a right: Harm aggravated by inaccurate information on the Internet. *Pediatrics, 109*(3), 522–523.

Cunningham, J. A., van Mierlo, T., & Fournier, R. (2008). An online support group for problem drinkers: AlcoholHelpCenter.net. *Patient Education and Counseling, 70*(2), 193–198. doi:10.1016/j.pec.2007.10.003

Dale, J. R., Williams, S. M., & Bowyer, V. (2012). *What is the effect of peer support on diabetes outcomes in adults?*. A systematic review: Diabet Med. doi:10.1111/j.1464-5491.2012.03749.x.

deBronkart, D. (2011). *TED Talks: Meet e-Patient Dave*. TEDxMaastricht. Retrieved from http://www.ted.com/talks/dave_debronkart_meet_e_patient_dave.html

Demiris, G. (2006). The diffusion of virtual communities in health care: concepts and challenges. *Patient Education and Counseling, 62*(2), 178–188. doi:10.1016/j.pec.2005.10.003

Dickerson, S. S., Flaig, D. M., & Kennedy, M. C. (2000). Therapeutic connection: Help seeking on the Internet for persons with implantable cardioverter defibrillators. *Heart and Lung, 29*(4), 248–255. doi:10.1067/mhl.2000.108326

Duggan, M., & Smith, A. (2014). *Social media update 2013 Pew Internet and American Life Project*. Washington, D.C.: Pew Research Center.

Eichhorn, K. C. (2008). Soliciting and providing social support over the internet: An investigation of online eating disorder support groups. *Journal of Computer-Mediated Communication, 14*(1), 67–78. doi:10.1111/j.1083-6101.2008.01431.x

Ellison, N., Steinfield, C., & Lampe, C. (2007). The benefits of Facebook "friends": Exploring the relationship between college students' use of online social networks and social capital. *Journal of Computer-Mediated Communication, 12*(3), article 1.

Emmons, K. M., Barbeau, E. M., Gutheil, C., Stryker, J. E., & Stoddard, A. M. (2007). Social influences, social context, and health behaviors among working-class, multi-ethnic adults. *Health Education and Behavior Journal, 34*(2), 315–334. doi:10.1177/1090198106288011

Eysenbach, G. (2005). The law of attrition. *Journal of Medical Internet Research, 7*(1), e11. doi:10.2196/jmir.7.1.e11

Eysenbach, G. (2008). Medicine 2.0: Social networking, collaboration, participation, apomediation, and openness. *Journal of Medical Internet Research, 10*(3), e22. doi:10.2196/jmir.1030

Eysenbach, G., Kohler, C., Yihune, G., Lampe, K., Cross, P., & Brickley, D. (2001). A framework for improving the quality of health information on the world-wide-web and bettering public (e-)health: The MedCERTAIN approach. *Medinfo, 10*(Pt 2), 1450–1454.

Eysenbach, G., Powell, J., Englesakis, M., Rizo, C., & Stern, A. (2004). Health related virtual communities and electronic support groups: Systematic review of the effects of online peer to peer interactions. *BMJ, 328*(7449), 1166. doi:10.1136/bmj.328.7449.1166

Eysenbach, G., Powell, J., Kuss, O., & Sa, E. R. (2002). Empirical studies assessing the quality of health information for consumers on the world wide web: A systematic review. *JAMA, 287*(20), 2691–2700.

Ferguson, T., & The e-Patient Scholars Working Group. (2007). e-patients: How they can help us heal health care.

Ferri, M., Amato, L., & Davoli, M. (2006). Alcoholics Anonymous and other 12-step programmes for alcohol dependence. *Cochrane Database Syst Rev*(3), CD005032. doi:10.1002/14651858.CD005032.pub2

Fox, S. (2011). Peer-to-peer healthcare. http://pewinternet.org/Reports/2011/P2PHealthcare.aspx. Archived at: http://www.webcitation.org/69cRxwJlK.

Fox, S., & Brenner, J. (2012). *Family Caregivers Online.* Washington, DC: Pew Internet & American Life Project.

Fox, S., & Duggan, M. (2013). Health Online 2013: Pew Research Center's Internet & American Life Project.

Fox, S., & Jones, S. (2009). The social life of health information: Americans' pursuit of health takes places within a widening network of both online and offline sources. http://www.pewinternet.org/∼/media//Files/Reports/2009/PIP_Health_2009.pdf. Archived at: http://www.webcitation.org/67LNe4tne

Frost, J. H., & Massagli, M. P. (2008). Social uses of personal health information within PatientsLikeMe, an online patient community: What can happen when patients have access to one another's data. *Journal of Medical Internet Research, 10*(3), e15. doi:10.2196/jmir.1053

Frost, J. H., Massagli, M. P., Wicks, P., & Heywood, J. (2008). How the Social Web Supports patient experimentation with a new therapy: The demand for patient-controlled and patient-centered informatics. *AMIA Annu Symp Proc*, 217–221.

George, D. R., Dellasega, C., Whitehead, M. M., & Bordon, A. (2013). Facebook-based stress management resources for first-year medical students: A multi-method evaluation. *Computers in Human Behavior, 29*(3), 559–562.

Graham, A. L., & Abrams, D. B. (2005). Reducing the cancer burden of lifestyle factors: Opportunities and challenges of the Internet. *Journal of Medical Internet Research, 7*(3), e26.

Graham, A. L., Bock, B. C., Cobb, N. K., Niaura, R., & Abrams, D. B. (2006a). Characteristics of smokers reached and recruited to an internet smoking cessation trial: A case of denominators. *Nicotine & Tobacco Research, 8*(Suppl 1), S43–S48.

Graham, A. L., Cha, S., Papandonatos, G. D., Cobb, N. K., Mushro, A., Fang, Y., et al. (2013). Improving adherence to web-based cessation programs: A randomized controlled trial study protocol. *Trials, 14*(48). doi:10.1186/1745-6215-14-48

Graham, A. L., Cobb, N. K., Papandonatos, G. D., Moreno, J. L., Kang, H., Tinkelman, D. G., et al. (2011a). A randomized trial of Internet and telephone treatment for smoking cessation. *Archives of Internal Medicine, 171*(1), 46–53. doi:10.1001/archinternmed.2010.451

Graham, A. L., & Papandonatos, G. D. (2008). Reliability of internet-versus telephone-administered questionnaires in a diverse sample of smokers. *Journal of Medical Internet Research, 10*(1), e8. doi:10.2196/jmir.987

Graham, A. L., Papandonatos, G. D., Bock, B. C., Cobb, N. K., Baskin-Sommers, A., Niaura, R., et al. (2006b). Internet- vs. telephone-administered questionnaires in a randomized trial of smoking cessation. *Nicotine & Tobacco Research, 8*(Suppl 1), S49–S57.

Graham, A. L., Papandonatos, G. D., Kang, H., Moreno, J. L., & Abrams, D. B. (2011b). Development and validation of the online social support for smokers scale. *Journal of Medical Internet Research, 13*(3), e69. doi:10.2196/jmir.1801

Granovetter, M. S. (1973). The strength of weak ties. *American Journal of Sociology, 78*(6), 1360–1380.

Greenberg, L., D'Andrea, G., & Lorence, D. (2004). Setting the public agenda for online health search: a white paper and action agenda. *Journal of Medical Internet Research, 6*(2), e18. doi:10.2196/jmir.6.2.e18

Griffiths, K. M., Calear, A. L., & Banfield, M. (2009a). Systematic review on Internet Support Groups (ISGs) and depression (1): Do ISGs reduce depressive symptoms? *Journal of Medical Internet Research, 11*(3), e40. doi:10.2196/jmir.1270

Griffiths, K. M., Calear, A. L., Banfield, M., & Tam, A. (2009b). Systematic review on Internet Support Groups (ISGs) and depression (2): What is known about depression ISGs? *Journal of Medical Internet Research, 11*(3), e41. doi:10.2196/jmir.1303

Groh, D. R., Jason, L. A., & Keys, C. B. (2008). Social network variables in alcoholics anonymous: A literature review. *Clinical Psychology Review, 28*(3), 430–450. doi:10.1016/j.cpr.2007.07.014

Gruder, C. L., Mermelstein, R. J., Kirkendol, S., Hedeker, D., Wong, S. C., Schreckengost, J. ... Miller, T. Q. (1993). Effects of social support and relapse prevention training as adjuncts to a televised smoking-cessation intervention. *Journal of Consulting and Clinical Psychology, 61*(1), 113–120.

Gustafson, D. H., Hawkins, R., Boberg, E., Pingree, S., Serlin, R. E., Graziano, F., et al. (1999). Impact of a patient-centered, computer-based health information/support system. *American Journal of Preventive Medicine, 16*(1), 1–9.

Gustafson, D. H., Hawkins, R., Pingree, S., McTavish, F., Arora, N. K., Mendenhall, J., et al. (2001). Effect of computer support on younger women with breast cancer. *Journal of General Internal Medicine, 16*(7), 435–445 (jgi00332 [pii]).

Heffner, R. (2012, July 4, 2012). The Lemon of Illness and the Demand for Lemonade: An Interview with Dr. Jessie Gruman. *Richard Heffner's Open Mind.* from http://www.thirteen.org/openmind/health/the-lemon-of-illness-and-the-demand-for-lemonade/2603/

Hill, W., Weinert, C., & Cudney, S. (2006). Influence of a computer intervention on the psychological status of chronically ill rural women: Preliminary results. *Nursing Research, 55*(1), 34–42. 00006199-200601000-00005 [pii].

Hoey, L. M., Ieropoli, S. C., White, V. M., & Jefford, M. (2008). Systematic review of peer-support programs for people with cancer. *Patient Education and Counseling, 70*(3), 315–337. doi:10.1016/j.pec.2007.11.016

Holt-Lunstad, J., Smith, T. B., & Layton, J. B. (2010). Social relationships and mortality risk: A meta-analytic review. *PLoS Med, 7*(7), e1000316. doi:10.1371/journal.pmed.1000316

House, J. S., & Kahn, R. L. (1985). Measures and concepts of social support. In S. Cohen & S. L. Syme (Eds.), *Social support and health* (pp. 83–108). Orlando: Academic Press.

House, J. S., Landis, K. R., & Umberson, D. (1988). Social relationships and health. *Science, 241*(4865), 540–545.

Houston, T. K., Cooper, L. A., & Ford, D. E. (2002). Internet support groups for depression: A 1-year prospective cohort study. *American Journal of Psychiatry, 159*(12), 2062–2068.

Hu, X., Bell, R. A., Kravitz, R. L., & Orrange, S. (2012). the prepared patient: Information seeking of online support group members before their medical appointments. *Journal of Health Communication.* doi:10.1080/10810730.2011.650828

Hwang, K. O., Ottenbacher, A. J., Graham, A. L., Thomas, E. J., Street, R. L, Jr., & Vernon, S. W. (2013). Online narratives and peer support for colorectal cancer screening: A pilot randomized trial. *American Journal of Preventive Medicine, 45*(1), 98–107. doi:10.1016/j.amepre.2013.02.024

Hwang, K. O., Ottenbacher, A. J., Green, A. P., Cannon-Diehl, M. R., Richardson, O., Bernstam, E. V., et al. (2010). Social support in an Internet weight loss community. *International Journal of Medical Informatics, 79*(1), 5–13. doi:10.1016/j.ijmedinf.2009.10.003

Hwang, K. O., Ottenbacher, A. J., Lucke, J. F., Etchegaray, J. M., Graham, A. L., Thomas, E. J., et al. (2011). Measuring social support for weight loss in an internet weight loss community. *Journal of Health Communication, 16*(2), 198–211. doi:10.1080/10810730.2010.535106

Hwang, K. O., Trickey, A. W., Graham, A. L., Thomas, E. J., Street, R. L., Jr., Kraschnewski, J. L., & Vernon, S. W. (2012). Acceptability of narratives to promote colorectal cancer screening in an online community. *Preventive Medicine, 54*(6), 405–407. doi:10.1016/j.ypmed.2012.03.018

Idriss, S. Z., Kvedar, J. C., & Watson, A. J. (2009). The role of online support communities: benefits of expanded social networks to patients with psoriasis. *Archives of Dermatology, 145*(1), 46–51. doi:10.1001/archdermatol.2008.529

Jain, V., & Raut, D. K. (2011). Medical literature search dot com. *Indian Journal of Dermatology Venereology and Leprology, 77*(2), 135–140. doi:10.4103/0378-6323.77451

Japuntich, S. J., Zehner, M. E., Smith, S. S., Jorenby, D. E., Valdez, J. A., Fiore, M. C., et al. (2006). Smoking cessation via the internet: A randomized clinical trial of an internet intervention as adjuvant treatment in a smoking cessation intervention. *Nicotine & Tobacco Research, 8*(Suppl 1), S59–67.

Johnsen, J. A., Rosenvinge, J. H., & Gammon, D. (2002). Online group interaction and mental health: An analysis of three online discussion forums. *Scandinavian Journal of Psychology, 43*(5), 445–449.

Joshi, M. P., Bhangoo, R. S., & Kumar, K. (2011). Quality of nutrition related information on the internet for osteoporosis patients: a critical review. *Technology and Health Care, 19*(6), 391–400. doi:10.3233/THC-2011-0643

Kaicker, J., Debono, V. B., Dang, W., Buckley, N., & Thabane, L. (2010). Assessment of the quality and variability of health information on chronic pain websites using the DISCERN instrument. *BMC Medicine, 8*, 59. doi:10.1186/1741-7015-8-59

Kang, S. H., & Bloom, J. R. (1993). Social support and cancer screening among older black Americans. *Journal of the National Cancer Institute, 85*(9), 737–742.

Kernot, J., Olds, T., Lewis, L. K., & Maher, C. (2013). Effectiveness of a facebook-delivered physical activity intervention for post-partum women: A randomized controlled trial protocol. *BMC Public Health, 13*, 518. doi:10.1186/1471-2458-13-518

Kontos, E. Z., Emmons, K. M., Puleo, E., & Viswanath, K. (2010). Communication inequalities and public health implications of adult social networking site use in the United States. *Journal of Health Communication, 15*(Suppl 3), 216–235. doi:10.1080/10810730.2010.522689

Korda, H., & Itani, Z. (2011). Harnessing Social Media for Health Promotion and Behavior Change. *Health Promotion Practice,* doi:10.1177/1524839911405850

Kownacki, R. J., & Shadish, W. R. (1999). Does Alcoholics Anonymous work? The results from a meta-analysis of controlled experiments. *Substance Use and Misuse, 34*(13), 1897–1916.

Kummervold, P. E., Gammon, D., Bergvik, S., Johnsen, J. A., Hasvold, T., & Rosenvinge, J. H. (2002). Social support in a wired world: Use of online mental health forums in Norway. *Nordic Journal of Psychiatry, 56* (1), 59–65. doi:10.1080/08039480252803945

Lazer, D., Pentland, A., Adamic, L., Aral, S., Barabasi, A. L., Brewer, D., et al. (2009). Social science. Computational social science. *Science, 323*(5915), 721–723. doi:10.1126/science.1167742

Leggatt-Cook, C., & Chamberlain, K. (2011). Blogging for weight loss: personal accountability, writing selves, and the weight-loss blogosphere. *Sociology of Health & Illness.* doi:10.1111/j.1467-9566.2011.01435.x

Lichtenstein, E., Glasgow, R. E., & Abrams, D. B. (1986). Social support in smoking cessation: In search of effective interventions. *Behavior Therapy, 17*(5), 607–619. doi:10.1016/S0005-7894(86)80098-3

Lorig, K. R., Laurent, D. D., Deyo, R. A., Marnell, M. E., Minor, M. A., & Ritter, P. L. (2002). Can a Back Pain E-mail Discussion Group improve health status and lower health care costs?: A randomized study. *Archives of Internal Medicine, 162*(7), 792–796.

May, S., & West, R. (2000). Do social support interventions ("buddy systems") aid smoking cessation? A review. *Tob Control, 9*(4), 415–422.

MayoClinic Admin. (2011). Mayo Clinic launches social network to connect global Mayo Clinic community. http://socialmedia.mayoclinic.org/2011/07/05/mayo-clinic-launches-social-network-to-connect-global-mayo-clinic-community/

Meier, A., Lyons, E. J., Frydman, G., Forlenza, M., & Rimer, B. K. (2007). How cancer survivors provide support on cancer-related Internet mailing lists. *Journal of Medical Internet Research, 9*(2), e12. doi:10.2196/jmir.9.2.e12

Mermelstein, R., Cohen, S., Lichtenstein, E., Baer, J. S., & Kamarck, T. (1986). Social support and smoking cessation and maintenance. *Journal of Consulting and Clinical Psychology, 54*(4), 447–453.

Mermelstein, R., Lichtenstein, E., & McIntyre, K. (1983). Partner support and relapse in smoking-cessation programs. *Journal of Consulting and Clinical Psychology, 51*(3), 465–466.

Moorhead, S. A., Hazlett, D. E., Harrison, L., Carroll, J. K., Irwin, A., & Hoving, C. (2013). A new

dimension of health care: systematic review of the uses, benefits, and limitations of social media for health communication. *Journal of Medical Internet Research, 15*(4), e85. doi:10.2196/jmir.1933

Murray, E., Lo, B., Pollack, L., Donelan, K., Catania, J., Lee, K., et al. (2003). The impact of health information on the Internet on health care and the physician-patient relationship: National U.S. survey among 1.050 U.S. physicians. *Journal of Medical Internet Research, 5*(3), e17. doi:10.2196/jmir.5.3.e17

Muthukumarasamy, S., Osmani, Z., Sharpe, A., & England, R. J. (2012). Quality of information available on the World Wide Web for patients undergoing thyroidectomy: Review. *Journal of Laryngology and Otology, 126*(2), 116–119. doi:10.1017/S0022215111002246

Namkoong, K., DuBenske, L. L., Shaw, B. R., Gustafson, D. H., Hawkins, R. P., Shah, D. V., et al. (2012). Creating a bond between caregivers online: Effect on caregivers' coping strategies. *Journal of Health Communication, 17*(2), 125–140. doi:10.1080/10810730.2011.585687

Napolitano, M. A., Hayes, S., Bennett, G. G., Ives, A. K., & Foster, G. D. (2013). Using Facebook and text messaging to deliver a weight loss program to college students. *Obesity (Silver Spring), 21*(1), 25–31. doi:10.1002/oby.20232

O'Grady, L., & Jadad, A. (2010, November 8). Shifting from shared to collaborative decision making: A change in thinking and doing. *Journal of Participatory Medicine, 2.*

Park, E. W., Schultz, J. K., Tudiver, F., Campbell, T., & Becker, L. (2004). Enhancing partner support to improve smoking cessation. *Cochrane Database of Systematic Reviews* (3), CD002928.

Peterson, G., Aslani, P., & Williams, K. A. (2003). How do consumers search for and appraise information on medicines on the Internet? A qualitative study using focus groups. *Journal of Medical Internet Research, 5* (4), e33. doi:10.2196/jmir.5.4.e33

Pew Internet & American Life Project. (2013). Demographics of internet users: *Pew Research Center's Internet & American Life Project Spring Tracking Survey, April 17–May 19, 2013.* Retrieved September 13, 2013, from http://www.pewinternet.org/Static-Pages/Trend-Data-%28Adults%29/Whos-Online.aspx . Archived at http://www.webcitation.org/6JedVxUVN

Poirier, J., & Cobb, N. K. (2012). Social influence as a driver of engagement in a web-based health intervention. *Journal of Medical Internet Research, 14*(1), e36. doi:10.2196/jmir.1957

Preyde, M., & Ardal, F. (2003). Effectiveness of a parent "buddy" program for mothers of very preterm infants in a neonatal intensive care unit. *CMAJ, 168*(8), 969–973.

PricewaterhouseCoopers, Health Research Institute. (2012). Social media "likes" healthcare from marketing to social business.

Rao, N. R., Mohapatra, M., Mishra, S., & Joshi, A. (2012). Evaluation of dengue-related health information on the internet. *Perspect Health Inf Manag, 9*, 1c.

Richardson, A., Graham, A. L., Cobb, N., Xiao, H., Mushro, A., Abrams, D., & Vallone, D. (2013). Engagement promotes abstinence in a web-based cessation intervention: cohort study. *Journal of Medical Internet Research, 15*(1), e14. doi:10.2196/jmir.2277

Rimer, B. K., Lyons, E. J., Ribisl, K. M., Bowling, J. M., Golin, C. E., Forlenza, M. J., & Meier, A. (2005). How new subscribers use cancer-related online mailing lists. *Journal of Medical Internet Research, 7*(3), e32. doi:10.2196/jmir.7.3.e32

Robinson, T. N., Patrick, K., Eng, T. R., & Gustafson, D. (1998). An evidence-based approach to interactive health communication: A challenge to medicine in the information age. Science Panel on Interactive Communication and Health. *JAMA, 280*(14), 1264–1269.

Schwarzer, R., & Satow, L. (2012). Online intervention engagement predicts smoking cessation. *Preventive Medicine.* doi:10.1016/j.ypmed.2012.07.006

Schwitzer, G. (2002). A review of features in Internet consumer health decision-support tools. *Journal of Medical Internet Research, 4*(2), E11. doi:10.2196/jmir.4.2.e11

Seeman, T. E. (1996). Social ties and health: The benefits of social integration. *Annals of Epidemiology, 6*(5), 442–451. S1047279796000956 [pii].

Selby, P., van Mierlo, T., Voci, S. C., Parent, D., & Cunningham, J. A. (2010). Online social and professional support for smokers trying to quit: an exploration of first time posts from 2562 members. *Journal of Medical Internet Research, 12*(3), e34. doi:10.2196/jmir.1340

Shahar, S., Shirley, N., & Noah, S. A. (2013). Quality and accuracy assessment of nutrition information on the Web for cancer prevention. *Informatics for Health and Social Care, 38*(1), 15–26. doi:10.3109/17538157.2012.710684

Shaw, B. R., McTavish, F., Hawkins, R., Gustafson, D. H., & Pingree, S. (2000). Experiences of women with breast cancer: exchanging social support over the CHESS computer network. *Journal of Health Communication, 5*(2), 135–159. doi:10.1080/108107300406866

Smithson, J., Sharkey, S., Hewis, E., Jones, R. B., Emmens, T., Ford, T., & Owens, C. (2011). Membership and boundary maintenance on an online self-harm forum. *Qualitative Health Research, 21*(11), 1567–1575. doi:10.1177/1049732311413784

Suarez, L., Lloyd, L., Weiss, N., Rainbolt, T., & Pulley, L. (1994). Effect of social networks on cancer-screening behavior of older Mexican-American women. *Journal of the National Cancer Institute, 86*(10), 775–779.

Suler, J. (2004). The online disinhibition effect. *Cyberpsychol Behav, 7*(3), 321–326. doi:10.1089/1094931041291295

Tang, T. S., Ayala, G. X., Cherrington, A., & Rana, G. (2011). A review of volunteer-based support interventions in diabetes. *Diabetes Spectrum, 24*, 85–98.

Tate, D. F., Wing, R. R., & Winett, R. A. (2001). Using Internet technology to deliver a behavioral weight loss program. *JAMA, 285*(9), 1172–1177.

Taylor, J. O., Gustafson, D. H., Hawkins, R., Pingree, S., McTavish, F., Wise, M., & Carter, M. (1994). The Comprehensive Health Enhancement Support System. *Quality Management in Health care, 2*(4), 36–43.

Valente, T. W. (1996). Social network thresholds in the diffusion of innovations. *Social Networks, 18*(1), 69–89.

Valente, T. W. (2012). Network interventions. *Science, 337*(6090), 49–53. doi:10.1126/science.1217330

Valle, C. G., Tate, D. F., Mayer, D. K., Allicock, M., & Cai, J. (2013). A randomized trial of a Facebook-based physical activity intervention for young adult cancer survivors. *Journal of Cancer Survivorship, 7*(3), 355–368. doi:10.1007/s11764-013-0279-5

van der Marel, S., Duijvestein, M., Hardwick, J. C., van den Brink, G. R., Veenendaal, R., Hommes, D. W., & Fidder, H. H. (2009). Quality of web-based information on inflammatory bowel diseases. *Inflammatory Bowel Diseases, 15*(12), 1891–1896. doi:10.1002/ibd.20976

van Uden-Kraan, C. F., Drossaert, C. H., Taal, E., Seydel, E. R., & van de Laar, M. A. (2009). Participation in online patient support groups endorses patients' empowerment. *Patient Education and Counseling, 74*(1), 61–69. doi:10.1016/j.pec.2008.07.044

Wald, H. S., Dube, C. E., & Anthony, D. C. (2007). Untangling the Web–the impact of Internet use on health care and the physician-patient relationship. *Patient Education and Counseling, 68*(3), 218–224. doi:10.1016/j.pec.2007.05.016

Wasserman, M., Baxter, N. N., Rosen, B., Burnstein, M., & Halverson, A. L. (2014). Systematic review of internet patient information on colorectal cancer surgery. *Diseases of the Colon & Rectum, 57*(1), 64–69. doi:10.1097/DCR.0000000000000011

Webel, A. R., Okonsky, J., Trompeta, J., & Holzemer, W. L. (2010). A systematic review of the effectiveness of peer-based interventions on health-related behaviors in adults. *American Journal of Public Health, 100*(2), 247–253. doi:10.2105/AJPH.2008.149419

WebMD Health Corp. (2010). WebMD announces new health social networking platform on WebMD.com. Retrieved from WebMD.com website: http://investor.shareholder.com/wbmd/releasedetail.cfm?ReleaseID=450474&CompanyID=WBMD

Weinert, C., Cudney, S., & Winters, C. (2005). Social support in cyberspace: The next generation. *Comput Inform Nurs, 23*(1), 7–15. 00024665-200501000-00004 [pii].

Weis, R., Stamm, K., Smith, C., Nilan, M., Clark, F., Weis, J., et al. (2003). Communities of Care and Caring: The case of MSWatch.com(R). *Journal of Health Psychology, 8*(1), 135–148. doi:10.1177/1359105303008001449

White, M., & Dorman, S. M. (2001). Receiving social support online: Implications for health education. *Health Education Research, 16*(6), 693–707.

Wicks, P., Keininger, D. L., Massagli, M. P., de la Loge, C., Brownstein, C., Isojarvi, J., & Heywood, J. (2012). Perceived benefits of sharing health data between people with epilepsy on an online platform. *Epilepsy & Behavior, 23*(1), 16–23. doi:10.1016/j.yebeh.2011.09.026

Wicks, P., Massagli, M., Frost, J., Brownstein, C., Okun, S., Vaughan, T. … Heywood, J. (2010). Sharing health data for better outcomes on PatientsLikeMe. *Journal of Medical Internet Research, 12*(2), e19. doi:10.2196/jmir.1549

Wikipedia (n.d.). (2012, September 11, 2012). On the Internet, nobody knows you're a dog. Retrieved October 13, 2012, from http://en.wikipedia.org/w/index.php?title=On_the_Internet,_nobody_knows_you%27re_a_dog&oldid=511879668

Wilson, C. T., & Brownell, K. D. (1978). Behavior therapy for obesity: Including family members in the treatment process. *Behavior Therapy, 9*, 943–945.

Winzelberg, A. J., Classen, C., Alpers, G. W., Roberts, H., Koopman, C., Adams, R. E., et al. (2003). Evaluation of an internet support group for women with primary breast cancer. *Cancer, 97*(5), 1164–1173. doi:10.1002/cncr.11174

Womble, L. G., Wadden, T. A., McGuckin, B. G., Sargent, S. L., Rothman, R. A., & Krauthamer-Ewing, E. S. (2004). A randomized controlled trial of a commercial internet weight loss program. *Obesity Research, 12*(6), 1011–1018. doi:10.1038/oby.2004.124

Wright, K. B., & Bell, S. B. (2003). Health-related Support Groups on the Internet: Linking empirical findings to social support and computer-mediated communication theory. *Journal of Health Psychology, 8*(1), 39–54. doi:10.1177/1359105303008001429

Yee, L., & Simon, M. (2010). The role of the social network in contraceptive decision-making among young, African American and Latina women. *Journal of Adolescent Health, 47*(4), 374–380. doi:10.1016/j.jadohealth.2010.03.014

Young, S. D., Cumberland, W. G., Lee, S. J., Jaganath, D., Szekeres, G., & Coates, T. (2013). Social networking technologies as an emerging tool for HIV prevention: A cluster randomized trial. *Annals of Internal Medicine, 159*(5), 318–324. doi:10.7326/0003-4819-159-5-201309030-00005

Zabinski, M. F., Wilfley, D. E., Calfas, K. J., Winzelberg, A. J., & Taylor, C. B. (2004). An interactive psychoeducational intervention for women at risk of developing an eating disorder. *Journal of Consulting and Clinical Psychology, 72*(5), 914–919. doi:10.1037/0022-006X.72.5.914

Zhao, S., Grasmuck, S., & Martin, J. (2008). Identity construction on Facebook: Digital empowerment in anchored relationships. *Computers in Human Behavior, 24*, 1816–1836.

Ziebland, S., & Wyke, S. (2012). Health and illness in a connected world: How might sharing experiences on the internet affect people's health? *Milbank Quarterly, 90*(2), 219–249. doi:10.1111/j.1468-0009.2012.00662.x

Zitter, R. E., & Fremouw, W. J. (1978). Individual versus partner consequation for weight loss. *Behavior Therapy, 9*, 808–813.

Decision-Making in the Age of Whole Genome Sequencing

Saskia C. Sanderson and Eric E. Schadt

Introduction

In 2001, the first human genome sequence was produced: it took 15 years and $3 billion (Lander et al. 2001; Venter et al. 2001; International Human Genome Sequencing Consortium 2004). Today, an entire human genome can be sequenced for less than $5000 (Drmanac et al. 2010). The cost of whole genome sequencing (WGS) is falling at a super Moore's law rate (National Research Council 2011). Technologies on the horizon like the IBM DNA transistor have theoretical sequencing limits in the hundreds of millions of bases per second per transistor. Packing millions of such transistors together in a single chip or handheld device could produce terabase and even petabase scale sequencing in seconds (Schadt et al. 2010). There seems to be little doubt that WGS could be routinely available to patients for a few dollars within the next 10 years.

Today, patients can obtain personal results from WGS, or "personal genome sequencing," in research studies like the MedSeq Project (www. genomes2people.org/g2p) and the Personal Genome Project (Church 2005; Lunshof et al. 2008; Angrist 2009; Lunshof et al. 2010). Consumers have obtained whole exome sequencing (WES) from direct-to-consumer (DTC) company 23andMe (http://blog.23andme.com/23andme-research/23 andme-moves-into-the-world-of-sequencing/), and Illumina's "MyGenome" app allows healthcare providers access to personal WGS results (www. illumina.com/company/events/understand-your-genome.html).

The rate of technological development has outpaced our ability to fully address important questions relating not only to the health, social, and economic implications of having easy access to one's genome, but also regarding patient education, understanding, and informed decision-making (Green and Guyer 2011; Brunham and Hayden 2012). Deciding whether to have personal WGS is complex, and involves considering scientific uncertainty, weighing up potential benefits and risks, understanding the range of possible results that could arise, and how such results may be used or interpreted by others (Green and Guyer 2011).

In clinical genetics, the gold standard for ensuring patients make informed decisions about genetic testing is in-person genetic counseling with a trained genetic counselor. The 2006 National Society of Genetic Counselors (NSGC) definition of genetic counseling is that genetic counseling "is the process of helping people understand and adapt to the medical, psychological and familial implications of genetic contributions to disease. This

S.C. Sanderson (✉)
Great Ormond Street Hospital and University
College London (UCL), London, UK
e-mail: saskia.sanderson@ucl.ac.uk

E.E. Schadt
Genetics and Genomic Sciences, Icahn School of
Medicine at Mount Sinai, New York, USA
e-mail: eric.schadt@mssm.edu

© Springer Science+Business Media New York 2016
M.A. Diefenbach et al. (eds.), *Handbook of Health Decision Science*,
DOI 10.1007/978-1-4939-3486-7_25

process integrates … interpretation of family and medical histories to assess the chance of disease occurrence or recurrence; education about inheritance, testing, management, prevention, resources and research; and counseling to promote informed choices and adaptation to the risk or condition" (Walker 2009, p. 7).

However, genetic counseling services are already stretched (Brunham and Hayden 2012). There are currently just over 4000 Board Certified Genetic Counselors and 33 Accredited Graduate Programs in Genetic Counseling in the US (http://www.abgc.net/About_ABGC/GeneticCounselors.asp; accessed 13 June 2016), yet hundreds of thousands of genomes are being sequenced presently and that number is growing at an exponential pace (while the training of genetic counselors is steady or at best growing at a linear pace). It would therefore be physically impossible for everyone getting sequenced to have even 5 min of time with a genetic counselor, let alone the hour or two it routinely takes to fully educate and counsel patients considering genetic testing at the present time.

Most DTC personal genomics companies provide little to no in-person genetic counseling (Dohany et al. 2012). For example, individuals purchasing personal genomics products from the DTC genetic testing company 23andme (www.23andme.com) are not required to have genetic counseling before, during, or after their purchase. Of note, Navigenics (www.navigenics.com), the one well-known DTC genetic testing company providing genetic information within a more traditional genetic counseling model, was bought by Life Technologies in 2012 (www.bloomberg.com/news/articles/2012-07-16/life-technologies-buys-navigenics-for-genetic-diagnostics; accessed 13 June 2016), supporting the suggestion that this is arguably not a sustainable model. It is vital that questions around the extent to which genetic counseling is a critical part of the genetic testing process, and whether novel educational and support systems can replace or enhance in-personal genetic counseling, are addressed.

In this chapter, we discuss how decision-making about genome sequencing may differ from decision-making about past health-related tests, review the limited evidence at present on decision-making about genome sequencing, discuss how the rate of evidence is growing exponentially and so decision-making is a moving target that we can expect to be constantly changing and very dynamic for the foreseeable future, and discuss the challenges and future directions for the field. We focus primarily on WGS in the context of "healthy" individuals, that is, individuals not selected specifically for having an initial disease or phenotype of interest. Although much of WGS being done today is, for example, to uncover the cause of an undiagnosed disease or to try to help treat a patient diagnosed with cancer, we anticipate that within the next few years WGS will not be restricted to individuals and families affected with rare genetic disorders and diseases, but that rather we are moving toward a future where every individual across society will have their genome sequenced. Relatedly, genomics research studies are growing in size and scope at a rapid pace. The evidence-based, double-blind randomized clinical trial paradigm is not adequate to handle all of the information coming and we therefore need a different paradigm, one that considers patient populations to be clinical trial populations, where medical evidence is built up in real time, with decision-making happening within adaptive designs that are constantly being updated as new data and results emerge. Patients and research participants will be required to make decisions about having WGS done and receiving results from it, acknowledging that the context in which they are having it done is constantly changing and evolving, and that therefore all of the future outcomes of the research or clinical procedures cannot be predicted at baseline. For the purposes of this chapter, we consider "healthy" individuals to include both research participants and future "healthy" "patients," given the lines between these two groups are arguably blurred.

Genome Sequencing and "Big Data"

From a data perspective and the impact of data on our daily lives, life was much simpler 30 years ago. Few computerized systems existed to store your personal information, the Internet was so primitive that most were not even aware it existed, handheld cellular phones were owned by only a privileged few thousand individuals, and DNA sequencing was carried out by running DNA out on gels. However, today we find ourselves in the midst of a big data revolution, a revolution permeating nearly every aspect of our lives. Electronic devices that consume much of our attention on a daily basis enable rapid transactions among individuals and between individuals and entire communities on unprecedented scales, where all of the information involved in these daily transactions can be seamlessly stored in digital form, whether the transactions involve cell phone calls, text messages, credit card purchases, emails, or visits to the doctor's office in which all tests carried out are digitized and entered into your electronic medical record.

The life and biomedical sciences have not stood on the sidelines of this revolution. There has been an incredible wave of new technologies in genomics—such as next-generation sequencing technologies (Eid et al. 2009), sophisticated imaging systems, and mass spectrometry-based flow cytometry (Bandura et al. 2009)—enabling data to be generated at very large scales. As a result we can monitor the expression of tens of thousands of protein- and noncoding genes simultaneously (Emilsson et al. 2008; Chen et al. 2012), score hundreds of thousands of Single-Nucleotide Polymorphisms (SNPs) in individual samples (Altshuler et al. 2008), sequence entire human genomes now for less than $5000 (Drmanac et al. 2010), and relate all of these data patterns to a great diversity of other biologically relevant information (clinical data, biochemical data, social networking data, etc.). Given technologies on the horizon like the IBM DNA transistor with theoretical sequencing limits in the hundreds of millions of bases per second per transistor (imagine millions of these transistors packed together in a single handheld device) (Schadt et al. 2010), we would not be talking in the future about Google rolling through neighborhoods with Wi-Fi sniffing equipment (Kravets 2010), but rather we would be talking about DNA sniffing equipment rolling

through neighborhoods sequencing everything they encounter in real time and then pumping such data into big data clouds to link with all other available information in the digital universe.

Keeping pace with these life sciences technology advances are information technology advances in which now more "classic" information-savvy companies like Microsoft, Amazon, Google, Facebook, Ebay, and Yahoo as well as a new breed of emerging big data mining companies such as Recorded Future, Factual, Locu, and Palantir have led the way in becoming masters of petabyte- and exabyte-scale datasets—linking pieces of data distributed over massively parallel architectures in response to user requests and presenting results to the user in a matter of seconds. Following these advances made in other disciplines, we are on track to access the same types of tools to tackle the big data problems now being faced by the life and biomedical sciences, especially as it relates to the interpretation of personal genomes, better informing a human genome by taking into account the digital universe of information, as opposed to the information that can be stored in the brain of a medical geneticist or genetic counselor. But large-scale data generation and big computer infrastructures are just two legs of the stool regarding what is needed to revolutionize our understanding of our own DNA. While the data revolution is driven by technologies that provide insights into how living systems operate, enabling decision-making at a hierarchy of levels (patients, physicians, expert researchers, physician scientists, big data mining firms, marketing firms, and lay individuals who simply want to better understand themselves), achieving understanding from such data that drives the most informed decisions will require that we tame the burgeoning information these technologies generate.

If we want to achieve understanding from the big genomics data, organize it, compute on it, build predictive models from it, then we must employ statistical reasoning beyond the more classic hypothesis testing of yesteryear. We have moved well beyond the idea that we can simply repeat experiments to validate findings generated in populations. While first instances of the

Central Dogma of Biology were incredibly simple, today, given the complex interplay of multiple dimensions of data (DNA, RNA, protein, metabolite, cellular, physiologic, ecologic and social structures more generally), a much more holistic view must be taken in which we embrace complexity in its entirety. Our emerging view of complex biological systems is one of a dynamic, fluid system that is able to reconfigure itself as conditions demand (Zerhouni 2003; Barabasi and Oltvai 2004; Han et al. 2004; Luscombe et al. 2004; Pinto et al. 2004).

Soon average individuals will have access to detailed information about their genetic makeup, the molecular states of different cell types and tissues sampled from their bodies, and more detailed, longitudinal collections of phenotypes informing on their weight, blood pressure, glucose and insulin levels, and a myriad of other clinical traits that inform on disease, disease risk, and drug response. Decisions motivated by interpretations of this information will be maximally informed if the right types of data are appropriately integrated and presented to us or our doctors in ways that maximize chances of assessing disease risk, detecting disease, or developing treatment strategies tailored to our particular disease subtype and individual genetic/environmental backgrounds. Already, there are powerful examples of how this new era of personalized medicine will change the way we are diagnosed and treated. A routine genetic test can indicate whether breast cancer patients will respond to treatment with Herceptin, and testing for certain changes in DNA that affect a gene needed to convert vitamin K into an active form required for proper blood clotting is being shown to assist doctors in assessing whether patients requiring an anticoagulant can tolerate a high dose of warfarin or whether a lower dose should be given to prevent what could be fatal side effects.

Just like the security analysts sifting through mountains of data to identify the next big threat, individuals concerned about their well-being, doctors who seek to treat these individuals, and researchers searching for causes and treatments of disease, will face their own "big data problem" as evolving technologies enable unprecedented, comprehensive views of our bodies at the genetic, molecular, and physiological levels. While many of us have grown up in the era of doctors wielding stethoscopes and thermometers as their primary tools to rapidly assess a patient's state of health, tomorrow's doctors will be faced with a myriad of "biological chips" and imaging technologies capable of monitoring variations in our DNA, variations in the activities of genes and proteins in our bodies that drive all cellular functions, and providing for resolution at the single-cell level of any organ in our bodies. There is a need to master the large-scale molecular data that underlies pathophysiological states, employ sophisticated mathematical algorithms capable of data integration, and leverage appropriate informatics infrastructure to apply these algorithms and translate the results into manageable bites of information that can be consumed by physicians and patients, if we hope to realize the dream of personalized medicine. Ultimately, through the use of advanced biomedical and informatics technologies, we will be able to enable different users of genomic information to become masters of this information.

How Does Decision-Making About Genome Sequencing Differ from Decision-Making About Other Health-Related Technologies?

The Changing Landscape of Actionable Variation in Genome-Wide Sequencing Data

The interpretation of genome-wide sequencing data to date has largely focused on variants that lead to changes in protein coding sequence. On average, comparing a given individual's genome assembled from WGS data to a common reference sequence will result in the identification of three to four million small nucleotide sequence variants, 30,000–50,000 of which will fall within the protein coding part of genes (Biesecker 2012, p. 394). While perhaps a majority of these protein coding variants will not be of clinical significance or of importance to the individual, many of these variants will be of clinical or personal significance, with current estimates demonstrating that most individuals who have been sequenced harbor three to eight actionable variants (Speicher et al. 2010; c. f. Biesecker 2012). While these protein coding variants may seem large in volume, these investigations to date have not paid significant attention to the vast number of variants that fall outside of gene regions (the case for the vast number of variants, including those associated with disease) nor is the sequence data generated today able to comprehensively characterize structural variations given the short-read nature of next-generation sequencing (NGS) technologies. Existing studies of gene expression data have associated many thousands of sequence variants with the expression levels of genes, and these variants have also been shown to be enriched for disease-associated alleles from the genome-wide association studies (GWAS). Layer on top of the work coming out of the ENCODE project in which roughly 80 % of the genome has been shown to be actively bound by proteins in tissue and development specific ways (Bernstein et al. 2012), and the expectation is that the vast majority of variants that are either actionable on their own or comprising multivariate models that well predict phenotypes of interest, will be regulatory in nature. Thus, the sheer volume of data produced by WGS is unprecedented, and the types of results that an individual may receive through WGS are unpredictable and open-ended. This has important implications for decision-making about WGS that are discussed further below.

Unpredictability of Diseases/Traits for Which Information May Be Uncovered

Individuals making decisions about having WGS done are not making a decision about receiving information about one disease or trait, but rather about whether to receive information about an undefined, unpredictable number and types of diseases and traits. This therefore differs from most other types of decision-making in the health arena, which tend to be disease-specific. For example, factors influencing a man's decision about whether to go ahead with prostate-specific androgen (PSA) testing for prostate cancer risk may include his perceived or actual risk of developing the disease, his family history of the disease, and his fear of the disease, as well as his perceptions or understandings of the benefits versus limitations of the test itself. The man in this scenario may weigh up how he would feel in response to receiving high risk results for prostate cancer based on PSA testing, and what he would do with this information about his prostate cancer risk. Similarly, a woman making a decision about *BRCA1/2* genetic testing for breast cancer risk, may factor in her personal and family history of breast cancer, her feelings about breast cancer, how a positive or negative *BRCA1/2* test result would make her feel, and what she would do with that result. In contrast, an individual considering how he or she might feel in response to results from WGS, has to consider how they would feel getting results potentially pertaining to a vast array of diseases or traits. Cassa et al. (2012) estimated the number of published disease-associated variants that met the criteria for disclosure to genomics research participants according to published guidelines. Based on their analysis, Cassa et al. (2012) estimated that investigators following these guidelines may be responsible for disclosing over 11,000 variants to each participant.

A specific assay like *BRCA1/2* testing leads to a single result that may inform with high accuracy what one's lifetime risk of developing breast cancer is given mutations in these genes. Such results can be useful to the individual since if they are determined to be at high risk, they may choose to have more routine and thorough exams for early detection or mastectomy or oophorectomy, and it may tune physicians into the increased risk so they are more thoughtful about the interpretation of related exam results. With WGS there may not be any particular condition of interest, but rather a desire to better understand oneself more generally, for example, risk of many different diseases, risk of nondisease-related traits that may lead to lifestyle changes, ancestry, and other types of personal information that today we can only imagine. Therefore, not only must an individual accept that they could uncover significant risk for any known disease, but also that other unanticipated results may arise, such as learning that your ancestry as determined by sequence data is not consistent with the ancestry your family considers as truth. In the context of understanding one's risk of a particular disease given WGS data, the results likely will not be as clear as a *BRCA1/2* test because the information half-life is very short, i.e., what is known about a specific genetic variant or disease today may be vastly different from that which is known about that variant or disease tomorrow. This makes it difficult to establish and apply guidelines on how to interpret the many hundreds of variants that may be associated with a given disease (Fabsitz et al. 2010; Cassa et al. 2012). How to assess the risk of a disease in the context of hundreds of variants, interactions between those variations and with the environment, and what actions to take given a particular risk score or diagnosis are all similarly complex. All of these factors exemplify that WGS as a diagnostic represents a very different scenario compared to more classic molecular diagnostic assays, with a different set of accompanying challenges for the individual and the researchers/clinicians facilitating that decision.

individual who has a strong family history of breast cancer and who has opted for *BRCA1/2* genetic testing may respond very differently to being told they have a mutation in *BRCA1/2* compared to an individual who learns that they have a very high risk of breast cancer through WGS. While such a discovery may be disturbing, at least there are actions one can take to enable early detection of breast cancer when treatment options and effectiveness are optimal. However, cases will exist in which a significant risk of disease will come to light, but for which little can be done to prevent and/or treat the disease at present. Carriers of the ApoE-e4 allele represent perhaps one of the more obvious cases in which a relatively common allele is strongly predictive of your risk for early-onset Alzheimer's, but for which no preventive treatment can be prescribed at this time.

Of course, positive benefits in a disease context could potentially be realized as well from knowledge of one's sequence data if one is identified as *not* having an increased risk of disease. Knowledge that disease-associated alleles segregating in your family are not represented in your genome may provide for a number of benefits including more informed decisions relating to reproduction, reduced stress and anxiety regarding risk of particular diseases, and more informed diagnoses relating to existing conditions, to name just a few.

Implications for Family Members

Patient May not Have Phenotype/Family History of Disease About Which Information Is Produced

In the case of most existing genetic tests such as genetic tests for Huntington's disease, breast cancer, and rare Mendelian disorders, eligibility for testing is determined by the individual having a personal or family history of the disease in question. However, in the case of WGS, particularly with "healthy" individuals, such eligibility criteria are not necessarily applied. This has implications for how prepared the individual may be for the results from WGS. For example, an

Although many genetic tests have implications for family members, this is arguably particularly important in the case of WGS because of the sheer number of results that could be obtained. Learning of one's genetic susceptibility to disease has direct implications for family members who may or may not want to know of such risks. For example, learning that you are an ApoE-e4 homozygote and so at significantly increased risk for early-onset Alzheimer's disease, will have direct implications for your parents and siblings, who may have no desire to learn of such a risk they can do nothing about. These implications go beyond disease risk for family members, since ancestry (Halder et al. 2008), political beliefs (Hatemi and McDermott 2012), and even being religious or not (Koenig et al. 2005) have genetic components that will increasingly be elucidated as more individuals are sequenced. Thus there is the potential for sequencing data to impact your social network in ways again that most may not anticipate.

Identifiability

Protecting an individual's right to privacy in medicine and research has always been a topic of significant discussion and concern, the primary focus being on the protection of information that is more obviously personally identifiable. DNA information collected on individuals has been of particular concern, given even with anonymized data or de-identified data it will be possible to link such data to a given individual as genetic databases proliferate (McGuire and Gibbs 2006). For example, in 2004, "Lin and colleagues demonstrated that an individual can be uniquely identified with access to just 75 single-nucleotide polymorphisms (SNPs) from that person" (Lin et al. 2006; c.f. McGuire and Gibbs 2006). Thus, decision-making about WGS differs from decision-making about simpler disease-specific tests such as the PSA test because the same promises about protection of privacy and confidentiality cannot, or should not, be made, and the individual needs to take this into account.

As sequencing technologies advance, we will increasingly realize that protecting and ensuring privacy regarding an individual's DNA will not be possible, thus necessitating an even larger focus on educating individuals up front that this will be the case. Equally important will be ensuring individuals are not discriminated against based on DNA information. The protection of personally identifiable information is intertwined with our collective expectation of keeping personal information private. For example, your social security number or data contained within your medical record are both forms of data that are personally identifiable and

for which you have a reasonable expectation of privacy. In contrast, although a photograph taken of your face is also clearly personally identifiable, in this case you have no reasonable expectation of privacy in public given we communicate in public by recognizing features such as faces and facial expressions, and given your image is easily acquired via cameras or video recorders.

However, today we are in a state of transition as we figure out collectively how to both understand the information that is personally identifiable and determine what reasonable expectation of privacy we have regarding such data. The social networking revolution has changed our expectations of privacy regarding a great diversity of personal data. Many individuals today disclose highly personal information on the web, loosening our expectations regarding what information should be kept private. Social networking sites like Facebook and Google have ridden this wave and slowly weakened any expectation of privacy we may have regarding information provided to their sites; buried within the consents users click through without ever reading, is their explicit approval to allow these companies to leverage for whatever purpose they deem appropriate any and all personal information, emails, likes and dislikes, political leanings, religious beliefs, and photographs and videos of highly personal scenes in which facial and scene recognition algorithms can be employed to understand your behaviors, your age, your gender, your friends, types of places you frequent, and the types of products you buy. These highly personal data are most commonly used by high-end data analytics firms to better target you with advertising to which you are most likely to respond. The same wants to share all levels of personal details exists in the scientific arena as well, with WGS and deep molecular profiling carried out now on several scientists who have openly disclosed all data with name attached (Ashley et al. 2010; Dewey et al. 2011; Chen et al. 2012).

While continuing to make assurances that we can protect an individual's privacy when DNA are collected as part of a research study, expanding laws, locking down relevant databases, and creating greater regulatory burdens to further protect privacy represent one set of options. Such steps are likely in vain though as the costs of technologies that can generate high-dimensional data on an individual continue to fall at super Moore's laws rates and as our ability to process big data increases exponentially, as discussed above. In fact, we demonstrated that it is possible to derive genotypic barcodes that can uniquely distinguish among individuals in very large populations, from non-DNA sources (Schadt et al. 2012). Given this growing inability to protect peoples' privacy regarding high-dimensional data that can be easily collected about them, it is imperative to consider alternative strategies. This is especially so if the courts ultimately rule there can be no reasonable expectation of privacy for genomic data, since the ability to acquire your DNA and to sequence it may become as easy and cheap as snapping a photograph of your face. Therefore, we must begin to not only better inform individuals regarding WGS data and their personal privacy, but we must ensure appropriate protections are in place to prevent discrimination based on these data. In the United States, the Genetic Information Nondiscrimination Act and Americans with Disabilities Act provide for many such protections, but as individuals become more empowered to share their data to achieve greater medical benefit from it, and as we move to more seamlessly map between DNA and more easily acquired high-dimensional phenotypic data to predict with greater ease a greater diversity of human behaviors and disease risks, laws must also evolve to ensure the rights of patients are protected (Schadt 2012).

Resource not a Test

Perhaps most important, is the point made eloquently by Biesecker that WGS "is a resource, not a test" (Biesecker 2012). Biesecker highlights that whole genome results are "overwhelming for both the clinician and the patient or research subject," and that we must "disabuse ourselves of the concept that the [WGS] is a unitary diagnostic test" (p. 397). Rather, Biesecker argues, "the burden and challenge of interpreting the

potential results should be distributed over the lifetime of the patient/research subject. By changing this approach, one is freed from the apparent obligation to return the results of the entire assay in temporal proximity to its generation … Taken further, a [WGS] dataset can be viewed as a health-care resource that can be interrogated by the patient and clinician in situations where it could be of potential use to the patient, when both agree to this use" (p .397). This paradigm shift has significant implications for decision-making by the individual. Again, rather than making a decision about whether to receive disease-specific test results at a single moment in time, a future patient deciding about WGS may instead be making a decision to have their genomic data generated and then used or stored in many different ways, potentially and to varying degrees controlled by them.

Current Evidence on Decision-Making About Whole Exome/Genome Sequencing

Early studies examined decision-making about clinical and research genetic tests for single diseases such as Huntington's disease (Codori et al. 1994; van der Steenstraten et al. 1994; Creighton et al. 2003), breast cancer, e.g., (Lerman et al. 1996), and Alzheimer's disease (Roberts et al. 2003; Roberts et al. 2004). These studies tended to show that patients' interest in receiving personal results depended on the characteristics of the test and disease (e.g., how predictive of the disease the test is, and how preventable or treatable the disease is), and on individual characteristics (e.g., anticipated ability to cope with adverse results, disease-specific worry) (reviewed in Lerman et al. 2002). Studies such as the Multiplex study at NIH (McBride, Alford et al. 2009; Hensley Alford, McBride et al. 2011; Reid et al. 2012) and the Coriell Personalized Medicine Collaborative (Gollust et al. 2012) have examined decision-making around genetic testing for several SNPs associated with several diseases at a time. Additionally, studies have examined decision-making around DTC genetic tests such as the Navigenics genetic test (Bloss et al. 2010; Bloss et al. 2011). This body of research to date has tended to suggest that individuals who seek out personal genomic information are primarily motivated by general curiosity, and because they believe it will lead to health improvements (e.g., Gollust et al. 2012). Evidence also suggests that there could be significantly lower uptake of genomic information among non-White populations (e.g., Bloss et al. 2011; Hensley Alford et al. 2011), and that uptake is higher among individuals who are more confident in their ability to understand genetics, and who have more health habits to change (McBride et al. 2009). However, even the studies such as Multiplex (McBride et al. 2009; Hensley Alford et al. 2011; Reid et al. 2012), Coriell (Gollust et al. 2012) and Scripps-Navigenics (Bloss et al. 2010; Bloss et al. 2011) do not begin to get into the myriad of novel challenges arising from WGS, such as the unpredictability of the results, the volume of data produced, and the identifiability of the data with its accompanying implications for privacy or its lack thereof.

Research on decision-making around actual WGS is really only just beginning to emerge. Perhaps the most informative study to date is the ClinSeq project (Biesecker et al. 2009; Facio et al. 2011, 2012; Kaphingst et al. 2012). The initial recruits into the ClinSeq project were individuals with varying levels of cardiovascular disease risk; however, the majority of the close to 1000 participants are healthy subjects. ClinSeq participants sign a broad informed consent, agreeing to have their DNA used for multiple research purposes, up to and including genome sequencing. Facio et al. (2011) examined motivations for participating in the genomics research among a sample of 322 ClinSeq participants: the primary motivations were altruism, and to learn about their own genetic risks of disease (Facio et al. 2011). Facio et al. (2012) then examined interest in receiving personal results from sequencing among a different sample of 311 ClinSeq participants: most wanted to obtain their results, and the main reason given was prevention, including changing lifestyle. Participants had a belief in the value of even uninterpretable information (Facio et al. 2012). Kaphingst et al. (2012) examined the impact of the informed

consent procedure on knowledge about genome sequencing in the same 311 ClinSeq participants: they found that knowledge was higher after informed consent than before, and that there were significant differences in knowledge between racial/ethnic and educational attainment groups (Kaphingst et al. 2012). These socioeconomic differences are particularly notable given the majority of participants were white, educated, high-income individuals.

In one small study on patients' attitudes toward actual WGS (Tabor et al. 2012), two families each comprising two parents, and two to three children, were interviewed about their experiences and opinions relating to WGS. Both families were affected with Miller syndrome. Outcomes assessed in the qualitative interviews included opinions on informed consent, motivations and expectations, privacy concerns, and perspectives on return of results. There were few concerns about privacy expressed, although it was noted that these families have different attitudes toward privacy given they already feel like their privacy is limited due to the visible characteristics of the affected family members' Miller syndrome. A range of preferences regarding return of results were expressed. They had strong preferences about how results should be returned, wanting both flexibility of the results return process, and options for the types of results to be returned. Tabor et al. (2012) suggest that "web-based tools that facilitate participant management of their individual research results could accommodate … [a] framework for results return that allows explicitly for participant preferences and enables modifications to preferences over time." Most of the family members interviewed felt that the informed consent procedure was too long and cumbersome (Tabor et al. 2012).

The published empirical research on how patients and research participants make decisions about WGS will undoubtedly explode over the next few years, but is currently limited. In the meantime, it is arguably helpful to turn to non-traditional sources of insights into people's decision-making about WGS and WES. The first individuals to have their entire genomes sequenced and published were James Watson

(Wheeler et al. 2008) and Craig Venter (Levy et al. 2007). Since then, a handful of people in the world have received their personal results from WES/WGS: they have received considerable media and social media attention as a consequence. These include the 10 individuals who had their genomes sequenced as part of the Personal Genome Project pilot (PGP-10) at Harvard led by Church (2005) (Ball et al. 2012), and the individuals who received the raw data and rudimentary interpretation of their WES data from DTC company 23andme (www.23andme.com). Many of these individuals have been writing or talking about their experiences with this in the media or social media such as Twitter (see Fig. 25.1).

These are not, in general, the average person on the street. Many have a professional interest in genetics and genomics. The PGP-10 includes Harvard professor Steven Pinker, genetics professor Misha Angrist, Harvard-educated Esther Dyson, and journalist John Lauerman. The individuals receiving 23andMe exome sequence results include an Associate Professor in biology and bioinformatics (Jung Choi, see https://

jchoigt.wordpress.com/2012/07/02/a-first-look-at-my-exome-variants-from-23andme/) and the Vice President of Golden Helix Inc. (Gabe Rudy, see http://blog.goldenhelix.com/grudy/my-23and me-exome-trios-arrived-sneak-peek/).

Many of these individuals have been interviewed about their motivations and experiences of WES/WGS in the media, or have blogged about it in the social media. Examination of these interviews, blogs, and articles can be enlightening.

However, while providing interesting anecdotal evidence, it is not possible to extrapolate from this highly self-selected group of primarily educated, white, male, and often extremely wealthy individuals to the rest of the population. Research examining the motivations, views, and experiences of individuals from a wider range of backgrounds, including Hispanic and African American individuals, and those from lower socioeconomic status groups, is vitally needed. Moreover, the Personal Genome Project was notable for its rigorous entrance examination to ensure that potential participants understood key genetics and sequencing concepts. The PGP has gone to great efforts to develop a new model of informed consent and education for WGS research. However, it excludes individuals who are unable or unwilling to take and pass the entrance exam, which clearly creates a problem of unequal access across society to the benefits potentially afforded from WGS moving forward. Given the paradigm shift in the genome sequencing age, new models and methods of educating and obtaining informed consent from individuals considering participating in WGS research, or obtaining WGS results for personal clinical or other use, are needed. These methods must be accessible and relevant to individuals from a range of educational and cultural backgrounds.

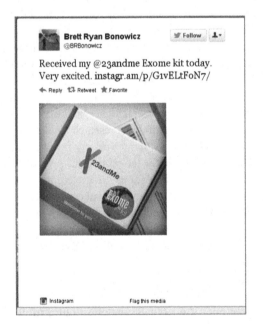

Fig. 25.1 One individual's post on Twitter about having received his DTC exome sequencing kit (Brett Ryan Bonowicz, BRBonwicz. "Received my @23andme Exome kit today. Very excited." 2 October, 2012, 9.28pm. Tweet)

Interventions to Aid Decision-Making About Genome Sequencing

The traditional approach to helping patients make informed decisions about receiving personal genetic results involves intensive, one-on-one genetic counseling. However, this is unsustainable as genome sequencing becomes commonplace. Patient decision aids may be one helpful approach to increase informed decision-making about personal WGS. Patient decision aids prepare people to participate in "close call" decisions that involve weighing benefits, harms, and scientific uncertainty (O'Connor et al. 2009). Patient decision aids are widely used to help patients make complex decisions related to their health and health care, and can come in a variety of formats, including pamphlets, brochures, videos and interactive computer-based formats.

In a recent systematic review of decision aids for people facing health treatment or screening decisions, patient decision aids were shown to perform better than usual care interventions in terms of leading to greater knowledge, lower decisional conflict relating to both feeling uninformed and feeling unclear about personal values (O'Connor et al. 2009). For example, in a large randomized controlled trial an interactive computer program was more effective than standard genetic counseling for increasing knowledge of breast cancer and genetic testing among women at low risk of carrying a *BRCA1* or *BRCA2* mutation (Green et al. 2004).

Additionally, another recent systematic review focusing specifically on computerized patient decision aids showed that computerized patient decision aids performed better than standard consultations/education regarding improved knowledge, lower decisional conflict, and greater satisfaction with the decision-making process than standard education (Sheehan and Sherman 2012). Computerized decision aids have the advantage of readily tailoring information to individual user characteristics, enabling feedback to reinforce comprehension, incorporating interactive and advanced visual features to facilitate participant involvement, and disseminating information easily (Sheehan and Sherman 2012).

The International Patient Decision Aids (IPDAS) Collaboration was established at the 2nd International Shared Decision Making conference in 2003. The IPDAS objective was to develop a set of quality criteria for patient decision aids. The retained criteria were in the following domains: systematic development process; providing information about options; presenting probabilities; clarifying and expressing values; using patient stories; guiding/coaching; disclosing conflicts of interest; providing Internet access; balanced presentation of options; using plain language; basing information on up-to-date evidence; and establishing effectiveness (Elwyn et al. 2006).

The IPDAS Collaboration strongly endorsed the *values clarification technique* of describing the physical, emotional, and social effects of options to help patients to explore "experienced utility" (Elwyn et al. 2006). Values clarification exercises have been developed as part of a decision aid for the treatment of early-stage prostate cancer (Feldman-Stewart et al. 2006), and as part of a computerized decision aid for low literate and naive computer users, newly diagnosed with early-stage breast cancer, recruited from two urban public hospitals (Jibaja-Weiss et al. 2006).

Jibaja-Weiss and Volk (2007) posit that even interactive computerized decision aids are often heavily reliant on written information, health and digital literacy, and advocate for using entertainment education (or "edutainment") as a means of promoting informed decision-making among patients with low health literacy (Jibaja-Weiss and Volk 2007). Edutainment is the process of purposely designing and implementing media that incorporate educational messages within an entertaining format, and to date has largely focused on using a "'soap opera" format. Computerized entertainment education has been used to aid decision-making about prostate cancer screening among men with low health literacy (Volk et al. 2008), and to aid decision-making about breast cancer surgery among women with low healthy literacy (Jibaja-Weiss et al. 2011).

At the Icahn School of Medicine at Mount Sinai (ISMMS) in New York City, we and colleagues developed a novel animated video about WGS that was developed specifically to be accessible to individuals from a range of socioeconomic and racial/ethnic backgrounds, using elements of the entertainment education process (Sanderson et al. 2016). The video was designed to be used as a general public education resource and is publicly available on YouTube. It was also designed to be useful as a communication and educational tool for genetic counselors interacting with patients or research participants considering having personal WGS done (see Fig. 25.2). The video was developed in an iterative manner. To develop the initial draft script, we drew on publicly available sources about genetics and genome sequencing, including the "Help Me Understand Genetics" handbook by the U.S. National Library of Medicine (http://ghr.nlm.nih.gov/handbook.pdf), the education section of the NHGRI website (http://www.genome.gov), and the Personal Genetics Education Project website at Harvard (www.pged.org), and also involved experts from a range of relevant backgrounds, including genetic counselors and other genetics experts. An early draft of the script was piloted with 10 racially/ethnically diverse patients at an outpatient clinic at MSSM. In addition, an online text and example graphics version was piloted with 173 racially/ethnically diverse individuals recruited through an online market research company. The draft animation was then developed with a Manhattan-based animation and design company, and then shown to four Hispanic and African-American community consultants. Revisions were made in light of the feedback we received, and the next draft of the animation was shown to 22 individuals in three focus groups. The individuals were recruited from communities surrounding ISMMS, and were primarily Hispanic and African-American. Revisions were subsequently made in light of this next feedback (Sanderson et al. 2016), and the final animation is freely available on YouTube (see https://www.youtube.com/watch?v=IXamRS85hXU&hd=1). We subsequently used the animation with participants recruited into the HealthSeq project at ISMMS in which they were offered personal results from WGS (Sanderson et al. 2016). The animation we developed is an example of a new generation of efforts to use new media to educate the public, and to aid healthcare providers as they strive to help patients and research participants understand personal genomics. Another example of an animation designed to explain about developments in genomics is the short animation explaining what the ENCODE project is in lay terms, funded by Illumina and created by Cartoonbrew (www.cartoonbrew.com/tag/dc-turner). This animation is also available on YouTube.

In summary, genetic counseling services to aid decision-making about genetic testing and genome sequencing are already stretched. Patients are likely to ask their primary healthcare providers for help interpreting their genomic test results, even if obtained outside the clinic setting.

Fig. 25.2 A still from a 10-min animation explaining what whole genome sequencing is

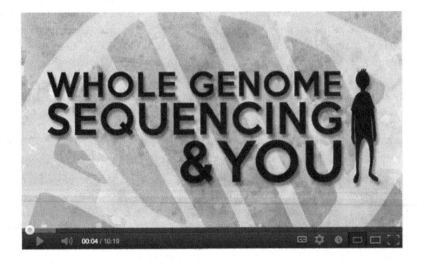

New and innovative models to educate patients and facilitate informed decision-making are needed. Patient decision aids such as animations and interactive media may go some way to improving informed decision-making without leading to undue burden on the healthcare system (e.g., by insisting on hours of one-on-one genetic counseling per patient). However, important questions remain about how best to achieve this, and evidence-based innovative interventions are urgently needed to create a genomics-literate public capable of making informed decisions about WGS without putting unnecessary burden on them or their healthcare providers.

Privacy and Open Informed Consent

Informed consent forms one of the cornerstones of research involving human. The standard practice for enrolling participants in a research study include fully informing potential participants on all aspects of a study including the aims of the study, risks, benefits, costs, and protection of personal privacy. The origins of modern day informed consent for medical research can be traced to the Nuremberg Code in 1947 in an effort to protect participants in research studies. However, the omics revolution combined with a far more open data sharing mentality permeating many aspects of society today (see section on identifiability above) are driving a new generation of informed consents that put the study participant's ability to openly share data generated on them front and center. Classic consents that ensure or even guarantee the privacy of the individual are being challenged by these new consents that aim to educate participants on what the data collected on them can say and the degree to which it can or cannot be protected, while simultaneously empowering the individual to take a more vested interest in research outcomes as well as giving them more control over sharing of their own data with others and with scientists in particular (Box 1).

This "open informed consent" movement is evolving to accommodate the view that many patients want to share their data generated for research with others, to further enable the scientific community to solve problems relating to their condition without being unnecessarily hampered by restrictive rules that prevent, in the name of privacy, a patient from benefiting more directly from data they contribute. The portable legalized consent (PLC—http://weconsent.us/) now approved for use by Sage Bionetworks is just such a step in this direction. The PLC seeks to appropriately educate research subjects and then enable them to have more control over the use of data generated on them for research or other purposes. The PLC not only provides for more informed study participants that better understand the risks and rewards involved in making their data available to others, but it has the potential to facilitate a more productive research environment as research subjects become entitled to not only receive the data generated on them (it is nearly inexplicable that research subjects have not had this right before) but to share it with any others who are willing to follow commonsense rules regarding use of the data. Educating research participants appropriately on what data collected on them can say and the degree to which it can or cannot be protected, and then empowering research participants to have a more vested interest in outcomes and the ability to empower other scientists with *their* data, is definitely a step in the right direction.

Challenges and Recommendations

The age of genome sequencing is bringing with it a complete paradigm change in how we think about patients' and research participants' decision-making about whether to obtain personal WGS, whether to participate in WGS research, and receiving personal results from WGS. No longer can we provide individuals with information about one disease and one test, measure their feelings about that disease and the test being offered, assess at one time point whether or not they take up the offer of that test for that disease, and assess the outcomes of that decision in a simple linear fashion. Informed consent documents and procedures for WGS will need to emphasize that privacy cannot be guaranteed, and that the purposes for which the sequence data will be used cannot be predetermined. Both of these messages are in direct opposition to current approaches to informed consent. Traditional genetic counseling models involving hours of in-person counseling will need to be replaced or enhanced with innovative media-based interventions that are accessible to individuals across society. The results from WGS will not be returned to individuals at one single moment in time; rather, interpretation of WGS data for any given individual will be a continuous, dynamic process over time. This poses significant challenges for researchers and clinicians alike, for whom new models of research and clinical practice will be needed to adapt to this changing landscape and timeline of interaction with patients and research participants. As Holly Tabor and colleagues suggest, the return of results to patients/research participants will likely need to utilize dynamic web-based platforms that can incorporate and be responsive to patients/research participants' preferences regarding the types of information they would like to receive over time (Tabor et al. 2012). In addition, a new generation of researchers and healthcare providers will be needed who are genomics savvy and able to deal with the deluge of genomic information that is coming. This includes social and behavioral science researchers who will need a deep understanding of WGS in order to be able to work with others to develop the information and educational materials, to develop the methods for returning the results to patients/research participants, and to assess decision-making among individuals who are offered personal WGS, as well as the cognitive, emotional, and behavioral outcomes of those decisions. In addition, WGS is leading us to an age where genomics will no longer be just about disease and illness, but will touch every aspect of people's lives, providing information on their ancestry, their health behaviors, their mood, and their psychological functioning. Appropriately dynamic, evolving and preference-sensitive

informed consent models, educational interventions, and return of results delivery formats are going to be needed if the promise of genomics is truly to be delivered.

Box 1. Current Generation, Open and Interoperable Informed Consents (from Schadt 2012)
Current Generation Informed Consents

- Often single study focused
- Top-down unidirectional researcher–participant (research subject) relationship
- Protecting the participant considered among the chief aims
- Data generation on study participants usually an integral part of the consent
- Data ownership and terms of use driven by the investigator and/or hosting institution
- Study participants are counseled to ensure they understand all aspects of the study, although no evidence of understanding is sought or required
- In most cases, anonymity, privacy, and confidentiality are guaranteed as key conditions for a participant's consent.

"Open Consents" for public resources: The Personal Genome Project Consent (Church 2005; Lunshof et al. 2008)
Open consent differs from classic informed consent in the following ways:

- Data ownership and terms of use of data no longer driven by study investigator
- Data are published to the web and made available without restriction
- Single study focused, but has broad and open-ended scope (data sharing as an aim)
- Participants agree to reciprocal interaction with researchers
- Participants must pass an exam to ensure they possess basic genetic literacy, are informed about the public nature of the study, understand the possibility of reidentification, and that some risks are unknown and unpredictable.

Interoperable and Open Consents: The Portable Legal Consent (PLC) (http://weconsent.us/) **Based upon the PGP consent, but altered in the following important ways:**

- The PLC can be used across any number of studies
- If variations of the same PLC form guarantee the same freedoms and create no more than the same obligations, it can be certified as interoperable across the PLC network
- Fully digital, requires no input from a physician or other health/research professional
- Requires users sign terms of a contract to ensure compliance with data use terms
- Intended for data already generated, to enable open access of data across many studies.

Summary Box

- Whole genome sequencing (WGS) could be routinely available to patients for a few dollars within the next 10 years.
- The volume of data produced by WGS is unprecedented, and the types of results that an individual may receive through WGS are unpredictable and open-ended.
- This has important implications for decision-making about WGS: decisions have to take account of the unpredictability of the results, the volume of data produced, and the identifiability of the data with its accompanying implications for privacy or its lack thereof.
- The traditional, intensive, one-on-one genetic counseling approach to helping patients make informed decisions about receiving personal genetic results is likely to be unsustainable as WGS becomes commonplace.
- New and innovative models to educate patients and facilitate informed decision-making are needed: animations and interactive media may be valuable resources fulfilling this need.

- A new generation of genomics-savvy social and behavioral science researchers is needed to develop the educational materials and methods for returning results to patients and research participants; to assess decision-making among individuals who are offered personal WGS; and to assess the cognitive, emotional, and behavioral outcomes of those decisions.

References

Altshuler, D., Daly, M. J., et al. (2008). Genetic mapping in human disease. *Science, 322*(5903), 881–888.

Angrist, M. (2009). Eyes wide open: The personal genome project, citizen science and veracity in informed consent. *Personalized Medicine, 6*(6), 691–699.

Ashley, E. A., Butte, A. J., et al. (2010). Clinical assessment incorporating a personal genome. *Lancet, 375*(9725), 1525–1535.

Ball, M. P., Thakuria, J. V., et al. (2012). A public resource facilitating clinical use of genomes. *Proceedings of the National Academy of Sciences of the United States of America, 109*(30), 11920–11927.

Bandura, D. R., Baranov, V. I., et al. (2009). Mass cytometry: Technique for real time single cell multi-target immunoassay based on inductively coupled plasma time-of-flight mass spectrometry. *Analytical Chemistry, 81*(16), 6813–6822.

Barabasi, A. L., & Oltvai, Z. N. (2004). Network biology: understanding the cell's functional organization. *Nature Reviews Genetics, 5*(2), 101–113.

Bernstein, B. E., Birney, E., et al. (2012). An integrated encyclopedia of DNA elements in the human genome. *Nature, 489*(7414), 57–74.

Biesecker, L. G. (2012). Opportunities and challenges for the integration of massively parallel genomic sequencing into clinical practice: Lessons from the ClinSeq project. *Genetics in Medicine, 14*(4), 393–398.

Biesecker, L. G., Mullikin, J. C., et al. (2009). The ClinSeq Project: piloting large-scale genome sequencing for research in genomic medicine. *Genome Research, 19*(9), 1665–1674.

Bloss, C. S., Ornowski, L., et al. (2010). Consumer perceptions of direct-to-consumer personalized genomic risk assessments. *Genetics in Medicine, 12*(9), 556–566.

Bloss, C. S., Schork, N. J., et al. (2011). Effect of direct-to-consumer genomewide profiling to assess disease risk. *New England Journal of Medicine, 364*(6), 524–534.

Brunham, L. R., & Hayden, M. R. (2012). Medicine. Whole-genome sequencing: the new standard of care? *Science, 336*(6085), 1112–1113.

Cassa, C. A., Savage, S. K., et al. (2012). Disclosing pathogenic genetic variants to research participants: Quantifying an emerging ethical responsibility. *Genome Research, 22*(3), 421–428.

Chen, R., Mias, G. I., et al. (2012). Personal omics profiling reveals dynamic molecular and medical phenotypes. *Cell, 148*(6), 1293–1307.

Church, G. M. (2005). The personal genome project. *Molecular Systems Biology, 1*(2005), 0030.

Codori, A. M., Hanson, R., et al. (1994). Self-selection in predictive testing for Huntington's disease. *American Journal of Medical Genetics, 54*(3), 167–173.

International Human Genome Sequencing Consortium. (2004). Finishing the euchromatic sequence of the human genome. *Nature, 431*(2011), 931–945.

National Research Council (2011). *Toward precision medicine: Building a knowledge network for biomedical research and a new taxonomy of disease.* Washington DC: National Academy of Sciences.

Creighton, S., Almqvist, E. W., et al. (2003). Predictive, pre-natal and diagnostic genetic testing for Huntington's disease: The experience in Canada from 1987 to 2000. *Clinical Genetics, 63*(6), 462–475.

Dewey, F. E., Chen, R., et al. (2011). Phased whole-genome genetic risk in a family quartet using a major allele reference sequence. *PLoS Genetics, 7*(9), e1002280.

Dohany, L., Gustafson, S., et al. (2012). Psychological distress with direct-to-consumer genetic testing: A case report of an unexpected BRCA positive test result. *Journal of Genetic Counseling, 21*(3), 399–401.

Drmanac, R., Sparks, A. B., et al. (2010). Human genome sequencing using unchained base reads on self-assembling DNA nanoarrays. *Science, 327*(5961), 78–81.

Eid, J., Fehr, A., et al. (2009). Real-time DNA sequencing from single polymerase molecules. *Science, 323*(5910), 133–138.

Elwyn, G., O'Connor, A., et al. (2006). Developing a quality criteria framework for patient decision aids: Online international delphi consensus process. *BMJ, 333*(7565), 417.

Emilsson, V., Thorleifsson, G., et al. (2008). Genetics of gene expression and its effect on disease. *Nature, 452*(7186), 423–428.

Fabsitz, R. R., McGuire, A., et al. (2010). Ethical and practical guidelines for reporting genetic research results to study participants: Updated guidelines from a national heart, lung, and blood institute working group. *Circulation: Cardiovascular Genetics, 3*(6), 574–580.

Facio, F. M., Brooks, S., et al. (2011). Motivators for participation in a whole-genome sequencing study: Implications for translational genomics research. *European Journal of Human Genetics, 19*(12), 1213–1217.

Facio, F. M., Eidem, H., et al. (2012). Intentions to receive individual results from whole-genome sequencing among participants in the ClinSeq study. *European Journal of Human Genetics, 21*(3), 261–265.

Feldman-Stewart, D., Brennenstuhl, S., et al. (2006). An explicit values clarification task: Development and validation. *Patient Education and Counseling, 63*(3), 350–356.

Gollust, S. E., Gordon, E. S., et al. (2012). Motivations and perceptions of early adopters of personalized genomics: Perspectives from research participants. *Public Health Genomics, 15*(1), 22–30.

Green, E. D., & Guyer, M. S. (2011). Charting a course for genomic medicine from base pairs to bedside. *Nature, 470*(7333), 204–213.

Green, M. J., Peterson, S. K., et al. (2004). Effect of a computer-based decision aid on knowledge, perceptions, and intentions about genetic testing for breast cancer susceptibility: A randomized controlled trial. *JAMA, 292*(4), 442–452.

Halder, I., Shriver, M., et al. (2008). A panel of ancestry informative markers for estimating individual biogeographical ancestry and admixture from four continents: Utility and applications. *Human Mutation, 29*(5), 648–658.

Han, J. D., Bertin, N., et al. (2004). Evidence for dynamically organized modularity in the yeast protein–protein interaction network. *Nature, 430*(6995), 88–93.

Hatemi, P. K., & McDermott, R. (2012). The genetics of politics: Discovery, challenges, and progress. *Trends in Genetics, 28*(10), 525–533.

Hensley Alford, S., McBride, C. M., et al. (2011). Participation in genetic testing research varies by social group. *Public Health Genomics, 14*(2), 85–93.

Jibaja-Weiss, M. L., Volk, R. J., et al. (2006). Preliminary testing of a just-in-time, user-defined values clarification exercise to aid lower literate women in making informed breast cancer treatment decisions. *Health Expectations, 9*(3), 218–231.

Jibaja-Weiss, M. L., & Volk, R. J. (2007). Utilizing computerized entertainment education in the development of decision aids for lower literate and naive computer users. *Journal of Health Communication, 12*(7), 681–697.

Jibaja-Weiss, M. L., Volk, R. J., et al. (2011). Entertainment education for breast cancer surgery decisions: a randomized trial among patients with low health literacy. *Patient Education and Counseling, 84*(1), 41–48.

Kaphingst, K., Facio, F., et al. (2012). Effects of informed consent for individual genome sequencing on relevant knowledge. *Clinical Genetics, 82*(5), 408–415.

Koenig, L. B., McGue, M., et al. (2005). Genetic and environmental influences on religiousness: Findings for retrospective and current religiousness ratings. *Journal of Personality, 73*(2), 471–488.

Kravets, D. (2010). Privacy in peril: Lawyers, nations clamor for Google Wi-Fi data. *Wired Magazine.*

Lander, E. S., Linton, L. M., et al. (2001). Initial sequencing and analysis of the human genome. *Nature, 409*(6822), 860–921.

Lerman, C., Croyle, R. T., et al. (2002). Genetic testing: Psychological aspects and implications. *Journal of Consulting and Clinical Psychology, 70*(3), 784–797.

Lerman, C., Narod, S., et al. (1996). BRCA1 testing in families with hereditary breast-ovarian cancer. A prospective study of patient decision making and outcomes. *JAMA, 275*(24), 1885–1892.

Levy, S., Sutton, G., et al. (2007). The diploid genome sequence of an individual human. *PLoS Biology, 5* (10), e254.

Lin, Z., Altman, R. B., et al. (2006). Confidentiality in genome research. *Science, 313*(5786), 441–442.

Lunshof, J. E., Bobe, J., et al. (2010). Personal genomes in progress: from the human genome project to the personal genome project. *Dialogues in Clinical Neuroscience, 12*(1), 47–60.

Lunshof, J. E., Chadwick, R., et al. (2008). From genetic privacy to open consent. *Nature Reviews Genetics, 9* (5), 406–411.

Luscombe, N. M., Babu, M. M., et al. (2004). Genomic analysis of regulatory network dynamics reveals large topological changes. *Nature, 431*(7006), 308–312.

McBride, C. M., Alford, S. H., et al. (2009). Characteristics of users of online personalized genomic risk assessments: Implications for physician-patient interactions. *Genetics in Medicine, 11*(8), 582–587.

McGuire, A. L., & Gibbs, R. A. (2006). Genetics. No longer de-identified. *Science, 312*(5772), 370–371.

O'Connor, A. M., Bennett, C. L., et al. (2009). Decision aids for people facing health treatment or screening decisions. *The Cochrane Database of Systematic Reviews, 3*, CD001431.

Pinto, S., Roseberry, A. G., et al. (2004). Rapid rewiring of arcuate nucleus feeding circuits by leptin. *Science, 304*(5667), 110–115.

Reid, R. J., McBride, C. M,. et al. (2012). Association between health-service use and multiplex genetic testing. *Genetics in Medicine, 14*(10), 852–859.

Roberts, J. S., Barber, M., et al. (2004). Who seeks genetic susceptibility testing for Alzheimer's disease? Findings from a multisite, randomized clinical trial. *Genetics in Medicine, 6*(4), 197–203.

Roberts, J. S., LaRusse, S. A., et al. (2003). Reasons for seeking genetic susceptibility testing among first-degree relatives of people with Alzheimer disease. *Alzheimer Disease and Associated Disorders, 17* (2), 86–93.

Sanderson, S. C., Suckiel, S. A., Zweig, M., Bottinger, E. P., Jabs, E. W., Richardson, L. D. (2016). Development and preliminary evaluation of an online educational video about whole-genome sequencing for research participants, patients, and the general public. *Genetics in Medicine, 18*(5), 501–512.

Sanderson, S. C., Linderman, M. D., Suckiel, S. A., Diaz, G. A., Zinberg, R. E., Ferryman, K., Wasserstein, M., Kasarskis, A., Schadt, E. E. (2016). Motivations, concerns and preferences of personal genome sequencing research participants: Baseline findings from the HealthSeq project. *European Journal of Human Genetics, 24*(1),14–20.

Schadt, E. E. (2012). The changing privacy landscape in the era of big data. *Molecular Systems Biology, 8*, 612.

Schadt, E. E., Turner, S., et al. (2010). A window into third-generation sequencing. *Human Molecular Genetics, 19*(R2), R227–R240.

Schadt, E. E., Woo, S., et al. (2012). Bayesian method to predict individual SNP genotypes from gene expression data. *Nature Genetics, 44*(5), 603–608.

Sheehan, J., & Sherman, K. A. (2012). Computerised decision aids: A systematic review of their effectiveness in facilitating high-quality decision-making in various health-related contexts. *Patient Education and Counseling, 88*(1), 69–86.

Speicher, M. R , Geigl, J. B., et al. (2010). Effect of genome-wide association studies, direct-to-consumer genetic testing, and high-speed sequencing technologies on predictive genetic counselling for cancer risk. *Lancet Oncology, 11*(9), 890–898.

Tabor, H. K., Stock, J., et al. (2012). Informed consent for whole genome sequencing: A qualitative analysis of participant expectations and perceptions of risks, benefits, and harms. *American Journal of Medical Genetics Part A, 158A*(6), 1310–1319.

van der Steenstraten, I. M., Tibben, A., et al. (1994). Predictive testing for Huntington disease: Nonparticipants compared with participants in the Dutch program. *American Journal of Human Genetics, 55* (4), 618–625.

Venter, J. C., Adams, M. D., et al. (2001). The sequence of the human genome. *Science, 291*(5507), 1304–1351.

Volk, R. J., Jibaja-Weiss, M. L., et al. (2008). Entertainment education for prostate cancer screening: A randomized trial among primary care patients with low health literacy. *Patient Education and Counseling, 73*(3), 482–489.

Walker, A. P. (2009). The practice of genetic counseling. In W. S. Uhlmann, J. B. Yashar (Eds.),. *A Guide to genetic counseling* (pp. 1–35). Hoboken, New Jersey: Wiley.

Wheeler, D. A., Srinivasan, M., et al. (2008). The complete genome of an individual by massively parallel DNA sequencing. *Nature, 452*(7189), 872–876.

Zerhouni, E. (2003). Medicine. The NIH roadmap. *Science, 302*(5642), 63–72.

Index